Manual of
Veterinary Clinical Chemistry:
A Case Study Approach

Leslie C. Sharkey, DVM, PhD, DACVP   M. Judith Radin, DVM, PhD, DACVP

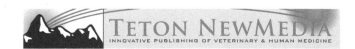

TETON NEWMEDIA
INNOVATIVE PUBLISHING OF VETERINARY & HUMAN MEDICINE

Executive Editor: Carroll C. Cann
Development Editor: Susan L. Hunsberger
Creative Director: Sue Haun www.fiftysixforty.com
Production Manager: Mike Albiniak www.fiftysixforty.com

Teton NewMedia
P.O. Box 4833
Jackson, WY 83001

1-888-770-3165
www.tetonnm.com

Printed in the United States of America

Print Number 5 4 3 2 1

    Library of Congress Cataloging-in-Publication Data on file.

ISBN 1-59161-018-4

Preface

Our goal is to provide a practical and engaging resource for veterinary students, residents and practitioners to develop and practice skills in interpretation of clinical chemistry data, using a case-based approach. The clinical chemistry profile is an important tool for the preliminary evaluation of the health of veterinary patients. Many texts describe the characteristics of individual tests, however there are few resources to assist practitioners in developing the organizational and interpretive skills needed to use this tool effectively.

The examples used in this text have been drawn from actual clinical cases reviewed by the authors and are organized using a broad systems approach with increasing complexity to the examples in each chapter. Because the interpretation of clinical chemistry data depends heavily on the clinical context, brief histories and physical examination findings are included along with other clinicopathologic data such as CBC, urinalysis, cytology or fluid analysis. Some cases also have figures that illustrate important findings on the physical examination, imaging studies, or microscopic evaluation of patient samples that students may find particularly helpful. Keys discussing the interpretation of individual analytes follow the clinical presentation. At the end of each case, a summary is given for each patient that includes a description of follow up tests and response to treatment.

Important diagnostic considerations that we have emphasized include the effects of age and artifacts that might be over-interpreted as indicating disease and the impact of the statistical principles that we use to define "normal." We have made an effort to include broad representation of common domestic species to make the book as useful as possible to a broad audience. In each chapter, there are "classic textbook" examples of disease processes. However, because these cases have been drawn from the patient populations at our hospitals, some patients have not "read the book" and should provide a diagnostic challenge that we hope is both entertaining and enlightening. Multiple cases of some common diseases are included to illustrate the variety of clinicopathologic findings that can be associated with the same diagnosis depending on individual patient factors. We also include diagnostic dilemmas in which different diseases may present with similar clinical signs and laboratory data. The summary sections of these cases compare and contrast several different cases in the book to illustrate how a clinician might approach distinguishing these diseases.

For many of these cases, the diagnosis was confirmed using ancillary tests or by biopsy or necropsy. We acknowledge that the interpretation of the data for each case in this book may be only one of several potentially correct interpretations. Mechanisms for abnormalities are the consensus of two board certified clinical pathologists based on the existing literature at the time the text was written, but these may be modified as veterinary science evolves. We hope that you will enjoy using the cases in this book to hone your interpretive skills in clinical chemistry.

Dedication

To Pamela Chen, a wonderful friend and a great spirit - L. Sharkey

To Jamie Diamond, my husband and true friend and to Joey Diamond, my intrepid explorer. - M.J. Radin

Acknowledgements

We would like to acknowledge the contributions of the many veterinarians, veterinary students, technicians, and medical technologists at Tufts University, the University of Minnesota, and The Ohio State University. Their hard work is the basis of this book.

Table of Contents

How to use the Manual of Veterinary Clinical Chemistry: A Case Study Approach

Unlike many other clinical pathology tests that are performed by diagnostic laboratories, clinical chemistry profile reports do not come with interpretations from the laboratory that generated them. The purpose of this book is to assist the veterinary student, veterinary resident, or veterinary practitioner in developing his or her skills in laboratory data interpretation and clinical reasoning. Although short introductory segments to each chapter provide a brief review of pertinent tests and a guide to their interpretation, this book is NOT an exhaustive textbook of clinical chemistry and use of this manual requires some background knowledge of clinical chemistry and veterinary medicine. The authors recommend that the reader have a classical text reference to accompany this volume, and several excellent potential resources are listed below.

Fundamentals of Veterinary Clinical Pathology
SL Stockham, MA Scott, eds., Blackwell Publishing, Ames, IA

Fluid, Electrolyte, and Acid Base Disorders in Small Animal Practice
SP DiBartola ed., Saunders Elsevier, St. Louis, MO.

Veterinary Hematology and Clinical Chemistry
MA Thrall, ed., Lippincott Williams &Wilkins, Philadelphia, PA.

Canine and Feline Endocrinology and Reproduction
EC Feldman, RW Nelson, eds., W.B. Saunders, St. Louis, MO

Large Animal Internal Medicine
BP Smith, ed., Mosby, St. Louis, MO.

Equine Internal Medicine
SM Reed, WM Bayly, RB McEachern, DC Sellon, eds., W.B. Saunders, St. Louis, MO.

Laboratory urinalysis and hematology, for the small animal practitioner
CA Sink, BF Feldman, Teton NewMedia, Jackson, WY.

Urinalysis, A clinical guide to compassionate patient care.
CA Osborne, JB Stevens, Bayer.

The first chapter provides a sample method for the review of clinical chemistry data, with an overview of the principles for the development of reference ranges and guidelines for integrating laboratory data with other clinical information. Subsequent chapters are based on tests of various organ systems, however "look a like" diseases with clinical chemistry abnormalities that appear to suggest one system while originating in another will also be included in that section (for example, a patient with an elevated serum alkaline phosphatase level secondary to an endocrinopathy or bone disease may be presented in the liver enzyme chapter).

Each chapter contains multiple cases from a variety of species that are designated Level 1, Level 2, or Level 3 based on the level of difficulty of the interpretation. It is recommended that the reader begin with introductory Level 1 cases and work forward. Although each case can stand on its own and the reader is not obligated to work consecutive cases, the order was carefully chosen to emphasize differentiating diseases with potentially similar laboratory data. Ancillary hematology, urinalysis, coagulation profile, and cytology data are also provided for each case, along with radiographs if available. Each case contains an interpretation section where all abnormalities are reviewed, and a subsequent section where all abnormalities are integrated into the clinical picture for final diagnosis and recommendations for further testing. When known, the clinical outcome of the case is provided since all of the cases presented here are real, live patients. This book is designed to provide the reader with an ENJOYABLE and PRACTICAL resource for improving skills in clinical chemistry interpretation.

The diagnostic plans and treatment information described for these cases are informational/historical only and should not be considered recommendations for any of the described conditions.

Abbreviations

A/G ratio - Albumin/globulin ratio
ALP - Alkaline Phosphatase
ALT - Alanine Aminotransferase
Anion Gap - (sodium + potassium) - (chloride + bicarbonate)
APTT - Activated Partial Thromboplastin Time
AST - Aspartate Aminotransferase
Bili - Bilirubin
BUN - Blood Urea Nitrogen
CBC - Complete Blood Count
CK - Creatine Kinase
cPLI - Canine Pancreatic Lipase Immunoreactivity
CT - Computed Axial Tomography (CAT or CT scan)
DIC - Disseminated Intravascular Coagulation
DSH - Domestic short haired
EDTA - Ethylenediaminetetra-acetic acid
FDP - Fibrin Degradation Products
FeLV - Feline Leukemia Virus
FIV - Feline Immunodeficiency Virus
GGT - Gamma Glutamyl Transferase
HPF - High Power Field
HC03 - Bicarbonate
Heme - Indicates presence of RBCs and/or hemoglobin in urine
IgG - Immunoglobulin G
LDH - Lactate Dehydrogenase
MCHC - Mean Corpuscular Hemoglobin Concentration
MCV - Mean Corpuscular Volume
PCV - Packed Cell Volume
PT - Prothrombin Time
PTH - Parathyroid Hormone
PTHrP - Parthyroid Hormone Related Protein
RBC - Red Blood Cell
SDH - Sorbitol Dehydrogenase
TLI - Trypsin Like Immunoreactivity
WBC - White Blood Cell

Chapter 1

Developing a Plan for Interpretation

Indications for the Clinical Chemistry Profile

The clinical chemistry profile is an integral component of the minimum database for most patients. Blood may be drawn for performing a clinical chemistry profile for multiple reasons including

1. Screening for disease in apparently healthy individuals (pre-anesthetic screens or geriatric profiles).

2. Assessing the severity of disease: the magnitude of deviation from the reference range of an analyte may be related to the severity of organ damage or dysfunction, but this is not the case for all tests.

3. Resolving differential diagnoses.

4. Development of prognosis.

5. Determining drug toxicities.

6. Evaluating response to therapy using serial testing.

Because all tests have false positives, false negatives, and laboratory artifacts that could impact the results, a diagnosis or prognosis can rarely be made on the basis of any single test result. Conversely, disease can rarely be completely ruled out based on a single normal test result. To arrive at a correct diagnosis, all laboratory test results must be analyzed along with the patient's history, physical examination findings, imaging studies, and the results of other diagnostic procedures.

Step 1: Is the blood work abnormal or is the patient abnormal?

There are various reasons for laboratory results to fall outside of reference ranges, and some of these have nothing to do with the presence of disease in a patient.

1. "Normally abnormal values" and how reference intervals are generated

Because the results of many clinical chemistry assays depend on the types of reagents and analyzers that are used, reference intervals should be generated within each laboratory whenever possible. The use of published reference intervals is sometimes unavoidable, especially with uncommon species, but methodologic differences may cause normal patients to have test results that fall outside these published values. Specific reference intervals also need to be developed for patients of certain ages (i.e., neonatal), reproductive status (i.e., pregnant or lactating), or breeds. Keep in mind that human laboratories may accept veterinary samples, but may not have species specific reference intervals.

Reference intervals are generated by measuring an analyte in the blood of a population of apparently healthy animals. The mean value is calculated, and the reference range is set as the mean plus or minus two standard deviations if the data are normally distributed. The practical consequence of this is that approximately 5% of "normal" patients will have results that fall outside of the reference interval (Figure 1-1). For example, the statistical probability that a completely normal patient will have all normal results on a serum biochemical profile containing 12 tests is only 54%!

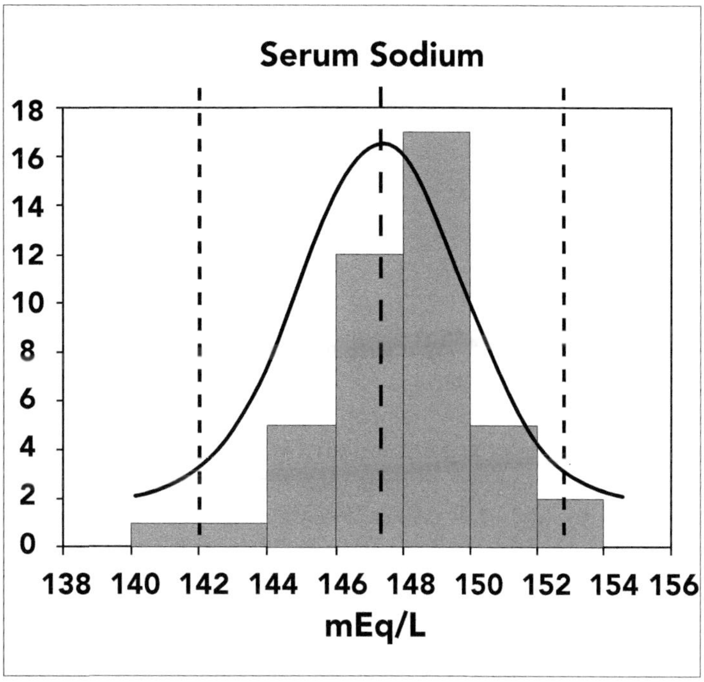

Serum Sodium

Figure 1-1. How reference intervals are calculated: In this example, serum sodium was measured in 43 normal dogs. The number of dogs with each sodium concentration is indicated by the bars. The mean (heavy dashed line) and reference interval (lightly dashed lines or ± 2SD) are calculated. Notice that values from 2 of 43 normal dogs are outside of the reference interval. You can expect 5% of normal patients to have a serum chemistry value that falls outside the reference interval.

2. Accuracy and precision in the laboratory.

Accuracy and precision are required to ensure that abnormal values truly reflect the status of the patient and are not the result of poor laboratory technique. Accuracy is the agreement between the laboratory result and its "true" value, and precision is the agreement between replicate measurements (Figure 1-2).

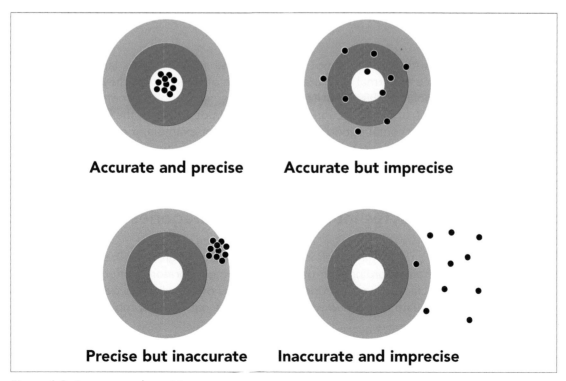

Accurate and precise **Accurate but imprecise**

Precise but inaccurate **Inaccurate and imprecise**

Figure 1-2. Accuracy and precision.

3. The probability of disease being present in a patient with an abnormal test result also depends on the sensitivity and specificity of the test and the prevalence of disease in the population.

Diagnostic sensitivity is a measure of the frequency of a positive or abnormal test result in the presence of disease.

Diagnostic specificity is a measure of the frequency of a negative or normal test result in the absence of disease.

While sensitivity and specificity reflect the accuracy of a test, they are determined using highly selected populations (all diseased for sensitivity or all free of the disease for specificity). The clinician is probably more interested in the positive predictive value of a test, which is the percentage of patients with a positive test that actually have the disease. Positive predictive value takes into account the prevalence of the disease. Be aware that tests are often evaluated at universities or large referral centers, where the prevalence of disease may be quite different from your clinical practice.

4. Laboratory artifacts or errors in the collection and processing of samples may cause a normal patient to have abnormal laboratory data. It is beyond the scope of this book to list all possible artifacts and errors, however these should ALWAYS be considered when the laboratory data seems incongruous with the clinical presentation of the patient. Hemolysis, icterus, and lipemia of samples may cause artifactual abnormalities of laboratory tests due to interference with test methodology. Leaving serum samples unspun may result in hypoglycemia due to in vitro consumption of glucose by cells in the blood sample. Leakage of electrolytes or enzymes out of cells and into serum may also be a problem. Collection of samples soon after eating can result in lipemia or elevation of serum glucose, cholesterol, and triglycerides. Certain types of medications may have physiological effects that result in laboratory abnormalities, or they or their metabolites may directly interfere with assay methodology.

5. Normal clinical chemistry profiles do not rule out disease. In some cases, laboratory parameters only become abnormal very late in the course of disease (i.e., they lack sensitivity). Good examples of this are BUN and creatinine, which only become elevated when approximately 75% of renal function is already lost. In other cases, the routine clinical chemistry profile does not contain good tests for disease. For example, there are no tests specific for pulmonary or cardiovascular disease on routine serum biochemical profiles, although hypoxia or hypoperfusion may cause secondary abnormalities that are detected by performing a serum biochemical profile.

Step 2: Group analytes into meaningful categories for interpretation

Many clinical chemistry profiles have their individual tests already grouped in some logical order on the report, often according to organ system. Some laboratories offer mini-profiles at lower cost that are specific for liver or kidney disease. It is often helpful to generate your own lists of tests to evaluate as a group when trying to rule out certain problems. For example:

Renal Disease	Liver Disease	Electrolyte Disturbances	Hydration Status
BUN	Bilirubin	Sodium	Packed Cell Volume
Creatinine	ALP	Chloride	Total Protein
Phosphorus	GGT	Potassium	Albumin
Calcium	ALT/SDH	Anion Gap	BUN/Creatinine
Sodium	Albumin	Bicarbonate	Urine Specific Gravity
Chloride	Cholesterol		Physical Exam
Postassium	Triglycerides		
Bicarbonate			
Albumin			
Amylase			
Urine Specific Gravity			

Evaluation of laboratory data is similar to the approach to the physical examination, taking a history, or evaluation of radiographs. It is not so important exactly what approach you utilize, as it is to develop a consistent method with which you are comfortable. A thorough and methodical approach will ensure that nothing is missed, and the process will become more efficient, which is always important in busy practices.

Step 3: Integrate the clinical chemistry data in the context of clinical information

If your patient has clinical chemistry abnormalities, but appears healthy, follow the outline in Figure 1-3. Interpretation of some laboratory data as normal or abnormal depends on clinical information. For example, isosthenuria in a well-hydrated patient that just consumed a large amount of water may be normal. Isosthenuria in a dehydrated patient that is also azotemic indicates the potential for significant impairment of renal function. Hyperglycemia in a calm cat is more suggestive for diabetes mellitus than hyperglycemia in a cat that is growling, hissing, and swatting at anything that moves in the examination room!

All possible causes of deranged laboratory data should be considered on the initial list of differential diagnoses, however some can likely be ruled out based on history and physical examination findings, while the remainder can be prioritized as more or less likely based on clinical information. Using the example of feline hyperglycemia, a thin cat with a history of polyuria/polydipsia and weight loss is more likely to have diabetes mellitus than a cat with a similar degree of hyperglycemia that was anxious during the clinic visit but has no clinical signs or history compatible with diabetes.

Step 4: Try to explain all problems and abnormalities of laboratory data with one primary problem.

This is a standard technique for developing diagnoses for patients. Keep in mind that occasional patients, particularly geriatric ones, may have more than one primary problem. To quote Dr. Bob Hamlin at The Ohio State University, "just because you have a headache, it doesn't mean you can't have diarrhea."

In most cases, complexities in blood work merely reflect problems that occur secondarily to the primary process. For example, liver enzyme elevations or urinary tract infections may be associated with diabetes mellitus. Many diseases may result in laboratory evidence of dehydration (increased packed cell volume, total protein, and/or albumin). Animals that have been hit by cars may have elevations of liver enzymes because of traumatic hepatocellular damage or hypoperfusion secondary to shock without primary liver disease.

Step 5: Use the clinical chemistry profile to guide the choices of further diagnostic work up.

Achieving an accurate diagnosis for a patient almost always requires a combination of clinical history, physical examination findings, some type of laboratory work, imaging studies, and possibly other testing. The serum biochemical profile may show evidence of a problem, for example electrolyte disturbances, and then the clinician must review clinical data for a cause. Based on the history and physical, the veterinarian may choose to perform imaging of the abdomen, a parvo test, an ACTH level, or other tests to help determine the underlying problem.

The sensitivity and specificity of many tests are improved by performing them on the appropriate population of patients. For example, 95% or more of dogs with hyperadrenocorticism have increased ALP. Because dexamethasone suppression and ACTH stimulation testing can be difficult to interpret, a practitioner can maximize the performance of these tests by performing them on "high risk" patients with appropriate clinical signs and laboratory data that also suggests the likelihood of hyperadrenocorticism.

Laboratory and clinical data can also aid in prioritizing possible diagnostic procedures when there are financial limitations or when some testing options are more invasive than others. For example, hyperthyroid cats often have increased liver enzymes, but no primary liver disease. As a result, if a cat is losing weight, is tachycardic, and has a palpable nodule in its neck, it may be more appropriate to run a T4 level than to schedule a liver biopsy.

Step 6: Practice!!!!

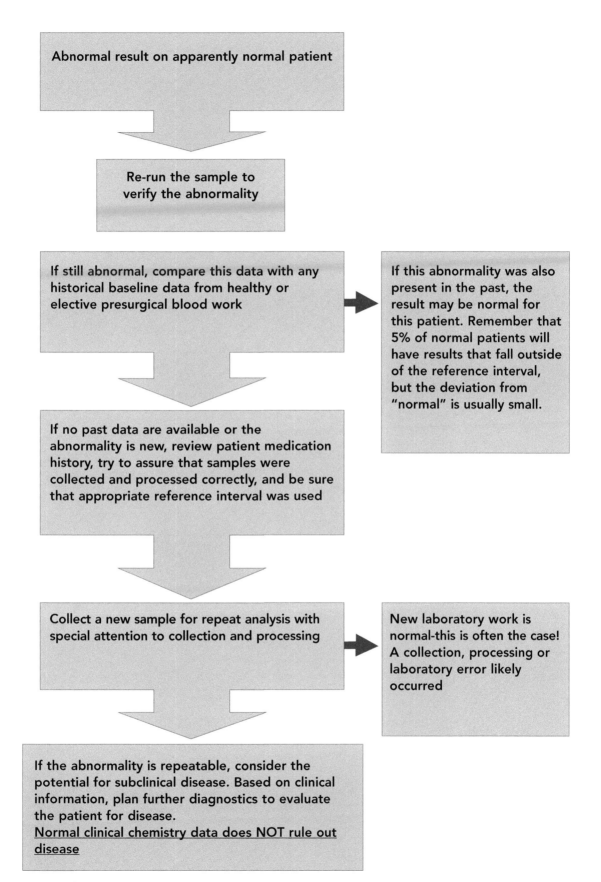

Figure 1-3.

Chapter 2

Liver Enzyme Elevations

Hepatobiliary disease can be difficult to diagnose because it often presents with nonspecific signs such as depression, weight loss, anorexia, diarrhea, and vomiting. Laboratory testing can be performed to determine if liver disease is the cause of these clinical signs, however interpretation of the results can be complicated because no consistent laboratory abnormalities are found in <u>all</u> patients with liver disease, and extrahepatic problems can also result in laboratory data that can be compatible with hepatobiliary disease.

The following are general tips to guide the interpretation of liver enzymes:

1. Elevations in serum enzyme activities are relatively sensitive but not specific for liver disease.

2. A thorough review of the patient history for medications, metabolic disorders, or other extrahepatic processes that could induce liver enzymes should be completed prior to costly or invasive work ups for primary liver disease.

3. Severe liver parenchymal loss can occur, yet liver enzyme concentrations in the circulation may be within normal limits.

4. The degree of enzyme elevation is not always prognostic, but often reflects the severity of insult and the numbers of cells affected.

5. Liver enzyme activity in the blood cannot be used to evaluate hepatic function. Serum bile acids or blood ammonia levels are generally recommended.

6. There may be discordance between the degree of enzyme elevations and the severity of histologic changes reported in biopsy specimens. Biochemical abnormalities may occur without morphologic changes in the hepatocytes that are observable at the light microscopic level. Conversely, enzymes may not be elevated despite marked parenchymal loss if active hepatocellular leakage is no longer occurring, for example with cirrhosis.

7. Decreases in liver enzyme levels in the blood over time may indicate improvement in the underlying disease, resolution of the enzyme-inducing process, or scarcity of viable hepatocytes. Liver enzyme activities below the reference interval are generally not considered to be diagnostically significant.

8. Various other laboratory abnormalities in the complete blood count, coagulation tests, and the serum biochemical profile may be present depending on the type, extent, and duration of liver disease.

9. Once extrahepatic causes for liver enzyme elevations have been ruled out clinically or by the use of further laboratory testing, liver enzyme values can be used to categorize the general process as:

• Hepatocellular damage (increased serum ALT, AST in small animals; increased serum SDH, AST in large animals)
• Cholestasis (increased serum ALP, GGT, bilirubin in small animals; increased serum GGT, bilirubin in large animals)
• Decreased liver function (increased serum bile acids, bilirubin, ammonia or fibrin degradation products; prolonged PT or PTT, decreased serum albumin, cholesterol, urea, glucose)
• A combination of the above.

It should be recognized that hepatocellular damage will lead to swelling of hepatocytes and secondary cholestasis, and that bile acids accumulating during cholestasis are toxic to hepatocytes. Either chronic or severe hepatocellular damage or cholestasis can ultimately impair liver function. The primary process is often reflected by relatively greater deviations in laboratory values than the secondary processes, but late in the course of the disease, it may not be possible to determine the initiating cause. While blood tests can suggest that hepatic disease is likely, a specific diagnosis almost always requires cytology or biopsy of liver tissue.

Guide for Evaluating the Cases in This Chapter

Review medication history, physical examination findings, and laboratory data to rule out extrahepatic conditions listed in Table 2-1

Hint! Not all of the patients presented in this chapter have hepatobiliary disease.

Step 1

If hepatobiliary disease is the cause of laboratory abnormalities, decide which processes are likely to be occurring in this patient: hepatocellular damage, cholestasis, and/or decreased liver function. Additional tests of liver function may be needed.

Step 2

When possible, determine which process is the predominant one: hepatocellular damage, cholestasis, or decreased liver function.

Step 3

Choose appropriate additional testing as needed to determine a specific diagnosis.

Hint: Remember that the liver is integrally involved in hemostasis! Don't forget to evaluate coagulation status prior to invasive procedures such as biopsy.

Step 4

Table 2-1
Some extrahepatic causes for increased concentrations of serum liver enzyme levels or bilirubin

Drug Induction
    Corticosteroids (canine): ALP, GGT, ALT, AST
    Anticonvulsants (phenobarbital, phenytoin, primidone): ALT, ALP, AST, GGT
Endocrinopathies
    Hyperthyroidism (cats): ALP, ALT
    Hypothyroidism (dogs): ALP
    Diabetes mellitus: ALP
    Hyperadrenocorticism (dogs): ALP, ALT, GGT, AST
Hypoxia/Hypotension: ALT, ALP, GGT, AST, LDH
Secondary to damaged bowel, toxic enteritis: ALT, AST, SDH
Muscle damage: AST, ALT (if severe), LDH
Neoplasia (primary or metastatic)
Increased Bone Remodeling (rapid bone growth, neoplasia, osteomyelitis): ALP (bone isoform)
Other
    Systemic infections
    Hemolysis: Bilirubin
    Pregnancy (cats): ALP (placental isoform)
    Colostrum fed neonates (dogs, lambs, calves): GGT
    Pancreatitis
    Anorexia: bilirubin (indirect) in horses

Liver Case 1 – Level 1

"Spunky" is a 10-week-old male Rottweiler puppy presenting for unproductive retching after which he "coughed" up a small piece of glass. He has had no diarrhea and has been appropriately vaccinated. Spunky is bright and responsive in the examination room and has good body condition. No abnormalities are found on physical examination.

White blood cell count:	10.8 x 10^9/L	(4.9-16.8)
Segmented neutrophils:	6.2 x 10^9/L	(2.8-11.5)
Band neutrophils:	0 x 10^9/L	(0-0.3)
Lymphocytes:	3.8 x 10^9/L	(1.0-4.8)
Monocytes:	0.5 x 10^9/L	(0.1-1.5)
Eosinophils:	0.3 x 10^9/L	(0-1.4)
WBC morphology: Appears within normal limits		

Hematocrit:	↓ 28%	(39-55)
Red blood cell count:	↓ 4.14 x 10^{12}/L	(5.8-8.5)
Hemoglobin:	↓ 9.2 g/dl	(14.0-19.1)
MCV:	67.0 fl	(60.0-75.0)
MCHC:	33.0 g/dl	(33.0-36.0)
RBC morphology: Appears within normal limits		
Platelets: Clumped, but appear adequate in number		

Glucose:	111 mg/dl	(67.0-135.0)
BUN:	23 mg/dl	(8-29)
Creatinine:	0.6 mg/dl	(0.6-2.0)
Phosphorus:	↑ 9.3 mg/dl	(2.6-7.2)
Calcium:	↑ 12.6 mg/dl	(9.4-11.6)
Magnesium:	2.0 mEq/L	(1.7-2.5)
Total Protein:	5.5 g/dl	(5.5-7.8)
Albumin:	3.2 g/dl	(2.8-4.0)
Globulin:	2.3 g/dl	(2.3-4.2)
A/G Ratio:	1.5	(0.7-2.1)
Sodium:	147 mEq/L	(142-163)
Chloride:	108 mEq/L	(106-126)
Potassium:	5.4 mEq/L	(3.8-5.4)
HCO3:	26 mEq/L	(15-28)
Anion Gap:	18.4 mEq/L	(15-25)
Total Bili:	<0.10 mg/dl	(0.10-0.30)
ALP:	↑ 560 IU/L	(20-320)
GGT:	4 IU/L	(2-10)
ALT:	20 IU/L	(18-86)
AST:	39 IU/L	(16-54)
Cholesterol:	279 mg/dl	(82-355)
Triglycerides:	158 mg/dl	(30-321)
Amylase:	541 IU/L	(409-1203)

Interpretation

CBC: The mild normocytic normochromic anemia is actually within published reference intervals for a puppy of Spunky's age. Total protein at the low end of the reference interval is also appropriate for a young puppy and is due to low globulin levels, but under other circumstances might suggest blood loss. This data illustrates the need to verify appropriate reference intervals for pediatric patients. Given Spunky's history of apparently ingesting glass, the PCV should be monitored along with careful observation for any signs of blood loss, especially via the gastrointestinal tract.

Serum Biochemical Profile
Hyperphosphatemia with hypercalcemia: This combination in a young, large breed dog is most likely normal during this period of rapid skeletal growth. Differential diagnoses for hyperphosphatemia with concurrent hypercalcemia in adult dogs include renal failure, vitamin D toxicosis, and hypoadrenocorticism. Spunky's other laboratory data and his clinical history are not supportive of any of these diagnoses.

Mildly increased ALP (1.5x): As indicated in the introduction, there are many hepatic and extrahepatic causes of increased ALP in the dog. In young, growing dogs, mild increases in ALP are normal and associated with bone growth. ALP allows mineral to be deposited in bone (Kronenberg). A complete medical history should include questions about exposure to any medications that could induce ALP.

Case Summary and Outcome
Normal findings for a young large breed dog

This combination of "abnormalities" constitutes normal physiology in this patient, who is very unlikely to have liver disease. Spunky was discharged with no further problems.

Kronenberg HM. NPT2a-the key to phosphate homeostasis. New Eng J Med 2002;347:1022-1024.

Liver Case 2 – Level 1

"Bandit" is a 1.5-year-old spayed female Labrador Retriever that was presented after the owners observed her being struck on her left thorax by a truck. The dog was thrown in the air, landed, and initially did not move. After a few minutes, she rose and started walking, but her front legs collapsed. At this point she lay on the grass crying. She has been treated in the past for pyoderma, but is not currently on any medications.

On physical examination, Bandit has bruising in the left axillary region, an abrasion on the medial aspect of the left radius and ulna, and a swelling on the thoracic wall caudal to the point of the left elbow. She is lame and painful on her left front leg, but otherwise, appears bright and alert. Radiographs of the chest, abdomen and left leg show only a mild pneumothorax. She was admitted to the hospital for observation.

White blood cell count:	8.1 x 10⁹/L	(4.9-16.9)
Segmented neutrophils:	6.8 x 10⁹/L	(2.8-11.5)
Band neutrophils:	0 x 10⁹/L	(0-0.3)
Lymphocytes:	↓ 0.5 x 10⁹/L	(1.0-4.8)
Monocytes:	0.6 x 10⁹/L	(0.1-1.3)
Eosinophils:	0.2 x 10⁹/L	(0-1.3)
WBC morphology: Appears within normal limits		

Hematocrit:	45%	(37-55)
Red blood cell count:	6.59 x 10¹²/L	(5.5-8.5)
Hemoglobin:	15.9 g/dl	(12.0-18.0)
MCV:	68.1 fl	(60.0-77.0)
MCHC:	34.0 g/dl	(31.0-34.0)
RBC morphology: Appears within normal limits		
Platelets:	227.0 x 10⁹/L	(181.0-525.0)

Plasma is clear and colorless.

Glucose:	88 mg/dl	(67.0-135.0)
BUN:	18 mg/dl	(8-29)
Creatinine:	1.1 mg/dl	(0.6-2.0)
Phosphorus:	3.1 mg/dl	(2.6-7.2)
Calcium:	10.9 mg/dl	(9.4-11.6)
Magnesium:	1.9 mEq/L	(1.7-2.5)
Total Protein:	5.9 g/dl	(5.5-7.8)
Albumin:	3.7 g/dl	(2.8-4.0)
Globulin:	2.3 g/dl	(2.3-4.2)
A/G ratio:	1.6	(0.7-1.6)
Sodium:	148 mEq/L	(142-163)
Chloride:	112 mEq/L	(111-129)
Potassium:	4.1 mEq/L	(3.8-5.4)
HCO3:	24 mEq/L	(15-28)
Anion Gap:	16.1 mEq/L	(15-25)
Total Bili:	0.03 mg/dl	(0.10-0.30)
ALP:	79 IU/L	(12-121)
GGT:	6 IU/L	(2-10)
ALT:	↑ 1505 IU/L	(18-86)

AST:	↑ 1411 IU/L	(16-54)
Cholesterol:	39 mg/dl	(30-321)
Triglycerides:	178 mg/dl	(30-321)
Amylase:	578 IU/L	(409-1203)

Urinalysis: Cystocentesis

Appearance: Dark yellow and hazy	Sediment:
Specific gravity: 1.044	RBC: 5-10 /high power field
pH: 9.0	WBC: Occasional
Protein: 30 mg/dl	
Glucose/ketones: negative	Occasional epithelial cells
Bilirubin: 1+	No bacteria seen
Heme: 3+	1+ fat droplets and debris

Interpretation

CBC: The release of endogeneous corticosteroids due to the stress of the injuries could produce a lymphopenia.

Serum Biochemical Profile

Increased ALT and AST (15-20x): Significant elevation of these two enzymes supports an interpretation of hepatocellular damage. The normal ALP and GGT indicates that cholestasis is not a factor in this case at this time. While ALT is relatively liver specific in small animal patients, AST could be compatible with some damage to muscle tissue or other organs. If muscle damage is very severe, ALT may increase due to leakage from muscle as well (Swenson). A serum CK level could be run to assess muscle damage, however, it is likely to be elevated in this case due to the trauma. The most likely cause for the Bandit's increased hepatocellular enzymes is trauma to the liver, though transient hypoperfusion of the liver due to shock following the accident could also be a factor.

Urinalysis: Bandit's urinalysis shows well-concentrated alkaline urine with small numbers of red and white blood cells. The presence of protein and heme are compatible with blood contamination from the cystocentesis procedure, or with hemorrhage secondary to trauma of the urogenital tract. Trace to 1+ (30 mg/dl) protein often is not significant when detected in a concentrated urine sample. However, false positive reactions for protein may be seen on urine dipstick results performed on alkaline urine. Carnivores generally have aciduria and alkaline urine may indicate the presence of urease positive bacteria. Transient alkaline urine may be observed postprandially.

Dogs have a low renal threshold for conjugated bilirubin and detection of a trace to 1+ bilirubin is not unusual, especially in concentrated urine. In the dog, bilirubin can be observed in the urine prior to any detectible rise in serum bilirubin concentrations.

Case Summary and Outcome

Bandit was discharged the next morning with medication for control of pain. She had an uneventful recovery.

Swenson CL, Graves TK. Absence of liver specificity for canine alanine aminotransferase (ALT). Vet Clin Pathol. 1997;26:26-28.

Liver Case 3 – Level 1

"Chewie" is a 6-year-old castrated male Bouvier who began showing signs of lameness in the left front limb approximately one month ago. The referring veterinarian initially diagnosed osteochondritis dessicans and prescribed a nonsteriodal anti-inflammatory drug. On presentation, Chewie is painful and has swelling in the region of his left proximal humerus.

White blood cell count:	5.8 x 10⁹/L	(4.9-16.8)
Segmented neutrophils:	4.1 x 10⁹/L	(2.8-11.5)
Band neutrophils:	0	(0-0.3)
Lymphocytes:	↓ 0.9 x 10⁹/L	(1.0-4.8)
Monocytes:	0.6 x 10⁹/L	(0.1-1.5)
Eosinophils:	↑ 0.2 x 10⁹/L	(0-0.1)
WBC morphology: Appears within normal limits		

Hematocrit:	48%	(39-55)
Red blood cell count:	7.78 x 10¹²/L	(5.8-8.5)
Hemoglobin:	16.7 g/dl	(14.0-19.1)
MCV:	60.9 fl	(60.0-75.0)
MCHC:	34.8 g/dl	(33.0-36.0)
RBC morphology: Appears within normal limits		
Platelets: Appear adequate in number		

Glucose:	99 mg/dl	(67.0-135.0)
BUN:	13 mg/dl	(8-29)
Creatinine:	1.2 mg/dl	(0.6-2.0)
Phosphorus:	3.9 mg/dl	(2.6-7.2)
Calcium:	11.1 mg/dl	(9.4-11.6)
Magnesium:	2.3 mEq/L	(1.7-2.5)
Total Protein:	6.8 g/dl	(5.5-7.8)
Albumin:	3.3 g/dl	(2.8-4.0)
Globulin:	3.5 g/dl	(2.3-4.2)
A/G ratio:	0.9	(0.7-2.1)
Sodium:	148 mEq/L	(142-163)
Chloride:	114 mEq/L	(106-126)
Potassium:	4.4 mEq/L	(3.8-5.4)
HCO3:	15 mEq/L	(15-28)
Anion Gap:	23.4 mEq/L	(15-25)
Total Bili:	0.20 mg/dl	(0.10-0.30)
ALP:	↑ 345 IU/L	(12-121)
GGT:	4 IU/L	(2-10)
ALT:	59 IU/L	(18-86)
AST:	27 IU/L	(16-54)
Cholesterol:	243 mg/dl	(82-355)
Triglycerides:	71 mg/dl	(30-321)
Amylase:	1200 IU/L	(409-1203)

Interpretation

CBC: The mild changes in lymphocyte and eosinophil numbers may be normal variation. Lymphopenia may be secondary to endogenous corticosteroid release or stress. However, the presence of a mild eosinophilia makes a steroid response less likely. Increases in eosinophils may be seen with parasitic disease or hypersensitivity reactions. The remainder of the CBC appears within normal limits.

Increased ALP (2.5x): This relatively mild elevation in ALP is quite nonspecific by itself. Due to the numerous causes for increased ALP in the dog, interpretation is heavily dependent on clinical information. In the context of Chewie's history and physical examination findings, increased ALP due to bone disease seems likely. While osteomyelitis is a possibility, so is osteosarcoma. As always, the possibility of endocrine disorders and exposure to medications that could induce increased ALP expression should be ruled out.

Case Summary and Outcome
Increased ALP secondary to bone disease

In contrast to Spunky (Case 1), Chewie is too old to expect ALP to be elevated due to normal skeletal growth. No medications that could induce ALP were given. While a lymphopenia may support a corticosteroid response, the lymphopenia observed in Chewie is very mild and the rest of the CBC is not consist with a stress or "steroid" leukogram. While some non-steroidal anti-inflammatory medications have been reported to cause liver failure in some dogs, this is associated with jaundice and elevations of not only ALP but also ALT and AST, which were not present in this patient.

Radiographs demonstrated a lytic lesion in the proximal humerus, however thoracic films were clear of evidence of metastatic disease. Please note that this does not rule out the presence of microscopic metastases, which are often present at the time of diagnosis of osteosarcoma. Cytologic evaluation of aspirates from the lytic lesion (Figure 2.1) were consistent with osteosarcoma. Chewie's limb was amputated, and biopsy showed osteosarcoma with areas of necrosis and hemorrhage. Dogs with osteosarcoma have shorter survival times and disease free intervals if the serum ALP is elevated at the time of diagnosis (Ehrhart, Kirpensteijn, Liptak). In this case, the serum biochemical profile helped support the clinical diagnosis and provided additional prognostic information.

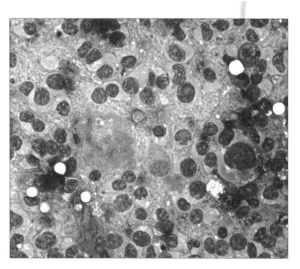

Figure 2-1. Smears of aspirates from a lytic bone lesion consisted of numerous round to oval to spindle shaped mesenchymal cells with abundant pale blue cytoplasm. Most cells had a single round to oval nucleus that was often eccentrically placed consistent with neoplastic osteoblasts. Features of malignancy such as anisocytosis and anisokaryosis were marked. Bright pink extracellular material compatible with osteoid was noted.

Ehrhart N, Dernell WS, Hoffmann WE, Weigel RM, Powers B, Withrow SJ. Prognostic importance of alkaline phosphatase activity in serum from dogs with appendicular osteosarcoma: 75 cases (1990-1996). J Vet Med Assoc. 1998;213:1002-1006.

Kirpenteijn J, Kik M, Rutteman GR, Teske E. Prognostic significance of a new histological grading system for osteosarcoma. Vet Pathol. 2002;39:240-246.

Liptak JM, Dernell WS, Ehrhart N, Withrow SJ. Canine appendicular osteosarcoma: diagnosis and palliative treatment. Comp Contin Ed. 2004;26:172-196.

Liver Case 4 – Level 1

"Beauty" is a 1.5-year-old miniature mare that presented with a history of a difficult labor of several hours duration. A partial fetotomy was performed in the field, but it could not be completed. On presentation, Beauty was painful with an elevated heart and respiratory rate.

White blood cell count:	↓ 1.6 x 10⁹/L	(5.9-11.2)
Segmented neutrophils:	↓ 0.7 x 10⁹/L	(2.3-9.1)
Band neutrophils:	0.1	(0-0.3)
Lymphocytes:	↓ 0.7 x 10⁹/L	(1.6-5.2)
Monocytes:	0.1 x 10⁹/L	(0-1.0)

WBC morphology: Moderately toxic neutrophils

Hematocrit:	42%	(30-51)
Red blood cell count:	7.91 x 10¹²/L	(6.5-12.8)
Hemoglobin:	14.8 g/dl	(10.9-18.1)
MCV:	51.8 fl	(35.0-53.0)
MCHC:	35.2 g/dl	(34.6-38.0)

RBC morphology: Appears within normal limits

Platelets: Appear adequate

Fibrinogen:	↑ 500 mg/dl	(100-400)

Glucose:	↑ 178 mg/dl	(6.0-128.0)
BUN:	23 mg/dl	(11-26)
Creatinine:	1.1 mg/dl	(0.9-1.9)
Phosphorus:	4.2 mg/dl	(1.9-6.0)
Calcium:	11.1 mg/dl	(11.0-13.5)
Total Protein:	7.0 g/dl	(5.6-7.0)
Albumin:	2.8 g/dl	(2.4-3.8)
Globulin:	4.2 g/dl	(2.5-4.9)
A/G Ratio:	0.7	(0.7-2.1)
Sodium:	139 mEq/L	(130-145)
Chloride:	99 mEq/L	(99-105)
Potassium:	3.5 mEq/L	(3.0-5.0)
HCO3:	31 mEq/L	(25-31)
Total Bili:	↑ 3.6 mg/dl	(0.30-3.0)
Direct Bili:	0.1 mg/dl	(0.0-0.5)
Indirect Bili:	↑ 3.5 mg/dl	(0.2-3.0)
GGT:	10 IU/L	(5-23)
AST:	↑ 1173 IU/L	(190-380)
CK:	↑ 39501 IU/L	(80-446)

Interpretation
CBC
Leukogram: Beauty has leukopenia characterized by neutropenia and lymphopenia. The toxic changes in the neutrophils and the increased fibrinogen indicate inflammation. Thus, the neutropenia is secondary to acute, overwhelming inflammation that is depleting the neutrophils in the peripheral blood. The lymphopenia is probably caused by release of endogenous corticosteroids secondary to stress in this patient.

Serum Biochemical Profile
Hyperglycemia: Stress is the most likely cause for hyperglycemia in this patient.

Hyperbilirubinemia with increased indirect bilirubin: Anorexia in horses will result in increased indirect bilirubin. Decreased liver function is another possibility, however we have no test results that specifically evaluate liver function here. Serum bile acids and blood ammonia can be performed as more specific tests of liver function. Sepsis can lead to decreased removal of bilirubin from the blood because endotoxin can inhibit hepatocellular uptake of bilirubin. The neutropenia with toxic changes is also compatible with sepsis. Hemolysis is an unlikely cause of hyperbilirubinemia in this patient, because she has a normal PCV.

Increased AST (30x) and CK (79x) with normal GGT: AST may increase with either hepatocellular damage or muscle damage, while the markedly increased CK is strong evidence for muscle damage. In combination with a normal GGT, the most likely source for the elevated AST in this patient is muscle.

Case Summary and Outcome
Acute overwhelming inflammation (sepsis and/or metritis), muscle trauma, anorexia, and stress.

Immediately after admission, Beauty was placed under general anesthesia in an effort to remove the fetus via controlled vaginal delivery, but the dead fetus was too large. She was taken to surgery for a cesarean section through a ventral midline approach. There were no surgical complications, and she was treated post-operatively with broad-spectrum intravenous antibiotics and Banamine®. Oxytocin was administered, and the uterus was flushed daily with dilute betadine and lactated ringer's solution for five days. Antibiotics were infused into the uterus three times. Beauty did develop mastitis after surgery that responded to antibiotic infusion, and several of her skin staples had to be removed for drainage of a mild infection of her incision. Beauty was discharged and had an uneventful recovery at home.

Beauty's case illustrates that the need to distinguish extrahepatic causes of enzyme elevations is important in the horse as well as in small animals. The measurement of SDH, which is more liver specific than AST in horses, will help the clinician distinguish increases in AST caused by hepatocellular damage versus increases caused by muscle damage. Anorexia-induced increases in bilirubin in horses can further complicate data interpretation. As noted previously, the possibility of sepsis as another potential cause for hyperbilirubinemia should be considered.

Liver Case 5 – Level 1

"Greta" is a 9-year-old female spayed German Shepherd dog with a history of watery stools. A previous work-up resulted in a diagnosis of inflammatory bowel disease, for which Greta has been treated with 20 mg of oral prednisone per day. This has resulted in improved clinical signs, however lately she has developed a distended abdomen, thin skin, and hair loss. She is also polyuric and polydipsic.

White blood cell count:	↑ 20.00 x 10⁹/L	(4.9-16.8)
Segmented neutrophils:	↑ 19.0 x 10⁹/L	(2.8-11.5)
Band neutrophils:	0	(0-0.3)
Lymphocytes:	↓ 0.6 x 10⁹/L	(1.0-4.8)
Monocytes:	0 x 10⁹/L	(0.1-1.5)
Eosinophils:	0.4 x 10⁹/L	(0-1.4)
WBC morphology: Appears within normal limits		
Hematocrit:	42%	(39-55)
Red blood cell count:	5.44 x 10¹²/L	(5.2-8.5)
Hemoglobin:	14.7 g/dl	(14.0-19.1)
MCV:	73.8 fl	(60.0-75.0)
MCHC:	35.0 g/dl	(33.0-36.0)
RBC morphology: Appears within normal limits		
Platelets:	525.0 x 10⁹/L	(181.0-525.0)
Glucose:	91 mg/dl	(67.0-135.0)
BUN:	12 mg/dl	(8-29)
Creatinine:	0.5 mg/dl	(0.5-2.0)
Phosphorus:	5.5 mg/dl	(2.6-7.2)
Calcium:	9.5 mg/dl	(9.4-11.6)
Magnesium:	2.3 mEq/L	(1.7-2.5)
Total Protein:	6.3 g/dl	(5.5-7.8)
Albumin:	3.0 g/dl	(2.8-4.0)
Globulin:	3.3 g/dl	(2.3-4.2)
A/G Ratio:	0.9	(0.7-2.1)
Sodium:	149 mEq/L	(142-163)
Chloride:	109 mEq/L	(106-126)
Potassium:	5.1 mEq/L	(3.8-5.4)
HCO3:	26 mEq/L	(15-28)
Anion Gap:	19.1 mEq/L	(15-25)
Total Bili:	<0.20 mg/dl	(0.10-0.30)
ALP:	↑ 464 IU/L	(20-320)
GGT:	↑ 163 IU/L	(2-10)
ALT:	↑ 329 IU/L	(18-86)
AST:	52 IU/L	(16-54)
Cholesterol:	114 mg/dl	(82-355)
Triglycerides:	80 mg/dl	(30-321)
Amylase:	453 IU/L	(409-1203)

Interpretation

CBC
Mature neutrophilic leukocytosis with lymphopenia: The mature neutrophilic leukocytosis could indicate inflammatory disease, however in the absence of toxic changes or a significant left shift, it may be more compatible with a corticosteroid leukogram. The lymphopenia supports this interpretation. Other elements of steroid-induced changes in the leukogram in dogs include a monocytosis and eosinopenia, neither of which are seen in this case. Some patients may not have all components of the steroid leukogram at once.

Serum Biochemical Profile
Increased ALP (25% increase) and GGT (16x increase): These enzymes are classically thought of as cholestatic enzymes. However, as is seen here, their production may be induced by corticosteroids in the absence of cholestatic disease. Note the serum bilirubin is within the reference interval.

Increased ALT (3-4x increase): This enzyme is used to detect hepatocellular damage, and will also increase with administration of corticosteroids.

Case Summary and Outcome
Steroid hepatopathy

Greta's liver enzymes were within the reference interval until her treatment with prednisone began. Although liver disease is possible, steroids are the most likely cause of the increased liver enzymes activities seen here. To confirm this interpretation, it is possible to measure the corticosteroid-induced isoenzyme of ALP, which is most often accomplished by levamisole inhibition. This test is based on the use of levamisole to suppress activity of the liver and bone isoenzymes in the serum sample. In dogs with normal serum ALP, the corticosteroid induced isoenzyme makes up about 5-20% of the total ALP. Because hepatobiliary disease has been reported in association with certain types of inflammatory bowel disease, the possibility of liver disease in Greta should remain on the list of differential diagnoses, especially if liver enzyme elevations persist following withdrawal of corticosteroid therapy. As always, the interpretation of elevated ALP in the dog depends significantly on history, clinical signs, and other laboratory work because of the numerous factors that can cause increased ALP.

In general, administration of corticosteroids causes greater increases in ALP than GGT, although the degree of increase depends on dose, method of administration, type of corticosteroid given, and individual sensitivity to the drug. Increases in ALT that are noted in patients with steroid hepatopathy may be related to areas of focal necrosis /cholestasis that are seen with the vacuolar hepatopathy induced by steroids.

Because of Greta's iatrogenic hyperadrenocorticism, her prednisone was tapered to a lower dose. Consequently, her inflammatory bowel disease worsened, so another immunosuppressive agent was added to her treatment. Two months after this change in her therapeutic protocol, her clinical signs were under good control. Her liver enzyme values had decreased but were still slightly elevated (ALP 217 IU/L, GGT 41 IU/L, ALT 118 IU/L).

Liver Case 6 – Level 1

"Rover" is a 13-year-old neutered male Siamese cross-bred cat with a history of weight loss with vomiting and diarrhea. On physical examination, Rover is tachycardic with a gallop rhythm. He is thin with an unkempt coat. Abdominal palpation is unremarkable.

White blood cell count:	7.5 x 10⁹/L	(4.5-15.7)
Segmented neutrophils:	5.8 x 10⁹/L	(2.1-10.1)
Lymphocytes:	↓ 1.3 x 10⁹/L	(1.5-7.0)
Monocytes:	0.2 x 10⁹/L	(0-0.9)
Eosinophils:	0.2 x 10⁹/L	(0.0-1.9)
WBC morphology: Appears within normal limits		

Hematocrit:	32%	(28-45)
Red blood cell count:	7.44 x 10¹²/L	(5.0-10.0)
Hemoglobin:	10.5 g/dl	(8.0-15.0)
MCV:	40.6 fl	(39.0-55.0)
MCHC:	32.8	(31.0-35.0)
RBC morphology: Appears within normal limits		
Platelets: Clumped, but appear adequate		

Glucose:	↑ 200 mg/dl	(70.0-120.0)
BUN:	25 mg/dl	(15-32)
Creatinine:	1.9 mg/dl	(0.9-2.1)
Phosphorus:	4.7 mg/dl	(3.0-6.0)
Calcium:	10.0 mg/dl	(8.9-11.6)
Total Protein:	7.8 g/dl	(6.0-8.4)
Albumin:	3.5 g/dl	(2.4-4.0)
Globulin:	4.3 g/dl	(2.5-5.8)
A:G Ratio	0.8	(0.7-1.6)
Sodium:	155 mEq/L	(149-163)
Chloride:	122 mEq/L	(119-134)
Potassium:	4.2 mEq/L	(3.6-5.4)
HCO3:	22 mEq/L	(13-22)
Total Bili:	0.2 mg/dl	(0.10-0.30)
ALP:	↑ 312 IU/L	(10-72)
ALT:	↑ 250 IU/L	(29-145)
AST:	↑ 159 IU/L	(12-42)
Cholesterol:	203 mg/dl	(77-258)
Triglycerides:	25 mg/dl	(25-191)
Amylase:	791 IU/L	(496-1874)

Urinalysis: (Method not indicated)

Appearance: Amber and opaque	Sediment:
Specific gravity: 1.045	0-5 RBC/high power field
pH: 7.0	No WBC seen
Protein: negative	No casts seen
Glucose/ketones: negative	No epithelial cells seen
Bilirubin: negative	No bacteria
Heme: negative	Trace fat droplets and debris

Interpretation

CBC
Lymphopenia: The mild lymphopenia here may be attributable to stress, however a mature neutrophilic leukocytosis does not accompany it to support a corticosteroid leukogram.

Serum Biochemical Profile
Hyperglycemia: Differentials include a stress response, post prandial effects, or diabetes mellitus. Both acute epinephrine release or more chronic corticosteroid release (stress) can cause hyperglycemia. Epinephrine induced hyperglycemia should be transient. The lymphopenia in the CBC supports a stress response. The degree of hyperglycemia is relatively mild, and while glucosuria and ketonuria are not present, this does not completely rule out diabetes mellitus. The clinical signs here are nonspecific and also do not help rule out diabetes. A serum fructosamine level would better reflect chronic glycemic control. Feline pancreatitis may be associated with either hyperglycemia or hypoglycemia.

Increased ALP (4x): Nonspecific induction of ALP is rare in the cat compared to the dog, so increased ALP is always considered significant in cats. Increased ALP will be seen with many feline liver diseases, in addition to hyperthyroidism and diabetes mellitus. In contrast, corticosteroids do not usually increase ALP in cats.

Increased ALT and AST (2-3x): As for dogs, these increases indicate hepatocellular damage associated with liver disease, hypoperfusion, or the effects of drugs, toxins, or hormones, including increased thyroid hormone. It is not possible to confirm a specific cause of the increased liver enzymes based on blood work alone.

Case Summary and Outcome
Liver enzyme elevations with mild hyperglycemia and lymphopenia.

In this case, hyperthyroidism should be the primary differential diagnosis. This is based on a combination of the clinical history (weight loss, tachycardia with gallop rhythm, vomiting and diarrhea) and the laboratory work. Most primary feline liver diseases will be associated with some degree of hyperbilirubinemia, which is absent here. While diabetes cannot be ruled out based on the initial laboratory data, the hyperglycemia is mild without significant abnormalities in the urinalysis. A diagnosis of hyperthyroidism must be confirmed by running a total T_4. Both hyperthyroidism and diabetes mellitus should be ruled out in cats presenting with liver enzyme elevations prior to performing more invasive diagnostic procedures such as liver aspirate or biopsy. In Rover's case, a diagnosis of hyperthyroidism was confirmed with a total T_4 of 9 µg/dl (normal is <2.5).

Liver enzyme elevations in hyperthyroid cats are most often reversible with control of their disease. The cause for the elevations is not clear, however malnutrition, cardiac complications, and direct toxic effects of thyroid hormone may be factors. Histologic lesions are generally mild and include fatty infiltration and hepatocellular degeneration and necrosis. There is some evidence that bone ALP contributes to the increased ALP in hyperthyroid cats.

Rover's hyperthyroidism was well controlled on a low dose of methimazole. His laboratory work was closely monitored over the first few months of therapy because of the possibility of hematologic side effects of the drug and because resolution of the hyperthyroidism can reveal previously subclinical renal insufficiency in some patients. Rover did not experience any reactions to the methimazole, nor did he develop azotemia, but his liver enzyme values normalized.

Liver Case 7 – Level 2

"Lady" is a 13-year-old spayed female American Eskimo dog who presented acutely recumbent and dull. Lady has a distended abdomen with a fluid wave, is febrile, and is tachycardic. Her mucus membranes are dull red with a capillary refill time (CRT) of 3.5 seconds. A large amount of fluid is collected during abdominocentesis. Lady's laboratory data include the following:

White blood cell count:	↓ 5.8 x 10⁹/L	(6.0-17.0)
Segmented neutrophils:	4.6 x 10⁹/L	(3.0-11.0)
Band neutrophils:	0.2 x 10⁹/L	(0-0.3)
Lymphocytes:	↓ 0.7 x 10⁹/L	(1.0-4.8)
Monocytes:	0.2 x 10⁹/L	(0.2-1.4)
Eosinophils:	0.1 x 10⁹/L	(0-1.3)
WBC morphology: Mild toxic change in neutrophils		

Hematocrit:	44%	(37-55)
Red blood cell count:	6.3 x 10¹²/L	(5.5-8.5)
Hemoglobin:	14.7 g/dl	(12.0-18.0)
MCV:	71.9 fl	(60.0-77.0)
MCHC:	33.4 g/dl	(31.0-34.0)
RBC morphology: Appears within normal limits		
Platelets:	↓ 127 x 10⁹/L	(250-450)

Slight hemolysis of plasma

Glucose:	92 mg/dl	(65.0-120.0)
BUN:	↑ 51 mg/dl	(8-33)
Creatinine:	↑ 1.7 mg/dl	(0.5-1.5)
Phosphorus:	6.0 mg/dl	(3.0-6.0)
Calcium:	10.5 mg/dl	(8.8-11.0)
Magnesium:	2.2 mEq/L	(1.4-2.7)
Total Protein:	7.0 g/dl	(5.2-7.2)
Albumin:	4.1 g/dl	(3.0-4.2)
Globulin:	2.9 g/dl	(2.0-4.0)
A/G Ratio:	1.4	(0.7-2.1)
Sodium:	149 mEq/L	(140-151)
Chloride:	106 mEq/L	(105-120)
Potassium:	3.9 mEq/L	(3.8-5.4)
HCO3:	18 mEq/L	(16-25)
Anion Gap:	↑ 28.9 mEq/L	(15-25)
Total Bili:	↑ 0.63 mg/dl	(0.10-0.50)
ALP:	↑ 2769 IU/L	(20-320)
ALT:	↑ 9955 IU/L	(10-95)
AST:	↑ 4847 IU/L	(15-52)
Cholesterol:	259 mg/dl	(110-314)
Triglycerides:	83 mg/dl	(30-300)
Amylase:	957 IU/L	(400-1200)

Abdominal fluid analysis (Figure 2-2)

Color: Dark red-brown	
Total Protein: 6.5 gm/dl	
Total Nucleated Cells: 33,600/µl	

Cytologic description: Smears contain large numbers of mildly degenerate neutrophils with intracellular and extracellular bacteria. Bacteria are large rods that sometimes have focal nonstaining areas suggestive for spore formation.

No urine could be collected on this patient.

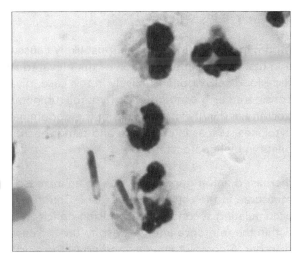

Figure 2-2. Cytology of abdominal fluid from Lady, case 7. Smears consisted of degenerate neutrophils with intracellular rod-shaped bacteria.

Interpretation
CBC
Leukogram: There is a mild leukopenia with lymphopenia and toxic changes in neutrophils. Corticosteroid effects could contribute to the lymphopenia, however other elements of the corticosteroid leukogram such as a neutrophilia and monocytosis are not evident. Toxic change in the neutrophils suggests an inflammatory process. Due to the acute presentation of the patient, further abnormalities of the CBC are expected to develop and a follow up CBC should be collected in the next 24 hours, or sooner if the clinical condition deteriorates.

Platelets: The mild thrombocytopenia is not of the severity that would be expected to result in spontaneous bleeding in the absence of platelet functional defects. Liver disease and/or a septic focus could contribute to the decreased platelet count and the mechanism is likely consumptive. Coagulation studies would help rule out the possibility of disseminated intravascular coagulation (DIC).

Serum Biochemical Profile
Mild Azotemia: A prerenal cause of the mild azotemia is suspected based on the clinical history, the absence of other abnormalities corroborating a primary renal problem (e.g. normal phosphorus, amylase, and hematocrit), and the suggestion of poor perfusion (prolonged CRT) and dehydration (albumin at the high end of the reference range). A concentrated urine specific gravity would help substantiate this interpretation, but a sample could not be obtained on this patient.

Marked elevation of ALT and AST: There is evidence for significant hepatocellular damage with hepatocellular enzyme elevations of approximately 100x the upper limit of the reference interval for both enzymes. Elevation of AST is less specific for liver and could indicate some muscle damage. A CK might help distinguish the source of the AST but is not clinically necessary in this case. Unfortunately, these enzyme elevations do not reveal the underlying cause of the hepatocellular damage, nor are they prognostic.

Moderate elevation of ALP: The most likely cause of the approximately 10-fold increase in ALP is mild cholestasis secondary to hepatocellular damage. This interpretation is supported by the relatively greater elevation in hepatocellular enzymes compared to cholestatic enzymes. Some degree of enzyme induction is possible, since we speculated about possible elements of a corticosteroid leukogram. Some reference laboratories offer measurement of the corticosteroid-induced ALP isoenzyme. As always, a complete drug history should be taken and other extrahepatic causes of liver enzyme elevations should be ruled out, especially in the dog (see Table 2-1).

Mild hyperbilirubinemia: The most likely cause for this finding is mild secondary cholestasis and fits with the interpretation of the elevated ALP. Hemolysis or a significant destruction of red blood cells appears unlikely in this case, given the normal hematocrit. Sepsis must be considered as a contributor to hyperbilirubinemia in this patient due to the presence of bacteria and inflammatory cells in the abdominal fluid. High levels of circulating inflammatory cytokines such as interleukin-6 and tumor necrosis factor directly inhibit the uptake of bilirubin by hepatocytes.

Increased anion gap: This is due to an increase in circulating anions that are not routinely measured in the chemistry panel (see Chapter 7). In this case, lactic acid is likely accumulating secondary to perfusion deficits in this dog. The fact that the bicarbonate is within the reference interval despite the increased anion gap suggests a mixed acid/base disorder. A complete understanding of the acid/base status of this patient would require arterial blood gas analysis.

Abdominocentesis: Septic suppurative exudate (see Figure 2-2)

Case Summary and Outcome

Severe hepatocellular damage with secondary mild cholestasis and mild/moderate prerenal azotemia, septic peritonitis.

Further investigation into the patient history revealed that the dog had been diagnosed with a large hepatocellular carcinoma at another clinic. The blood work was normal at that time. Twenty-four hours prior to presentation to the referral hospital, the liver tumor in the patient had been treated by administration of 12-15, ultrasound guided, intratumoral injections of 100% ethanol. Wedge biopsy sections of the liver showed remnants of the original liver tumor with areas of coagulation necrosis and acute suppurative portal hepatitis. The necrosis was likely the result of the ethanol injections. The patient died in the hospital.

Liver Case 8 – Level 2

"Patton" is a 2.5-year-old, intact male German Shepherd dog who presented for vomiting bile-tinged fluid, lethargy, and anorexia of 1 week duration. His condition had progressed to stumbling, blindness, and collapse. At the time of presentation, Patton is in severe shock and has a fever of 108°F. Abdominocentesis is collected with routine blood work.

White blood cell count:	↑ 19.4 x 10⁹/L	(6.0-17.0)
Segmented neutrophils:	↑ 17.6 x 10⁹/L	(3.0-11.0)
Band neutrophils:	0 x 10⁹/L	(0-0.300)
Lymphocytes:	↓ 0.8 x 10⁹/L	(1.0-4.8)
Monocytes:	0.8 x 10⁹/L	(0.150-1.350)
Eosinophils:	0.2 x 10⁹/L	(0-1.250)
Nucleated RBC/100 WBC:	3	

WBC morphology: Appears within normal limits

Hematocrit:	↓ 31%	(37-55)
Red blood cell count:	↓ 4.48 x 10⁶/ul	(5.5-8.5 x 10⁶)
Hemoglobin:	↓ 10.4 g/dl	(12.0-18.0)
MCV:	71.2 fl	(60.0-77.0)
MCHC:	33.5 g/dl	(31.0-34.0)

RBC morphology: Moderately increased anisocytosis, slightly increased polychromasia

Platelets:	↓ 134 x 10⁶/L	(250-450)

Platelet morphology: Small clumps are present, therefore the platelet count should be considered a minimum.

Plasma is icteric.

Glucose:	96 mg/dl	(65.0-120.0)
BUN:	8 mg/dl	(8-33)
Creatinine:	invalid due to hyperbilirubinemia	
Phosphorus:	4.0 mg/dl	(3.0-6.0)
Calcium:	10.4 mg/dl	(8.8-11.0)
Magnesium:	1.4 mEq/L	(1.4-2.7)
Total Protein:	5.7 g/dl	(5.2-7.2)
Albumin:	3.2 g/dl	(3.0-4.2)
Globulin:	2.5 g/dl	(2.0-4.0)
A/G Ratio:	1.3	(0.7-2.1)
Sodium:	141 mEq/L	(140-151)
Chloride:	↓ 100 mEq/L	(105-120)
Potassium:	↓ 3.7 mEq/L	(3.8-5.4)
HCO3:	↑ 27 mEq/L	(16-25)
Anion Gap:	17.7 mEq/L	(15-25)
Total Bili:	↑ 17.50 mg/dl	(0.10-0.50)
ALP:	↑ 11,168 IU/L	(20-320)
GGT:	↑ 40 IU/L	(2-10)
ALT:	↑ 622 IU/L	(10-95)
AST:	↑ 227 IU/L	(15-52)
Cholesterol:	↑ 470 mg/dl	(110-314)
Triglycerides:	83 mg/dl	(30-300)
Amylase:	910 IU/L	(400-1200)

Abdominal fluid: (Figure 2-3)

Pre-spin color: red and cloudy	
Post-spin: orange and clear	
Total protein: 5.2 gm/dl	
Total nucleated cells: 51,900/µl	

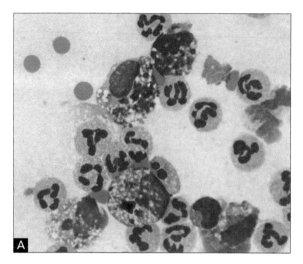

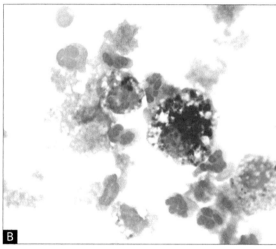

Figure 2-3A & B. A. Cytology of abdominal fluid from Patton, case 8. Smears consisted of nondegenerate neutrophils and foamy macrophages containing blue-green to black pigment. B. Golden yellow bile pigment occurs extracellularly in some areas. This is compatible with bile peritonitis.

Smears consist of many vacuolated macrophages containing abundant granular blue-green to black pigment. Smudges of golden yellow pigment occur extracellularly. Scattered non-degenerate neutrophils and occasional red blood cells are present in the background. An etiologic agent is not present.

Interpretation
CBC
Leukogram: Neutrophilic leukocytosis with lymphopenia and no morphologic abnormalities is consistent with corticosteroid-induced changes in the leukogram, although monocytosis is not present. Despite the absence of toxic changes or a left shift, inflammation is suspected in addition to corticosteroid effects based on the remainder of the data.

Erythrogram: Mild normocytic normochromic anemia. Possibilities include anemia of chronic disease (non-regenerative) or acute blood loss with insufficient time to produce a detectable change in red blood cell indices. Acute hemolysis is also possible. There is some morphologic evidence for an attempt at regeneration, including the increase in polychromasia and nucleated RBCs. Nucleated RBC's may be related to endothelial cell damage secondary to shock, although splenic dysfunction is also possible. A reticulocyte count should be done and successive CBC's should be monitored as needed.

Platelets: The presence of platelet clumps suggests that the platelet count may be artifactually low and should be repeated on a fresh sample. Such a mild thrombocytopenia is not of the degree expected to result in spontaneous bleeding in the absence of other pathology. Liver disease or severe inflammation could contribute to decreased platelets (the mechanism is likely consumptive), and coagulation studies would help rule out the possibility of disseminated intravascular coagulation.

Serum Biochemistry

Hypochloremia: In this patient, the hypochloremia is not accompanied by changes in serum sodium. Vomiting of gastric contents causes loss of chloride, and the chloride tends to vary inversely with bicarbonate (HCO3). (For full discussion of electrolyte evaluation, see Chapter 7)

Hypokalemia: Patton has several factors that could contribute to hypokalemia. Gastrointestinal loss through vomiting and/or diarrhea is an important cause. Decreased intake of potassium in anorectic patients can lead to hypokalemia, most often in combination with external losses. Cellular translocation should always be considered as a cause of abnormal potassium. The alkalemia in this patient could trigger a shift of potassium into the cells in exchange for hydrogen ion. (For full discussion of electrolyte evaluation, see Chapter 7)

Increased HCO3: This value indicates alkalosis, again related to loss of acid through vomiting of gastric contents.

Marked hyperbilirubinemia: The combination of dramatic elevations in ALP and GGT supports cholestasis as the cause for this abnormality. Although the patient is anemic, the decrement in hematocrit is small and there are no changes in RBC morphology to suggest a hemolytic mechanism. As noted for Lady (Case 7), sepsis may also impair hepatocellular uptake of bilirubin. Van den Burgh fractionation of bilirubin in small animal patients is not considered a reliable marker for hemolytic versus cholestatic hyperbilirubinemia because of rapid equilibration of the conjugated and unconjugated forms of bilirubin.

Marked increase in ALP and GGT: These elevations (roughly 35x and 4x the upper limit of the reference interval) are secondary to significant cholestasis in this patient. As always, contributions from extrahepatic causes of liver enzyme elevations must be considered.

Mild increase in ALT and AST: These elevations (roughly 5x the upper limit of the reference interval) are mild compared to the increases in the cholestatic enzymes. Based on the relative increases in enzymes, Patton likely has hepatocellular damage secondary to a primary cholestatic process.

Hypercholesterolemia: Patton most likely has hypercholesterolemia secondary to cholestasis. Hypercholesterolemia may also be seen in association with several endocrinopathies, nephrotic syndrome, pancreatitis, liver disease, as a post-prandial finding, and idiopathic hyperlipidemia.

Abdominocentesis: There is marked, mixed inflammation with pigment indicative of bile peritonitis (See Figure 2-3).

Case Summary and Outcome

Primary cholestasis with secondary hepatocellular damage. Electrolyte and acid/base abnormalities consistent with vomiting. Bile peritonitis.

This case is in contrast to Lady (Case 7), in which hepatocellular damage was the primary process as seen by the relatively greater elevation of hepatocellular enzymes versus cholestatic enzymes. In addition to enzyme changes, the marked hyperbilirubinemia and moderate hypercholesterolemia support a significant cholestatic process. In neither case do we have available tests of liver function.

Abdominal radiographs of Patton showed free gas in the abdomen highlighting the gall bladder. During exploratory surgery, an engorged necrotic gall bladder was seen and a rupture was present at the liver border, explaining the bile peritonitis. Histologically the perforation was accompanied by chronic suppurative inflammation and granulation tissue, but the cause for the rupture could not be determined. A recent study reports that gall bladder infarction may be a cause for ruptured gall bladder (Holt). Patients in that study had similar clinicopathologic abnormalities to this patient. After surgery, Patton was treated with multiple antibiotics and Reglan®. His clinical condition improved, however he remained blind in the right eye despite normal papillary light reflexes. The blindness was interpreted to be secondary to a central event, but the etiology was not investigated further.

Holt DE, Mehler S, Mayhew PD, Hendrick MJ. Canine gallbladder infarction: 12 cases (1993-2003). Vet Pathol 2004;41:416-418.

Liver Case 9 – Level 2

"Bruja" is a 14-year-old spayed female German shepherd mixed breed dog presenting for progressive anorexia, lethargy, and weakness. She has recently begun vomiting yellow-green, clear fluid at least 3 times a day. Bruja was spayed at the age of 6 months and has had intermittent drainage from the spay incision for the last 13 years that is antibiotic responsive. On presentation, Bruja is nervous, but appears depressed. The abdomen is distended with fluid and tender on palpation.

White blood cell count:	↑ 33.3 x 10⁹/L	(4.9-16.9)
Segmented neutrophils:	↑ 29.3 x 10⁹/L	(2.8-11.5)
Band neutrophils:	0	(0-0.3)
Lymphocytes:	2.7 x 10⁹/L	(1.0-4.8)
Monocytes:	1.0 x 10⁹/L	(0.1-1.5)
Basophils:	0.3 x 10⁹/L	(0-0.3)

WBC morphology: Slightly toxic neutrophils, a single mast cell is seen on scanning of the feathered edge

Hematocrit:	↓ 30%	(39-55)
Red blood cell count:	↓ 4.30 x 10¹²/L	(5.8-8.5)
Hemoglobin:	↓ 9.5 g/dl	(14.0-19.1)
MCV:	67.7 fl	(60.0-75.0)
MCHC:	↓ 31.7 g/dl	(33.0-36.0)

RBC morphology: No polychromasia noted

Platelets: Estimate of numbers not available due to clumping, macroplatelets seen

Plasma is icteric

Glucose:	95 mg/dl	(65.0-120.0)
BUN:	↑ 119 mg/dl	(8-33)
Creatinine:	↑ 4.5 mg/dl	(0.5-1.5)
Phosphorus:	↑ 8.1 mg/dl	(3.0-6.0)
Calcium:	9.5 mg/dl	(8.8-11.0)
Magnesium:	1.9 mEq/L	(1.4-2.7)
Total Protein:	5.5 g/dl	(5.2-7.2)
Albumin:	↓ 2.5 g/dl	(3.0-4.2)
Globulin:	3.0 g/dl	(2.0-4.0)
A/G Ratio:	0.8	(0.7-2.1)
Sodium:	144 mEq/L	(140-151)
Chloride:	↓ 102 mEq/L	(105-120)
Potassium:	3.9 mEq/L	(3.8-5.4)
HCO3:	17 mEq/L	(16-25)
Total Bili:	↑ 2.57 mg/dl	(0.10-0.50)
ALP:	↑ 677 IU/L	(20-320)
GGT:	5 IU/L	(1-10)
ALT:	↑ 126 IU/L	(10-95)
AST:	↑ 259 IU/L	(15-52)
Cholesterol:	288 mg/dl	(110-314)
Triglycerides:	274 mg/dl	(30-300)
Amylase:	↑ 8991 IU/L	(400-1200)

Abdominal fluid analysis:
Prespin color: red and cloudy
Postspin color: light red and clear
Total protein: 5.0 gm/dl
Total nucleated cell count: 214,560/µL

Cytologic description: 92% neutrophils, 8% large mononuclear cells. Neutrophils are markedly degenerate and toxic, with foamy basophilic cytoplasm and swollen poorly defined nuclei. Multiple large Döhle bodies are present in many cells. Scattered foamy macrophages are also present in a finely granular background containing occasional erythrocytes. Small numbers of large pale rod shaped intracellular bacteria are present.

Urine specific gravity: 1.039, other data not available

Interpretation
CBC
Leukogram: The mature neutrophilic leukocytosis with toxic change indicates inflammation. The presence of a single mast cell is not diagnostically significant in this case.

Erythrogram: The mild normocytic hypochromic anemia is difficult to classify. Anemia of chronic disease is nonregenerative, and usually normocytic normochromic. Rarely, hypochromia may be seen with chronic inflammation as this represents an iron supply limiting type of anemia. The hypochromia may also be associated with a mild or incipient regenerative response or possible iron deficiency. A reticulocyte count could be performed to evaluate marrow response to the anemia.

Serum Biochemical Profile

Azotemia with hyperphosphatemia: Considering the concentrated urine, the azotemia should be classified as pre-renal. Anorexia and vomiting may be the cause of dehydration.

Hypoalbuminemia: The degree of hypoalbuminemia is mild. Third space loss of albumin into the high protein abdominal effusion could contribute to hypoalbuminemia, although concurrent renal and gastrointestinal losses must be considered. Because albumin is produced by the liver, markedly decreased liver function could result in hypoalbuminemia, especially if combined with abnormal losses. Given the liver enzyme elevations, serum bile acids should be measured to evaluate liver function. Coagulation testing may be in order prior to any invasive procedures. Albumin is also a negative acute phase rectant, so the inflammation may decrease heptic production. Starvation can lead to hypoalbuminemia, but this patient's body condition appeared adequate and her history of anorexia was relatively acute.

Hypochloremia: In this case, the most likely cause of the mild hypochloremia with normal serum sodium levels is loss by vomiting.

Hyperbilirubinemia: As always, hemolysis and liver disease are the main differential diagnoses for hyperbilirubinemia. This patient is anemic, however she also has elevated liver enzymes. Septic patients may have hyperbilirubinemia in the absence of either of these conditions because endotoxin can directly impair hepatocellular uptake of bilirubin.

Increased ALP (2x): Elevated ALP in this patient is likely due to cholestasis, however enzyme induction and extrahepatic causes of increased ALP must also be considered.

Increased ALT (1.5x) and AST (5x): These changes are indicative of hepatocellular damage.

Elevated amylase: The increased amylase may be attributable to decreased GFR, however pancreatitis cannot be ruled out, especially considering the clinical signs in this patient.

Case Summary and Outcome

Cholestasis and hepatocellular damage, pre-renal azotemia, septic peritonitis. The possibility of pancreatitis needs to be further evaluated.

Abdominal radiographs revealed an enlarged liver with a large gas filled area compatible with a liver abscess (Figure 2-4). Bruja underwent exploratory surgery, but died during the procedure. Histologic sections of the liver revealed a chronic active pericholangiohepatitis with mild to moderate bridging fibrosis and micronodular hyperplasia. The abscessed tissue was not included in the submitted tissue. Micronodular hyperplasia is a common lesion in aged dogs. The cause for the other lesions is less clear, as is the possible relationship between the liver abscess and the chronic drainage from the spay incision.

In contrast to Lady and Patton (Cases 7 and 8), it cannot be determined if cholestasis or hepatocellular damage predominates using the laboratory data for this patient. This case is a good illustration of the failure of the degree of liver enzyme elevations to provide an accurate prognosis (Tip 4 in the introduction to the chapter). Despite the presence of significant liver pathology, enzyme abnormalities were relatively modest (Tip 6).

Hepatic abscesses are uncommon in the dog. In puppies, they may occur secondary to omphalophlebitis, while in adult dogs they are considered a complication of hematogenous spread from another septic process (Grooters). Clinical signs are nonspecific. Common laboratory findings in patients with hepatic abscesses include inflammatory leukograms and mild anemia, particularly if the process is chronic. There is often mild to marked thrombocytopenia, but since Bruja's platelets were clumped, we cannot determine if this abnormality was present in her case. Serum biochemical abnormalities include hyperbilirubinemia and elevated hepatocellular and cholestatic enzymes, as we see in this case. It should be noted that not all dogs with liver abscesses have elevated ALT or AST (Farrar), so normal hepatocellular enzymes do not exclude this condition. Nonspecific biochemical abnormalities associated with vomiting and diarrhea may also be present. Imaging studies are often helpful to distinguish hepatic abscesses from other causes of liver enzyme elevations, however it may be difficult to differentiate some lesions such as hepatic cysts, hematomas, and tumors from hepatic abscesses. Cytologic evaluation of aspirates from these masses can help differentiate these etiologies, however the potential to spread infection must be considered.

Farrar ET, Washabau RJ, Saunders HM. Hepatic abscesses in dogs: 14 cases (1982-1994). J Am Vet Med Assoc 1996;208:243-24.

Grooters AM, Sherding RG, Johnson SE. Hepatic abscesses in dogs. Compendium Cont Educ 1995;17:833-838.

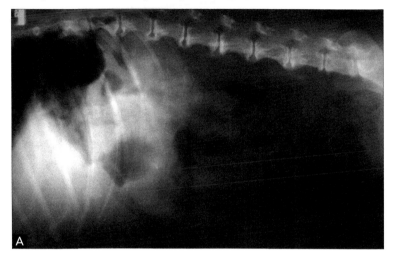

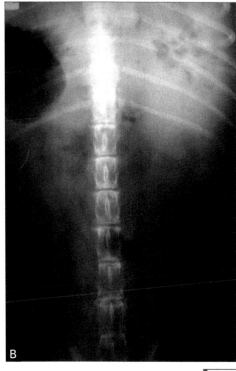

Figure 2-4A & B. A. Lateral radiograph of the abdomen of Bruja. A large gas filled area is compatible with a liver abscess. B. A ventrodorsal view.

Liver Case 10 – Level 2

"Dervish" is a 6-month-old Norwegian Forest cat with a history of pectus excavatum and intermittent episodes of coughing and wheezing. Four days after castration surgery, he became listless and febrile. After receiving supportive care (including fluid therapy) from the referring veterinarian, the cat was sent to the teaching hospital for further evaluation. On presentation, Dervish was wheezing and dypneic, had mydriasis, and exhibited decreased mentation.

White blood cell count:	↓ 1.8 x 10⁹/L	(5.5-19.5)
Segmented neutrophils:	↓ 0.1 x 10⁹/L	(2.5-12.5)
Lymphocytes:	↓ 1.1 x 10⁹/L	(1.5-7.0)
Monocytes:	0.5 x 10⁹/L	(0-0.9)
Basophils:	0.1 x 10⁹/L	(0-0.2)
WBC morphology: No significant abnormalities		
Hematocrit:	↓ 24%	(28-45)
Red blood cell count:	↓ 4.64 x 10¹²/L	(5.0-10.0)
Hemoglobin:	8.7 g/dl	(8.0-15.0)
MCV:	39.1 fl	(39.0-55.0)
MCHC:	↑ 36.3	(31.0-35.0)
Reticulocyte count: None seen		
RBC morphology: No abnormal findings		
Platelets: Appear adequate in number		

Plasma is icteric.

Glucose:	↑ 125 mg/dl	(70.0-120.0)
BUN:	↓ 11 mg/dl	(13-35)
Creatinine:	1.1 mg/dl	(0.6-2.0)
Phosphorus:	5.8 mg/dl	(3.0-7.0)
Calcium:	8.9 mg/dl	(8.6-11.0)
Magnesium:	1.7 mEq/L	(1.6-2.4)
Total Protein:	↓ 5.6 g/dl	(5.8-8.2)
Albumin:	2.7 g/dl	(2.5-4.0)
Globulin:	2.9 g/dl	(2.2-4.5)
A/G Ratio:	0.9	(0.7-1.6)
Sodium:	152 mEq/L	(142-153)
Chloride:	120 mEq/L	(108-128)
Potassium:	4.7 mEq/L	(3.5-5.2)
HCO3:	19.7 mEq/L	(13-27)
Anion Gap:	17 mEq/L	(8-19)
Total Bili:	↑ 1.14 mg/dl	(0.10-0.50)
ALP:	↑ 480 IU/L	(12-121)
ALT:	↑ 1862 IU/L	(18-86)
AST:	↑ 1148 IU/L	(16-54)
Cholesterol:	166 mg/dl	(80-255)
Triglycerides:	100 mg/dl	(20-100)
Amylase:	580 IU/L	(409-1203)

Urinalysis: Free catch

Appearance: Amber and opaque	Sediment:
Specific gravity: 1.010	0-5 RBC/high power field
pH: 7.0	No WBC seen
Protein: negative	Rare granular casts
Glucose/ketones: negative	Occasional epithelial cells
Bilirubin: 2+	1+ bilirubin crystals
Heme: trace	1+ fat droplets

Coagulation Panel

PT:	↑ 46.7s	(6.2-9.3s)
APTT:	↑ 38.4s	(8.9-16.3s)

Interpretation

CBC

Leukogram: The leukopenia is characterized by neutropenia and lymphopenia. Differentials for the neutropenia include consumptive processes such as acute severe inflammation in which tissue demand for neutrophils exceeds marrow production, immune-mediated destruction (rare), and/or decreased production. The concurrent presence of a nonregen-erative anemia could indicate some bone marrow disease, however the degree of anemia is more compatible with anemia of chronic disease. Lymphopenia may be due to stress (corticoteroid effects), although viral infection is another possibility that might also explain damage to other hematopoietic precursors.

Erythrogram: Mild normocytic anemia. The most likely cause for this, as indicated above, would be anemia of chronic disease. The elevated MCHC should be interpreted as artifact. Increases in MCHC may be due to intravascular hemolysis, ex vivo rupture of red blood cells due to sample handling, lipemia, or Heinz bodies.

Serum Biochemical Profile

Hyperglycemia: There is a mild hyperglycemia present. This is most likely due to stress or glucose-containing fluid administration.

Decreased BUN: Decreased production secondary to hepatic insufficiency or dietary protein restriction may lower BUN. Because liver enzyme activities are elevated and coagulation times are prolonged, a decreased BUN in this case suggests hepatic insufficiency and the need for liver function tests. Given the low specific gravity of the urine, increased excretion as a result of diuresis could also contribute to the low BUN in this patient. This patient has been treated with fluids, calling into question the significance of the urine specific gravity as an indicator of renal concentrating ability. Serum creatinine is normal, suggesting that renal function is adequate.

Hypoproteinemia: Although the total protein is low, both albumin and globulins are within reference ranges. The albumin is at the lower end of the reference range and should be monitored. If liver function tests support decreased liver function, albumin may continue to drop, however liver dysfunction must be severe for this to occur.

Hyperbilirubinemia: The degree of hyperbilirubinemia is mild, and is compatible with decreased liver function and/or some degree of cholestasis. The latter conclusion is supported by the increased ALP. The leukopenia and fever suggest that sepsis must be ruled out as a cause for decreased bilirubin uptake by hepatocytes. Hemolytic disease is less likely to be a major contributor because of the mildly decreased PCV and the lack of erythrocyte morphological changes indicating a mechanism for hemolysis. In addition, most significant hemolytic disease results in a regenerative response. Hemolytic anemia may initially appear nonregenerative if the CBC is performed within the first few days of onset. It takes at least 3 days after the onset of anemia before a significant reticulocytosis can be detected.

Increased ALP: There is a 4-fold elevation in ALP, compatible with cholestasis. Increases in ALP are more specific for cholestasis in cats than dogs, because nonspecific enzyme induction is less common. As a result, smaller increases in ALP are considered significant in cats compared to dogs. In this case, cholestasis is probably secondary to a more significant hepatocellular insult (see below).

Increased ALT and AST: The 20-fold increase in ALT and AST support hepatocellular injury as the primary problem in Dervish. While there may be some degree of hypoxia because of the anemia and respiratory disease, other causes of hepatocellular damage should be investigated.

Urinalysis: Dervish is isosthenuric, however it is difficult to assess his renal function for several reasons. He has had fluid therapy as part of his supportive regime, which will decrease his urine specific gravity. In addition, other data suggest that decreased liver function may suppress his BUN. Polyuria/polydypsia is frequent in dogs with liver disease, but is seen less often in cats. When present, polyuria/polydipsia may be associated with hepatic encephalopathy, which likely explains the impaired mentation observed in Dervish. In dogs with hepatic encephalopathy, abnormal neurotransmitters increase stimulation of the pituitary, leading to hypercortisolism and an increased osmotic threshold for antidiuretic hormone release. The 2+ bilirubin and bilirubin crystals are secondary to the hyperbilirubinemia.

Coagulation: Both the PT and APTT are markedly prolonged, consistent with defective secondary hemostasis. In combination with the clinical signs and low BUN, prolonged clotting times suggest the possibility of decreased liver function and appropriate testing should be done. Dervish also may have significant inflammatory disease and/or sepsis, as supported by the fever and leukopenia, so he may be predisposed to the development of disseminated intravascular coagulation (DIC). Platelets appear adequate, making DIC less likely at this time. Measurement of fibrin degradation products would help sort this out.

Case Summary and Outcome
Marked hepatocellular damage with mild secondary cholestasis, defective secondary hemostasis. Severe neutropenia with nonregenerative anemia suggestive for inflammation.

Dervish has decreased liver function based on a plasma ammonia level of 48.0 µM/L (Reference Interval 0-24). Bile acids are another test of liver function. In general, bile acids are often the test of choice to evaluate liver function because they are more sensitive than blood ammonia levels and require less finicky handling. Samples for bile acid measurement do not have to be kept on ice, or run within 30 minutes, as do samples for blood ammonia. However, bile acids are of less use in patients with increased bilirubin due to cholestasis and may be more useful in those with equivocal liver enzyme levels, normal bilirubin or suspected hemolysis. Additionally, post-prandial bile acid levels are preferred over fasted for the detection of decreased liver function in cats. Unfortunately, Dervish's diminished neurologic function interfered with eating. Ammonia is the only toxin implicated in hepatic encephalopathy that can be measured clinically, and was a good choice in this case.

While Cases 7 and 8 (Lady and Patton) certainly had significant liver disease, there was little evidence on the serum biochemical profile of decreased liver function. Indicators of decreased liver function on routine blood work are subtle and nonspecific. Due to the remarkable reserve of liver function in animals, these abnormalities occur very late in disease or with fulminant acute processes, once the majority of organ function is lost. Clues to decreased liver function on routine laboratory work include decreased BUN, decreased creatinine (less often), decreased urinary concentrating ability, hypoalbuminemia, hypoglycemia, hypocholesterolemia, and prolonged clotting times. Evidence for decreased liver function may occur simultaneously with evidence of hepatocellular damage such as enzyme elevations, however liver enzyme levels are NOT always abnormal in patients with decreased liver function. Despite the loss of the majority of functional hepatic mass, liver enzyme values are rarely below reference range in these patients. If liver enzyme levels are markedly high at presentation and begin to drop over time, the patient may be improving, or alternatively, may be losing functional hepatic mass.

Dervish was treated for hepatic encephalopathy and improved following administration of intravenous fluids, antibiotics, and vitamin K for his coagulopathy. He was discharged from the hospital without liver biopsy, so the cause for his liver disease was not identified. Abdominal ultrasound was normal, and serologic testing for FeLV, FIV, and toxoplasmosis was negative. Liver enzyme values eventually normalized, but Dervish has remained blind. The consulting opthalmologist diagnosed central retinal degeneration, a possible inherited condition. Dervish was given valium at the time of neutering, which has been reported to cause fulminant hepatic failure in some cats (Center). However the cats in that published report received repeated oral dosing. Other underlying factors such portovascular anomalies were also considered.

Dervish has had waxing and waning neutropenia for over 2 years, with evidence of myeloid hyperplasia on repeated bone marrow samples. Episodes of neutropenia are associated with fever and opportunistic bacterial infections which respond to antibiotics. The cause for neutropenia has not been determined.

Center SA, Elston TH, Rowland PH, Rosen DK, Reitz BL, Brunt JE, Rodan I, House J, Bank S, Lynch LR, Dring LA, Levy JK. "Fulminant hepatic failure associated with oral administration of diazepam in 11 cats" JAVMA 1996;209: 618-621.

Liver Case 11 – Level 2

"Squid" is an 11-year-old, spayed female domestic shorthaired cat with a history of lethargy, anorexia, and weight loss. She presented dehydrated and weak with icteric mucus membranes. Her liver is enlarged and can be palpated approximately 4 cm past the last costal cartilage. The margins of the liver are rounded. On survey radiographs of the abdomen, both kidneys appear to be normal sized, but 4 radio-opaque cystic calculi are seen.

Glucose:	88 mg/dl	(70.0-120.0)
BUN:	↓ 10 mg/dl	(15-32)
Creatinine:	1.1 mg/dl	(0.9-2.1)
Phosphorus:	4.2 mg/dl	(3.0-6.0)
Calcium:	↓ 8.5 mg/dl	(8.9-11.6)
Total Protein:	↓ 4.8 g/dl	(6.0-8.4)
Albumin:	↓ 2.1 g/dl	(2.4-4.0)
Globulin:	2.7 g/dl	(2.5-5.8)
A/G Ratio:	0.8	(0.5-1.4)
Sodium:	149 mEq/L	(149-163)
Chloride:	119 mEq/L	(119-134)
Potassium:	3.6 mEq/L	(3.6-5.4)
HCO3:	22 mEq/L	(13-22)
Anion Gap:	11.6 mEq/L	(9-21)
Total Bilirubin:	Invalid due to lipemia	
ALP:	↑ 997 IU/L	(10-72)
GGT:	<3.0 IU/L	(0-5)
ALT:	↑ 249 IU/L	(29-145)
AST:	↑ 287 IU/L	(12-42)
Cholesterol:	203 mg/dl	(77-258)
Triglycerides:	↑ 1134 mg/dl	(25-191)
Amylase:	791 IU/L	(496-1874)

Urinalysis: Sampling method was not indicated

Appearance: Amber and opaque	Sediment:
Specific gravity: 1.009	0-5 RBC/high power field
pH: 7.0	Occasional WBC seen
Protein: negative	No casts seen
Glucose/ketones: negative	No epithelial cells seen
Bilirubin: 1+	No bacteria
Heme: trace	Trace fat droplets and debris

Interpretation

CBC: Data are not available on this patient.

Serum Biochemistry Profile

Decreased BUN with normal serum creatinine: This could be compatible with decreased production secondary to diminished liver function or, less likely, starvation. Given the isosthenuria, diuresis could contribute.

Hypoproteinemia with hypoalbuminemia: In combination with the low BUN, decreased hepatic production of albumin is the most likely cause of the hypoalbuminemia. Starvation/protein malnutrition also should be considered a differential diagnosis. Other differentials for hypoalbuminemia include excessive losses through such routes as the kidney, gastrointestinal tract, or exudative skin lesions. The history and physical examination do not include significant cutaneous losses or diarrhea, and the urine protein is negative. Neither is hemorrhage described, although a packed cell volume is needed to help rule out hemorrhage. Loss of protein through hemorrhage, exudative cutaneous lesions, or the gastrointestinal tract generally include loss of both albumin and globulins, which does not appear to be the case here. It should be noted that many hepatic diseases in cats are associated with an acute phase reaction, resulting in increased globulins. Hepatic lipidosis is an exception and is often not associated with hyperglobulinemia (Center).

Hypocalcemia: The hypocalcemia is likely secondary to the hypoalbuminemia (see Chapter 6). Formulas to correct total serum calcium for the degree of hypoalbuminemia have been derived for the normal dog, but have not been validated for use in healthy or ill cats.

Increased ALP (12x), normal GGT: Although the bilirubin value was not valid due to the lipemia, the finding of icteric mucous membranes, bilirubin in the urine, and increased ALP suggest cholestasis. The 12-fold increase in ALP in Squid is very significant. Because of lower tissue concentrations and shorter half-life of ALP in the cat, even elevations as little as 2-3 fold are considered an important indicator of cholestasis. Enzyme induction is less common in cats, and there is no history of this patient receiving any medications. A packed cell volume would help rule out a hemolytic component to the icterus. Most liver diseases in cats cause elevation of both ALP and GGT, with the exception of hepatic lipidosis in which ALP may disproportionately increase compared to GGT. Based on these enzyme levels, hepatic lipidosis should be a primary differential diagnosis in this patient. Because hepatic lipidosis may be a primary or secondary disorder, the patient should be thoroughly evaluated for any other underlying diseases.

Increased ALT and AST: The mild, 2-fold increase in these enzymes indicates that some degree of hepatocellular damage is occurring.

Hypertriglyceridemia: Triglyceride concentrations are variable in hepatic lipidosis. Mobilization of peripheral fat stores to the liver and inadequate liver processing of lipid can increase triglyceride concentration in the blood.

Urinalysis: Squid is isosthenuric. As mentioned in the previous case (Dervish, Case 10), liver disease may be associated with polyuria and polydipsia, and subsequently poorly concentrated urine. Primary impaired renal concentrating ability also is possible and further assessment is warranted. Unlike in dogs, bilirubin is not detected in urine from normal cats. As indicated above, the presence of bilirubin in the urine is due to hyperbilirubinuria. Only conjugated bilirubin passes the glomerular filter.

Case Summary and Outcome
Feline hepatic lipidosis

Similar to Dervish's blood work (Case 10), Squid's results suggest a combination of cholestasis, hepatocellular damage, and decreased liver function. As noted above, the high ALP and normal GGT should prioritize a diagnosis of hepatic lipidosis in this case. This interpretation is further supported in Squid's case by the hepatomegaly and a history of anorexia and weight loss. Liver biopsy or cytology is required to confirm the impression given by the blood work. Both are adequate tests to detect markedly vacuolated hepatocytes compatible with hepatic lipidosis, but biopsy is the preferred procedure for ruling out concurrent diseases that may trigger secondary hepatic lipidosis. Because liver disease is a common cause of coagulopathies in the cat and because several results here (low BUN, hypoalbuminemia, and icterus) suggest the potential for decreased liver function, coagulation studies should be performed prior to any invasive procedures, and prophylactic vitamin K therapy should be considered. Liver function tests such as ammonia or bile acids are not likely to alter clinical management and are not a high priority in hepatic lipidosis patients that are icteric (Griffin).

Squid received vitamin K prior to aspiration of her liver. Cytology of her liver was consistent with hepatic lipidosis and characterized by sheets of hepatocytes distorted by the presence of numerous, small to large-sized, discrete cytoplasmic vacuoles (see Figure 2-5). Bile pigment was present intracellularly and between cells, forming bile plugs. Numerous erythrocytes and lipid vacuoles with scattered leukocytes were present in the background. Squid was discharged with a feeding tube. She did well at home and recovered uneventfully.

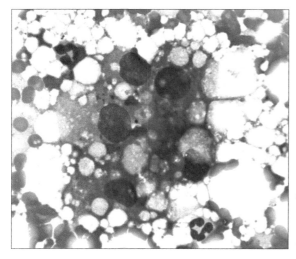

Figure 2-5. Cytology smears of the liver aspirate from Squid, Case 11. The sample contained markedly vacuolated hepatocytes consistent with hepatic lipidosis.

Center SA, Crawford MA, Guida L. A retrospective study of 77 cats with severe hepatic lipidosis: 1975-1990. J Vet Intern Med 1993;7:349-359.

Griffin B. Feline hepatic lipidosis: pathophysiology, clinical signs, and diagnosis. Compendium 2000;22:847-856.

Liver Case 12 – Level 2

"Binar" is a 1.5-year-old castrated male tabby cat with copper eyes. He is an indoor cat and is up to date on all vaccinations. There are no other pets in the household. Binar presents with seizures that are refractory to treatment with intravenous valium. Following collection of blood samples, he is placed under general anesthesia for control of seizure activity. When he recovers from general anesthesia, he shows a variety of neurologic signs including mental dullness, head pressing, stumbling, and hypermetria. The owners are not aware of any access to toxins. The physical exam is otherwise normal.

White blood cell count:	8.8 x 10⁹/L	(4.5-15.7)
Segmented neutrophils:	6.8 x 10⁹/L	(2.1-10.1)
Lymphocytes:	1.7 x 10⁹/L	(1.5-7.0)
Monocytes:	0.2 x 10⁹/L	(0-0.9)
Eosinophils:	0.1 x 10⁹/L	(0.0-1.9)

WBC morphology: No significant abnormalities

Hematocrit:	32%	(28-45)
Red blood cell count:	7.44 x 10¹²/L	(5.0-10.0)
Hemoglobin:	10.5 g/dl	(8.0-15.0)
MCV:	40.6 fl	(39.0-55.0)
MCHC:	32.8	(31.0-35.0)

RBC morphology: Within normal limits
Platelets: Clumped, cannot estimate

Glucose:	112 mg/dl	(70.0-120.0)
BUN:	↓ 9 mg/dl	(15-32)
Creatinine:	↓ 0.7 mg/dl	(0.9-2.1)
Phosphorus:	4.5 mg/dl	(3.0-6.3)
Calcium:	↓ 8.7 mg/dl	(8.9-11.5)
Magnesium:	2.1 mEq/L	(1.9-2.6)
Total Protein:	↓ 4.7 g/dl	(6.0-8.4)
Albumin:	↓ 2.3 g/dl	(2.4-3.9)
Globulin:	↓ 2.4 g/dl	(2.5-5.8)
A/G Ratio:	0.9	(0.7-1.6)
Sodium:	150 mEq/L	(149-164)
Chloride:	120 mEq/L	(119-134)
Potassium:	3.6 mEq/L	(3.6-5.4)
HCO3:	20 mEq/L	(13-22)
Anion Gap:	14 mEq/L	(9-21)
Total Bili:	0.2 mg/dl	(0.10-0.30)
ALP:	15 IU/L	(10-72)
ALT:	↑ 150 IU/L	(29-145)
AST:	↑ 45 IU/L	(12-42)
Cholesterol:	211 mg/dl	(77-258)
Triglycerides:	47 mg/dl	(25-191)
Amylase:	593 IU/L	(496-1874)

Urine was not available on this patient

Interpretation

CBC: No abnormalities.

Serum Biochemical Profile

Decreased BUN and Creatinine: Considering the concurrently low serum albumin and neurologic signs, BUN may be decreased secondary to impaired production with hepatic insufficiency in this patient. Dietary protein restriction also may lower BUN. Diuresis is frequently a cause of a decreased serum creatinine. However, a low serum creatinine also may be seen in thin animals with poor muscle mass such as may occur with malnutrition or cachexia.

Hypoproteinemia with hypoalbuminemia and hypoglobulinemia: Considering the low BUN and creatinine and neurologic signs, decreased hepatic production of albumin should be considered an important differential diagnosis, but it does not account for the border-line low globulin level. As was pointed out for Squid (Case 11), liver disease in cats may be associated with decreased albumin production, however hyperglobulinemia is a relatively consistent feature. Low BUN and serum creatinine with hypoalbuminemia may also characterize severe starvation accompanied by muscle wasting, but this is not suggested by the clinical history, nor does it explain the hypoglobulinemia. Differentials for decreases in both fractions of proteins (panhypoproteinemia) could include excessive losses through the gastrointestinal tract or into body cavities, exudative cutaneous lesions, or hemorrhage. The history does not include diarrhea or significant cutaneous losses. Urine protein data is not available for Binar, so renal loss could not be assessed. There is no history of hemorrhage, and the packed cell volume is within reference range.

Hypocalcemia: The hypocalcemia is likely secondary to the low albumin level in the blood (see Chapter 6). Formulas to correct total serum calcium for the degree of hypoalbuminemia have been derived for the normal dog, but have not been validated for use in healthy or ill cats.

Minimal increases in ALT and AST: The history of seizures in this patient suggests that transient hepatocellular hypoxia/hypoperfusion during the seizure could contribute to the elevation of hepatocellular enzymes. In combination with the other laboratory abnormalities, however, the potential for more significant primary liver disease should be considered. Because the degree of elevation of ALT and AST is roughly proportional to the number of hepatocytes injured and the severity of the injury, the mild elevations could suggest that there is minimal hepatic mass present.

Case Summary and Outcome

Portosystemic shunt

Postprandial bile acids were 54 µmol/L, supporting decreased liver function. A dye study revealed a portoazygous shunt.

Binar's case illustrates the possibility of marked liver disease in the absence of dramatic enzyme elevations. This is in contrast to Dervish and Squid (Cases 10 and 11), both of whom had decreased liver function associated with marked enzyme elevations and hyperbilirubinemia. This made the diagnosis of liver disease more obvious based only on routine laboratory testing. Hepatic encephalopathy should be considered in any patient with signs of diffuse cerebral disease, especially in young cats because idiopathic epilepsy is rare. There is a possible association between congenital portovascular anomalies and copper colored eyes in cats. A mild microcytic anemia is more consistently a feature of portosystemic shunts in the dog than the cat. The same is true for ammonium urate crystalluria, polyuria/polydipsia, and hypoalbuminemia, although Binar did have low serum protein. When present, liver enzyme elevations are generally mild with portosystemic shunts, especially in cats. Fasting bile acids and sometimes fasting ammonia will be within the reference range in some patients because there may be sufficient functional hepatic mass to extract these substances from the blood given adequate time. However postprandial bile acids are almost always significantly elevated and are considered a good screening test for the disease. As noted in the discussion of Dervish (Case 10), ammonia is the only toxin implicated in hepatic encephalopathy that can be measured clinically, but sample handling requirements usually limit its use in private practice.

Binar had a coil surgically placed in his shunt, which attenuated flow through the vessel and improved his liver function. He was continued on medical management of his condition and returned to the care of his referring veterinarian.

Liver Case 13 – Level 2

"Rocky" is an 8-year-old, neutered male Boxer, who was previously healthy and was not being treated with any medications. Rocky's owner was out of town for one week. When the owner arrived home, Rocky was noted to be lethargic, and he became progressively more so over the next 2 days. At this time, the owner noticed discolored urine. On presentation, the dog is weak and collapses on entering the clinic. His mucous membranes are pale and yellow, and his temperature is 102°. His pulse is 160/minute and bounding and an arrhythmia is noted. Respirations are 44/minute.

White blood cell count:	↑ 28.4 x 10⁹/L	(4.9-17.0)
Segmented neutrophils:	↑ 23.3 x 10⁹/L	(3.0-11.0)
Band neutrophils:	↑ 1.7 x 10⁹/L	(0-0.3)
Lymphocytes:	1.4 x 10⁹/L	(1.0-4.8)
Monocytes:	↑ 2.0 x 10⁹/L	(0.1-1.3)
Eosinophils:	0 x 10⁹/L	(0-1.250)
Nucleated RBC/100 WBC:	19	
WBC morphology: No significant abnormalities		

Hematocrit:	↓ 7%	(37-55)
Red blood cell count:	Not reported	(5.5-8.5 x 10¹²/L)
Hemoglobin:	↓ 4.5 g/dl	(12.0-18.0)
MCV:	Not reported	(60.0-77.0)
MCHC:	Not reported	(31.0-34.0)

RBC morphology: Erythrocyte agglutination is observed and confirmed by saline dilution (see Figure 2-6). Moderately increased anisocytosis and polychromasia

Platelets:	↓ 103.0	(181.0-525.0 x 10⁹/L)

Plasma is icteric.

Glucose:	134 mg/dl	(67.0-135.0)
BUN:	↑ 53 mg/dl	(8-29)
Creatinine:	invalid due to hyperbilirubinemia	
Phosphorus:	3.9 mg/dl	(2.6-7.2)
Calcium:	9.5 mg/dl	(9.4-11.6)

Magnesium:	2.4 mEq/L	(1.7-2.5)
Total Protein:	↓ 4.8 g/dl	(5.5-7.8)
Albumin:	3.3 g/dl	(2.8-4.0)
Globulin:	↓ 1.5 g/dl	(2.3-4.2)
A/G Ratio:	↑ 2.2	(0.7-1.6)
Sodium:	142 mEq/L	(142-163)
Chloride:	112 mEq/L	(111-129)
Potassium:	3.8 mEq/L	(3.8-5.4)
HCO3:	23 mEq/L	(15-28)
Anion Gap:	10.8 mEq/L	(8-19)
Total Bili:	↑ 56.5 mg/dl	(0.10-0.50)
ALP:	↑ 270 IU/L	(12-121)
ALT:	↑ 392 IU/L	(18-86)
AST:	↑ 235 IU/L	(16-54)
Cholesterol:	230 mg/dl	(82-355)
Triglycerides:	178 mg/dl	(30-321)
Amylase:	1052 IU/L	(409-1203)

Urinalysis: Free catch

Appearance: Amber and opaque	Sediment:
Specific gravity: 1.026	0-5 RBC/high power field
pH: 7.0	No WBC seen
Protein: 30 mg/dl	Rare granular casts
Glucose/ketones: negative	Occasional epithelial cells
Bilirubin: 3+	No bacteria
Heme: 3+	1+ fat droplets and debris

Coagulation panel

PT:	↑ 9.7s	(6.2-9.3s)
APTT:	14.2s	(8.9-16.3s)
Fibrinogen:	300 mg/dl	(100-300)
FDP:	↑ >20 µg/ml	(<5)

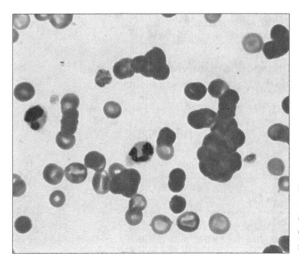

Figure 2-6. The blood film from Rocky, Case 13, contained large aggregates of erythrocytes that did not disperse on addition of saline to the sample.

Interpretation

CBC

Leukogram: Neutrophilic leukocytosis with a regenerative left shift and monocytosis. The left shift indicates significant inflammation, which could also explain the monocytosis. Sources of inflammation in this patient include immune-mediated hemolytic anemia and possible liver lesions.

Erythrogram: Severe anemia. Agglutination precludes reporting of indices to characterize the anemia, however the presence of anisocytosis and polychromasia suggests some degree of regeneration. A reticulocyte count should be performed to quantitate the response. The nucleated red blood cells are likely part of the regenerative response. However, hypoxic damage to the endothelial cells of the bone marrow and spleen could impair the ability of these organs to regulate the passage of only mature cells into the circulation.

Platelets: A mild thrombocytopenia is present, but is not of the degree expected to result in spontaneous bleeding in the absence of other pathology. Inflammation and early disseminated intravascular coagulation could contribute to decreased platelets through increased consumption. Immune-mediated destruction is possible as well. As many as one third to one half of dogs with immune-mediated hemolytic anemia also have immune-mediated thrombocytopenia.

Serum Biochemical Profile

Increased BUN: The cause of the azotemia needs to be determined as prerenal, renal, or postrenal. Creatinine cannot be reported to assist in interpretation because high bilirubin interferes with the creatinine reaction, causing a falsely low result. A prerenal component seems likely. The urine is somewhat concentrated. However, since there is no evaluation of hydration status, it is difficult to tell if the urine should be expected to be maximally concentrated (e.g. specific gravity greater than 1.030).

Hypoproteinemia with hypoglobulinemia: The cause for this is unclear, since significant inflammation would be expected to increase globulins through increased production of both immunoglobulins and acute phase reactants. Widespread inflammation could lead to increased capillary permeability and loss of protein into the interstitium. (See Chapter 4 for more information on evaluation of proteins)

Severe hyperbilirubinemia: The data on this patient suggest hemolysis as the cause for the hyperbilirubinemia. The severe, likely regenerative anemia with relatively mild increases in ALP make cholestasis a less likely etiology for this abnormality. A reticulocyte count may be performed to quantitate the regenerative response, but because it takes several days after an acute hemolytic event for the bone marrow to start releasing increased numbers of reticulocytes, a significant reticulocytosis may not initially be detected.

Mild increase in ALP: An approximately 2 fold elevation in ALP can be difficult to interpret in canine patients. In the absence endocrinopathies or a history of the use of medications that induce ALP production, hepatic hypoxia seems the most likely cause for this elevation.

Mild to moderate increases in ALT and AST: The 4-5 fold increases in hepatocellular enzymes are slightly greater than the elevation noted for ALP. Given the clinical history, a contributing cause for the hepatocellular damage is hypoxia of the hepatocytes along with ischemic liver lesions that are often described in patients with immune-mediated hemolytic anemia.

Coagulation Panel: The combination of >20 µg/ml FDPs and the thrombocytopenia indicates that this patient is at risk for the development of disseminated intravascular coagulation. Although only PT is mildly prolonged at this time, coagulation times should be monitored. Liver disease may be associated with increased FDPs because of impaired hepatic clearance.

Case Summary and Outcome

Immune mediated hemolytic anemia with secondary liver enzyme elevations due to hepatic hypoxia.

Rocky had a degree of hyperbilirubinemia comparable to Patton (Case 8), however Rocky also had severe anemia and mildly increased ALP indicating that hemolysis rather than cholestasis caused the hyperbilirubinemia. In patients with immune-mediated hemolytic anemia, hyperbilirubinemia exceeding 5 mg/dL has been shown to correlate with a less favorable prognosis and is associated with increased risk for thrombosis (Carr). Increased ALP has also been shown to be a risk factor for thromboembolic complications (Johnson), which are common in patients with immune-mediated hemolytic anemia. There were slightly greater elevations in hepatocellular enzymes than cholestatic indicators, but compared to the previous cases (Lady and Patton, Cases 7 and 8), it is more difficult this time to determine whether hepatocellular damage or cholestasis is the predominant pattern due to concurrent hemolysis. Hemorrhagic, ischemic, and cholestatic liver lesions have been demonstrated in necropsy studies of dogs with immune-mediated hemolytic anemia, and these lesions were more severe in patients with higher bilirubin levels (McManus).

This patient was Coombs test positive at 1+, and received a blood transfusion along with corticosteroids, azothiaprine, gastroprotectants, and intravenous fluids. Rocky was released from the hospital with a guarded to poor prognosis. He did well at home for 2 weeks, at which point he returned to the hospital with decreased appetite. He was icteric with marked hepatosplenomegaly, had a heart murmur and had increased respiratory effort. He stabilized over night in the intensive care unit, but by the next morning, he had profuse abdominal effusion that was characterized as a septic suppurative exudate and was euthanized. At necropsy, the liver showed evidence of steroid hepatopathy. In addition, Rocky had severe membranoproliferative glomerulonephritis and hemoglobin nephropathy secondary to the immune-mediated hemolytic anemia.

Carr AP, Panciera DL, Kidd L. Prognostic factors for mortality and thromboembolism in canine immune-mediated hemolytic anemia: a retrospective study of 72 dogs. J Vet Intern Med 2002;16:504-509.

Johnson LR, Lappin MR, Baker DC. Pulmonary thromboembolism in 29 dogs; 1985-1995. J Vet Intern Med. 1999;13:338-345.

McManus PM, Craig LE. Correlation between leukocytosis and necropsy findings in dogs with immune-mediated hemolytic anemia: 34 cases (1995-1999). J Am Vet Med Assoc 2001;218:1308-1313.

Liver Case 14 – Level 2

"Peach" is a 10-year-old male llama that presented for evaluation of facial pruritis and dermatitis. This was reported after the llama was turned out onto new pasture. Physical examination revealed bilateral suppurative excoriation of the bases of both ears, a crusted hyperkeratotic muzzle, bilateral chemosis with severe mucopurulent conjunctivitis, and severe generalized facial edema. The remainder of the physical was unremarkable, except the llama had a somewhat low body condition score.

White blood cell count:	↑ 35.3 x 10⁹/L	(7.5-21.5)
Segmented neutrophils:	↑ 30.7 x 10⁹/L	(4.6-16.0)
Band neutrophils:	0	(0-0.3)
Lymphocytes:	2.5 x 10⁹/L	(1.0-7.5)
Monocytes:	↑ 1.4 x 10⁹/L	(0.1-0.8)
Eosinophils:	0.7 x 10⁹/L	(0.0-3.3)
WBC morphology: No abnormal findings		
Hematocrit:	31%	(29-39)
Red blood cell count:	7.91 x 10¹²/L	(6.5-12.8)
Platelets: Adequate		
RBC morphology: No abnormal findings		
Fibrinogen:	↑ 500 mg/dl	(100-400)
Glucose:	↑ 320 mg/dl	(90-140.0)
BUN:	30 mg/dl	(13-32)
Creatinine:	1.9 mg/dl	(1.5-2.9)
Phosphorus:	5.3 mg/dl	(4.6-9.8)
Calcium:	10.0 mg/dl	(8.0-10.0)
Total Protein:	↑ 8.4 g/dl	(5.5-7.0)
Albumin:	3.5 g/dl	(3.5-4.4)
Globulin:	↑ 4.9 g/dl	(1.7-3.5)
A/G Ratio:	↓ 0.7	(1.4-3.3)
Sodium:	147 mEq/L	(147-158)
Chloride:	116 mEq/L	(106-118)
Potassium:	5.8 mEq/L	(4.3-5.8)
HCO3:	15 mEq/L	(14-28)
Total Bili:	↑ 0.4 mg/dl	(0.0-0.1)
ALP:	↑ 3118 IU/L	(30-780)
GGT:	↑ 1272 IU/L	(5-29)
SDH:	↑ 150 IU/L	(14-70)
AST:	↑ 356 IU/L	(110-250)
CK:	319 IU/L	(30-400)

Interpretation

CBC: Neutrophilic leukocytosis with monocytosis and increased fibrinogen indicate inflammation, which is compatible with the described facial lesions.

Serum Biochemical Profile

Hyperglycemia: Stress is a likely cause for hyperglycemia in this llama, although it should be appreciated that camelids have low circulating baseline insulin levels and a poor pancreatic response to hyperglycemia (Cebra 2001). Some authors recommend relatively more aggressive monitoring and treatment of hyperglycemia in llamas than in other species due to this physiological limitation (Cebra 2000).

Hyperproteinemia with hyperglobulinemia: As discussed in the CBC results, these findings are most compatible with inflammation. Both immunoglobulins and acute phase reactants can contribute to increased globulins. Mechanisms are discussed in Chapter 4. In patients with inflammatory disease the increase in globulins is usually polyclonal, reflecting enhanced production of multiple types of proteins. The albumin is at the low end of the reference range, though not technically abnormal at this time. Decreased liver function could depress production, and there is some evidence in other species that albumin is a negative acute phase reactant. Alternatively, albumin may be lost via the exudative skin lesions in this patient, or may be associated with a chronically poor nutritional status.

Hyperbilirubinemia: There are several potential etiologies for the mild hyperbilirubinemia in this case. Causes for increased serum bilirubin include hemolysis, cholestasis, decreased liver function, and sepsis. Hemolysis cannot be completely ruled out in this patient, however the serum was not hemolyzed and the PCV is in the low normal range. Cholestasis and decreased liver function are possible, although no specific tests of liver function have been performed on this patient. The neutrophilic leukocytosis could indicate a septic process, but is not specific for infectious disease, but rather indicates inflammation. The presence of a septic process was later confirmed.

Increased AST, SDH, ALP and GGT: Increased AST and SDH with normal CK is most compatible with hepatocellular damage. ALP and GGT will increase with hepatobiliary disease, including cholestasis. While the increase in GGT is most remarkable, it is difficult to determine what process is predominating in this patient based on the laboratory data presented here.

Case Summary and Outcome
Hepatobiliary disease with inflammation and hyperglycemia

A liver biopsy was performed to help achieve a specific diagnosis and prognosis in this patient. Sections of liver tissue were characterized by mild to moderate portal fibrosis with mild infiltrates of lymphocytes and plasma cells as well as scattered neutrophils. Three punch biopsies of the dermal lesions revealed epidermal ulceration, intra-epidermal pustules and severe superficial pyoderma compatible with a bacterial etiology. Peach was treated with intravenous antibiotics, corticosteroids to reduce inflammation in the face, Banamine® for pain management, and a keratolytic antimicrobial shampoo. Within 24 hours the facial edema resolved and the patient was comfortable and resumed eating. Peach was discharged, but died 2 weeks later. At necropsy, persistent pyoderma was noted. In addition, there were 2-3 gallons of peritoneal fluid accompanied by variably-sized, white nodules that were scattered throughout the liver, kidney, pericardium, and pleura. There was serous atrophy of pericardial fat, and the pericardium contained 1 mm diameter white nodes and areas were thickened and rough. Small white foci were occasionally noted throughout the pleura. On histologic examination, the white nodules were embolic foci of intense suppurative inflammation that were often centered on blood vessels. The lesions in the heart and kidney were thought to be the cause of death, and that the primary septic focus was the skin lesions.

For this patient, hepatitis due to disseminated bacterial infection was the likely cause of the laboratory abnormalities. Hepatic disease in camelids is often a consequence of malnutrition or metabolic disorders, which could also have contributed in this case, given the poor body condition of the animal. Other causes of liver disease that have been reported for llamas are similar to those for other species and include lipidosis, toxicity, and neoplasia.

As for other species, liver biopsy is often required for a specific diagnosis of hepatobiliary disease. While the collection of percutaneous biopsy specimens has been shown to be safe in camelids with minimal subsequent changes in clinical laboratory parameters (Anderson), it is unclear how well diagnoses based on these small biopsy specimens correlate with samples collected during abdominal exploratory or at necropsy. In small animal patients, there is some evidence that significant discordance between diagnoses exists depending on the method of biopsy collection, possibly due to sampling bias (Cole). That may be why the original biopsy sample did not reveal the systemic bacterial infection apparent at necropsy, although it cannot be determined if that process was present at the time of biopsy or developed after discharge.

Anderson DE and Silveira F. Effects of percutaneous liver biopsy in alpacas and llamas. Am J Vet Res 60:1423-1425, 1999.

Cebra CK, Tornquist SJ, Van Saun RJ, Smith BB. Glucose tolerance testing in llamas and alpacas. Am J Vet Res 62:682-686, 2001.

Cebra CK. Hyperglycemia, hypernatremia, and hyperosmolarity in 6 neonatal llamas and alpacas. J Am Vet Med Assoc 217:1701-1704, 2000.

Cole TL, Center SA, Flood SN, Rowland PH, Valentine BA, Warner KL, Hollis HN. Diagnostic comparison of needle and wedge biopsy specimens of the liver in dogs and cats. J Am Vet Med Assoc 220:1483-1490, 2002.

Liver Case 15 – Level 3

"Stella" is a nine-year-old miniature mare who presented for weakness, depression, and colic. Her mucous membranes are pale and yellow, she has weak pulses, and rapid shallow breathing. She is thin, with poor body condition. Owners report that she has been anorexic and has lost weight since foaling several days ago. The owner noted passage of brown urine before Stella was led to the trailer for transport to the hospital. No feces have been found in her stall for 2 days, but she has normal gut sounds in all four quadrants.

White blood cell count:	↑ 12.5 x 10⁹/L	(5.9-11.2)
Segmented neutrophils:	↑ 10.4 x 10⁹/L	(2.3-9.1)
Band neutrophils:	0	(0-0.3)
Lymphocytes:	2.0 x 10⁹/L	(1.6-5.2)
Monocytes:	0.1 x 10⁹/L	(0-1.0)

WBC morphology: No abnormal findings

Hematocrit:	↓ 10%	(30-51)
Red blood cell count:	↓ 1.53 x 10¹²/L	(6.5-12.8)
Hemoglobin:	↓ 3.6 g/dl	(10.9-18.1)
MCV:	↑ 64.0 fl	(35.0-53.0)
MCHC:	36.0 g/dl	(34.6-38.0)

RBC morphology: Numerous Heinz bodies present, slightly increased anisocytosis (Figure 2-7).

Platelets: Adequate

Fibrinogen:	300 mg/dl	(100-400)

Glucose:	123 mg/dl	(6.0-128.0)
BUN:	↑ 37 mg/dl	(11-26)
Creatinine:	1.2 mg/dl	(0.9-1.9)

Phosphorus:	2.5 mg/dl	(1.9-6.0)
Calcium:	11.6 mg/dl	(11.0-13.5)
Total Protein:	↑ 8.1 g/dl	(5.6-7.0)
Albumin:	2.9 g/dl	(2.4-3.8)
Globulin:	↑ 5.2 g/dl	(2.5-4.9)
A/G Ratio:	↓ 0.6	(0.7-2.1)
Sodium:	131 mEq/L	(130-145)
Chloride:	↓ 93 mEq/L	(99-105)
Potassium:	4.3 mEq/L	(3.0-5.0)
HCO3:	↓ 19 mEq/L	(25-31)
Total Bili:	↑ 10.3 mg/dl	(0.30-3.0)
Direct Bili:	0.4 mg/dl	(0.0-0.5)
Indirect Bili:	↑ 9.9 mg/dl	(0.2-3.0)
GGT:	↑ 56 IU/L	(5-23)
AST:	↑ 2064 IU/L	(190-380)
CK:	↑ 568 IU/L	(80-446)
LDH:	↑ 3614 IU/L	(160-500)
Ammonia:	↑ 203 umol/L	(0-55)
Triglycerides:	↑ 700 mg/dl	(9-52)

Urinalysis: Free catch	Sediment:
Appearance: Amber and cloudy	WBC: 0-2/hpf
Specific gravity: 1.030	RBC: 0-2/hpf
Heme: 4+	Rare epithelial cells seen
pH: 8.0	4+ calcium carbonate crystals (>50/low power field)
Protein: 4+ (>500 mg/dl)	No bacteria, mucus or casts seen
Glucose, Bilirubin, Ketones: Negative	

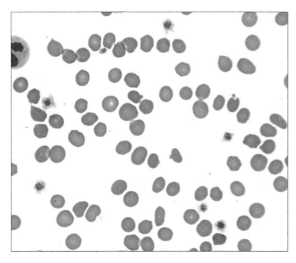

Figure 2-7. Blood film from Stella, Case 15, includes erythrocytes with Heinz bodies and scattered platelets (Wright Geimsa stain, 1000x).

Interpretation

CBC

Leukogram: Stella has a mild neutrophilic leukocytosis. This could be compatible with stress (although lymphopenia is not seen), or inflammation. There are no toxic changes in the neutrophils nor a left shift, and fibrinogen is within reference range, suggesting that inflammation is either very mild or acute. The hyperglobulinemia on the serum biochemical profile supports inflammation.

Erythrogram: Stella has a severe anemia. In the equine, reticulocytes are not released into the circulation during regenerative responses, so it is not generally possible to categorize anemias as regenerative or nonregenerative based on a single CBC. The presence of Heinz bodies provide a possible explanation for the source of the anemia, as they reflect oxidative damage to the red blood cell. When Heinz bodies are observed in the blood of horses, the clinician should consider ingestion of plants such as onions, *Brassica* species, or wilted red maple leaves (*Acer rubrum*) or exposure to drugs such as phenothiazines or methylene blue. On further questioning of the owners, it was discovered that Stella had access to red maple leaves.

Serum Biochemical Profile

Increased BUN: This is likely prerenal as the urine is adequately concentrated.

Hyperproteinemia with hyperglobulinemia: The increased globulins may reflect increases in either immunoglobulins or acute phase reactants. Regardless, it suggests inflammation. Albumin appears normal at this time, indicating that dehydration is not the primary explanation for the hyperproteinemia, however concurrent losses of albumin cannot be ruled out and may mask the effects of dehydration.

Hypochloremia with low normal sodium and low bicarbonate: The low chloride is disproportionate to the change in sodium and is occurring in combination with low bicarbonate, an indicator of metabolic acidosis. Because chloride generally varies inversely with bicarbonate (which is NOT the case here), the data support a mixed acid/base disorder. An arterial blood gas is required for complete evaluation of the acid/base status of this patient.

Hyperbilirubinemia with increased indirect bilirubin: In contrast to small animal patients in which fractionation of bilirubin does not often yield much diagnostic information, bilirubin fractionation can be of use in the horse. Increases in indirect (unconjugated) bilirubin in the horse include hemolysis, liver failure, and anorexia. In this case, there is evidence that all three could contribute to the hyperbilirubinemia. Increases in direct (conjugated) bilirubin in the horse rarely make up greater than 25% of the total bilirubin, and suggest biliary obstruction.

Increased GGT: Increases in this enzyme reflect hepatobiliary disease or cholestasis. Increases are seen in periparturient mares and miniature breed horses with fatty liver syndromes.

Increased AST (5x), LDH (7x) and CK (125% of normal): Increases in AST and LDH can indicate liver or muscle damage. Because the CK is also elevated, but more modestly increased than AST and LDH, liver damage is likely responsible for the majority of the enzyme elevation, with a smaller effect of muscle damage. It should be remembered that none of these enzymes are considered tests of liver function.

Hyperammonemia: This test does evaluate liver function, which appears to be impaired.

Hypertriglyceridemia: Hyperlipidemia is not common in the horse, but can occur in miniature breed horses and ponies with fatty liver syndrome. In this disease, decreased caloric intake causes mobilization of fat with accumulation of lipid in the plasma and liver. Decreased liver function often results.

Urinalysis: The urine is no longer brown, and is adequately concentrated. A positive reaction for blood may occur on urine test strips with the presence of either intact red blood cells, free hemoglobin, or myoglobin. The strong positive reaction for blood combined with small numbers of erythrocytes reported on the sediment exam suggests that hemoglobin or myoglobin was responsible for this result unless significant lysis of erythrocytes occured in vitro in the urine sample. Calcium carbonate crystals are a normal finding in equine urine, especially if the diet includes alfalfa hay.

Case Summary and Outcome

Red Maple leaf toxicity resulting in severe hemolytic anemia secondary to Heinz body formation, hepatocellular damage and decreased liver function, hyperlipidemia, and possible mixed acid/base abnormalities.

Stella received blood transfusions to help improve her tissue oxygenation. She responded to Banamine® and butorphanol to control signs of colic. Because of the potential for hemoglobin nephropathy, she was treated with fluids and diuretics. Because of her neurologic signs and decreased liver function, Stella also received lactulose, vitamins B and K, and oral dextrose. She also was encouraged to eat. Five days after admission, Stella's blood ammonia was normal, her liver enzymes were decreasing, and her hematocrit was steady. She was discharged with instructions to limit the protein in her diet to 12% to control signs of hepatic encephalopathy and to examine pastures carefully to prevent any further access to wilted red maple leaves.

Stella's laboratory abnormalities reflect the complexity of her multiple medical problems. Like Rocky (Case 13), hypoxia secondary to an acute hemolytic event may have damaged hepatocytes, which were further impaired by the fatty liver syndrome. It is not possible to determine if anorexia secondary to the hemolytic event precipitated the hyperlipidemia, or if it was a pre-existing, smoldering condition secondary to foaling complications. Concurrent muscle and liver hypoxia contributed to elevated enzyme levels in the blood. Muscle damage similarly can complicate interpretation of increased liver enzymes in small animal patients (see Bandit, Case 2). As noted above, Stella had all three common causes of increased indirect bilirubin, and the relative contributions of each cannot be determined. The acid/base abnormalities are incompletely characterized, however acidosis secondary to tissue hypoxia with the metabolic acidosis that characterizes fatty liver may be combined with respiratory alkalosis secondary to the tachypnea.

Liver Case 16 – Level 2

"Skipper" is a 15-year-old mare with a several week history of elevated liver enzymes and bilirubin associated with jaundice, intermittent fevers, and decreased appetite. She has lost weight and has some muscle loss through her haunches and withers. She has multiple abrasions to her right fetlock and pastern which have been oozing blood–tinged fluid for the past week. Her vital signs are normal, but her sclera and gums are yellow. She is moderately depressed, but is alert and interested in her environment when stimulated.

White blood cell count:	9.0×10^9/L	(5.9-11.2)
Segmented neutrophils:	7.0×10^9/L	(2.3-9.1)
Band neutrophils:	0	(0-0.3)
Lymphocytes:	1.6×10^9/L	(1.6-5.2)
Monocytes:	0.4×10^9/L	(0-1.0)
WBC morphology: No abnormal findings		

Hematocrit:	51%	(30-51)
Red blood cell count:	10.7×10^{12}/L	(6.5-12.8)
MCV:	47.2 fl	(35.0-53.0)
MCHC:	38.0 g/dl	(34.6-38.0)
Platelets:	↓ $79.0 \times 10^{12} \times 10^9$	(83.0-271.0)
RBC morphology: Rouleaux present		

Fibrinogen:	↑ 600 mg/dl	(100-400)

Glucose:	110 mg/dl	(6.0-128.0)
BUN:	12 mg/dl	(11-26)
Creatinine:	invalid due to hyperbilirubinemia	
Phosphorus:	2.7 mg/dl	(1.9-6.0)
Calcium:	12.0 mg/dl	(11.0-13.5)
Total Protein:	↑ 8.0 g/dl	(5.6-7.0)
Albumin:	2.7 g/dl	(2.4-3.8)
Globulin:	↑ 5.3 g/dl	(2.5-4.9)
A/G Ratio:	↓ 0.5	(0.7-2.1)
Sodium:	135 mEq/L	(130-145)
Chloride:	99 mEq/L	(99-105)
Potassium:	3.4 mEq/L	(3.0-5.0)
HCO3:	29 mEq/L	(25-31)
Total Bili:	↑ 11.7 mg/dl	(0.30-3.0)
Direct Bili:	↑ 1.70 mg/dl	(0.0-0.5)
Indirect Bili:	↑ 10.00 mg/dl	(0.2-3.0)
ALP:	↑ 2151 IU/L	(109-352)
GGT:	↑ 1344 IU/L	(5-23)
SDH:	↑ 7.1 IU/L	(2-6)
AST:	367 IU/L	(190-380)
CK:	108 IU/L	(80-446)

Coagulation Profile

PT:	11.1s	(10.9-14.5)
APTT:	56.6s	(54.7-69.9)

Interpretation

CBC

Increased Fibrinogen: High fibrinogen levels suggest inflammation, which in this case is corroborated by hyperglobulinemia on the serum biochemical profile. While there are no changes in the leukogram at this time, fibrinogen in large animal patients is a more sensitive indicator of inflammation than the leukogram.

Thrombocytopenia: Thrombocytopenia is associated with liver disease. The cause is often thought to be consumptive, and related to endothelial damage within a highly vascular organ. Another proposed mechanism is generalized immune activation that can be seen when Kupffer cell function is impaired and the body is subjected to higher than normal levels of toxins and bacteria from the improperly filtered portal circulation.

Serum Biochemical Profile

Hyperproteinemia with hyperglobulinemia: The increased globulins may reflect increases in either immunoglobulins or acute phase reactants. Regardless, it suggests inflammation. Albumin appears normal at this time, indicating that dehydration is not the primary explanation for the hyperproteinemia, however concurrent losses or decreased production of albumin cannot be ruled out and may mask the effects of dehydration. In this case, because there is evidence of liver disease, decreased hepatic production of albumin is a possibility as well.

Hyperbilirubinemia with increased direct and indirect bilirubin: Increases in indirect (unconjugated) bilirubin in the horse include hemolysis, liver failure, and anorexia. Because the hematocrit is within reference ranges, hemolysis is an unlikely contributor, but both anorexia and liver disease are likely. Increased direct bilirubin is also present, suggesting some degree of cholestasis.

Increased ALP (8x) and GGT (47x): Increases in these enzymes reflect hepatobiliary disease or cholestasis.

Increased SDH: Increased SDH supports a diagnosis of hepatocellular disease.

Coagulation profile: Clotting times are normal at this time. Decreased liver function must be severe to cause impaired production of coagulation factors, but animals with liver disease may have prolonged clotting times because the liver also produces plasmin activators and inhibitors and the liver is responsible for clearance of activated coagulation factors, fibrinolytic enzymes, and the breakdown products of coagulation.

Case Summary and Outcome

Cholestatic liver disease with mild inflammation

Hepatic ultrasound was performed to help guide liver biopsy collection once the normal coagulation test results were received. On ultrasound, the liver was diffusely inhomogeneous, but there was no evidence of biliary obstruction. Liver biopsy specimens revealed mild to moderate bridging fibrosis, bile duct proliferation, and mild nodular hyperplasia. This was thought to be suggestive of some form of chronic toxic hepatitis, however a specific cause was never determined. There was a suggestion that the ulcerated lesions on Skipper's fetlock and pastern could be related to photosensitization from concurrent liver disease, however these lesions were not biopsied for confirmation. The patient was discharged with symptomatic therapy.

Similarly to Stella (Case 15), Skipper was anorectic, contributing to the increased indirect bilirubin. In contrast to Stella, however, there was no evidence of hemolysis to further complicate interpretation of increased indirect bilirubin. In addition, Skipper had increased direct bilirubin, suggesting a significant cholestatic component to her liver disease that was not evident for Stella. Skipper's AST and CK were within reference ranges, indicating that concurrent muscle damage was not a factor in this case as it was for Stella. Specific tests of liver function were not performed for Skipper, but are recommended given her history. At this time her liver function appears adequate to produce sufficient coagulation proteins, but this is a very insensitive measure of liver function.

Liver Case 17 – Level 3

"Flower" is a 6-month-old Morgan colt presenting with decreased mentation and a delayed menace response. According to the owner, the colt has had red urine for 10 days. The diet consists of soft timothy hay and 12% Blue Seal sweet feed, however the colt has been anorectic for the last week, The body condition is adequate. The patient is housed with 30 other horses including 2 healthy foals, who have access to each other and a common pasture. On physical examination, the foal is weak, has a splayed stance, and sways when standing. There is increased respiratory effort, with an evident heave line. A Coggin's test for equine infectious anemia was negative. Supportive therapy consisting of intravenous fluids and antibiotics were provided during the first five days of hospitalization.

	Day 1	Day 5	
White blood cell count:	↑ 15.7 x 10⁹/L	↑ 17.9	(5.9-11.2)
Segmented neutrophils:	↑ 9.3 x 10⁹/L	↑ 11.5	(2.3-9.1)
Band neutrophils:	0	0	(0-0.3)
Lymphocytes:	↑ 6.7 x 10⁹/L	↑ 5.9	(1.6-5.2)
Monocytes:	0.7 x 10⁹/L	0.5	(0-1.0)
WBC morphology: No abnormal findings			
Hematocrit:	45%	↓ 24	(30-51)
Red blood cell count:	11.9 x 10¹²/L	↓ 5.47	(6.5-12.8)
Hemoglobin:	15.6 g/dl	↓ 8.6	(10.9-18.1)
MCV:	38.0 fl	44	(35.0-53.0)
MCHC:	34.2 g/dl	35.8	(34.6-38.0)
RBC morphology: Normal			
Platelets: Adequate			
Plasma is icteric on both days 1 and 5			
Fibrinogen:	100 mg/dl	100	(100-400)
Glucose:	82 mg/dl	↓ 39	(60.0-128.0)
BUN:	↓ 5 mg/dl	↓ 5	(11-26)
Creatinine:	Invalid due to increased bilirubin		
Phosphorus:	5.2 mg/dl	4.6	(1.9-6.0)
Calcium:	11.0 mg/dl	11.5	(11.0-13.5)
Total Protein:	↓ 5.3 g/dl	↓ 3.7	(5.6-7.0)
Albumin:	↓ 2.1 g/dl	↓ 2.1	(2.4-3.8)
Globulin:	2.8 g/dl	↓ 1.6	(2.5-4.9)
A/G Ratio:	0.9	1.3	(0.7-2.1)
Sodium:	130 mEq/L	130	(130-145)

Chloride:	99 mEq/L	99	(99-105)
Potassium:	5.0 mEq/L	3.8	(3.0-5.0)
HCO3:	↓ 23 mEq/L	↓ 21	(25-31)
Anion Gap:	13 mEq/L	14	(7-15)
Total Bili:	↑ 17.2 mg/dl	↑ 20.5	(0.30-3.0)
Direct Bili:	↑ 2.9 mg/dl	↑ 5.6	(0.0-0.5)
Indirect Bili:	↑ 14.3 mg/dl	↑ 14.9	(0.2-3.0)
ALP:	↑ 1565 IU/L	↑ 1544	(109-352)
GGT:	↑ 30 IU/L	↑ 95	(5-23)
AST:	↑ 4936 IU/L	↑ 12033	(190-380)
LDH:		↑ 20895 IU/L	(160-500)
SDH:		↑ 160 IU/L	(2-6)
CK:	201 IU/L	↑ 1722	(80-446)
Ammonia:		↑ 97 umol/L	(7-49)

Urinalysis: Day 1 Free catch

Appearance: Brown and cloudy	Sediment:
Specific gravity: 1.026	0-5 RBC/hpf
pH: 6.5	Occasional WBC
Protein: 500 mg/dl	Occasional squamous epithelial cells and bilirubin crystals
Glucose: 3+	
Bilirubin: 3+	
Heme: 3+	

Coagulation profile: Day 1

PT:	↑ 35.5s	(9.4-12.4)
APTT:	↑ >120s	(41.8-64.7)
FDP:	Negative	

Interpretation
CBC
Leukogram: The leukograms on both days 1 and 5 are characterized by a mild, mature neutrophilic leukocytosis and mild mature lymphocytosis. Potential causes of these changes include a stress leukogram, with corticosteroid effects contributing to the neutrophilia and excitement (epinephrine) causing the lymphocytosis. Mild inflammation is also possible, however there is no morphologic evidence of toxic change or left shift of the neutrophils. Antigenic stimulation also may promote lymphocytosis.

Erythrogram: On day 5, there is a moderate normocytic normochromic anemia. The significant decrease in hematocrit over 5 days suggests loss of red blood cells. Hemorrhage is possible and supported by the low albumin and globulins, however there is no clinical evidence of bleeding. Hemolysis is possible, and is supported by the icteric plasma, however the plasma was icteric prior to the development of anemia and may be related to anorexia or liver disease. Red blood cell morphology is normal and does not provide additional information as to the possible causes of red blood cell losses. Unfortunately, because horses do not release immature erythrocytes into the circulation, a reticulocyte count cannot be used to determine if there is a regenerative response. The increase in MCV over time supports regeneration.

Serum Biochemical Profile

Hypoglycemia: The most common cause of hypoglycemia is failure to process the sample appropriately, leading to utilization of glucose by cells in the blood sample. Therefore, it is always appropriate to verify hypoglycemia by drawing another sample with careful attention to sample handling. A sample should be spun and the serum obtained as soon as the clot forms, to avoid glucose utilization by blood cells. Drawing the sample into a tube containing sodium fluoride may also be used to prevent glucose consumption. There are many other less common causes of hypoglycemia. Decreased liver function is a possible, but rare cause of hypoglycemia, however, it is compatible with other laboratory data for this patient that suggest liver disease. The patient is anorectic, however the adequate body condition does not support starvation as a cause for hypoglycemia, which is unusual even with profoundly low food intake (See Chapter 6, Case 16). Tumors that produce either insulin (insulinoma) or, more commonly, insulin-like growth factors also may be associated with hypoglycemia. The age of the patient makes paraneoplastic hypoglycemia very unlikely. Sepsis is another potential cause for hypoglycemia, however the leukogram is more compatible with mild compensated inflammation than sepsis.

Decreased BUN: The most likely cause of low BUN in this patient is decreased liver function. Other causes could include starvation, polyuria, and overhydration.

Panhypoproteinemia with slightly elevated A:G ratio: Decreased production of albumin due to liver failure is supported by other findings on the serum biochemical profile and the concurrent coagulopathy. Other causes are decreased production secondary to starvation, however this is unlikely with a normal body condition. Increased loss of protein, primarily by hemorrhage or gastrointestinal losses, is also a good possibility because of approximately equal losses of albumin and globulins by Day 5.

The possibility of hemorrhage as a cause for protein loss is supported by the anemia seen on Day 5. Although there is no history of diarrhea, the patient should be tested for endoparasites as well as ectoparasites. Renal protein loss seems less likely because globulin proteins often remain within reference interval in patients with protein losing nephropathy. However, proteinuria was noted on the urinalysis, and a urine protein/creatinine ratio should be determined to clarify potential renal losses of protein. Confirmation of proteinuria is especially important because heme proteins may falsely increase urine protein measurement by dipstick methods.

Decreased HCO3: Low bicarbonate indicates acidemia, but blood gas analysis is required for complete evaluation. Given the clinical information, acidemia may be due to lactic acidosis secondary to perfusion deficits and hypoxia/anemia could contribute. Typically, an acidemia caused by accumulation of lactic acid should increase the anion gap, since lactic acid is an unmeasured anion. In this case, the low albumin may lower the anion gap. The sum of the increase in anion gap due to lactic acidosis and the decrease in anion gap due to the hypo-albuminemia may result in a normal value. This is a good illustration of how multiple abnormalities may combine to produce an analyte value that falls within the reference interval.

Marked direct and indirect hyperbilirubinemia: Anorexia in horses will cause an increase in the indirect bilirubin of up to 6-8 mg/dl. The anemia in this horse on day 5 indicates that hemolysis also could contribute to increased bilirubin. This horse also has strong evidence for liver disease, including decreased liver function, which will cause increases in both direct and indirect bilirubin.

Increased ALP and GGT (4-5x): Hepatobiliary disease will cause increased ALP and GGT in horses. Rapid bone growth in young animals may contribute to increased ALP, however in this patient liver disease is the more likely cause.

Increased AST, LDH, and SDH: Hepatocellular damage will cause elevations in all of these enzymes, however AST and LDH may be nonspecific and muscle damage will contribute to increases as well. In this case, the CK is initially within the reference interval until the patient develops significant anemia. It seems likely therefore, that at least on day 1, the increased AST is due to liver damage.

Hyperammonemia: Increased blood ammonia indicates decreased liver function, or rarely, urea cycle disorders.

Urinalysis: The brown color of the urine and the 3+ Heme reaction is compatible with hemoglobinuria secondary to intravascular hemolysis, although hematuria and myoglobinuria can produce similar results. Hemolysis is suspected because numbers of red blood cells in the sediment appear low for the intensity of the heme reaction. Red cells can occasionally lyse in vitro. The presence of bilirubin crystals indicates bilirubinuria secondary to extravascular hemolysis and/or liver disease. Aciduria may be attributable to anorexia and metabolic acidosis. In this case, the urine is somewhat concentrated, with a specific gravity of 1.026. Liver failure may lead to suboptimal urinary concentrating ability because of lack of urea for generation of gradient for concentration, among other mechanisms. The presence of pigments in the urine may interfere with colorimetric assessment of glucose in the urine, resulting in a false positive.

Coagulation panel: Marked prolongation of the PT and APTT indicate a secondary hemostatic defect of both the intrinsic and extrinsic pathways or the common pathway. This is compatible with markedly decreased liver function. Disseminated intravascular coagulation (DIC) is a differential diagnosis, however platelet numbers are within the reference interval, and FDP's are not elevated. Fibrinogen (100 mg/dl) might be low due to impaired synthesis secondary to liver dysfunction. Low fibrinogen is less often a feature of DIC in large animals compared to small animals because of the capacity of domestic large animal species to produce abundant fibrinogen. The history was negative for exposure to warfarin-type anticoagulants, which may produce similar prolongation of the PT and APTT.

Case Summary and Outcome

Decreased liver function with evidence of hepatocellular damage and cholestasis. Possible hemolytic anemia secondary to liver failure, or hemorrhage related to a coagulapathy resulting from liver disease.

On day 6 of hospitalization, the colt began moaning, lying down, and looking at his flanks, although gut sounds were normal. He continued to pass red-brown urine, and his PCV dropped to 10%. Later that day he developed epistaxis. His coagulation parameters normalized after transfusions of blood and fresh frozen plasma, and no further bleeding was noted. The next day he became more obtunded and ataxic, developed ventral edema, and had a precipitous fall in his PCV. He was euthanized due to lack of response to therapy and poor prognosis. At necropsy, the foal's liver was small, and histologic examination revealed severe portal and midzonal chronic active necrotizing hepatitis with intrahepatic cholestasis. Grossly, the kidneys showed green/brown discoloration. Histologically, there was moderate multifocal, subacute tubular necrosis and pigmented granular casts, compatible with hemoglobin nephropathy.

The cause of the liver disease in Flower was never confirmed, however potential differentials should include infectious disease such as Tyzzer's disease, immune-mediated disease such as Theiler's disease (although unlikely in this young animal), exposure to hepatotoxins, or a congenital hepatopathy. This foal was related to the foals reported to have Morgan foal hepatopathy (McConnico), a congenital liver disease analogous to hyperammonemia-hyper-ornithinemia-homocitrullinuria syndrome in people.

This case should be compared with Stella (Case 15), who also had concurrent hemolysis and liver disease. In both these cases, the combination of anorexia, liver disease, and severe hemolysis complicated the interpretation of the laboratory work. These cases are in contrast to Skipper (Case 16), whose laboratory abnormalities were more easily attributable to liver disease because of her normal hemogram.

Severe acute anemia will often cause hepatocellular damage secondary to poor oxygenation of tissues. As seen with both this foal and Stella, muscle tissue may also suffer hypoxic damage. Therefore, it may be difficult to interpret the elevation of enzymes that occur in both tissues, such as AST and LDH. The Heinz bodies present in Stella's blood suggested a mechanism for the hemolysis. For Flower, the normal red blood cell morphology made it more difficult to determine the cause for the anemia. No agglutination was observed to suggest immune-mediated mechanisms, although a Coomb's test was not performed. Red blood cell parasites were not detected on microscopic examination of blood films. The brown urine suggested intravascular hemolysis, but a cause could not be found. The presumptive cause for hemolysis in this patient was liver failure, however hemolysis was not described in the Morgan foal hepatopathy report. A hemolytic syndrome associated with increased erythrocyte fragility has been described as a near terminal event in horses with severe liver failure.

McConnico RS, Duckett WM, Wood PA Persistent hyperammonemia in two related Morgan weanlings JVIM 1997;11:264-266.

Liver Case 18 – Level 2

"Hilda" is a 10-year-old spayed female Doberman presenting for lethargy, vomiting, and anorexia. She had a gastric dilatation volvulus 3 months ago and has been on carprofen for arthritis for the past 2 years. She has also been on phenylpropanolamine for urinary incontinence and is a carrier for the von Willebrands trait. Hilda has been anorectic for several days. She will drink water, though she vomits it up afterwards. She has become progressively more lethargic to the point of not rising more than once a day. She has watery diarrhea once a day. The dog frequently receives high fat treats such as Danish pastries, cheesecake, bread and butter, and cat food.

On physical examination, Hilda is dull and lethargic with sunken eyes. She has mild conjunctivitis, and her sclera are yellow. Auscultation is within normal limits, and her capillary refill time is less than two seconds. Temperature, pulse and respirations are normal. She has several large lipomatous masses.

White blood cell count:	13.5 x 10⁹/L	(6.0-17.0)
Segmented neutrophils:	↑ 12.3 x 10⁹/L	(3.0-11.5)
Band neutrophils:	0	(0-0.3)
Lymphocytes:	↓ 0.7 x 10⁹/L	(1.0-4.8)
Monocytes:	0.5 x 10⁹/L	(0.150-1.350)
Plasma appearance: icteric		
WBC morphology: Within normal limits		
Hematocrit:	41%	(37-55)
Red blood cell count:	6.56 x 10¹²/L	(5.5-8.5)
Hemoglobin:	15.2 g/dl	(12.0-18.0)
MCV:	64.9 fl	(60.0-77.0)
MCHC:	↑ 37.1 g/dl	(31.0-34.0)
RBC morphology: Within normal limits		
Platelets: Appear slightly decreased		
Glucose:	↑ 168 mg/dl	(65.0-120.0)
BUN:	↑ 169 mg/dl	(8-33)
Creatinine:	↑ 8.6 mg/dl	(0.5-1.5)
Phosphorus:	↑ 16.3 mg/dl	(3.0-6.0)
Calcium:	10.1 mg/dl	(8.8-11.0)
Magnesium:	2.1 mEq/L	(1.4-2.7)
Total Protein:	6.5 g/dl	(5.2-7.2)
Albumin:	3.2 g/dl	(3.0-4.2)
Globulin:	3.3 g/dl	(2.0-4.0)
A/G Ratio:	1.0	(0.7-2.1)
Sodium:	140 mEq/L	(140-151)
Chloride:	↓ 82 mEq/L	(105-120)
Potassium:	4.3 mEq/L	(3.8-5.4)
HCO3:	20 mEq/L	(16-25)
Anion Gap:	↑ 42.3 mEq/L	(15-25)
Total Bili:	↑ 20.52 mg/dl	(0.10-0.50)
ALP:	↑ 4410 IU/L	(20-320)
GGT:	10 IU/L	(1-10)
ALT:	↑ 189 IU/L	(10-95)

AST:	↑ 285 IU/L	(15-52)
Cholesterol:	308 mg/dl	(110-314)
Triglycerides:	121 mg/dl	(30-300)
Amylase:	↑ 1683 IU/L	(400-1200)
Lipase:	↑ 3486 IU/L	(120-258)
Ammonia:	2.0 uM/L	(<32)

Coagulation profile

PT:	8.7s	(5.9-9.1)
APTT:	14.8s	(12.2-18.6)

Urine specific gravity: 1.012, other data not available

Interpretation

CBC

Leukogram: Hilda has a mild mature neutrophilia with lymphopenia, possibly due to corticosteroid effects. Mild inflammation cannot be ruled out.

Platelets: If no clumps are seen, there may be thrombocytopenia. An automated or manual count should be performed to quantitate platelet numbers.

Serum Biochemical Profile

Marked azotemia with hyperphosphatemia: These values suggest decreased glomerular filtration rate. In combination with the isosthenuric urine, the azotemia can be classified as renal. A prerenal component secondary to dehydration may exacerbate the renal azotemia.

Hypochloremia: The history indicates that chloride could be lost via vomiting of gastric contents. Acid/base abnormalities also may contribute to hypochloremia, however the HCO3 is within the reference interval for this patient. Arterial blood gas is required for full evaluation of acid/base disturbances.

Increased anion gap: A likely source of unmeasured anions in this patient could be uremic acids. Lactic acidosis may occur in dehydrated patients with impaired tissue perfusion.

Hyperbilirubinemia: In the absence of anemia or other evidence for significant hemolysis and given the liver enzyme elevations, cholestasis is the cause for the hyperbilirubinemia.

Increased ALP (13-15x): If there is no apparent cause for enzyme induction, increased ALP is interpreted as evidence for cholestasis. The GGT is at the upper limit of the reference range and should be monitored for increases.

Increased ALT and AST (2x and 6x): Hepatocellular damage is occurring concurrently with cholestasis and could be secondary to the damaging effects of bile on the hepatocytes.

Increased amylase and lipase: Given the history of vomiting and diarrhea along with a high fat diet, pancreatitis is possible. Clinicians should be aware, however, that decreased glomerular filtration rate (GFR) can result in increased amylase and lipase. Generally, decreased GFR will cause relatively minor elevations in pancreatic enzymes, often 2-4x the upper limit of the reference range.

Case Summary and Outcome
Renal azotemia with cholestasis and hepatocellular damage, possible pancreatitis

As has been stated previously, the serum biochemical profile can rarely point to the specific cause of liver disease. In this case, there is evidence of cholestasis and hepatocellular damage, however the available laboratory indicators of liver function (blood ammonia, coagulation times, serum albumin) are normal. The combination of renal azotemia and elevated liver enzymes in canine patients should trigger the suspicion of leptospirosis in areas where this disease occurs. Unlike dogs with leptospirosis, clinical signs are generally mild or inapparent in infected cats, despite inflammation in the kidney and liver.

Initial leptospirosis titers for Hilda were negative, but convalescent titers were 1:6,400 for *L. pomona* and 1:1,600 for *L. bratislava*. Titers are often negative during acute illness, and a four fold or greater increase in titers support a diagnosis of leptospirosis. Replication of the leptospire organism causes liver and kidney damage, and renal colonization can be long term. In the liver, the toxins produced by the organisms may cause subcellular damage that is not reflected by histologic changes. Intrahepatic cholestasis results from inflammation in the liver.

Hilda was hospitalized for several weeks for treatment for leptospirosis and for supportive care while her renal function returned. She was discharged to the care of her referring veterinarian.

Liver Case 19 – Level 3
"Lily" is a 7-year-old spayed female domestic short haired cat who presented with a one day history of severe lethargy and anorexia. According to the owner, Lily is drinking a lot and has been lying next to the water bowl. Her litter box was very wet this morning, but another cat does share the litter box. Lily is an indoor cat that eats "strange" things such as lemon grass, aloe, and pieces of plastic. The owner reports that she was normal until yesterday, with a normal appetite and the cat has not lost weight. On physical examination, Lily was febrile, icteric, and had a painful abdomen. A cranial abdominal mass was palpated.

White blood cell count:	↓ 4.0 x 10⁹/L	(4.5-15.7)
Segmented neutrophils:	↓ 1.8 x 10⁹/L	(2.1-10.1)
Band neutrophils:	↑ 0.8 x 10⁹/L	(0-0.3)
Lymphocytes:	↓ 1.3 x 10⁹/L	(1.5-7.0)
Monocytes:	0.1 x 10⁹/L	(0-0.9)

WBC morphology: Neutrophils have moderate cytoplasmic basophilia and vacuolization. They often contain large Dohle bodies.

Hematocrit:	↓ 26%	(28-45)
Red blood cell count:	↓ 4.36 x 10¹²/L	(5.0-10.0)
Hemoglobin:	↓ 7.5 g/dl	(8.0-15.0)
MCV:	40.6 fl	(39.0-55.0)
MCHC:	32.8	(31.0-35.0)

RBC morphology: Within normal limits

Platelets: Clumped, but appear adequate

Glucose:	↑ 312 mg/dl	(70.0-120.0)
BUN:	32 mg/dl	(15-32)

Creatinine:	1.0 mg/dl	(0.9-2.1)
Phosphorus:	3.0 mg/dl	(3.0-6.0)
Calcium:	↓ 8.1 mg/dl	(8.9-11.6)
Total Protein:	6.6 g/dl	(6.0-8.4)
Albumin:	3.9 g/dl	(2.4-4.0)
Globulin:	2.7 g/dl	(2.5-5.8)
A/G Ratio:	1.4	(0.5-1.4)
Sodium:	↓ 145mEq/L	(149-163)
Chloride:	↓ 111 mEq/L	(119-134)
Potassium:	↓ 3.2 mEq/L	(3.6-5.4)
HCO3:	15 mEq/L	(13-22)
Total Bili:	↑ 9.0 mg/dl	(0.10-0.30)
ALP:	↑ 376 IU/L	(10-72)
GGT:	5 IU/L	(0-5)
ALT:	↑ 338 IU/L	(29-145)
AST:	↑ 517 IU/L	(12-42)
Cholesterol:	119 mg/dl	(77-258)
Triglycerides:	394 mg/dl	(25-191)
Amylase:	754 IU/L	(496-1874)

Urinalysis: Not available

Interpretation
CBC
Leukogram: This patient is leukopenic with a left shift and toxic change characteristic of marked inflammation. The lymphopenia suggests an overlapping stress leukogram.

Erythrogram: A mild normocytic normochromic anemia is compatible with a nonregenerative anemia associated with chronic disease. A reticulocyte count should be performed to quantify any regenerative response.

Serum Biochemical Profile
Hyperglycemia: Differential diagnoses include stress hyperglycemia, post-prandial effects, endocrinopathies such as diabetes mellitus or hyperthyroidism, or pancreatitis. Blood glucose levels >300 mg/dl have been seen in stressed cats in the absence of diabetes mellitus, and stress hyperglycemia may be exaggerated in sick cats (Rand). A urinalysis is not available, but this degree of hyperglycemia may result in glucosuria regardless of the initiating cause.

Hypocalcemia:
Differentials for hypocalcemia associated with a normal serum albumin and normal phosphorus concentrations include pancreatitis and malabsorption. Other causes of hypocalcemia such as renal failure and hypoparathyroidism are usually, but not always, associated with hyperphosphatemia. See Chapter 6 on calcium and phosphorus for a more complete discussion of mineral metabolism.

Hyponatremia and hypochloremia: Electrolyte abnormalities will be discussed more thoroughly in Chapter 7. In this case, the hyponatremia likely reflects osmotic shifts in water secondary to the hyperglycemia. Renal, cutaneous, and third space losses are possible. Computation of a corrected chloride (111 mEq/L x 156 mEq/L ÷ 145 mEq/L = 119 mEq/L chloride, within the reference interval) shows that changes in chloride are proportional to changes in sodium and are also probably attributable to the fluid shifts.

Hypokalemia: Hypokalemia may reflect decreased intake in anorexic patients, or increased losses via the kidney or gastrointestinal tract, or third space losses. Decreased intake is most likely to result in hypokalemia in combination with some type of loss. In this patient, anorexia and increased losses through polyuria are contributory. Transcellular shifts of potassium secondary to acid/base abnormalities also will occur; acidosis may cause a shift of potassium outside of the cell in exchange for hydrogen ion.

Hyperbilirubinemia: Major rule outs for hyperbilirubinemia include hepatobiliary disease and hemolysis. In combination with the serum enzyme elevations, liver disease is strongly suspected. The anemia here is mild and nonregenerative, suggesting that a clinically significant hemolytic event is unlikely.

Increased ALP (5x): Potential causes for this elevation include cholestasis or endocrinopathies such as diabetes mellitus or hyperthyroidism. As was discussed in Rover's case (Case 6), nonspecific elevations in ALP are rare in the cat, so increased ALP is always considered significant. Increases in ALP secondary to diabetes mellitus usually are <500 IU/L, as seen here. While hyperglycemia provides some evidence for diabetes mellitus, the hyper-bilirubinemia indicates high potential for cholestasis. An increased ALP with normal GGT should flag hepatic lipidosis as a potential differential diagnosis, however other liver diseases cannot be ruled out.

Increased ALT and AST (2x and 10x): These enzymes indicate hepatocellular damage and support similar differential diagnoses listed for increased ALP.

Case Summary and Outcome

Hepatocellular injury and cholestasis; hyperglycemia; decreased electrolytes; inflammatory disease with mild non-regenerative anemia.

Abdominal ultrasound of Lily revealed a mild abdominal effusion. The abdominal mass proved to be an enlarged hypoechoic pancreas surrounded by bright peripancreatic fat. Lily was diagnosed with pancreatitis, and this was interpreted to be the inflammatory focus that caused the neutropenia with left shift and toxic changes. Lily was treated with broad spectrum antibiotics, intravenous fluids, and insulin. An esophagotomy tube was placed for nutritional support. A liver biopsy was recommended if her liver enzymes did not normalize. Unfortunately, Lily was euthanized at her referring veterinarian's practice a month later.

Serum liver enzyme concentrations are often increased in patients with pancreatitis, possibly secondary to exposure of the liver to toxic byproducts of pancreatic inflammation or secondary to ischemia. In cats with pancreatitis, hyperbilirubinemia may reflect severe hepatocellular damage or intrahepatic or extrahepatic obstruction of bile flow. Hyperglycemia can be secondary to hyperglucagonemia and stress, however, some cats are transiently or permanently diabetic after developing pancreatitis due to damage to islet cells in the pancreas. The hypocalcemia is also explained by pancreatitis. The mechanism resulting in hypocalcemia secondary to pancreatitis is uncertain but may relate to saponification of peripancreatic fat or increased calcium uptake by muscle. Because pancreatitis in cats is frequently associated with non-pancreatic conditions such as inflammatory bowel disease, diabetes mellitus, or neoplasia, interpretation of blood work can be complex in these cases (Simpson). Because Lily never had a liver biopsy, the possibility of primary liver disease cannot be ruled out, though the combination of pancreatitis and diabetes mellitus are sufficient to explain her laboratory abnormalities.

This case should be compared with Rover (Case 6), the hyperthyroid cat with hyperglycemia and elevated liver enzymes associated with hyperthyroidism. Lily's hyperbilirubinemia helps support more significant hepatic pathology than was expected for Rover. The normal amylase in spite of ultrasound evidence for pancreatic disease should be noted in this case. Amylase is a poor test for pancreatitis in cats, and cases of suspected pancreatitis should have samples submitted for lipase or trypsin-like immunoreactivty (TLI) that will be discussed in more detail in a later chapter.

Rand JS, Kinnaird E, Baglioni A, Blackshaw J, Priest J. Acute stress hyperglycemia in cats is associated with struggling and increased concentrations of lactate and norepinephrine. J Vet Intern Med 2002;16:123-132.

Simpson K. The emergence of feline pancreatitis. J Vet Intern Med 2001;15:327-328.

Liver Case 20 – Level 3

"Calvin" is a 4-month-old neutered male ferret that presented for vomiting, anorexia, and lethargy. His owner reports that Calvin is drinking more, and his abdomen appears painful when he is held. He has previously been healthy. On presentation, Calvin is recumbent and is non-responsive until picked up. He appears weak, and has urinated on himself in the carrier. He has pale mucous membranes and does appear painful in his abdomen on palpation. Ausculation is within normal limits.

Glucose:	144 mg/dl	(95-205)
BUN:	↑ 165 mg/dl	(7-40)
Creatinine:	↑ 1.5 mg/dl	(0.3-0.8)
Phosphorus:	↑ 20.7 mg/dl	(4.8-8.7)
Calcium:	↓ 6.0 mg/dl	(8.4-10.7)
Total Protein:	↓ 4.2 g/dl	(5.2-7.3)
Albumin:	↓ 1.5 g/dl	(2.8-4.0)
Globulin:	2.7 g/dl	(2.3-3.8)
Sodium:	128 mEq/L	(128-159)
Chloride:	↓ 86 mEq/L	(105-120)
Potassium:	↑ 7.7 mEq/L	(4.3-6.0)
HCO3:	25 mEq/L	(16-28)
Total Bili:	↑ 0.2 mg/dl	(0-0.1)
ALP:	↑ 119 IU/L	(30-90)
ALT:	↑ 1543 IU/L	(40-175)
AST:	↑ 1190 IU/L	(35-150)
Cholesterol:	149 mg/dl	(85-204)

Interpretation

CBC: Not available

Serum Biochemical Profile

Azotemia: Complete interpretation of the significance of this finding requires a urine specific gravity, which is not available. Pre-renal and renal azotemia are most likely since the ferret is urinating. It should be noted that serum creatinine is even less sensitive an indicator of renal dysfunction in ferrets than it is in dogs and cats, and this value will rarely exceed 2.0 or 3.0, even in ferrets with histologic evidence of end stage renal failure.

Hyperphosphatemia and hypocalcemia: *This combination of abnormalities may be present in patients with renal failure, although primary hypoparathyroidism and nutritional secondary hyperparathyroidism are possible.* The hyperphosphatemia is attributable to decreased glomerular filtration rate (GFR), while the hypocalcemia may be exacerbated by the hypoalbuminemia. Because a fraction of serum calcium is complexed with albumin, hypoalbuminemia may lead to decreases in total serum calcium, while ionized calcium will often be normal. Formulas generated for correction of serum calcium for low albumin have been generated for the dog, but cannot be extrapolated to other species.

Hypoproteinemia with hypoalbuminemia and normal globulin: In general, this pattern may be seen with increased losses of protein via the kidney or secondary to decreased production of albumin by the liver. It is not possible to evaluate renal losses without a urine sample. Decreased total protein is a common finding in sick or geriatric ferrets, primarily as a reflection of prolonged anorexia or inflammation in the bowel.

Hypochloremia and hyperkalemia: Low chloride may reflect losses due to vomiting. Decreased GFR may lead in impaired renal excretion of potassium. Transcellular shifts may occur with acid/base abnormalities, although the HCO3 is within reference range. Hypochloremia and hyperkalemia may be seen with hypoadrenocorticism, however adrenal disease in ferrets is generally secondary to a hyperfunctional gland rather than a hypofunctional one.

Hyperbilirubinemia, increased ALP (mild) with marked increase in ALT and AST (approximately 10x): The relatively greater elevation in hepatocellular enzymes compared to cholestatic enzymes suggests hepatocellular insult as the primary process, with mild secondary cholestasis. With the exception of liver tumors, primary hepatic disease is rare in ferrets (Hoefer). Anorexia, with resultant mobilization of fat stores to the liver, will cause hepatocellular swelling and increased liver enzymes in ferrets, however the increase in ALT seen in this patient is somewhat greater than the increases of up to 800 IU/L that have been noted in anoretic ferrets. The potential for toxicity should always be considered because of the mischevious nature of ferrets.

Case Summary and Outcome
Hepatocellular damage with mild secondary cholestasis, azotemia, and hypoproteinemia.

Possible differential diagnoses in this ferret include gastritis and ulceration, renal failure, ingestion of a gastrointestinal foreign body with prerenal azotemia, hepatic neoplasia, and toxicity. Further inquiry into the history of this patient revealed that the owner had found a fragment of a 200 mg tablet of ibuprofen on the floor of her apartment the evening of onset of clinical signs. Due to their curious nature, ferrets can be at risk for exposure to toxins, and they have been known to pry tops off of bottles of medication or to chew open containers.

While the pharmacologic properties of ibuprofen have not been thoroughly studied in the ferret, acute renal insufficiency, liver disease, and hypoalbuminemia have been reported in human cases of ibuprofen intoxication. Ibuprofen inhibits prostaglandin synthesis, and can decrease renal blood flow and GFR. Renal and gastrointestinal signs dominate in dogs with ibuprofen toxicity, while very high doses may result in central nervous system signs. This ferret presented with decreased mentation. A recent study of ibuprofen ingestion in ferrets reported that 93% of affected animals had neurologic signs, while 55% had gastrointestinal signs such as anorexia, vomiting, gagging, diarrhea or melena (Richardson). Signs of renal insufficiency were also reported. Ferrets appear to be even more sensitive to the toxic effects of ibuprofen than are cats.

Calvin was treated with intravenous fluids and gastroprotectants. After one day of therapy, his mentation improved and he began eating and drinking, but he was still weak when handled. After 2 days of therapy, he was bright and responsive and no longer had pain on abdominal palpation. By days three and four after presentation, Calvin's laboratory work began to normalize, indicating an improving prognosis. He was discharged on the fourth day, with instructions to have his blood work rechecked in 2 weeks. Calvin had an uneventful recovery.

	Day 3	Day 4	
Glucose:	134 mg/dl	96	(95-205)
BUN:	25 mg/dl	40	(7-40)
Creatinine:	0.5 mg/dl	↑ 1.0	(0.3-0.8)
Phosphorus:	6.4 mg/dl	8.7	(4.8-8.7)
Calcium:	↓ 8.1 mg/dl	9.6	(8.4-10.7)
Total Protein:	↓ 5.0 g/dl	5.5	(5.2-7.3)
Albumin:	↓ 2.2 g/dl	↓ 2.5	(2.8-4.0)
Globulin:	2.8 g/dl	3.0	(2.3-3.8)
Sodium:	QNS	157 mEq/L	(128-159)
Chloride:	QNS	115 mEq/L	(105-120)
Potassium:	QNS	3.7 mEq/L	(4.3-6.0)
HCO3:	QNS	27 mEq/L	(16-28)
Total Bili:	0.1 mg/dl	0.1	(0-0.1)
ALP:	37 IU/L	43	(30-90)
ALT:	↑ 648 IU/L	↑ 192	(40-175)
AST:	↑ 241	61	(35-150)

Hoefer HL. Gastrointestinal Diseases. In: Ferrets, Rabbits, and Rodents: Clinical Medicine and Surgery. 1997. E.V. Hillyer and K.E. Quesenberry, W. B. Saunders Co. Philadelphia. Pp 26-36.

Richardson JA, Balabuszko RA. Ibuprofen ingestion in ferrets: 43 cases. J of Vet Emerg Crit Care 2001;11:53-59.

Liver Case 21 – Level 3

"Snoopy" is a 6-year-old spayed female Bassett cross who presents with an eight day history of diarrhea. No blood has been noticed in the stools, and there has been no change in appetite or behavior. Four days ago, the diarrhea worsened to a liquid consistency with mucus. Since then, she has been lethargic. Two days ago, Snoopy appeared to have labored breathing, and she regurgitated once last night. On physical examination, Snoopy is febrile and has a distended abdomen.

White blood cell count:	↓ 3.6 x 10⁹/L	(4.9-16.9)
Segmented neutrophils:	↓ 1.7 x 10⁹/L	(2.8-11.5)
Band neutrophils:	0	(0-0.3)
Lymphocytes:	1.5 x 10⁹/L	(1.0-4.8)
Monocytes:	0.4 x 10⁹/L	(0.1-1.5)

WBC morphology: A few reactive lymphocytes are seen on scanning.

Hematocrit:	39%	(39-55)
Red blood cell count:	6.01 x 10¹²/L	(5.8-8.5)
Hemoglobin:	↓ 13.4 g/dl	(14.0-19.1)
MCV:	65.8 fl	(60.0-75.0)
MCHC:	34.4 g/dl	(33.0-36.0)

RBC morphology: Appears within normal limits
Platelets: Appear moderately decreased

Glucose:	↓ 43 mg/dl	(65.0-120.0)
BUN:	33 mg/dl	(8-33)
Creatinine:	0.9 mg/dl	(0.5-1.5)
Phosphorus:	6.0 mg/dl	(3.0-6.0)
Calcium:	10.4 mg/dl	(8.8-11.0)
Magnesium:	2.6 mEq/L	(1.4-2.7)
Total Protein:	↑ 8.5 g/dl	(5.2-7.2)
Albumin:	↓ 2.2 g/dl	(2.8-4.2)
Globulin:	↑ 6.3 g/dl	(2.0-4.0)
A/G Ratio:	↓ 0.3	(0.7-2.1)
Sodium:	141 mEq/L	(140-151)
Chloride:	↓ 99 mEq/L	(105-120)
Potassium:	↓ 3.7 mEq/L	(3.8-5.4)
HCO3:	18 mEq/L	(16-25)
Total Bili:	↑ 0.90 mg/dl	(0.10-0.50)
ALP:	↑ 417 IU/L	(20-320)
GGT:	10 IU/L	(1-10)
ALT:	↑ 1915 IU/L	(10-95)
AST:	↑ 710 IU/L	(15-52)
Cholesterol:	165 mg/dl	(110-314)
Triglycerides:	70 mg/dl	(30-300)
Amylase:	575 IU/L	(400-1200)
Ammonia:	↑ 144 µmol/L	(0-46)

Coagulation Profile:

PT:	↑ 20s	(5.9-9.1)
APTT:	↑ >120s	(12.2-18.6)

Interpretation

CBC: Snoopy has leukopenia with a neutropenia, a borderline normocytic normochromic anemia, and an apparent thrombocytopenia. A manual platelet count is recommended to quantitate the low count. Sepsis with disseminated intravascular coagulation may cause the neutropenia, thrombocytopenia and prolonged coagulation times. If extramarrow causes of the pancytopenia are not found, a bone marrow aspirate and biopsy should be considered to investigate this problem.

Serum Biochemical Profile

Hypoglycemia: Sample handling should always be considered a possible cause of hypoglycemia secondary to continuing consumption of glucose by cells in unspun blood samples. There are many other less common causes of hypoglycemia. In this patient, liver failure is a likely cause of true hypoglycemia. This interpretation is supported by multiple other laboratory abnormalities compatible with liver dysfunction including hypoalbuminemia, hyperbilirubinemia, elevated liver enzymes and hyperammonemia. Sepsis could be an issue given the neutropenia and suggestion of disseminated intravascular coagulation (thrombocytopenia with prolonged clotting times). Paraneoplastic hypoglycemia should be considered in this patient as well if there is evidence of organomegaly or mass lesions.

Hyperproteinemia with hypoalbuminemia and hyperglobulinemia: Mechanisms for hypoalbuminemia may include decreased hepatic production, increased losses through the gut, kidney, third space or cutaneous lesions and/or secondary to malnutrition/starvation. Because only approximately one third of liver function is required to maintain production of albumin, impaired hepatic function will more readily result in hypoalbuminemia if there is concurrent protein loss. In Lucy's case, decreased production by a poorly functioning liver is possibly compounded by losses through the gastrointestinal tract as a result of diarrhea. Albumin production by the liver will also be decreased if there is hyperglobulinemia, possibly as a compensatory change during an acute phase inflammatory response. Hyperglobulinemia can be seen associated with increased production of acute phase reactants by the liver during inflammation, by increased production of immunoglobulins secondary to antigenic stimulation, or by autonomous antibody production by neoplastic lymphocytes or plasma cells. Serum protein electrophoresis may be performed to distinguish reactive hyperglobulinemia (usually polyclonal) from paraneoplastic hyperglobulinemia (usually monoclonal). Polyclonal gammopathy has been reported in canine and feline patients with chronic liver disease, possibly related to decreased Kupffer cell function. This leads to increased exposure of the body to antigens normally cleared from the portal blood. The development of autoantibodies has also been described in association with chronic liver disease. In Snoopy, the decrease in albumin combined with the marked increase in globulins resulted in a low A:G ratio.

Mild hypochloremia and hypokalemia: These electrolyte changes are attributable to gastrointestinal losses, and possibly decreased intake of potassium secondary to anorexia.

Hyperbilirubinemia: In the absence of evidence for hemolysis, the mild hyperbilirubinemia supports a diagnosis of liver disease. The relatively greater increases in ALT and AST compared to ALP support severe hepatocellular damage rather than primary cholestatic disease. In this case, hyperbilirubinemia may occur secondary to hepatocellular swelling with blocking of canaliculi or failure by damaged hepatocytes to clear and process bilirubin. In this case, it is likely a combination of both mechanisms. Impaired bilirubin uptake by hepatocytes secondary to the effect of endotoxin also may play a role.

Increased ALP (mild, 125% of normal): In combination with the hyperbilirubinemia and elevations of other liver enzymes, cholestasis is probably the cause of the elevation in ALP.

Increased ALT and AST: The 15-20 fold increases in these enzymes are compatible with significant hepatocellular damage, and are more significant than the mild increase in ALP.

Coagulation profile: There is prolongation of both the PT and APTT, supporting significant impairment of secondary hemostasis. Failure to produce coagulation factors may occur secondary to significant hepatic parenchymal loss. Given the thrombocytopenia, the potential for DIC should be considered. This coagulopathy will have to be addressed prior to any biopsy procedures.

Case Summary and Outcome
Hepatocellular damage and decreased liver function

Snoopy was treated with fresh frozen plasma to help normalize her clotting factors, and was given antibiotics due to her fever and neutropenia. Further diagnostic tests included a liver aspirate and bone marrow aspirate. Many large lymphoblasts mixed with small clusters of vacuolated hepatocytes were seen on the cytology of her liver aspirate (see Figure 2-8). Her bone marrow aspirate included many hypercellular particles, consisting of 66% large lymphoblasts similar to those seen in the liver aspirate. Lucy had granulocytic, erythroid, and megakaryocytic hypoplasia. Cytology of the liver and bone marrow were consistent with a diagnosis of lymphoma.

Lucy underwent chemotherapy for her lymphoma, and her liver function transiently improved. She remained persistently neutropenic and intermittently was thrombocytopenic and/or anemic. After two months of therapy, Lucy was euthanized after developing abdominal pain and effusion, respiratory distress, and anorexia.

In this case, diffuse infiltration of the liver by neoplastic cells resulted in impaired liver function. Clinical pathology findings associated with either primary or metastatic neoplasia of the liver are quite variable and do not show a consistent pattern. Some patients present with multiple laboratory abnormalities associated with liver disease, while others may have completely normal blood work. Because serum biochemical data rarely leads to a specific classification of the liver disease, liver cytology or preferably biopsy is required to establish the presence of neoplasia.

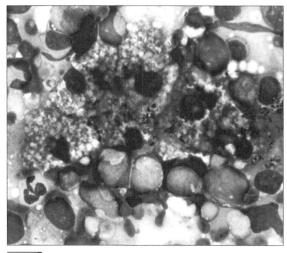

Figure 2-8. Liver aspiration cytology from Snoopy, Case 21. The specimen included sheets of vacuolated hepatocytes and numerous large lymphoblasts. Wrights stain, 1000x.

Overview

Step 1: For many cases, extrahepatic processes were the primary or secondary cause of laboratory abnormalities that are compatible with liver disease. Bone growth (Case 1), neoplasia (Case 3), muscle damage (Cases 2, 4, 15, 17), drug treatment (Case 5), endocrinopathy (Case 6), hypoxia/hypotension (Cases 2, 13, 15), and other gastrointestinal disease (Case 19) were represented in these case studies. Always consider extrahepatic causes of laboratory abnormalities that may suggest hepatobiliary disease.

Step 2: Using laboratory indicators, categorize the patient as having significant hepatocellular damage (Cases 2, 7, 8, 9, 10, 11, 13, 14, 15, 17, 18, 19, 20, 21), cholestasis (Cases 7, 8, 9, 10, 11, 13, 14, 15, 16, 17, 18, 19, 20, 21) or decreased liver function (Cases 10, 11, 12, 15, 17, 21). Please note the significant overlap; many patients have more than one process occurring in the diseased liver.

Step 3: Using the relative increases in laboratory parameters that indicate hepatocellular damage (Case 7, 21), cholestasis (Case 8, 16) and decreased liver function (Case 12), attempt to prioritize which process is likely to be the primary issue. This is not possible in all cases (Cases 9, 10, 11, 13, 19).

Step 4: For ALL of these cases, information in addition to what could be obtained from routine laboratory work alone was required for specific diagnosis and treatment of patients. In almost all cases, the history and physical were strong indicators of the cause of disease (Cases 1, 2, 4, 5, 7, 15, 20), while many required additional laboratory testing (Cases 6, 7, 18), imaging studies (Cases 3, 9, 12, 19), and/or cytology/biopsy (Cases 3, 8, 11, 14, 16, 21). This reinforces the concept that laboratory data must be interpreted within the context of clinical information.

Chapter 3

Tests of the Gastrointestinal System and
Carbohydrate Metabolism

The serum biochemical profile includes the measurement of multiple analytes that assist with the diagnosis of gastrointestinal disease, including pancreatic enzymes, cholesterol, triglycerides, and glucose. As we saw in the chapter on liver enzymes, diseases of other organ systems also may cause abnormal results for these tests. Many metabolic and endocrine disorders may influence parameters that are included in this section. In addition, significant gastrointestinal disease may occur in a patient with normal laboratory data. Specific diagnosis of gastrointestinal disease often requires additional specialty laboratory testing that is not performed as part of the routine biochemical profile (for example, trypsin-like immunoreactivity or cobalamine/Vitamin B12 levels). As always, other diagnostic modalities such as imaging studies and cytology or biopsy are often required for confirmation of diagnosis.

Guidelines for Interpretation of Serum Amylase and Lipase

1. Pancreatitis should be ruled out in patients with increased serum amylase or lipase, however the sensitivity and specificity of these tests for pancreatic disease are not optimal. The degree of enzyme elevation does not correlate with the severity of histologic changes in the pancreas.

2. Decreased glomerular filtration rate can increase the serum amylase and lipase up to two to three times the upper limit of the reference range.

3. Dexamethasone treatment may increase serum lipase concentrations. In contrast, serum amylase may decrease in healthy dogs treated with corticosteroids (Williams).

4. Serum amylase and lipase may increase with extrapancreatic pathology, including intestinal and hepatic disease.

5. Neither serum amylase nor lipase is a good indicator of pancreatitis in cats (Gerhardt).

6. Serum and abdominal fluid amylase and lipase are frequently increased in New World camelids presenting for pancreatic necrosis (Pearson).

7. Pancreatitis is rare in cattle and horses. Serum and abdominal fluid amylase and lipase may be elevated, however these values also may be increased secondary to enteritis.

8. As was described for serum liver enzyme levels, amylase and lipase values that fall below the reference range are not considered clinically significant and do not indicate pancreatic insufficiency.

The interpretation of cholesterol, triglycerides, and glucose is much more complex than that of the pancreatic enzymes.

Interpretation of Serum Cholesterol

1. There are many causes of hypercholesterolemia.

2. Some drugs may alter serum cholesterol levels (L-asparaginase, azathioprine, corticosteroids, methimazole, and others) so a careful medication history should be taken.

3. Hypocholesterolemia is not common and may occur secondary to hypoadrenocorticism, protein-losing enteropathy, severe prolonged liver failure, or malnutrition.

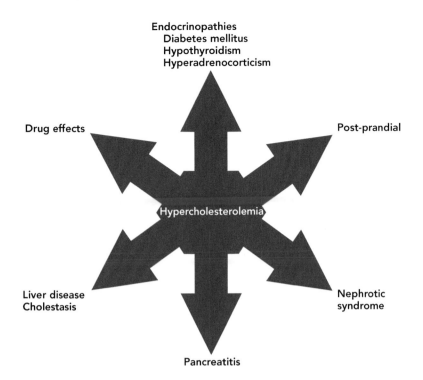

Endocrinopathies
Diabetes mellitus
Hypothyroidism
Hyperadrenocorticism

Drug effects

Post-prandial

Hypercholesterolemia

Liver disease
Cholestasis

Nephrotic
syndrome

Pancreatitis

Interpretation of Serum Triglycerides

1. Increased serum triglycerides cause a milky appearance to the serum or plasma (lipemia). Increased serum cholesterol will not do this.

2. Post-prandial effects are the most common cause of elevated triglycerides and should always be ruled out first.

3. Causes for hypertriglyceridemia are similar to those listed above for hypercholesterolemia.

4. Only rarely have drugs been reported to influence serum triglyceride levels.

5. Idiopathic syndromes associated with hyperlipidemia (hyperlipidemia is either increased cholesterol and/or triglycerides) have been reported.

6. Low serum triglycerides are generally not considered clinically important.

Interpretation of Serum Glucose

<u>A note on methodology:</u> Although the focus of this manual is on interpretation of data rather than the technical aspects of assays, the use of small, portable glucometers is common and therefore worth mentioning. There are many types of these analyzers, and a thorough review is beyond this chapter; however recent research has shown that data from these glucometers appears to slightly underestimate glucose levels determined by reference methods in most cases. The differences are most often small, and not clinically significant, but are greatest at very high blood glucose concentrations. The interested reader is referred to several articles (Wess and Reusch, Wess, and Cohn).

Hypoglycemia

1. **Always rule out artifactual hypoglycemia first,** especially if the patient does not appear to have clinical signs associated with hypoglycemia. Serum or plasma should be separated from cells within 30 minutes of sample collection to avoid consumption of glucose by cells

within the sample. High leukocyte or platelet counts in the blood may accelerate the consumption of glucose within the sample. Collection of samples into tubes containing sodium fluoride will prevent consumption of glucose by the cells.

2. Sepsis is a common cause of hypoglycemia.

3. Various neoplasms will cause excessive uptake of glucose by tissues due to the production of abnormal insulin like growth factors (mesenchymal, epithelial, or hematopoietic tumors; especially large tumors occurring in the chest or abdomen) or the production of insulin (beta cell tumors).

4. Hypoglycemia may occur with hepatic insufficiency as a result of impaired gluconeogenesis and/or failure to clear insulin.

5. Juvenile hypoglycemia is seen in pigs or small breed dogs due to impaired gluconeogenesis.

6. Less common causes of hypoglycemia are starvation, malabsorption, or glycogen storage diseases.

Hyperglycemia

1. Post-prandial effects may result in mild hyperglycemia just as they can contribute to increased cholesterol and triglycerides.

2. Stress (corticosteroid effects) and excitement (epinephrine release) will increase serum glucose concentrations. Increases in serum glucose related to stress may overlap with those observed in diabetes mellitus, especially in cats (Rand), and can potentially result in glucosuria. Sympathoadrenal response to head trauma can also result in hyperglycemia (Syring).

3. Diabetes mellitus is an important cause of hyperglycemia, but must be differentiated from the previous two common causes.

4. Administration of corticosteroids or dextrose containing solutions will increase blood glucose.

5. Endocrinopathies such as hyperadrenocorticism and hyperthyroidism can be associated with hyperglycemia.

6. Some drugs, such as xylazine, may cause hyperglycemia. This is an important consideration if a difficult patient must be anesthetized to obtain a blood sample.

Cohn LA, McCaw DL, Tate DJ, Johnson JC. Assessment of five portable blood glucose meters, a point-of-care analyzer, and color test strips for measuring blood glucose concentration in dogs. J Am Vet Med Assoc 2000:216;198-202

Gerhardt A, Steiner JM, Williams DA, Kramer S, Fuchs C, Janthur M, Hewicker-Trautwein M, Nolte I. Comparison of the sensitivity of different diagnostic tests for pancreatitis in cats. J Vet Intern Med. 2001;15:329-333.

Pearson EG, Snyder SP. Pancreatic necrosis in New World camelids: 11 cases (1990-1998). J Am Vet Assoc. 2000;217:241-244.

Rand JS, Kinnaird E, Baglioni A, Blackshaw J, Priest J. Acute stress hyperglycemia in cats is associated with struggling and increased concentrations of lactate and norepinephrine. J Vet Intern Med 2002;16:123-132.

Syring RS, Otto CM, Drobatz KJ. Hyperglycemia in dogs and cats with head trauma: 122 cases (1997-1999). J Am Vet Med Assoc 2001;218:1124-1129)

Wess G. Evaluation of five portable glucose monitors for use in dogs. J Am Vet Med Assoc. 2000;216: 203-209.

Wess G, Reusch C. Assessment of five portable blood glucose meters for use in cats. Am J Vet Res 2000;61:1587-1592.

Williams DA. Diagnosis of canine and feline pancreatitis. In: Proceedings of the 2003 Meeting of the American College of Veterinary Pathologists. November 15-19, Banff, Alberta, Canada. pp 6-12.

GI Case 1 – Level 1

"Gilligan" is a 4-year-old neutered male German Shepherd mix that was presented for treatment of a broken lower canine tooth. Other than the fractured tooth, the physical examination is within normal limits, and Gilligan is not currently taking any medications.

White blood cell count:	14.4 x 10⁹/L	(4.9-16.8)
Segmented neutrophils:	10.3 x 10⁹/L	(2.8-11.5)
Band neutrophils:	0	(0-0.300)
Lymphocytes:	3.1 x 10⁹/L	(1.0-4.8)
Monocytes:	1.0 x 10⁹/L	(0.1-1.5)
Eosinophils:	0 x 10⁹/L	(0-1.440)
WBC morphology: Appears within normal limits		
The plasma is lipemic.		
Hematocrit:	50%	(39-55)
Red blood cell count:	7.27 x 10¹²/L	(5.8-8.5)
Hemoglobin:	17.2 g/dl	(14.0-19.1)
MCV:	70.8 fl	(60.0-75.0)
MCHC:	34.5 g/dl	(33.0-36.0)
RBC morphology: Appears within normal limits		
Platelets: Appear adequate		

Glucose:	90 mg/dl	(67.0-135.0)
BUN:	17 mg/dl	(8-29)
Creatinine:	1.1 mg/dl	(0.6-2.0)
Phosphorus:	4.3 mg/dl	(2.6-7.2)
Calcium:	10.7 mg/dl	(9.4-11.6)
Magnesium:	1.7 mEq/L	(1.7-2.5)
Total Protein:	7.0 g/dl	(5.5-7.8)
Albumin:	3.8 g/dl	(3.0-4.2)
Globulin:	3.2 g/dl	(2.3-4.2)
Sodium:	147 mEq/L	(142-163)
Chloride:	113 mEq/L	(106-126)
Potassium:	4.5 mEq/L	(3.8-5.4)
HCO3:	26 mEq/L	(15-28)
Anion Gap:	12.5 mEq/L	(8-19)
Total Bili:	0.1 mg/dl	(0.10-0.50)
ALP:	158 IU/L	(20-320)
GGT:	3 IU/L	(1-10)
ALT:	72 IU/L	(18-86)
AST:	43 IU/L	(16-54)
Cholesterol:	314 mg/dl	(110-314)
Triglycerides:	↑ 995 mg/dl	(30-321)
Amylase:	1003 IU/L	(409-1203)

Interpretation

CBC: All parameters are within normal limits.

Serum Biochemical Profile
Hypertriglyceridemia: In a healthy patient with no other abnormalities evident on physical

examination, history, or laboratory testing, elevated triglycerides most likely signifies post-prandial effects or idiopathic hyperlipidemia.

Case Summary and Outcome

Gilligan's owners were instructed to fast him overnight prior to the collection of the blood sample; however their 6-year-old son had fed the dog a large can of dog food three hours prior to the appointment. A serum biochemical profile performed on a fasted blood sample the next day did not contain laboratory abnormalities.

Hyperlipidemia is a general term used to describe the presence of excess lipid (cholesterol or triglycerides) in the blood. Only increased serum triglyceride concentrations cause hyperlipemia, which imparts the milky appearance to serum or plasma (Figure 3-1). Hypercholesterolemia may cause a slight haziness, but not the marked turbidity that is seen with increased triglycerides. Note the difference between hyperlipidemia and hyperlipemia: hyperlipemic samples are hyperlipidemic, but not all hyperlipidemic samples are hyperlipemic. Occasionally samples that are hyperlipidemic based on serum cholesterol and/or triglyceride measurements have a normal gross appearance.

The most common cause of lipemia in the dog is post-prandial effects. An eight to ten hour fast should be sufficient to clear the blood of lipids. Serum triglycerides may be significantly elevated after eating, however the increase in cholesterol is generally mild and often remains within the upper limit of the reference range. Patients with fasting hyperlipidemia should be evaluated for causes of secondary hyperlipidemia such as pancreatitis, diabetes mellitus, hypothyroidism, cholestasis, hypoadrenocorticism, and nephrotic syndrome. If hyperlipidemia is persistent despite fasting, and there is no evidence of concurrent diseases that elevate lipids, then primary idiopathic hyperlipidemia should be considered. Idiopathic hyperlipidemia is most commonly seen in miniature schnauzers and beagles, but occasionally has been reported in other breeds as well as mixed breed dogs.

The transport of lipids in the blood requires that they be associated with proteins to enhance solubility. These lipid protein complexes vary in size, density, electrical charge, composition, and metabolic function. The relative proportions of different types of complexes can be characterized by density centrifugation, electrophoretic mobility, chromatography, or chemical precipitation. These methods are not often available to the general practitioner, and more research is required before these tests are likely to be widely applied in clinical veterinary practice.

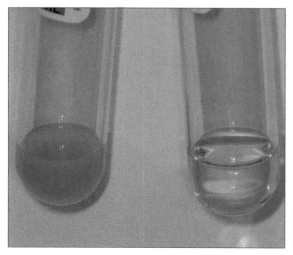

Figure 3-1. Lipemic serum is milky (tube on left), while normal serum is clear and straw colored (tube on right).

GI Case 2 – Level 1

"Marmalade" is a 15-year-old neutered male domestic short haired cat presenting for a routine check up and blood work. He has had slight weight loss since his last visit to the clinic two years ago. He occasionally has problems with hair-balls, and has recently seemed to have some difficulty eating dry cat food. His owner thinks he has a "bad tooth." Marmalade is crying and snarling in his carrier, and is swatting at you through the windows. When the carrier is opened, he defecates and urinates on the table and, to get to the point, requires general anesthesia for examination and phlebotomy. On physical examination, Marmalade does have an abscessed canine tooth, but the physical examination is otherwise normal.

White blood cell count:	↑ 25.5 x 10⁹/L	(4.5-15.7)
Segmented neutrophils:	↑ 15.8 x 10⁹/L	(2.1-10.1)
Lymphocytes:	↑ 8.3 x 10⁹/L	(1.5-7.0)
Monocytes:	↑ 1.2 x 10⁹/L	(0-0.850)
Eosinophils:	0.2 x 10⁹/L	(0.0-1.900)
WBC morphology: Appears within normal limits		

Hematocrit:	32%	(28-45)
Red blood cell count:	7.44 x 10¹²/L	(5.0-10.0)
Hemoglobin:	10.5 g/dl	(8.0-15.0)
MCV:	40.6 fl	(39.0-55.0)
MCHC:	32.8	(31.0-35.0)
RBC morphology: Appears within normal limits		
Platelets: Clumped, but appear adequate		

Glucose:	↑ 250 mg/dl	(70.0-120.0)
BUN:	25 mg/dl	(15-32)
Creatinine:	1.9 mg/dl	(0.9-2.1)
Phosphorus:	4.7 mg/dl	(3.0-6.0)
Calcium:	10.0 mg/dl	(8.9-11.6)
Total Protein:	7.8 g/dl	(6.0-8.4)
Albumin:	3.5 g/dl	(2.4-4.0)
Globulin:	4.3 g/dl	(2.5-5.8)
Sodium:	155 mEq/L	(149-163)
Chloride:	122 mEq/L	(119-134)
Potassium:	4.2 mEq/L	(3.6-5.4)
HCO3:	22 mEq/L	(13-22)
Anion Gap:	15.2 mEq/L	(9-21)
Total Bili:	0.2 mg/dl	(0.10-0.30)
ALP:	65 IU/L	(10-72)
ALT:	75 IU/L	(29-145)
AST:	32 IU/L	(12-42)
Cholesterol:	203 mg/dl	(77-258)
Triglycerides:	25 mg/dl	(25-191)
Amylase:	791 IU/L	(496-1874)

Urinalysis: Free catch

Appearance: Amber and opaque	Sediment:
Specific gravity: 1.045	0-5 RBC/high power field
pH: 7.0	No WBC seen
Protein: negative	No casts seen
Glucose/ketones: negative	No epithelial cells seen
Bilirubin: negative	No bacteria
Heme: negative	Trace fat droplets and debris

Interpretation

CBC: This patient has a mature neutrophilic leukocytosis, a mature lymphocytosis, and a monocytosis. The neutrophilia could be secondary to inflammation, epinephrine release or corticosteroid effects, however a lymphopenia would be expected in response to corticosteroids. The concurrent monocytosis indicates that inflammation from the abscessed tooth may be the cause. The lymphocytosis may occur secondary to antigenic stimulation. Given the circumstances of the clinic visit and absence of reactive morphologic changes, an epinephrine induced lymphocytosis is also possible.

Serum Biochemical Profile

Hyperglycemia: Based on the history, the primary rule out for hyperglycemia should be stress. Anesthesia can result in epinephrine release as well. Xylazine is a commonly used sedative/analgestic that interferes with insulin release and may result in a transient hyperglycemia which may be severe enough to cause a glucosuria. Post-prandial effects may be ruled out by determining the time of the last meal but are less likely with high protein, low carbohydrate cat foods. (Note that in Case 1, Gilligan had recently eaten, but had blood glucose levels within the reference interval) Diabetes remains on the list of differential diagnoses, however there is little support for this diagnosis based on clinical signs or laboratory data. Other laboratory abnormalities often associated with diabetes such as glucosuria, hypercholesterolemia, and elevated liver enzymes are absent.

Case Summary and Outcome

Marmalade's hyperglycemia was caused by a combination of stress and anesthesia. In some cases, repeat sampling when the cat is less stressed, or having the owner obtain blood at home will result in normal blood glucose determinations (Casella, Reusch). In Marmalade's case, however, any degree of handling with medical intent was not well received. The absence of glucosuria is helpful here, however stress induced hyperglycemia may result in blood glucose concentrations that exceed the renal threshold for reabsorption (approximately 200 mg/dl) for extended periods of time in anxious cats. A recent report showed that some healthy stressed cats had blood glucose concentrations in the diabetic range for as long as 90-120 minutes after the stressor (Rand).

The serum fructosamine test is available to help discriminate stress-induced hyperglycemia from diabetes mellitus. Serum fructosamine levels reflect the amount of plasma proteins that have undergone irreversible, non-enzymatic glycation in the presence of hyperglycemia. Fructosamine concentration is proportional to the blood glucose concentration over the life of the proteins in the serum, thus averaging the blood glucose concentration over the preceeding few weeks in the patient. This is a great advantage over blood glucose concentrations, which reflect only the immediate situation and may be altered by numerous variables. Serum fructosamine has been shown to be a useful test for differentiating stress hyperglycemia from diabetes and could be performed in patients where the clinical history and physical exam make this distinction less clear (Crenshaw).

Casella M, Wess G, Reusch CE. Measurement of capillary blood glucose concentrations by pet owners: a new tool in the management of diabetes mellitus. J Am Anim Hosp Assoc 2002; 38:239-245.

Crenshaw KL, Peterson ME, Heeb LA, Moroff SD, Nichols R. Serum fructosamine concentration as an index of glycemia in cats with diabetes mellitus and stress hyperglycemia. J Vet Intern Med 1996;10:360-364.

Rand JS, Kinnaird E, Baglioni A, Blackshaw J, Priest J. Acute stress hyperglycemia in cats is associated with struggling and increased concentrations of lactate and norepinephrine. J Vet Intern Med 2002;16: 123-132.

Reusch CE, Wess G, Casella M. Home monitoring of blood glucose concentration in the management of diabetes mellitus. Compendium 2001;23:544-555.

GI Case 3 – Level 1

"Gretchen" is a 12-year-old spayed female Cocker Spaniel presenting for head shaking. On physical exam, Gretchen has seborrhea and yeasty smelling ears, which are sensitive to manipulation. She also has significant dental disease. Gretchen's physical examination is otherwise normal. Routine blood work is performed prior to administering anesthesia to clean her teeth and ears.

White blood cell count:	↑ 19.8 x 10⁹/L	(4.9-16.8)
Segmented neutrophils:	↑ 16.2 x 10⁹/L	(2.8-11.5)
Band neutrophils:	0	(0-0.300)
Lymphocytes:	↓ 0.8 x 10⁹/L	(1.0-4.8)
Monocytes:	↑ 2.5 x 10⁹/L	(0.1-1.5)
Eosinophils:	0.3 x 10⁹/L	(0-1.440)
WBC morphology: Appears within normal limits		

Hematocrit:	42%	(39-55)
Red blood cell count:	5.8 x 10¹²/L	(5.8-8.5)
Hemoglobin:	14.0 g/dl	(14.0-19.1)
MCV:	73.4 fl	(60.0-75.0)
MCHC:	33.1 g/dl	(33.0-36.0)
RBC morphology: Appears within normal limits		
Platelets: Clumped but appear adequate		

Glucose:	↓ 40 mg/dl	(67.0-135.0)
BUN:	23 mg/dl	(8-29)
Creatinine:	0.6 mg/dl	(0.6-2.0)
Phosphorus:	6.0 mg/dl	(2.6-7.2)
Calcium:	10.6 mg/dl	(9.4-11.6)
Magnesium:	2.0 mEq/L	(1.7-2.5)
Total Protein:	5.5 g/dl	(5.5-7.8)
Albumin:	3.2 g/dl	(2.8-4.0)
Globulin:	2.3 g/dl	(2.3-4.2)
A/G Ratio:	1.5	(0.7-2.1)
Sodium:	147 mEq/L	(142-163)
Chloride:	108 mEq/L	(106-126)
Potassium:	↑ 5.5 mEq/L	(3.8-5.4)
HCO3:	26 mEq/L	(15-28)
Anion Gap:	18.5 mEq/L	(8-19)
Total Bili:	<0.10 mg/dl	(0.10-0.30)
ALP:	260 IU/L	(20-320)
GGT:	4 IU/L	(2-10)
ALT:	20 IU/L	(18-86)
AST:	39 IU/L	(16-54)
Cholesterol:	279 mg/dl	(82-355)
Triglycerides:	158 mg/dl	(30-321)
Amylase:	541 IU/L	(409-1203)

Interpretation

CBC: The leukogram is characterized by a mild mature neutrophilic leukocytosis, lymphopenia, and monocytosis compatible with a corticosteroid leukogram. This may be related to stress, or from the skin and dental disease. If corticosteroids have been administered to this dog orally or topically, medication could contribute to the changes in leukocytes. The neutrophilic leukocytosis may also reflect the inflammation of the ears or oral cavity.

Serum Biochemistry

Hypoglycemia: Because this patient does not have any clinical signs referable to hypoglycemia, laboratory artifact should be ruled out prior to invasive or expensive work-up for other conditions that cause hypoglycemia. Resubmission of a freshly collected sample with special attention to prompt separation of serum from cells is recommended.

Hyperkalemia: The significance of this mild deviation from the reference interval is unclear. Potassium may also leak from cells if there is a significant delay in separating the cells from the serum. In the absence of clinical signs, an individual analyte value that falls slightly outside the reference interval could be "normal" for this particular patient as a result of biological variation (see introductory chapter on the development of reference intervals). Repeat analysis may reveal that the analyte falls back into the reference interval. If repeat analysis shows a greater deviation from the reference interval or other accompanying abnormalities, further diagnostic work may be indicated.

Case Summary and Outcome:

Inquiry into the processing of this sample led to the discovery that there had been a significant delay between the collection of this sample and centrifugation, leading to consumption of glucose in the sample by cells. This patient did not have clinical or laboratory evidence of sepsis, liver failure, neoplasia, or nutritional deficits. Repeat sampling revealed normal serum glucose concentrations.

GI Case 4 – Level 1

"Kippy" is a 12-year-old neutered male poodle presenting for lethargy of two weeks duration and progressive abdominal distention. His appetite has been decreased for two days and he has vomited once. On physical examination, Kippy's abdomen is very distended and a fluid wave is palpable. His hair coat is sparse and he has numerous subcutaneous masses. He has a low-grade fever. Abdominal ultrasound revealed a very large abdominal mass that encompasses a large portion of the abdominal cavity and is compressing the stomach and bladder. The mass appears to arise from the liver, is attached by a pedicle, and contains numerous cystic structures.

White blood cell count:	↑ 35.5 x 10⁹/L	(4.9-16.8)
Segmented neutrophils:	↑ 28.8 x 10⁹/L	(2.8-11.5)
Band neutrophils:	↑ 1.1 x 10⁹/L	(0-0.3)
Lymphocytes:	2.8 x 10⁹/L	(1.0-4.8)
Monocytes:	1.4 x 10⁹/L	(0.1-1.5)
Eosinophils:	1.4 x 10⁹/L	(0-1.4)
WBC morphology: Neutrophils have mild toxic change		

Hematocrit:	↓ 17%	(39-55)
Red blood cell count:	↓ 2.40 x 10¹²/L	(5.8-8.5)
Hemoglobin:	↓ 5.4 g/dl	(14.0-19.1)
MCV:	↑ 76.1 fl	(60.0-75.0)
MCHC:	↓ 28.8 g/dl	(33.0-36.0)
Nucleated RBC/100 WBC	↑ 4	
Platelets:	↓ 77.0 x 10⁹/L	(181-525)

Glucose:	↓ 52 mg/dl	(67.0-135.0)
BUN:	20 mg/dl	(8-29)
Creatinine:	1.1 mg/dl	(0.6-2.0)
Phosphorus:	5.4 mg/dl	(2.6-7.2)
Calcium:	9.8 mg/dl	(9.4-11.6)
Magnesium:	2.5 mEq/L	(1.7-2.5)
Total Protein:	5.5 g/dl	(5.5-7.8)
Albumin:	3.0 g/dl	(2.8-4.0)
Globulin:	2.5 g/dl	(2.3-4.2)
A/G Ratio:	1.2	(0.7-2.1)
Sodium:	146 mEq/L	(142-163)
Chloride:	117 mEq/L	(106-126)
Potassium:	5.4 mEq/L	(3.8-5.4)
HCO3:	16 mEq/L	(15-28)
Anion Gap:	18.4 mEq/L	(8-19)
Total Bili:	0.30 mg/dl	(0.10-0.30)
ALP:	121 IU/L	(20-320)
GGT:	4 IU/L	(2-10)
ALT:	18 IU/L	(18-86)
AST:	↑ 85 IU/L	(16-54)
Cholesterol:	249 mg/dl	(82-355)
Triglycerides:	107 mg/dl	(30-321)
Amylase:	↑ 2630 IU/L	(409-1203)

Interpretation

CBC: Kippy has a neutrophilic leukocytosis with a left shift and toxic change, indicating significant inflammation. His anemia is macrocytic hypochromic, therefore likely regenerative, although a reticulocyte count is required to quantitate the response. The increased numbers of nucleated erythrocytes may have entered the circulation as part of a regenerative response or as a result of endothelial insult (i.e. hypoglycemia, hypoxia, endotoxemia) or abnormality of hematopoietic tissues. Moderate thrombocytopenia is likely due to increased consumption of platelets; decreased production is less likely based on the good activity in the other hematopoietic cell types. The cause of increased consumption cannot be determined on the basis of this data alone; however platelets may be adhering to damaged endothelium or may be consumed as a result of early DIC. A coagulation profile would help clarify the status of hemostasis in this patient.

Serum Biochemical Profile

Hypoglycemia: Artifactual hypoglycemia was ruled out in this case by repeated measurement in properly processed samples. Because of the large pedunculated liver mass, paraneoplastic hypoglycemia should be considered. Sepsis is a possible cause of hypoglycemia in this case based on the marked inflammatory leukogram and the thrombocytopenia. Cultures of blood, urine, and any suspicious lesions could help evaluate this possibility. Starvation induced hypoglycemia is relatively uncommon and is usually associated with very long periods of food deprivation and poor body condition, which were not noted here.

Increased AST: As an isolated finding, the increased AST is of limited diagnostic value. Hypoxia of tissues secondary to anemia could contribute to the elevation. The relation of this value to the liver mass is unclear given the normal ALT.

Increased amylase: Increases in amylase are most often associated with pancreatic or intestinal pathology or with decreased glomerular filtration rate. In this case, pancreatic and intestinal disease cannot be ruled out. The absence of azotemia makes decreased GFR an unlikely cause for the hyperamylasemia. A less common but potential cause for increased serum amylase is hepatic neoplasia, which is compatible with the clinical signs and history in this patient. (See Cases 13 and 14 in this chapter).

Case Summary and Outcome

Kippy was treated with intravenous fluids and antibiotics, and a twelve-pound mass was surgically removed from Kippy's abdomen (Figure 3-2). Histologic examination revealed a low-grade hepatocellular carcinoma with areas of coagulation necrosis and hemorrhage. The subcutaneous masses were lipomas. Kippy recovered from surgery and was discharged. Blood work repeated five days after surgery showed resolution of the hypoglycemia and improvement of the hematologic abnormalities, eliminating concern for other potential causes of the hypoglycemia. Note that the clinical chemistry data for Gretchen (Case 4) and Kippy are almost identical, and yet Gretchen's hypoglycemia was artifactual and of no diagnostic significance, while Kippy's hypoglycemia was the result of serious underlying disease. The comparison of the two cases highlights the need to interpret clinical chemistry data in the context of the history and other laboratory data, both of which were suspicious for significant disease in Kippy's case.

Tumor associated hypoglycemia has been reported in people and dogs, and possibly in horses (Bagley, Baker, Beaudry). Mesenchymal, epithelial, and hematopoietic tumors may cause hypoglycemia. Mesenchymal and epithelial tumors are often large and occur in the chest or abdomen. Although these tumors could consume substantial amounts of glucose, another mechanism has been shown to be the critical factor causing hypoglycemia. In many cases, these tumors secrete incompletely processed insulin-like growth factor II (IGF-II), a hormone that causes hypoglycemia by activating the insulin receptor (Le Roth). Normally,

IGF-II is produced in the liver. After secretion into the circulation, IGF-II forms a complex with a binding protein which limits the biological activity. In contrast, the abnormally processed IGF-II produced by tumors does not complex with the binding protein, and therefore it is free to interact with the insulin receptor to inhibit glucose production by the liver, thus increasing peripheral uptake of glucose by other tissues.

A retrospective study of dogs with massive hepatocellular carcinoma showed that the majority of patients had elevations in three or more serum liver enzyme activities, and that elevations in serum ALT and AST were negative prognostic indicators (Liptak). Despite this, overall mortality was low and no local recurrence was noted after surgical removal of the tumor, even when the tumor was incompletely excised. Tumor associated hypoglycemia was only noted in two of 48 dogs.

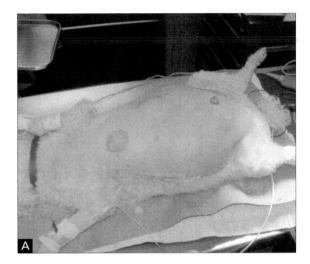

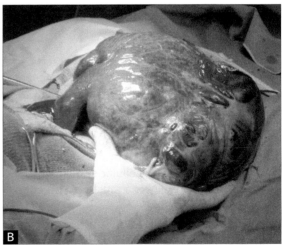

Figure 3-2A & B. A. This photograph of Kippy just prior to surgery demonstrates his distended abdomen with multiple subcutaneous lipomas. B. A gross photo taken at surgery of Kippy's large hepatocellular carcinoma.

Bagley RS, Levy JK, Malarkey DE. Hypoglycemia associated with intra-abdominal leiomyoma and leiomyosarcoma in six dogs. J Am Vet Med Assoc 1996;208;69-71.

Baker JL, Aleman M, Madigan J. Intermittent hypoglycemia in a horse with anaplastic carcinoma of the kidney. J Am Vet Med Assoc 2001;218: 235-237.

Beaudry D, Knapp DW, Montgomery T, Sandusky GS, Morrison WB, Nelson RW. Hypoglycemia in four dogs with smooth muscle tumors. J Vet Intern Med 1995;9:415-418.

Le Roth D. Tumor induced hypoglycemia. New England Journal of Medicine. 1999;341: 757-758.

Liptak JM, Dernell WS, Monnet E, Powers BE, Bachand AM, Kenney JG, Withrow SJ. Massive hepatocellular carcinoma in dogs: 48 cases (1992-2002). J Am Vet Med Assoc 2004;225:1225-1230.

GI Case 5 – Level 1

"Ides" is a 4-year-old castrated male ferret. The owner has the impression that Ides has been slightly weak and quiet for several weeks. He says that Ides collapsed and had a seizure over the weekend. Ides presents to you on emergency with another episode of collapse. His face is smeared with saliva, and he is recumbent and minimally responsive.

Complete blood count results performed at the referring veterinarian's office were within reference intervals.

Glucose:	↓ 30 mg/dl	(95-205)
BUN:	27 mg/dl	(7-40)
Creatinine:	0.4 mg/dl	(0.3-0.8)
Phosphorus:	6.1 mg/dl	(4.8-8.7)
Calcium:	9.6 mg/dl	(8.4-10.7)
Total Protein:	7.3 g/dl	(5.2-7.3)
Albumin:	3.5 g/dl	(2.8-4.0)
Globulin:	3.8 g/dl	(2.3-3.8)
Sodium:	154 mEq/L	(128-159)
Chloride:	109 mEq/L	(105-120)
Potassium:	5.1 mEq/L	(4.3-6.0)
HCO3:	27 mEq/L	(16-28)
Total Bili:	0.2 mg/dl	(0-0.7)
ALP:	115 IU/L	(30-120)
ALT:	↑ 554 IU/L	(82-289)
AST:	↑ 170 IU/L	(35-150)
Cholesterol:	149 mg/dl	(85-204)
Triglycerides:	25 mg/dl	(10-32)

Interpretation

Serum Biochemical Profile

Hypoglycemia: This sample was processed correctly, and in combination with the clinical signs, true hyperglycemia is considered to be present in this patient. Although there are numerous potential causes for hypoglycemia, ferrets with blood glucose concentrations lower than 60 mg/dl are likely to have insulinomas due to the prevalence of this tumor in this species.

Mildly increased in ALT and AST: With the exception of liver tumors, primary hepatic disease is rare in ferrets. In ferrets, repeated bouts of hypoglycemia will mobilize fat stores to the liver, causing hepatocellular swelling and increased liver enzymes. The possibility of metastasis of an insulinoma must also be considered.

Case Summary and Outcome

This patient was initially managed conservatively with medical therapy, which included frequent feedings and prednisone. Although this regime will frequently control clinical signs for a period of time, Ides continued to have periods of lethargy and weakness, but no further episodes of collapse. Ides was eventually taken to surgery, and three firm pancreatic nodules were palpated and removed, and a liver biopsy was performed. Histologic examination of tissues revealed multiple benign insulinomas and glycogen infiltration of hepatocytes with no evidence of metastatic disease. Ides was discharged and recovered uneventfully. Like Kippy, the remainder of the clinical chemistry profile was relatively unremarkable despite the presence of neoplasia. This may be the case with many types of tumors. When measured, patients with insulinoma have normal to high insulin levels associated with hypoglycemia, while patients with other malignancies that cause hypoglycemia often have appropriately low circulating insulin.

Insulinomas are one of the most common tumors in middle-aged ferrets, and they may be present concurrently with other common tumors of ferrets such as adrenal tumors. Clinical signs result from pronounced hypoglycemia secondary to continuous hyperinsulinemia. The normal counter-regulatory mechanisms that increase blood glucose concentrations in hypoglycemic animals (the stimulation of hepatic gluconeogenesis and glycogenolysis by glucagon, cortisol, epinephrine, and growth hormone) are not fully operational in ferrets with insulinoma. A blood glucose value of <60 mg/dl in the absence of clinical signs or laboratory abnormalities suggesting another cause for hyperglycemia is considered diagnostic. Measurement of blood glucose should be performed on multi-test automated biochemistry analyzers to avoid the wide variation of results that may be obtained by the use of hand-held glucometers at low serum glucose values. Insulin levels may be measured, and are normal or elevated in the presence of hypoglycemia. Some authors advocate the use of suggestive clinical signs and intermittent hypoglycemia for diagnosis without measurement of serum insulin values because these values may be normal in some ferrets with insulinoma. Definitive diagnosis requires histologic examination of pancreatic nodules, which may be difficult to detect without surgery. As noted above, initially medical management alone may be sufficient to control clinical signs. Surgery generally does result in some amelioration of clinical signs and/or improved medical management for 2-6 months after surgery. However, surgical treatment is often not curative because of the frequent presence of microscopic insulinomas that are not identified and removed.

Pilny AA, Chen S. Ferret insulinoma: diagnosis and treatment. Compendium 2004;29:722-728.

Williams BH. Controversy and Confusion in Interpretation of Ferret Clinical Pathology. http://www.afip.org/ferrets. Updated 2002.

GI Case 6 – Level 1

"Russell" is a 10-year-old neutered male Jack Russell Terrier presenting for work-up of possible liver disease. He has suffered four brief seizures in the last several months that appear to be associated with food consumption. The seizure episodes last about five minutes and they consist of trembling and the appearance of not be being mentally "present"; he does not paddle or lose control of his bladder or bowel. Russell is otherwise healthy, and on physical examination, he is bright, alert, and responsive with no abnormalities noted. On abdominal radiographs, Russell's liver appears to be small. This impression is confirmed with ultrasonography, however the liver is thought to be architecturally and texturally normal. No splenic or renal abnormalities are noted, however a nodule is identified in the left limb of the pancreas.

White blood cell count:	12.0 x 10⁹/L	(4.1-13.3)
Segmented neutrophils:	10.0 x 10⁹/L	(2.1-11.2)
Band neutrophils:	0	(0-0.3)
Lymphocytes:	1.5 x 10⁹/L	(1.0-5.1)
Monocytes:	0.5 x 10⁹/L	(0.1-1.2)
Eosinophils:	0.0 x 10⁹/L	(0-1.4)
WBC morphology: Appears within normal limits		

Hematocrit:	40%	(39-55)
Red blood cell count:	↓ 5.60 x 10¹²/L	(5.71-8.29)
Hemoglobin:	14.5 g/dl	(14.0-19.1)
MCV:	72.4 fl	(64.0-73.0)
MCHC:	36.0 g/dl	(33.6-36.6)
Platelets:	420 x 10⁹/L	(160-425)

Glucose:	↓ 41 mg/dl	(80.0-125.0)
BUN:	20 mg/dl	(6-24)
Creatinine:	1.1 mg/dl	(0.6-2.0)
Phosphorus:	5.4 mg/dl	(2.2-6.6)
Calcium:	9.8 mg/dl	(9.4-11.6)
Magnesium:	2.1 mEq/L	(1.4-2.2)
Total Protein:	5.5 g/dl	(4.7-7.3)
Albumin:	3.0 g/dl	(2.5-3.7)
Globulin:	2.5 g/dl	(2.3-4.2)
A/G Ratio:	1.2	(0.7-2.1)
Sodium:	145 mEq/L	(142-151)
Chloride:	119 mEq/L	(108-121)
Potassium:	5.4 mEq/L	(3.6-5.6)
HCO3:	16 mEq/L	(15-26)
Anion Gap:	15.4 mEq/L	(6-16)
Total Bili:	0.30 mg/dl	(0.10-0.30)
ALP:	↑ 270 IU/L	(1-145)
GGT:	4 IU/L	(0-7)
ALT:	18 IU/L	(5-65)
AST:	52 IU/L	(10-56)
Cholesterol:	249 mg/dl	(115-300)
Amylase:	630 IU/L	(409-1203)

Coagulation Panel		
PT:	6.4s	(5.6-7.8)
APTT:	7.6s	(8.9-13.7)
FDPs:	<5 ug/ml	(<5)

Interpretation

CBC: The CBC is unremarkable except for a mild decrease in the RBC count. This may indicate a developing mild anemia of chronic disease since the hematocrit is at the low end of the reference interval. Alternatively, these values may be normal for this patient as a result of normal biological variation. Repeat blood work could be considered to determine if there is a decreasing trend in the erythrocyte values.

Serum Biochemical Profile

Hypoglycemia: Once processing errors were ruled out, true hypoglycemia was suspected based on the "seizure" episodes. The pancreatic nodule is of concern, and insulinoma should be considered. Simultaneous measurement of glucose and insulin levels under fasted conditions are recommended. Impaired gluconeogenesis associated with liver failure can cause hypoglycemia (see Chapter 2, Case 21), although this is relatively uncommon. Other laboratory abnormalities associated with markedly decreased liver function include hypoalbuminemia, hypocholesterolemia, prolonged PT and APTT and occasionally mild hyperbilirubinemia, but none of these supporting abnormalities are observed in this case. Because none of measured parameters on the clinical chemistry profiles are sensitive or specific for the detection of decreased liver function, measurement of serum bile acids and/or blood ammonia are recommended because of the small liver. Remember that normal liver enzyme levels in the blood do not rule out liver disease. Clinical and laboratory findings make sepsis extremely unlikely.

Mild increase in ALP: This is an extremely non-specific finding in the dog (see Chapter 2). Corticosteroids and other drugs may induce elevations in ALP, however Russell does not have a corticosteroid leukogram, nor does he have a history of taking any medications. In the absence of other physical or laboratory evidence of liver disease, the significance of this elevation is unclear. Repeat sampling in 4-6 weeks is recommended, or sooner if the clinical condition changes.

Coagulation Profile: Within normal limits

Case Summary and Outcome

An aspirate smear of the liver was evaluated and found to be normal. Simultaneous fasting glucose and insulin levels were performed. Insulin was 48.8 IU/ml with a fasting glucose was 56 mg/dl, compatible with insulinoma. Normally insulin should be 2-25 IU/ml when glucose is between 70-100. Russell was treated with corticosteroids, frequent meals and avoidance of strenuous exercise until his tumor was surgically removed and confirmed to be an insulinoma by histologic examination of biopsy specimens. Unfortunately, resection was incomplete. Russell continued to do well at home on corticosteroid therapy for 18 months, after which he presented again after a low glucose measurement at the referring veterinarian's clinic. This laboratory abnormality was not associated with clinical signs that the owner had noticed. Repeat blood work at this time confirmed the low glucose and revealed a corticosteroid leukogram and elevated ALP, which may be attributed to corticosteroid treatment, though other causes cannot be ruled out.

Although thoracic radiographs were clear of metastases, abdominal ultrasound showed multiple liver nodules. Cytology of these nodules revealed small numbers of normal hepatocytes with sheets and small clusters of cells indicative of a neuroendocrine tumor compatible with insulinoma (Figure 3-3). Fasting insulin level measured on the same serum as the 18-month serum biochemical profile was 264 IU/ml, compatible with recurrence of disease. Russell was discharged from the hospital on medical therapy with a guarded prognosis.

This case was initially referred in for evaluation of liver disease, which was never definitively ruled out, however seemed unlikely to be the primary cause of the clinical signs given the preponderance of evidence. Russell's small liver and "neurologic signs" could have been compatible with poor hepatic function, but as noted above, other supportive laboratory data were lacking. The clinical presentation and laboratory findings were similar to the same disease in Ides, the ferret in the previous case. Interestingly, despite the confirmed presence of metastatic disease in the liver, hepatic enzyme changes were minimal and likely related to the corticosteroid therapy. This is similar to Kippy, who had an extremely large liver tumor and mostly unremarkable liver enzyme data.

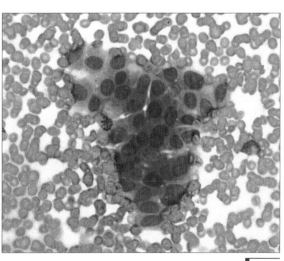

Figure 3-3. Smears consist of small clusters of uniform oval to polyhedral cells characterized by moderate to marked amounts of pale blue cytoplasm. Cells have one or two small round to oval nuclei. These findings were considered to be compatible with metastatic insulinoma.

GI Case 7 – Level 1

"Yap Yap" is a 6-month-old West Highland White terrier presenting with a history of foreign body ingestion (she passed a knee-high nylon stocking in the stool). Yap Yap continued to have intermittent vomiting after passing the stocking, so blood work was performed.

White blood cell count:	14.0 x 10⁹/L	(4.0-15.5)
Segmented neutrophils:	8.5 x 10⁹/L	(2.0-10.0)
Band neutrophils:	0 x 10⁹/L	(0-0.3)
Lymphocytes:	4.5 x 10⁹/L	(1.0-4.5)
Monocytes:	0.6 x 10⁹/L	(0.2-1.4)
Eosinophils:	0.2 x 10⁹/L	(0-1.2)
Basophils:	↑ 0.2 x 10⁹/L	(0)

WBC morphology: Appears within normal limits

Hematocrit:	↓ 30%	(37-60)
Red blood cell count:	↓ 4.36 x 10¹²/L	(5.5-8.5)
Hemoglobin:	↓ 10.0 g/dl	(12.0-18.0)
MCV:	70.0 fl	(60.0-77.0)
MCHC:	32.9 g/dl	(31.0-34.0)

RBC morphology: Within normal limits

Platelets: Appear adequate

Glucose:	↓ 78 mg/dl	(90.0-140.0)
BUN:	↓ 6 mg/dl	(8-33)
Creatinine:	0.5 mg/dl	(0.5-1.5)
Phosphorus:	6.6 mg/dl	(5.0-9.0)
Calcium:	10.4 mg/dl	(8.8-11.0)
Total Protein:	↓ 3.9 g/dl	(4.8-7.2)
Albumin:	↓ 1.8 g/dl	(3.0-4.2)
Globulin:	2.0 g/dl	(2.0-4.0)
Sodium:	145 mEq/L	(140-151)
Chloride:	115 mEq/L	(105-120)
Potassium:	4.0 mEq/L	(3.8-5.4)
Total Bili:	0.10 mg/dl	(0.10-0.50)
ALP:	↑ 421 IU/L	(20-320)
ALT:	↑ 1320 IU/L	(10-95)
Cholesterol:	↓ 90 mg/dl	(110-314)
Amylase:	↓ 386 IU/L	(400-1200)

Urinalysis: Voided

Appearance: Yellow and clear	Sediment: inactive

Specific gravity: 1.010

pH: 7.5

Negative for protein, glucose, ketones, bilirubin, heme

Interpretation

CBC: Yap Yap has a mild normocytic normochromic non-regenerative anemia compatible with chronic disease.

Serum Biochemical Profile

Hypoglycemia: Assuming appropriate sample collection and processing and considering the age of the patient, decreased liver function or potentially a congenital metabolic defect should be considered. There is no evidence of sepsis, and the patient's nutrition is adequate. Based on the age of the patient, neoplasia is very unlikely.

Decreased BUN: Hepatic insufficiency and dietary protein restriction may result in BUN below the reference range. Increased excretion with polyuria can contribute as well.

Hypoproteinemia with hypoalbuminemia: Hypoalbuminemia may result from decreased production, increased losses, or a combination of both causes. Some degree of intestinal protein loss is possible and suggested by the history, but decreased production secondary to poor liver function also may be a factor. This possibility is supported by the concurrent low BUN, hypocholesterolemia, and dilute urine. As seen with decreased BUN, starvation can trigger increased catabolism of serum albumin and may compromise production of this protein, but seems unlikely in this case. There is no significant renal loss of protein noted on the urinalysis, although given the dilute urine, a urinary protein:creatinine ratio could be performed as a more sensitive test for proteinuria.

Very mild increase in ALP: This minimal elevation may be attributable to numerous hepatic and extrahepatic processes (see Chapter 2). In a 6-month-old dog, bone isoenzyme should be considered, however YapYap is a small breed dog and is less likely than a larger dog to have increased bone ALP due to skeletal growth at this age. With the concurrent increase in ALT, a liver insult may be present and increased ALP can suggest a cholestatic component, although bilirubin is currently within reference intervals. Inflammatory processes of the intestine that might be expected with foreign body ingestion can involve the liver by either direct extension or via the portal blood. Enzyme induction by medications such as corticosteroids and anticonvulsants should be ruled out.

Increase in ALT: Elevation in ALT indicates some degree of hepatocellular damage, but is not specific for any particular cause. Hepatocellular damage may occur secondary to intestinal pathology and exposure of the liver to increased endotoxin, bacteria, and inflammatory mediators carried from damaged intestines by the portal circulation. Alternatively, primary liver disease is also possible. Hypoxia secondary to anemia is possible, but is less likely with mild or slowly developing anemias.

Hypocholesterolemia: Decreased liver function, protein losing enteropathy or severe malnutrition could diminish serum cholesterol. The combination of low serum glucose, BUN, albumin, and cholesterol is very suggestive for decreased liver function, however gastrointestinal protein loss cannot be ruled out given the history and low-normal globulin values.

Decrease in Amylase: A decrease in enzyme activity is not considered a clinically significant finding.

Urinalysis: Yap Yap is isosthenuric, but not azotemic. Interpretation of isosthenuria as physiologic or pathologic depends on clinical information such as hydration status. Because impaired ability to concentrate urine appears prior to azotemia, decreased renal function cannot be ruled out. Liver failure may also interfere with renal concentrating ability in the absence of pathology in the kidney.

Case Summary and Outcome

The combination of hypoglycemia, low BUN, hypoalbuminemia, and hypocholesterolemia in the absence of starvation or severe malnutrition suggests decreased liver function. PT and APTT were not evaluated, but may have been prolonged in this case because of diminished production of coagulation factors by the liver. Elevations in ALP and ALT also support hepatic pathology, but do not provide a specific diagnosis, nor are they liver function tests. Based on the suspicion of impaired liver function, serum bile acid levels were performed and confirmed decreased liver function: fasted: 62.9 µmol/L (reference interval = 0.0-5.0), post-prandial 197.7 µmol/L (reference interval = 5.0-25.0).

It was concluded that the isosthenuria was likely related to liver disease. Polyuria and polydipsia are a frequent signs of liver disease in dogs and may have contributed to the low urine specific gravity in this patient. Abnormal neurotransmitters overstimulate the pituitary, leading to increased ACTH secretion and hypercortisolism. As a result, the osmotic threshold for ADH release is increased so higher plasma osmolality is required to stimulated anti-diuresis. When patients become significantly dehydrated, the new threshold is reached so significant dehydration is not common. Reduced urea formation in the liver may also decrease urinary concentrating ability. Other poorly understood mechanisms probably contribute as well.

Imaging studies revealed a small liver and a portal-caval shunt, which was repaired with an ameroid constrictor ring. Wedge biopsy specimens collected at surgery revealed absence or atrophy of hepatic venules and proliferation of arterioles compatible with portosystemic shunt or microvascular dysplasia. Yap Yap appeared energetic and healthy prior to sugery, and the procedure and immediate post-operative recovery period were uneventful. Unfortunately, seven days after discharge, she presented for lethargy, anorexia, and a markedly distended abdomen. On physical examination, Yap Yap was quiet but responsive and had pale mucous membranes. Abdominal radiographs revealed poor abdominal detail, and ultrasound studies showed a thrombus near the ameroid constrictor with markedly decreased blood flow to the mesentery. Yap Yap died shortly after the procedure, no post-mortem examination was performed.

GI Case 8 – Level 1

"Freeze" is a one-day-old premature alpaca cria presenting with a history of seizures the previous day, increased respiration, dull mentation, and abrasions over both carpi and both hocks. Prior to referral, she was febrile and had been treated with subcutaneous fluids, antibiotics, and colostrum from her dam. On physical examination she is dull, recumbent, and febrile. (Note: neonatal reference intervals are published for the llama; see Fowler)

White blood cell count:	↓ 4.3 x 10⁹/L	(7.1-19.4)
Segmented neutrophils:	2.3 x 10⁹/L	(1.1-14.6)
Band neutrophils:	0.0 x 10⁹/L	(0-0.5)
Lymphocytes:	↓ 1.6 x 10⁹/L	(1.7-4.7)
Monocytes:	0.3 x 10⁹/L	(0.0-1.4)
Eosinophils:	0.1 x 10⁹/L	(0-1.1)
WBC morphology: No abnormalities noted		

Hematocrit:	↓ 23%	(24-35)
Hemoglobin:	10.3 g/dl	(10.1-14.9)
MCHC:	↑ 44.8	(39.4-44.1)
RBC morphology: Appears within normal limits		
Plasma is icteric.		

Platelets: Appear adequate

Glucose:	↓ 28 mg/dl	(94.0-170.0)
BUN:	↑ 158 mg/dl	(10-21)
Creatinine:	↑ 3.5 mg/dl	(1.1-2.9)
Phosphorus:	10.1 mg/dl	(7.1-11.1)
Calcium:	10.0 mg/dl	(9.4-10.6)
Total Protein:	5.8 g/dl	(5.1-6.7)
Albumin:	3.3 g/dl	(3.1-4.1)
Globulin:	2.5 g/dl	(1.4-3.4)
A/G Ratio:	1.3	(0.97-2.8)
Sodium:	149 mEq/L	(148-155)
Chloride:	109 mEq/L	(101-116)
Potassium:	5.6 mEq/L	(4.6-5.9)
HCO3:	30 mEq/L	(24-32)
Total Bili:	↑ 1.50 mg/dl	(0.0-0.60)
ALP:	532 IU/L	(342-975)
GGT:	↑ 548 IU/L	(8-29)
AST:	↑ 2113 IU/L	(168-482)
CK:	↑ 66129 IU/L	(13-130)

Interpretation

CBC

Leukogram: Freeze has a leucopenia with a mild lymphopenia, which could be compatible with a corticosteroid response. With the history of fever in a very young patient, acute viral infection with lympholysis is a differential.

Erythrogram: The hematocrit is just below the reference range. Because the reference range was not generated in the laboratory in which the patient values were generated, small deviations from the reference range are difficult to interpret. Crias have been noted to have a "physiologic anemia" after birth, which could be the result of shortened fetal red blood cell lifespan, decreased stimulus for erythrocyte production, and high blood oxygen affinity (Adams). The clinical interpretation of this value is unclear at this time, however any further decrement in this value could be important. The mild increase in MCHC also may be related to generation of reference intervals, however, intravascular or in vitro hemolysis may contribute.

Serum Biochemical Profile
Marked hypoglycemia: In the context of the clinical history of seizures, this value is likely accurate, however verification to rule out laboratory error is always appropriate. Because the patient is also febrile, sepsis is a primary differential diagnosis for hypoglycemia. Liver failure can result in impaired gluconeogenesis, and portovascular anomalies have been reported in alpaca crias (Ivany). Elevations in serum bilirubin and GGT support hepatic pathology. Serum bile acids and blood ammonia can be evaluated to assess liver function. Ill or anorexic neonates of many species are predisposed to the development of hypoglycemia, possibly due to limited energy reserves or immaturity of gluconeogenic systems (Lawler). This appears to be less common in camelids, who often develop hyperglycemia when stressed in the neonatal period (Cebra). Mechanistically, adult llamas and alpacas appear to have a weak insulin response and slow cellular uptake of glucose that promotes hyperglycemia (Cebra et al).

Increased BUN and creatinine: Based on the clinical history, fluid intake is likely to have been low since birth, and pre-renal azotemia is suspected. Interpretation of the azotemia should be done in concert with urinalysis; however urine specific gravity is often low in animals on an all milk diet (Adams).

Hyperbilirubinemia: Hemolysis, liver disease, and sepsis are all possible contributors to this abnormality. The patient has clinical signs or laboratory abnormalities that could be compatible with all three causes, so a single precipitating factor cannot be identified at this time.

Elevated serum GGT: In adult ruminants and camelids, increased serum GGT is an indicator of hepatic pathology. In some species serum GGT activity may increase in neonatal animals because colostrum contains large amounts of GGT, which is absorbed through the neonatal gut. In calves and lambs, but not crias, serum GGT has been advocated as an indicator of passive transfer status (Johnston, Tessman). In this case, the concurrent hyperbilirubinemia indicates that liver disease should not be dismissed at this point.

Elevated AST and CK: These increases likely reflect muscle damage secondary to the seizure activity.

Case Summary and Outcome
Freeze was treated with diazepam and phenobarbital for the seizures. Antibiotic and fluid therapy was continued, along with nasogastric feedings. Over the next few days the enzyme values normalized, the azotemia resolved, and the cria was normoglycemic. Both blood ammonia and serum bile acid tests were normal, suggesting normal liver function. Her increased liver enzyme values at the time of admission are interpreted to be associated with poor perfusion/hypoxia and endotoxemia. The specific cause of the hypoglycemic episode could not be determined, however sepsis was considered to be the most likely cause. Blood and urine cultures could have been performed, although previous therapy with antibiotics would likely have suppressed bacterial growth. Freeze was nursing well, gaining weight, and had no further signs of neurologic disease at the time of discharge.

Adams MA and Garry F. Llama Neonatology. Vet Clin North Am-Food Animal. 1994;10:209-227.

Cebra CK. Hyperglycemia, hypernatremia, and hyperosmolarity in six neonatal llamas and alpacas. J Am Vet Med Assoc. 2000;217:1701-1704.

Cebra CK, Tornquist SJ, Van Saun RJ, and Smith BB. Glucose tolerance testing in llamas and alpacas. Am J Vet Res. 2001;62:682-686.

Fowler ME and Zinkl JG. Reference ranges for hematologic and serum biochemical values in llamas (Lama glama). Am J Vet Res. 1989;50:2049-2053.

Ivany JM, Anderson DE, Birchard SJ, Matoon JR, Neubert BG. Portosystemic shunt in an alpaca cria. J Am Vet Med Assoc. 2002;220:1696-1699.

Johnston NA, Parish SM, Tyler JW, Tillman CB. Evaluation of serum γ-glutamyltransferase activity as a predictor of passive transfer status in crias. J Am Vet Med Assoc. 1997;211:1165-1166.

Lawler DF and Evans RH. Nutritional and environmental considerations in neonatal medicine. In: Kirk's Current Veterinary Therapy XII. JD Bonagura ed. 1995. W.B. Saunders Company, Philadelphia PA. pp 37-40.

Tessman RK, Tyler JW, Parish SM, Johnson DL, Gant RG, Grasseschi HA. Use of age and serum γ-glutamyltransferase activity to assess passive transfer status in lambs. J Am Vet Med Assoc 1997;211:1163-1164.

GI Case 9 – Level 2

"Maya" is a 6-month-old intact female DSH cat that was obtained by the owners from a family friend. One week ago, the owners noticed that Maya was lethargic, and last night she stopped eating and drinking. Today, they found Maya limp on the kitchen floor. Maya is an exclusively indoor cat, but is unvaccinated. She lives with another indoor cat who has been vaccinated. On physical examination, Maya is very depressed, is recumbent, and has dry mucous membranes. She has watery yellow stool around her rectum, and vomits a large amount of clear, brown-tinged fluid. Her peripheral pulses are weak and she is hypothermic. A jugular catheter is placed for fluid therapy, and there is greater than expected bleeding from the catheterization site. Her body condition is adequate and FeLV/FIV tests are negative.

White blood cell count:	↓ 0.2 x 10⁹/L	(4.5-15.7)
WBC morphology: Only five lymphocytes are present on the blood smear		

Hematocrit:	↓ 26%	(28-45)
Red blood cell count:	↓ 5.93 x 10¹²/L	(6.8-10.0)
Hemoglobin:	↓ 8.7 g/dl	(10.5-14.9)
MCV:	44.5 fl	(39.0-56.0)
MCHC:	33.5	(31.0-35.0)
Platelets: Clumped		

Glucose:	↓ 25 mg/dl	(70.0-120.0)
BUN:	32 mg/dl	(15-32)
Creatinine:	1.9 mg/dl	(0.9-2.1)
Phosphorus:	5.7 mg/dl	(3.0-6.0)
Calcium:	↓ 6.7 mg/dl	(8.9-11.6)
Total Protein:	↓ 1.7 g/dl	(6.0-8.4)
Albumin:	↓ 1.0 g/dl	(2.4-4.0)
Globulin:	↓ 0.7 g/dl	(2.5-5.8)
Sodium:	↓ 143 mEq/L	(149-163)
Chloride:	120 mEq/L	(119-134)
Potassium:	↓ 3.2 mEq/L	(3.6-5.4)
HCO3:	15 mEq/L	(13-22)
Total Bili:	↑ 0.7 mg/dl	(0.10-0.30)
ALP:	10 IU/L	(10-72)
ALT:	45 IU/L	(29-145)
AST:	35 IU/L	(12-42)
Cholesterol:	77 mg/dl	(77-258)
Triglycerides:	29 mg/dl	(25-191)
Amylase:	590 IU/L	(496-1874)

Interpretation

CBC: Maya's leukogram is characterized by a severe leucopenia (Figure 3-4). Too few leukocytes were present on the blood film for an accurate differential cell count, however a severe neutropenia is present. A normocytic, normochromic anemia is present. The anemia is more severe than it appears to be because Maya is significantly dehydrated, and hemoconcentration increases the hematocrit. Platelet numbers cannot be evaluated due to clumping.

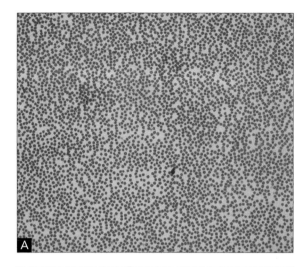

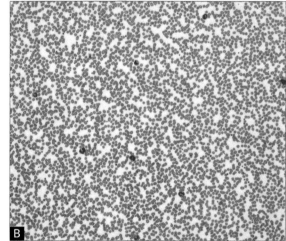

Figure 3-4A & B.
A. Representative field from Maya's blood film showing severe leucopenia. B. Similar field from a cat with a normal leukocyte count for comparison.

Serum Biochemical Profile

Marked hypoglycemia: Artifactual hypoglycemia was ruled out by confirming appropriate collection and processing of the sample. The hypoglycemia is severe enough to result in clinical signs, which could include mental dullness or seizures. In combination with the severe neutropenia, sepsis is an important differential diagnosis for the hypoglycemia in this patient. Maya is too young to prioritize neoplasia, and her good body condition makes starvation unlikely. Inadequate gluconeogenesis secondary to liver failure is possible since no specific tests of liver function have been performed and Maya is hypoalbuminemic, hyperbiliru-binemic, has low normal serum cholesterol, and has abnormal bleeding secondary to catheter placement. Abnormal bleeding may alternatively be explained by diminished platelet function associated with hypothermia, or disseminated intravascular coagulation (DIC).

Hypocalcemia: Because of extensive binding of calcium to albumin, low total calcium levels in the blood may be explained by hypoalbuminemia. Correction formulas have been developed for the dog, but are not applicable to the cat. Low total calcium caused by hypoproteinemia is not typically associated with clinical signs of hypocalcemia, however if there is any question, the biologically active ionized fraction of calcium should be determined.

Panhypoproteinemia: Low levels of both albumin and globulin proteins indicate plasma loss. Hemorrhage is a common cause, however Maya has no history of external blood loss. Plasma may also be lost via exudation or extravasation through compromised gut wall and skin or in association with parasitism. In Maya's case, increased capillary permeability associated with endotoxemia or gastrointestinal losses seem most likely. (See Chapter 4 for further discussion of abnormalities in protein)

Mild hyponatremia: Hyponatremia in dehydrated patients is often attributable to increased losses, especially if combined with hypotonic fluid replacement by drinking water. Maya is likely to have lost sodium through her compromised gastrointestinal tract, however other sources of loss include third space, renal, and cutaneous losses.

Mild hypokalemia: As with sodium, gastrointestinal losses of potassium are likely to contribute to the hypokalemia. Decreased intake also may be a factor in anorectic patients. Like sodium, potassium may be lost into effusions or through the kidney or skin. Transcellular shifts in patients with acid/base disorders also may influence serum potassium levels, but Maya's HCO3 is within the reference interval at this time. Arterial blood gas is required for full assessment of acid/base status in any patient.

Mild hyperbilirubinemia: Increased bilirubin often reflects inadequate uptake of bilirubin by hepatocytes, and is most often associated with liver disease or hemolysis. Although Maya is mildly anemic, no icterus or hemolysis are noted on examination of her plasma that would support significant hemolysis. All liver enzymes are within reference range, however liver enzyme levels are not adequate tests of liver function, and serum bile acid determinations are required for further evaluation of hepatic function. As indicated in the interpretation of hypoglycemia, the low albumin and cholesterol could be compatible with decreased liver function, however the predominance of clinical and laboratory data suggest endotoxemia as the cause for the hyperbilirubinemia. Endotoxin decreases hepatocellular uptake of bilirubin, and may cause mild to moderate hyperbilirubinemia.

Case Summary and Outcome

Because of Maya's clinical signs, unvaccinated status, and profound leukopenia, feline panleukopenia was suspected. A canine parvo test was positive, and she was treated with intravenous fluids and crystalloids and placed in an incubator. Dopamine was administered to support blood pressure, and she was treated with broad-spectrum antibiotics. Unfortunately, despite aggressive therapy, Maya died the next day.

Feline panleukopenia is characterized by damage to the intestinal villi, resulting in malabsorptive diarrhea and increased permeability of the gut wall. Viral replication in hematopoietic tissues causes leukopenia, which is often profound and parallels the severity of clinical disease. The combination of intestinal compromise and leukopenia leads to secondary bacteremia and endotoxemia and is rapidly fatal. Disseminated intravascular coagulation may occur secondary to sepsis, although cats are less likely to have clinically detectable abnormal bleeding than dogs with similar laboratory parameters. Blood clotting is also impaired when the body temperature is low. The cause for the bleeding around the catheterization site was not resolved because coagulation testing was not performed in this patient.

Both Freeze (Chapter 3, Case 8) and Maya have histories of febrile illness, hypoglycemia, and hyperbilirubinemia, although Maya's clinical presentation and laboratory data more clearly indicate sepsis. In contrast, Freeze appeared to have had a less severe illness with resultant better outcome. Both sepsis and liver disease can cause hyperbilirubinemia. Both may occur simultaneously in the patient, in which case it may not be possible to determine which is the major contributor to the increased bilirubin levels in the blood. See Chapter 2 Case 9 (dog), Chapter 2 Case 14 (llama), and Chapter 2 Case 21 (dog).

GI Case 10 – Level 1

"Bursley" is a 4-year-old intact male Pit Bull presenting with a 2 month history of progressive behavioral changes consisting of aggression (grumpy when moved), dull attitude, hypodypsia, and poor appetite associated with weight loss of 15 pounds. On presentation, Bursley is depressed, and he appears to fall asleep while standing up. He has a thin hair coat over the dorsal midline, and his testicles are reduced in size. Bursley has bilaterally depressed conscious proprioceptive deficits in both the front and the rear. His pulse is 48 beats per minute with no pulse deficits, respirations are 16 per minute, and the capillary refill time is >3 seconds.

White blood cell count:	↓ 4.4 x 10⁹/L	(6.0-17.0)
Segmented neutrophils:	↓ 2.4 x 10⁹/L	(3.0-11.0)
Band neutrophils:	0 x 10⁹/L	(0-0.3)
Lymphocytes:	1.5 x 10⁹/L	(1.0-4.8)
Monocytes:	0.2 x 10⁹/L	(0.2-1.4)
Eosinophils:	0.2 x 10⁹/L	(0-1.3)
Basophils:	0.1 x 10⁹/L	(0)

WBC morphology: Mild toxic change in neutrophils

Hematocrit:	↓ 36%	(37-55)
Red blood cell count:	↓ 5.02 x 10¹²/L	(5.5-8.5)
Hemoglobin:	↓ 11.7 g/dl	(12.0-18.0)
MCV:	71.2 fl	(60.0-77.0)
MCHC:	32.5 g/dl	(31.0-34.0)

Platelets:	222.0 x 10⁹/L	(200.0-450.0)

Glucose:	105 mg/dl	(65.0-120.0)
BUN:	9 mg/dl	(8-33)
Creatinine:	0.7 mg/dl	(0.5-1.5)
Phosphorus:	3.9 mg/dl	(3.0-6.0)
Calcium:	10.6 mg/dl	(8.8-11.0)
Magnesium:	1.7 mEq/L	(1.4-2.7)
Total Protein:	↑ 7.4 g/dl	(5.2-7.2)
Albumin:	↑ 4.5 g/dl	(3.0-4.2)
Globulin:	2.9 g/dl	(2.0-4.0)
A/G Ratio:	1.6	(0.7-2.1)
Sodium:	150 mEq/L	(140-151)
Chloride:	112 mEq/L	(105-120)
Potassium:	4.2 mEq/L	(3.8-5.4)
HCO3:	21 mEq/L	(16-25)
Anion Gap:	21.2 mEq/L	(15-25)
Total Bili:	0.17 mg/dl	(0.10-0.50)

ALP:	162 IU/L	(20-320)
ALT:	31 IU/L	(10-95)
AST:	27 IU/L	(15-52)
Cholesterol:	↑ 363 mg/dl	(110-314)
Triglycerides:	37 mg/dl	(30-300)
Amylase:	486 IU/L	(400-1200)

Urinalysis: Cystocentesis

Appearance: Yellow and clear   Sediment: inactive

Specific gravity: 1.020

pH: 7.0

Negative for protein, glucose, ketones, bilirubin, heme

Interpretation

CBC: Bursley has a mild leukopenia with neutropenia with toxic changes that suggests inflammation. There is a mild normocytic normochromic, apparently nonregenerative, anemia, compatible with chronic disease or hypothyroidism. Mild hemoconcentration may mask a slightly lower PCV.

Serum Biochemical Profile

Hyperproteinemia with hyperalbuminemia: Hyperalbuminemia is not the result of overproduction by the liver, but does reflect hemoconcentration. Bursely's owners report that he is drinking less water than is usual and dehydration is noted on the physical examination, which support hemoconcentration as the cause for the increased albumin and hyperproteinemia.

Hypercholesterolemia: There are numerous potential causes for hypercholesterolemia (see introduction to this chapter), however several can be ruled out in this case based on the history and laboratory data. Bursley has not eaten recently and is not taking medications, ruling out these as likely contributors to this abnormality. Pancreatitis or liver disease are less likely based on Bursley's history (no vomiting, diarrhea, or icterus) and normal serum activites of liver and pancreatic enzymes. Endocrinopathies can be associated with hypercholesterolemia, specifically diabetes mellitus, hyperadrenocorticism, and hypothyroidism. The absence of hyperglycemia or glucosuria makes diabetes unlikely. The alopecia might support hyperadrenocorticism, however 95% of dogs with this condition have increased ALP, which is not present here. Based on the clinical presentation and laboratory data, hypothyroidism seems probable, although further testing is required to confirm this diagnosis.

Case Summary and Outcome

Thyroid test results for Bursley included a low basal T4 (<1.0 µg/dl, reference interval 1.0-4.4), and decreased free T4 (0.44 ng/dl, reference inverval 0.8-2.0). Thyroid stimulating hormone (TSH) levels were low, suggesting secondary hypothyroidism. A CT scan showed a large enhancing mass in the region of the pituitary. Options for therapy included radiation therapy and symptomatic therapy including thyroid hormone supplementation, however the owner elected euthanasia due to the poor prognosis and economic constraints. At necropsy, a 2.2 cm soft, pale yellow mass replaced the pituitary gland and expanded into the hypothalamus. Histologically, the mass was identified as a pituitary chromophobe adenoma.

Secondary hypothyroidism is uncommon, and accounts for less than 5% of clinical cases of hypothyroidism. The mild nonregenerative anemia is a classic abnormality described in hypothyroid dogs, however it is not present in all cases. Decreased serum erythropoietin levels, diminished oxygen demand by peripheral tissues, and impaired iron uptake have been proposed as contributing factors to the anemia. The white blood cell count is variable in these patients. More than 75% of hypothyroid dogs will have fasting hypercholesterolemia in their serum biochemical profiles. Fasting hypertriglyceridemia may also be seen, but was not observed in this patient. While both cholesterol production and degradation are impaired by hypothyroidism, degradation is more effected. Thyroid hormone is necessary for the activation of lipoprotein lipase, for the expression of low density lipoprotein (LDL) receptors, and for hepatic uptake of cholesterol from the circulation.

GI Case 11 – Level 1

"Salvatore" is a 10-year-old neutered male Maltese presenting for hemoptysis and extensive petechia on the trunk and abdomen. Although his physical examination was otherwise within normal limits, he had a dry, non-productive cough during the examination. Thoracic radiographs and abdominal ultrasound failed to identify further abnormalities.

White blood cell count:	↑ 19.7 x 10⁹/L	(4.9-16.8)
Segmented neutrophils:	↑ 16.1 x 10⁹/L	(2.8-11.5)
Band neutrophils:	0	(0-0.3)
Lymphocytes:	1.8 x 10⁹/L	(1.0-4.8)
Monocytes:	1.2 x 10⁹/L	(0.1-1.5)
Eosinophils:	0.6 x 10⁹/L	(0-1.4)
Nucleated RBC/100 WBC	↑ 7	
WBC morphology: Appears within normal limits		

Hematocrit:	↓ 35%	(39-55)
Red blood cell count:	not available	(5.8-8.5)
Hemoglobin:	↓ 11 g/dl	(14.0-19.1)
MCV:	66.6 fl	(60.0-75.0)
MCHC:	↓ 31.4 g/dl	(33.0-36.0)
RBC morphology: Slightly increased polychromasia and anisocytosis		
Platelets:	↓ 16 x 10⁹/L	(181-525)

Glucose:	↑ 146 mg/dl	(67.0-135.0)
BUN:	21 mg/dl	(8-29)
Creatinine:	0.6 mg/dl	(0.6-2.0)
Phosphorus:	4.1 mg/dl	(2.6-7.2)
Calcium:	11.1 mg/dl	(9.4-11.6)
Magnesium:	2.2 mEq/L	(1.7-2.5)
Total Protein:	6.6 g/dl	(5.5-7.8)
Albumin:	3.8 g/dl	(2.8-4.0)
Globulin:	2.8 g/dl	(2.3-4.2)
A/G Ratio:	1.4	(0.7-2.1)
Sodium:	157 mEq/L	(142-163)
Chloride:	122 mEq/L	(106-126)
Potassium:	3.8 mEq/L	(3.8-5.4)
HCO3:	21 mEq/L	(15-28)
Anion Gap:	17.8 mEq/L	(12-23)
Total Bili:	0.10 mg/dl	(0.10-0.30)
ALP:	300 IU/L	(20-320)
GGT:	5 IU/L	(2-10)
ALT:	58 IU/L	(18-86)
AST:	44 IU/L	(16-54)
Cholesterol:	234 mg/dl	(82-355)
Triglycerides:	144 mg/dl	(30-321)
Amylase:	1200 IU/L	(409-1203)

Interpretation

CBC: Salvatore's hematology data includes a mild mature neutrophilic leukocytosis, and a mild normocytic hypochromic anemia with increased numbers of nucleated erythrocytes and severe thrombocytopenia. The neutrophilic leukocytosis may be due to inflammation, and the anemia secondary to chronic disease. If a healthy baseline hematocrit is available for comparison, it might be possible to determine how significant a deviation this hematocrit is from the patient's normal hematocrit. Because of the severe thrombocytopenia and clinical evidence of a coagulopathy, blood loss anemia is likely. Blood loss anemias are generally regenerative if given sufficient time, so this bleeding may be relatively acute (<3-5 days). There are marginal signs of regeneration (low MCHC, increased polychromsia and anisocytosis), however a reticulocyte count is needed to quantitate the response. Increased numbers of nucleated erythrocytes in the circulation may occur as part of a regenerative response or may be associated with some type of endothelial damage or lesions in the hematopoietic organs. Severe thrombocytopenia in a relatively healthy patient with minimal changes in other hematopoietic lines suggests immune-mediated thrombocytopenia, although infectious causes such as tick-borne diseases should also be considered.

Serum Biochemical Profile

Hyperglycemia: On the day of presentation, Salvatore has mild hyperglycemia could be compatible with stress.

Case Summary and Outcome

Immune-mediated thrombocytopenia was presumptively diagnosed based on the marked thrombocytopenia and the absence of other causes of decreased platelets. Serologic tests for tick borne diseases such as Rocky Mountain Spotted Fever and Ehrlichial organisms were negative. Salvatore was treated with immunosuppressive doses of corticosteroids. His clinical condition improved, and subsequent blood samples were collected 14 days after initiation of therapy.

Laboratory data obtained 14 days after initiation of corticosteroid treatment:

White blood cell count:	↑ 20.4 x 10⁹/L	(4.9-16.8)
Segmented neutrophils:	↑ 16.5 x 10⁹/L	(2.8-11.5)
Band neutrophils:	0	(0-0.3)
Lymphocytes:	↓ 0.5 x 10⁹/L	(1.0-4.8)
Monocytes:	↑ 3.4 x 10⁹/L	(0.1-1.5)
Eosinophils:	0	(0-1.4)
Nucleated RBC/100 WBC	1	
WBC morphology: Appears within normal limits		

Hematocrit:	↓ 37%	(39-55)
Red blood cell count:	↓ 5.15 x 10¹²/L	(5.8-8.5)
Hemoglobin:	↓ 12.9 g.dl	(14.0-19.1)
MCV:	71.6 fl	(60.0-75.0)
MCHC:	34.9 g/dl	(33.0-36.0)
RBC morphology: Slightly increased polychromasia and anisocytosis		
Platelets:	↑ 644 x 10⁹/L	(181-525)

Glucose:	98 mg/dl	(67.0-135.0)
BUN:	22 mg/dl	(8-29)
Creatinine:	0.6 mg/dl	(0.6-2.0)

Phosphorus:	4.3 mg/dl	(2.6-7.2)
Calcium:	11.0 mg/dl	(9.4-11.6)
Magnesium:	2.5 mEq/L	(1.7-2.5)
Total Protein:	6.7 g/dl	(5.5-7.8)
Albumin:	3.8 g/dl	(2.8-4.0)
Globulin:	2.9 g/dl	(2.3-4.2)
A/G Ratio:	1.3	(0.7-2.1)
Sodium:	146 mEq/L	(142-163)
Chloride:	106 mEq/L	(106-126)
Potassium:	4.3 mEq/L	(3.8-5.4)
HCO3:	26 mEq/L	(15-28)
Anion Gap:	18.3 mEq/L	(8-19)
Total Bili:	0.10 mg/dl	(0.10-0.30)
ALP:	↑ 2258 IU/L	(20-320)
GGT:	↑ 46 IU/L	(2-10)
ALT:	↑ 491 IU/L	(18-86)
AST:	42 IU/L	(16-54)
Cholesterol:	↑ 360 mg/dl	(82-355)
Triglycerides:	↑ 1291 mg/dl	(30-321)
Amylase:	833 IU/L	(409-1203)

CBC
Day 14: By this time, Salvatore's leukogram is characteristic for a corticosteroid leukogram and includes a mature neutrophilic leukocytosis, lymphopenia, and monocytosis. Superimposed inflammation could account for a portion of the neutrophilic leukocytosis and monocytosis. Salvatore still has mild anemia, however the thrombocytopenia has resolved, and a rebound thrombocytosis is evident.

Serum Biochemical Profile Day 14
Increased ALP, GGT, and ALT: The majority of the increase in ALP and GGT is likely due to corticosteroid induction of these enzymes (please see Chapter 2 for complete discussion of these parameters), although some degree of cholestasis may accompany the vacuolar hepatopathy associated with corticosteroid effects on the liver. The increased ALT could be the result of focal hepatocellular necrosis or cholestasis secondary to corticosteroid treatment. Canine ALT has a longer half life than AST, which may explain the discrepancy between the values.

Hypercholesterolemia and hypertriglyceridemia: Increased lipolysis stimulated by corticos-teroids causes increased cholesterol and triglyceride levels in the blood.

Salvatore was weaned off of his corticosteroids and recovered well. The serum biochemical abnormalities resolved after discontinuation of prednisone. Increases in endogenous corticos-teroids or treatment with pharmacologic doses of corticosteroids may have multiple metabolic effects that could cause abnormalities in the serum biochemical profile. The occurrence of both clinical signs and laboratory abnormalities related to corticosteroid treatment can vary dramatically between individual animals on similar doses of hormone. The increases in liver enzymes, cholesterol and triglycerides observed in this patient are not always present in patients with hypercortisolism (See Chapter 2, Case 5). While liver enzyme elevations are often present, the degree of increase is not consistent. Treatment with corti-costeroids can also increase serum bile acids. Additional possible abnormalities associated with corticosteroids include mild hyperglycemia secondary to insulin resistance. Occasionally glucosuria may accompany the hyperglycemia if the renal threshold for reabsorption of glucose is exceeded (about 200 mg/dl for the dog). Less commonly, BUN may be decreased secondary to glucocorticoid stimulated diuresis; diuresis also decreases urine specific gravity in some patients. Rarely, serum phosphate may be decreased due to increased losses in the urine.

GI Case 12 – Level 2

"Kazoo" is a 7-year-old neutered male yellow Labrador who began vomiting four days ago. Abdominal radiographs suggested the presence of a foreign body in his stomach, and a tennis ball was removed via gastrotomy. He was discharged two days after surgery, and presented this morning groggy and unresponsive. On physical examination, Kazoo is thin, markedly dehydrated, and hypothermic. His mucous membranes are injected, and he appears to have fluid in his abdominal cavity.

White blood cell count:	↑ 48.1 x 10⁹/L	(4.9-16.8)
Segmented neutrophils:	↑ 36.2 x 10⁹/L	(2.8-11.5)
Band neutrophils:	0	(0-0.3)
Lymphocytes:	3.6 x 10⁹/L	(1.0-4.8)
Monocytes:	↑ 2.1 x 10⁹/L	(0.1-1.5)
Eosinophils:	↑ 6.2 x 10⁹/L	(0-1.4)
WBC morphology: Neutrophils are slightly toxic and occasional reactive lymphocytes are seen.		

Hematocrit:	↓ 34%	(39-55)
Red blood cell count:	↓ 4.89 x 10¹²/L	(5.8-8.5)
Hemoglobin:	↓ 11.5 g/dl	(14.0-19.1)
MCV:	69.3 fl	(60.0-75.0)
MCHC:	33.8 g/dl	(33.0-36.0)
Platelets:	↓ 136 x 109/L	(181-525)

Glucose:	↓ 52 mg/dl	(67.0-135.0)
BUN:	↑ 44 mg/dl	(8-29)
Creatinine:	↑ 3.2 mg/dl	(0.6-2.0)
Phosphorus:	5.9 mg/dl	(2.6-7.2)
Calcium:	10.4 mg/dl	(9.4-11.6)
Magnesium:	1.9 mEq/L	(1.7-2.5)
Total Protein:	↓ 3.8 g/dl	(5.5-7.8)
Albumin:	↓ 2.0 g/dl	(3.0-4.2)
Globulin:	↓ 1.8 g/dl	(2.3-4.2)
A/G Ratio:	1.1	(0.7-2.1)
Sodium:	148 mEq/L	(142-163)
Chloride:	117 mEq/L	(106-126)
Potassium:	4.5 mEq/L	(3.8-5.4)
HCO3:	20 mEq/L	(15-28)
Anion Gap:	15.5 mEq/L	(8-19)
Total Bili:	0.20 mg/dl	(0.1-0.3)
ALP:	67 IU/L	(12-121)
GGT:	<3 IU/L	(2-10)
ALT:	72 IU/L	(18-86)

AST:	↑ 336 IU/L	(16-54)
Cholesterol:	↓ 32 mg/dl	(110-314)
Triglycerides:	76 mg/dl	(30-321)
Amylase:	1044 IU/L	(409-1203)

Coagulation data:

PT:	↑ 14.6s	(6.2-9.3)
APTT:	↑ 33.4s	(8.9-16.3)
FDP:	↑ ≥20 µg/ml	(<5)

Abdominal fluid analysis:

Pre-spin color: red	Total protein: 3.7 gm/dl
Pre-spin turbidity: opaque	Total nucleated cells: 37,400/µL
Post spin color: straw	
Post spin turbidity: clear	

Direct smears contain 86% nondegenerate neutrophils, 3% mature lymphocytes, 10% large mononuclear cells, and 1% eosinophils. No etiologic agents are present.

Interpretation

CBC
Leukogram: The leukogram is characterized by a mature neutrophilic leukocytosis, monocytosis, and eosinophilia. The neutrophils are toxic, indicating systemic inflammation. Occasional reactive lymphocytes are compatible with antigenic stimulation. Hypersensitivity disorders and parasitic diseases should be included as differential diagnoses for the increased eosinophils, in addition to mast cell tumor and lymphoma (both tumors can stimulate the production and recruitment of eosinophils in some cases). Despite the poor condition of the patient, the lymphopenia and eosinopenia compatible with a stress leukogram are absent. Eosinophilia in extremely stressed or ill patients can be compatible with hypoadrenocorticism.

Erythrogram: The mild normocytic normochromic anemia is likely nonregenerative and suggests anemia of chronic disease.

Thrombocytopenia: Both decreased production and increased consumption could contribute to the decreased platelet counts. The activity of the myeloid lineage argues against a generalized bone marrow disorder and lack of production, however the nonregenerative anemia could suggest marrow compromise. Hemorrhage, vascular abnormalities, disseminated intravascular coagulation (DIC) and immune mediated-destruction all accelerate platelet destruction. The prolongation of PT and APTT and increase of FDPs support DIC as the most likely cause for the thrombocytopenia. Primary immune mediated thrombocytopenia is usually associated with much lower platelet numbers than those documented here (See Case 11 in this chapter).

Serum Biochemical Profile
Hypoglycemia: All samples were processed appropriately, so laboratory error was ruled out. The clinical information, inflammatory leukogram, and presence of DIC are compatible with sepsis as a cause for the hypoglycemia. Considering the leukogram data, hypoadrenocorticism may also be a cause for Kazoo's hypoglycemia. Corticosteroids from the adrenal gland increase hepatic gluconeogenesis and decrease glucose uptake and utilization in peripheral tissues. Consequently, hypoglycemia may result from inadequate corticosteroid production

due to inadequate hepatic gluconeogenesis and increased insulin sensitivity. The combination of hypoglycemia, hypoalbuminemia, hypocholesterolemia, and prolonged coagulation times are also compatible with decreased liver function, which should be evaluated by fasted and post-prandial bile acid testing. The clinical history describes the patient as thin, and he has probably not had normal food intake for awhile, so nutritional compromise could contribute to hypoglycemia in this case as well, although this is a rarely a cause of low blood glucose.

Azotemia: Prerenal azotemia is likely because Kazoo is markedly dehydrated. A renal component cannot be ruled out without a urine specific gravity.

Panhypoproteinemia: A proportional decrease in albumin and globulins suggests protein loss via hemorrhage, cutaneous lesions, the gastrointestinal tract or third space loss. Significant protein could be lost into the abdominal effusion in this patient, and a poor nutritional plane and increased protein catabolism after surgery could complicate Kazoo's protein metabolism. Vigorous fluid resuscitation may exacerbate the hypoproteinemia. As noted in the section on hypoglycemia, the combination of low glucose, albumin, cholesterol, and prolonged coagulation times could reflect poor liver function. Starvation can contribute to hypoalbuminemia, and may be an issue in this case relative to poor body condition and a period of anorexia.

Moderately increased AST: Because this enzyme is present in multiple tissues, the interpretation of increased AST can be unclear. Because the ALT is within the reference interval, elevated AST is best interpreted here as a potential indicator of muscle damage. Muscle damage is likely secondary to the poor perfusion status of this animal. Increased AST could also be iatrogenic and related to invasive procedures like surgery, however serum AST levels would be expected to normalize several days after the procedure. Measurement of creatine kinase (CK) could help confirm muscle origin for AST, but this information is not critical to the diagnosis for this patient. Because Kazoo has multiple laboratory abnormalities that are compatible with diminished liver function, hepatocellular damage also could increase the AST. Generally, hepatocellular damage is accompanied by increases in ALT, however patients with decreased liver function may have too few remaining hepatocytes to release sufficient enzyme to elevate serum levels, or appreciable hepatocellular damage may no longer be occurring (i.e. port-systemic shunts or cirrhosis). Please see Chapter 2 on liver enzymes for a more complete discussion of this topic.

Hypocholesterolemia: As noted above, decreased liver function should be ruled out as a cause of the hypocholesterolemia in this patient. Another differential diagnosis in this patient is hypoadrenocorticism. Keep in mind that not all Addisonians have the classical electrolyte abnormalities. In particular, patients with glucocorticoid dependent hypoadrenocorticism often have hypocholesterolemia (Lifton). The absence of adequate amounts of cortisol in the circulation may alter cholesterol absorption from the gut, or may depress hepatic production by failing to appropriately suppress the metabolic rate, particularly during illness.

Coagulation data: Prolongation of both the PT and the APTT demonstrate deficiencies of secondary coagulation involving both the extrinsic and intrinsic or the common pathways. This abnormality in combination with the moderate thrombocytopenia and the presence of fibrin degradation products is diagnostic for DIC. Decreased liver function may contribute to the prolongation of the PT and APTT secondary to diminished production of coagulation factors and poor liver function can be associated with increased FDPs because of impaired clearance by the liver. Conversely, DIC can be associated with liver disease secondary to a number of mechanisms including impaired clearance of activated clotting factors, altered production of pro- and anticoagulants, and endothelial cell activation within a markedly vascular sinusoidal organ. Sepsis and cardiovascular collapse with poor tissue perfusion may also result in DIC.

Abdominal fluid analysis: Kazoo's abdominal fluid is an exudate characterized by suppurative inflammation. The recent abdominal surgery may explain some or all of the inflammation. While there is no direct evidence of a bacterial cause (no organisms are seen and the neutrophils are nondegenerate), sepsis should be suspected due to the patient's poor clinical condition and DIC. A culture of the fluid is strongly recommended.

Case Summary and Outcome

At the time of presentation, Kazoo's clinical signs were suggestive for sepsis, and thoracic radiographs were supportive of pneumonia. Kazoo slowly improved on intravenous antibiotics and fluids, however his progress was slower than expected. Because of the combination of poor clinical response with persistent eosinophilia, hypocholesterolemia, and apparent difficulties maintaining adequate blood glucose concentrations, Kazoo was evaluated for hypoadrenocorticism. An ACTH stimulation test revealed a resting cortisol value of 0.21 µg/dl (reference interval 2-6) and a post ACTH cortisol level of <0.20 µg/dl (reference interval 6-18), supporting a diagnosis of hypoadrenocorticism. Kazoo was discharged on oral antibiotics and oral prednisone with the recommendation that his owners try to fatten him up. All serum biochemical abnormalities had resolved on re-evaluation of the patient several weeks after therapy, so work up for potential liver failure was not pursued.

Primary hypoadrenocorticism results from loss of approximately 85-90% of both adrenal cortices. Secondary hypoadrenocorticism due to lesions in the hypothalamic-pituitary axis resulting in ACTH deficiency is rare. Immune mediated destruction of the adrenal glands is the suspected cause of hypoadrenocorticism in many patients, although granulomatous disease, infarction, trauma, metastatic disease, and iatrogenic causes are also possible. Patients with hypoadrenocorticism often have nonspecific signs such as weakness and give the impression of severe illness. Vague gastrointestinal signs may be present. Although most patients with hypoadrenocorticism have insufficiency of all zones of the adrenal cortex, classical laboratory abnormalities on the serum biochemical profile including hyponatremia, hypochloremia, and hyperkalemia reflect the mineralocorticoid deficiency. Because these abnormalities are not consistently present in all patients with hypoadrenocorticism, ACTH stimulation testing is recommended for the evaluation of patients with suggestive presentations (Peterson). Kazoo is in the minority of patients in which the destruction of all cortical zones is not equal, resulting in evidence of glucocorticoid insufficiency, but not mineralocorticoid deficiency. Although hypoadrenocorticism may have an insidious onset with a waxing and waning presentation, a stressful event may precipitate clinical signs of hypoad-renocorticism. The stress of the tennis ball foreign body and surgery likely resulted in the abrupt onset of clinical signs in this patient. It is probable that signs of mineralocorticoid deficiency will eventually develop, and Kazoo should be monitored with this in mind.

Like Bursley (Case 10) and Salvatore (Case 11), an endocrinopathy led to abnormalities in glucose and cholesterol homeostasis, reinforcing the important role of hormones in modulating metabolism. As we saw with Maya (Case 9) and Freeze (Case 8), any patient with signs of sepsis should be monitored for hypoglycemia. These patients tend to present with more severe signs of illness than patients presenting with hypoglycemia associated with neoplasia (see Cases 4, 5, and 6, Kippy, Ides, and Russell). Depression caused by severe illness may be indistinct from clinical signs of hypoglycemia in septic patients. Kazoo's endocrinopathy predisposed him to have hypoglycemia in response to periods of anorexia or increased glucose utilization that would normally be bridged by hepatic gluconeogenesis. It is not possible to know whether Kazoo was also septic, since cultures were not performed. He did not have hyperbilirubinemia, as do some septic patients.

Lifton SJ, King LG, Zerbe CA. Glucocorticoid deficient hypoadrenocorticism in dogs: 18 cases (1986-1995). J Am Vet Med Assoc 1996;209:2076-2081.

Peterson ME, Kintzer PP, Kass PH. Pretreatment and laboratory findings in dogs with hypoadrenocorticism: 225 cases (1979-1993). J Am Vet Med Assoc 1996;208:85-91.

GI Case 13 – Level 1

"Shorty" is an 11-year-old spayed female domestic shorthaired cat presenting with a history of several weeks of inappetance. During the past week, she has been anorexic, vomiting, and lethargic. Previous treatment consisting of a diet change and prednisone did not result in clinical improvement. On physical examination, Shorty has a left parasternal grade III/VI systolic heart murmur, is dehydrated, and has a firm, palpable cranial abdominal mass. The remainder of the physical examination is within normal limits. Abdominal radiographs show a cranial abdominal mass that could involve the liver, pancreas, or spleen. On ultrasound, the liver is diffusely nodular. The palpable mass is in or near the pancreas.

White blood cell count:	↑ 17.7 x 10⁹/L	(4.5-15.7)
Segmented neutrophils:	↑ 14.7 x 10⁹/L	(2.1-10.1)
Lymphocytes:	↓ 1.1 x 10⁹/L	(1.5-7.0)
Monocytes:	1.6 x 10⁹/L	(0-0.850)
Eosinophils:	0.3 x 10⁹/L	(0.0-1.900)
WBC morphology: No significant abnormalities		

Hematocrit:	36%	(28-45)
Red blood cell count:	7.51 x 10¹²/L	(5.0-10.0)
Hemoglobin:	11.5 g/dl	(8.0-15.0)
MCV:	48.4 fl	(39.0-55.0)
MCHC:	31.9	(31.0-35.0)
RBC morphology: No significant abnormalities		
Platelets: Clumped, but appear adequate		

Glucose:	↑ 142 mg/dl	(70.0-120.0)
BUN:	22 mg/dl	(15-32)
Creatinine:	1.0 mg/dl	(0.9-2.1)
Phosphorus:	3.7 mg/dl	(3.0-6.0)
Calcium:	9.6 mg/dl	(8.9-11.6)
Magnesium:	2.5 mEq/L	(1.9-2.6)
Total Protein:	7.3 g/dl	(6.0-8.4)
Albumin:	3.5 g/dl	(2.4-4.0)
Globulin:	3.8 g/dl	(2.5-5.8)
Sodium:	155 mEq/L	(149-163)
Chloride:	122 mEq/L	(119-134)
Potassium:	5.3 mEq/L	(3.6-5.4)
HCO3:	18 mEq/L	(13-22)
Total Bili:	0.2 mg/dl	(0.10-0.30)
ALP:	48 IU/L	(10-72)
ALT:	71 IU/L	(29-145)
AST:	41 IU/L	(12-42)

Cholesterol:	123 mg/dl	(77-258)
Triglycerides:	56 mg/dl	(25-191)
Amylase:	↑ 17,535 IU/L	(496-1874)
Lipase:	↑ 22,239 IU/L	(17-179)

Urinalysis: Cystocentesis

Appearance: Yellow and slightly cloudy	Sediment:
Specific gravity: >1.060	0-5 RBC/hpf
pH: 6.0	No WBC seen
Protein: negative	No casts seen
Glucose/ketones: negative	No epithelial cells seen
Bilirubin: negative	No bacteria seen
Heme: negative	Trace fat droplets and debris

Coagulation Profile

PT:	12.0s	(6.9-12.6)
APTT:	11.5s	(11.5-25.0)
FDP:	<5 µg/ml	(<5)

Interpretation

CBC: Shorty has a mild, mature neutrophilic leukocytosis and lymphopenia which is consistent with the history of having been treated with corticosteroids or may occur with stress.

Serum Biochemical Profile:
Hyperglycemia: The most likely cause for the mild hyperglycemia in this patient is stress, which is supported by the concurrent stress or corticosteroid leukogram. Diabetes mellitus cannot be ruled out, but is unlikely based on the mild elevation, normal urinalysis and absence of classic clinical history.

Marked hyperamylasemia and hyperlipasemia (10 and 125 x the upper limit of reference ranges, respectively): Both decreased glomerular filtration rates and the administration of corticosteroids have been reported to increased serum amylase and lipase levels up to 4x the upper limit of the reference range. Although Shorty has been treated with corticosteroids, renal function appears to be good. Shorty is not azotemic despite being dehydrated, and the urine is very concentrated. The marked elevations here are more compatible with primary pancreatic pathology, although many cats with pancreatic disease may have normal pancreatic enzyme levels.

Urinalysis: No significant abnormalities. The urine is appropriately concentrated for a dehydrated cat.

Coagulation profile: Normal

Case Summary and Outcome

Cytologic specimens of the pancreas and biopsies of the liver were obtained at the time of ultrasound examination. Cytology smears (Figure 3-5) were interpreted to be compatible with epithelial neoplasia, and metastatic pancreatic adenocarcinoma was identified on liver biopsy specimens. Despite the presence of tumor in the liver, liver enzyme data was unremarkable, as we have seen in Kippy (primary hepatocellular carcinoma-Case 4) and Russell (metastatic insulinoma-Case 6). A trypsin-like immunoreactivity test (TLI) was performed to support a diagnosis of primary pancreatic disease, and TLI was found to be elevated (305 µg/L, reference interval 12-82). Shorty was discharged with a grave prognosis and died at home several weeks later.

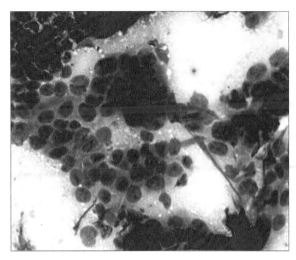

Figure 3-5. Smears collected from the pancreas consisted of amorphous debris and multiple sheets of epithelial cells The cells are characterized by scant slightly grainy basophilic cytoplasm. Each cell contains a single nucleus with coarse chromatin and a single large nucleolus. Anisocytosis and anisokaryosis are mild.

The laboratory work in this case is compatible with either pancreatitis or pancreatic neoplasia. Increased serum lipase can occur in dogs with pancreatic or hepatic neoplasia (Quigley). Unfortunately, serum amylase and lipase are less useful in cats than in dogs or people for the diagnosis of pancreatic disease, and other hematologic and biochemical abnormalities are nonspecific (Gerhardt). Some authors have suggested that serum amylase and lipase are actually of no diagnostic utility for pancreatitis in cats (Simpson, Williams). TLI has been proposed as a better alternative for the diagnosis of pancreatic disease in the cat, and was elevated in this patient. TLI is not increased in all feline patients with pancreatic pathology, however, and TLI may be elevated in cats with inflammatory bowel disease or gastrointestinal lymphoma (Swift). In this case, the presence of a mass and cytology suggested neoplasia rather than inflammation. Ultrasonography has been advocated as a test for pancreatitis in cats, but some reports suggest that imaging studies are less helpful than originally thought (Saunders).

Gerhardt A, Steiner JM, Williams DA, Kramer S, Fuchs C, Janthur M, Hewicker-Trautwein M, Nolte I. Comparison of the sensitivity of different diagnostic tests for pancreatitis in cats. J Vet Intern Med 2001;15:329-333.

Quigley KA, Jackson ML, Haines DM. Hyperlipasemia in 6 dogs with pancreatic or hepatic neoplasia: evidence for tumor lipase production. Vet Clin Path 2001;30:114-120).

Saunders HM, VanWinkle TJ, Drobatz K, Kimmel SE, Washabau RJ. Ultrasonagraphic findings in cats with clinical, gross pathologic, and histologic evidence of acute pancreatitic necrosis: 20 cases (1994-2001). J Am Vet Med Assoc 2002;221:1724-1730).

Simpson KW. Pancreatitis in cats. Proceedings 21st annual meeting American College of Veterinary Internal Medicine. June 4-8, 2003, Raleigh, NC. pp 29-31.

Swift NC, Marks SL, MacLachlan NJ, Norris CR. Evaluation of serum feline trypsin-like immunoreactivity for the diagnosis of pancreatitis in cats. J Am Vet Med Assoc 2000;217:37-42.

Williams DA. Diagnosis of canine and feline pancreatitis. Proceedings 54th annual meeting American College of Veterinary Pathologists. November 15-19, 2003, Banff, Alberta, Canada. pp 6-11.

GI Case 14 – Level 1

"Muffy" is a 10-year-old spayed female Shih Tzu presenting with a history of several days of depression, vomiting, and decreased appetite. She has had loose stool for approximately one month. On physical examination, Muffy seems uncomfortable when her abdomen is palpated.

White blood cell count:	8.1 x 10⁹/L	(6.0-16.3)
Segmented neutrophils:	6.1 x 10⁹/L	(3.0-11.0)
Band neutrophils:	0 x 10⁹/L	(0-0.3)
Lymphocytes:	↓ 0.9 x 10⁹/L	(1.0-4.8)
Monocytes:	0.9 x 10⁹/L	(0.2-1.4)
Eosinophils:	0.2 x 10⁹/L	(0-1.3)
WBC morphology: Within normal limits		

Hematocrit:	42%	(37-55)
Red blood cell count:	6.22 x 10¹²/L	(5.5-8.5)
Hemoglobin:	14.8 g/dl	(12.0-18.0)
MCV:	66.2 fl	(60.0-77.0)
MCHC:	33.2 g/dl	(31.0-34.0)
RBC morphology: Within normal limits		
Platelets: Clumped but appear adequate		

Glucose:	68 mg/dl	(65.0-120.0)
BUN:	9 mg/dl	(8-33)
Creatinine:	0.6 mg/dl	(0.5-1.5)
Phosphorus:	4.1 mg/dl	(3.0-6.0)
Calcium:	11.0 mg/dl	(8.8-11.0)
Magnesium:	1.7 mEq/L	(1.4-2.7)
Total Protein:	6.5 g/dl	(5.5-7.8)
Albumin:	3.3 g/dl	(2.8-4.0)
Globulin:	3.3 g/dl	(2.3-4.2)
A/G Ratio:	1.0	(0.7-2.1)
Sodium:	143 mEq/L	(140-151)
Chloride:	107 mEq/L	(105-120)
Potassium:	4.7 mEq/L	(3.8-5.4)
HCO3:	25 mEq/L	(16-28)
Anion Gap:	15.7 mEq/L	(12-23)
Total Bili:	0.2 mg/dl	(0.10-0.30)
ALP:	↑ 2,646 IU/L	(20-121)
GGT:	↑ 108 IU/L	(2-10)
ALT:	↑ 190 IU/L	(18-86)
AST:	↑ 233 IU/L	(15-52)
Cholesterol:	355 mg/dl	(82-355)
Triglycerides:	118 mg/dl	(30-321)
Amylase:	↑ 1489 IU/L	(400-1200)
Lipase:	↑ 31,731 IU/L	(20-189)

Interpretation

CBC: The mild lymphopenia is likely secondary to stress/corticosteroid response.

Serum Biochemical Profile

Mild increases in ALP and GGT: Increases in these enzymes suggest some degree of cholestasis. Since the bilirubin is within the reference interval, cholestasis may be mild. Many potential causes of increased ALP exist (see Chapter 2), and enzyme induction by some mechanisms may not increase bilirubin.

Mildly increased ALT and AST: Hepatocellular damage results in increased release of these enzymes from liver cells.

Mild increase in amylase, marked increase in lipase: Minor elevations in amylase and lipase may be present in patients with decreased glomerular filtration rates. Since this patient is not azotemic, this appears unlikely in this case. Intestinal disease may increase concentrations of these enzymes in the blood, and the Muffy's clinical signs support some type of intestinal disease. Pancreatitis is a major differential diagnosis in patients with marked elevations of serum amylase and lipase. Muffy's case is somewhat unusual in that the increase in amylase is mild, while the lipase levels are dramatically increased. This pattern has been reported in association with pancreatic and hepatic neoplasia (Quigley).

Case Summary and Outcome

On survey radiographs, Muffy had a diffuse nodular pattern in her lungs and a calcified mass in her abdomen. On ultrasound, the liver and spleen appeared normal. Multiple mineralized nodules could be visualized in the pancreas. Cytologic specimens of the pancreatic masses and some mesenteric nodules consisted of multiple clusters of tightly adherent atypical epithelial cells consistent with carcinoma, as well as crystalline material compatible with the mineralization. Surgical biopsy results were diagnostic for a poorly differentiated carcinoma, possible of endocrine or neuroendocrine origin. Muffy was treated with antibiotics, antacids, and metoclopramide, and began chemotherapy.

Pancreatitis is an important differential diagnosis in this case. Most dogs with pancreatitis will have some evidence of inflammation on the CBC, however a normal CBC does not completely rule out pancreatitis. Mild liver enzyme elevations are commonly associated with pancreatitis because of local inflammation or partial to complete obstruction of bile flow. While there is potential for hepatic metastases in Muffy, elevations of liver enzymes are not uniformly noted in patients with metastatic neoplasia in the liver (Shorty-Case 13, metastatic pancreatic carcinoma and Russell-Case 6, metastatic insulinoma). Trypsin-like immunoreactivity testing can be performed to help substantiate a diagnosis of pancreatitis, but was not needed in this case because of the differential elevation of lipase and amylase and the agreement of the cytology and biopsy results on the diagnosis of malignancy.

Quigley KA, Jackson ML, Haines DM. Hyperlipasemia in 6 dogs with pancreatic or hepatic neoplasia: evidence for tumor lipase production Vet Clin Path 2001;30:114-120.

GI Case 15 – Level 2

"Quasi" is a one-year-old neutered male German Shepherd cross presenting for vomiting, lethargy, and inappetence. A foreign body obstruction was suspected, but radiographs of the abdomen were inconclusive. Abdominal ultrasound revealed a 15 x 4 cm mass in the area of the pancreas with a moderate amount of abdominal effusion. Quasi is being treated with phenobarbital for idiopathic epilepsy, which is well controlled. Phenobarbital levels are in the therapeutic range.

White blood cell count:	↑ 27.2 x 10⁹/L	(4.9-16.8)
Segmented neutrophils:	↑ 22.9 x 10⁹/L	(2.8-11.5)
Band neutrophils:	0	(0-0.300)
Lymphocytes:	2.7 x 10⁹/L	(1.0-4.8)
Monocytes:	↑ 1.6 x 10⁹/L	(0.1-1.5)
Eosinophils:	0.0 x 10⁹/L	(0-1.440)

WBC morphology: Within normal limits

Hematocrit:	50%	(39-55)
Red blood cell count:	7.27 x 10¹²/L	(5.8-8.5)
Hemoglobin:	↑ 21.7 g/dl	(14.0-19.1)
MCV:	70.8 fl	(60.0-75.0)
MCHC:	↑ 43.4 g/dl	(33.0-36.0)

RBC morphology: Appears within normal limits
Platelets: Clumped but appear adequate
The plasma is moderately hemolyzed and markedly lipemic

Glucose:	90 mg/dl	(67.0-135.0)
BUN:	13 mg/dl	(8-29)
Creatinine:	0.7 mg/dl	(0.6-2.0)
Phosphorus:	4.0 mg/dl	(2.6-7.2)
Calcium:	10.1 mg/dl	(9.4-11.6)
Magnesium:	1.7 mEq/L	(1.7-2.5)
Total Protein:	5.7 g/dl	(5.5-7.8)
Albumin:	↓ 2.8 g/dl	(3.0-4.2)
Globulin:	2.9 g/dl	(2.3-4.2)
A/G Ratio:	1.0	(0.7-2.1)
Sodium:	↓ 137 mEq/L	(142-163)
Chloride:	↓ 103 mEq/L	(106-126)
Potassium:	4.0 mEq/L	(3.8-5.4)
HCO3:	26 mEq/L	(15-28)
Anion Gap:	12 mEq/L	(8-19)
Total Bili:	Bili, ALP, and GGT are invalid due to	
ALP:	hemolysis	
GGT:		
ALT:	↑ 121 IU/L	(18-86)
AST:	↑ 126 IU/L	(16-54)
Cholesterol:	↑ 355 mg/dl	(110-314)
Triglycerides:	↑ 1910 mg/dl	(30-321)
Amylase:	↑ 3383 IU/L	(409-1203)
Lipase:	↑ 2246 IU/L	(120-258)

Abdominal fluid analysis: Slightly lipemic fluid

Pre-spin color: light red	Total protein: 5.0 gm/dl
Pre-spin turbidity: opaque	Total nucleated cells: 73,800/µl
Post spin color: pink	PCV: 6%
Post spin turbidity: hazy	Cholesterol: 186 mg/dl
	Triglyceride: 319 mg/dl

Direct smears are of high cellularity. Cells are in good condition and consist of 84% nondegenerate neutrophils, 13% macrophages, and 3% mature lymphocytes. The macrophages contain abundant pale cytoplasm with clear vacuoles and occasional cellular debris. The background contains moderate numbers of erythrocytes and granular precipitate due to the high protein content of the fluid. No microorganisms or atypical cells are seen.

Coagulation

Platelets:	439.0 x 10⁹/L	(181-525)
PT:	6.3s	(5.9-9.1)
APTT:	15.6s	(12.2-18.6)

Interpretation

CBC: Quasi has a mature neutrophilic leukocytosis and monocytosis characteristic of an inflammatory leukogram. The increased hemoglobin concentration and MCHC is an artifact related to the hemolysis and/or lipemia, since erythrocytes do not overproduce hemoglobin and the hematocrit is within the reference interval.

Serum Biochemical Profile
Mild hypoalbuminemia: Both decreased production by the liver or increased losses can contribute to low albumin. Albumin is a negative acute phase reactant, which can limit hepatic production of this protein with inflammation. Marked liver failure is possible in this patient, however specific tests of liver function such as bile acids are required to further evaluate this possibility. Decreased production may be secondary to poor nutritional plane, which is not the case in this patient. Increased losses of albumin must also be considered, and the most likely site of protein loss for Quasi is into the abdominal effusion. The potential for renal loss of protein could be evaluated by performing a urinalysis and/or a urine protein:creatinine ratio. Gastrointestinal losses are more difficult to quantitate.

Mild hyponatremia and hypochloremia: Increased electrolyte losses or dilution secondary to retention of free water are common causes of electrolyte abnormalites. Sources of loss are similar to those for protein, and third space loss into the effusion is most likely in this patient. Gastrointestinal or renal losses are also possible. When inappropriate renal losses of electrolytes are suspected, urinary fractional excretions can be performed. Hyponatremia and hypochloremia due to decreased intake is uncommon in domestic animals.

Mildly elevated ALT and AST: Increases in these enzymes indicate some degree of hepatocellular damage. Because of the close anatomic proximity of the pancreas and liver and the vascular anatomy, hepatocellular damage in patients with pancreatitis is likely related to hepatic ischemia or toxins and inflammatory mediators originating in the inflamed pancreas. The potential for concurrent cholestasis is difficult to evaluate because hemolysis has invalidated relevent measurements. Primary hepatic pathology cannot be excluded at this time. The history of treatment with phenobarbital is important in this case because of the ability of this drug to cause microsomal enzyme induction, resulting in reversible increases in ALP (2-12 times normal) and ALT (2 to 5 times normal). Alternatively, phenobarbital may cause true hepatic injury in some animals. Signs of this include a greater increase in ALT than ALP or evidence of liver dysfunction such as increased serum bile acid concentrations, hypoalbuminemia, and/or hypocholesterolemia.

Hypercholesterolemia and hypertriglyceridemia: Fasting hyperlipidemia is commonly associated with pancreatitis. As seen here, the increase in triglycerides is often of a greater magnitude than the hypercholesterolemia. The elevated triglycerides impart a milky appearance to the serum, and predispose to *in vitro* hemolysis, so the plasma may have a "tomato soup" appearance. In some cases, hyperlipidemia may predispose the patient to pancreatitis, while in other cases it may occur secondary to decreased lipoprotein lipase activity with pancreatitis. Alternatively, some authors cite lipolysis of intra-abdominal fat by free pancreatic enzymes as a contributor. Hyperlipidemia also may be the result of eating a fatty meal, liver disease, idiopathic conditions, or endocrinopathies such as hyperadrenocorticism, hypothyroidism, or diabetes mellitus.

Elevated amylase and lipase: The combination of increased amylase and lipase should lead the clinician to consider pancreatitis as a differential diagnosis. Unfortunately, extrapancreatic sources of these enzymes exist, and greater than two-fold elevations can occur in patients with gastritis, diseases of the small intestine, and liver pathology. Decreased glomerular filtration rate can also increase serum concentrations of these enzymes up to 2-3 times the upper limit of the reference interval. Lipase is considered to be more specific for pancreatitis than amylase, although treatment with dexamethasone can increase lipase without parallel increases in amylase. Serum amylase and lipase activity within the reference interval does not rule out pancreatic inflammation. Pancreatic neoplasia may be associated with increases in serum amylase and lipase.

Abdominal fluid analysis: The fluid is an exudate with evidence of suppurative inflammation. The absence of degenerate changes in the neutrophils and bacteria supports sterile inflammation, a common finding in canine patients with pancreatitis.

Coagulation Profile: The coagulation profile in this patient is within normal limits. Systemic inflammation characteristic of severe acute pancreatitis can lead to endothelial cell damage from neutrophil proteases and oxidants. In some patients, the resulting endothelial cell activation and exposure of basement membrane collagen can trigger coagulation and lead to disseminated intravascular coagulation.

Case Summary and Outcome

During exploratory surgery an enlarged, inflamed pancreas and edematous peripancreatic fat were seen. The abdomen was flushed, and a jejunostomy tube was placed. Biopsy specimens demonstrated severe steatitis, however no actual pancreatic tissue was present in the sections. Hepatic changes included moderate capsulitis, but no parenchymal abnormalities. Quasi vomited intermittently for the first few days after surgery, but ultimately began eating solid food and was discharged.

Quasi has typical abnormalities in routine clinical pathology data suggestive for pancreatitis, including an inflammatory leukogram and fasting hyperlipidemia. When pancreatitis results in a significant abdominal effusion, protein and electrolytes may decreased because of third space loss. Note that the presence or absence of an identifiable mass lesion did NOT differentiate inflammation from neoplasia. In contrast to Muffy (Case 14-pancreatic carcinoma) who had marked increases in lipase with almost negligible changes in amylase, Quasi has elevations in both pancreatic enzymes.

There is no ideal widely available test for pancreatitis. For diagnosis, clinicians often rely on the presence of a combination of clinical signs and laboratory abnormalities compatible with the disorder. As was noted for this patient, an inflammatory leukogram, elevated liver enzymes, and hyperlipidemia (hypercholesterolemia and hypertriglyceridemia) are common findings. Depending on the duration and severity of disease, concurrent electrolyte, acid base and coagulation abnormalities along with pre-renal azotemia may be present. Some patients are hypocalcemic. In addition to the measurement of amylase and lipase, serum trypsin-like immunoreactivity (TLI) may be measured and tends to increase sooner and more proportional to severity than other enzymes. Since serum TLI is pancreas specific, it may have some advantages over amylase and lipase, however decreased glomerular filtration rate will increase TLI similar to amylase and lipase. Severe malnutrition and very high protein diets can also elevate TLI. TLI is an immunoassay, and differences in the enzyme structures make it necessary to have species-specific assays. New assays for the measurement of pancreatic lipase in dogs and cats are now being developed and validated. Initial data look promising, however further research is needed.

GI Case 16 – Level 2

"Nutmeg" is an 11-year-old spayed female, mixed breed Labrador Retriever presenting with a two week history of anorexia, followed by depression and weight loss. She has been treated with nutritional supplements for arthritis.

WBC:	↑ 35.4 x 10⁹/L	(6.0-17.6)
Segmented neutrophils:	↑ 29.1 x 10⁹/L	(2.8-11.5)
Band neutrophils:	↑ 0.7 x 10⁹/L	(0-0.3)
Lymphocytes:	2.1 x 10⁹/L	(1.0-4.8)
Monocytes:	↑ 3.5 x 10⁹/L	(0.1-1.5)
Eosinophils:	0 x 10⁹/L	(0-1.2)
WBC morphology: Appears within normal limits		
Nucleated RBC/100 WBC:	↑ 2	
Plasma appearance: Icteric		
Hematocrit:	↓ 31%	(39-55)
Red blood cell count:	↓ 4.98 x 10¹²/L	(5.5-8.5)
Hemoglobin:	↓ 11.0 g/dl	(12.0-18.0)
MCV:	68.5 fl	(60.0-77.0)
MCHC:	↑ 35.5 g/dl	(31.0-34.0)
RBC morphology: Moderately increased anisocytosis, rare spherocytes seen.		
Platelets:	↓ 56.0 x 10⁹/L	(181.0-525.0)
Glucose:	↓ 88 mg/dl	(90.0-140.0)
BUN:	25 mg/dl	(8-33)
Creatinine:	0.6 mg/dl	(0.5-2.0)
Phosphorus:	4.1 mg/dl	(2.6-6.2)
Calcium:	9.7 mg/dl	(8.8-11.0)
Magnesium:	1.7 mEq/L	(1.7-2.5)
Total Protein:	6.3 g/dl	(4.8-7.2)
Albumin:	3.6 g/dl	(2.8-4.0)
Globulin:	2.7 g/dl	(2.0-4.0)
Sodium:	146 mEq/L	(140-151)
Chloride:	107 mEq/L	(105-126)

Potassium:	4.2 mEq/L	(3.8-5.4)
HCO3:	17 mEq/L	(15-28)
Total Bili:	↑ 9.66 mg/dl	(0.10-0.50)
ALP:	↑ 15,126 IU/L	(20-320)
GGT:	↑ 479 IU/L	(1-10)
ALT:	↑ 910 IU/L	(10-95)
AST:	↑ 155 IU/L	(16-54)
Cholesterol:	291 mg/dl	(110-314)
Triglycerides:	258 mg/dl	(30-321)
Amylase:	↑ 1,470 IU/L	(400-1200)
Lipase:	↑ 2,223 IU/L	(120-258)

Coagulation		
PT:	7.6s	(6.2-9.3)
APTT:	11.6s	(8.9-16.3)
Fibrinogen:	400 mg/dl	(200-500)
FDPs:	<5 µg/ml	(<5)

Interpretation
CBC
Plasma: Icteric plasma can be caused by hemolysis or cholestasis. In general, hemolytic anemias are regenerative and icterus is associated with a lower PCV than is seen in this patient. With the increases in liver enzymes on the serum biochemical profile, cholestasis is more likely responsible for the icterus, however the potential for decreased red blood cell survival or hemolysis is suggested by the presence of spherocytes.

Leukogram: Nutmeg has a neutrophilic leukocytosis with a mild left shift. No toxic changes are noted despite evidence of inflammation. The monocytosis also supports inflammation or tissue necrosis.

Erythrogram: Nutmeg has a mild normocytic anemia. The increase in the MCHC is artifactual, as is always the case since erythrocytes cannot increase their hemoglobin content above the normal range. In this patient, the icteric plasma may account for this change, or there may be in vitro or in vivo hemolysis. Some degree of enhanced red blood cell destruction is indicated by the spherocytosis. The presence of spherocytes suggests an immune-mediated mechanism for red blood cell turnover and is often used to substantiate a diagnosis of immune-mediated hemolytic anemia when seen in large numbers. Low numbers of spherocytes can be associated with other illnesses, especially liver disease. Based on the indices, the anemia is likely nonregenerative. Hemolysis is usually associated with a regenerative response, but it may take 3-4 days for a regenerative response to become apparent following acute onset of red cell destruction. In this case there also may be marrow suppression from chronic disease/inflammation, blunting a regenerative response. Serial CBC's with reticulocyte counts should be performed to evaluate a bone marrow response. Small numbers of nucleated erythrocytes are a nonspecific finding and may accompany a regenerative response. Nucleated erythrocytes in the absence of a regenerative response may signal some type of endothelial cell insult with subsequent premature escape of developing red blood cells.

Thrombocytopenia: General mechanisms for thrombocytopenia include decreased production or increased destruction. The non-regenerative anemia combined with the thrombocytopenia could indicate a hypoproliferative marrow. However the leukocytosis suggests that at least some lineages are productive, and other explanations should be evaluated prior to considering a bone marrow aspirate. The presence of spherocytes can be associated with immune-mediated disease, thus immune-mediated destruction of platelets is also possible. Platelets may be consumed during coagulation and often decrease in disseminated intravascular coagulation (DIC). DIC is unlikely in this case given the otherwise normal coagulation panel and lack of FDPs. Clinical signs compatible with hemorrhage and consumption of platelets by this mechanism are lacking. Activation of endothelial cells for any reason, including hypoxia or severe systemic inflammation can trigger platelet adhesion. The liver is an extremely vascular organ, and hepatic endothelial cell activation could be sufficient to cause detectable thrombocytopenia. Severe acute pancreatitis is frequently associated with thrombocytopenia, likely due to systemic inflammation.

Serum Biochemical Profile

Mild hypoglycemia: This may be due to delay in processing of the sample or may be due to sepsis, hepatic insufficiency or neoplasia. This degree of hypoglycemia is unlikely to be associated with clinical signs and is of questionable clinical significance. Repeat analysis may reveal a value within the reference interval.

Increased bilirubin: See discussion of icteric plasma. The marked increases in ALP and GGT suggest that cholestasis is the most important contributor to the hyperbilirubinemia. Fractionation of bilirubin into direct and indirect is not considered reliable in distinguishing hemolysis from cholestasis as a cause for hyperbilirubinemia in small animals. In fact, mixed hyperbilirubinemia is very common.

Increased ALP and GGT: Elevation of both of these enzymes in an icteric dog strongly supports cholestasis, however both can increase in response to other causes such as exposure to corticosteroids. Increased ALP is a relatively non-specific finding because it is found in multiple tissues and can be induced by hormones and drugs. For a more complete discussion of extrahepatic causes of liver enzyme elevations, please see Chapter 2.

Increased serum ALT and AST: Mild to moderate increases in these enzymes may occur with hepatocellular damage, however AST is less tissue specific and muscle damage as well as hemolysis can increase this value. Elevations in these hepatocellular enzymes are of a relatively smaller magnitude than those in the cholestatic enzymes, which could suggest hepatocellular damage secondary to cholestasis or secondary to pancreatic disease (see amylase and lipase). Please note that none of these enzymes are considered indicators of liver function. Poor perfusion or hypoxia of hepatocytes secondary to anemia can injure hepatocytes, resulting in increased leakage of enzymes into the circulation.

Mild hyperamylasemia with hyperlipasemia: Both of these enzymes are considered to be markers of pancreatic damage, however they are not produced exclusively by that organ, thus decreasing their specificity for the diagnosis of pancreatic disease. Hyperamylasemia and hyperlipasemia are sometimes noted in patients with intestinal or liver disease. While decreased glomerular filtration rate can elevate amylase and lipase activities in the circulation, this patient is not azotemic. Currently, a suggestive constellation of clinical signs and laboratory abnormalities are used to substantiate the diagnosis of pancreatis. While a variety of other tests are undergoing evaluation for improving the ability to diagnose pancreatitis (see Jimbo, Case 22), at this point no single ideal test exists.

Case Summary and Outcome

After evaluation of initial clinical laboratory data, abdominal ultrasound was performed. The liver was markedly enlarged and diffusely hypoechoic, and the bile duct was distended.

Tortuous, distended tubular structures interpreted to be biliary ducts were seen throughout the parenchyma. The ultrasound impression of the pancreas was compatible with chronic pancreatitis and fibrosis. At surgery, the gall bladder was enlarged and contained sludged bile. A cholecystoduodenostomy was performed and the patient improved after the procedure with improvement of bile flow. Biopsy samples of the liver and pancreas collected at surgery showed moderate chronic cholangiohepatitis and steroid hepatopathy with moderate chronic lymphoplasmacytic and neutrophilic pancreatitis.

Serial serum biochemical profiles were collected during the period of hospitalization for supportive care after surgery.

	7 days post surgery	14 days post surgery	
Glucose:	105 mg/dl	↓87	(90.0-140.0)
BUN:	↓4 mg/dl	↓4	(8-33)
Creatinine:	0.5 mg/dl	0.5	(0.5-2.0)
Phosphorus:	4.1 mg/dl	5.0	(2.6-6.2)
Calcium:	9.4 mg/dl	10.2	(8.8-11.0)
Magnesium:	↓1.3 mEq/L	↓1.2	(1.7-2.5)
Total Protein:	5.0 g/dl	5.4	(4.8-7.2)
Albumin:	↓2.3 g/dl	2.8	(2.8-4.0)
Globulin:	2.7 g/dl	2.6	(2.0-4.0)
Sodium:	146 mEq/L	149	(140-151)
Chloride:	116 mEq/L	115	(105-126)
Potassium:	4.4 mEq/L	4.8	(3.8-5.4)
HCO3:	19 mEq/L	20	(15-28)
Total Bili:	↑5.62 mg/dl	↑1.50	(0.10-0.50)
ALP:	↑6,332 IU/L	↑4,265	(20-320)
GGT:	↑68 IU/L	↑40	(1-10)
ALT:	49 IU/L	24	(10-95)
AST:	↑149 IU/L	↑68	(16-54)
Cholesterol:	↑375 mg/dl	↑432	(110-314)
Triglycerides:	181 mg/dl	98	(30-321)
Amylase:	↑1,491 IU/L	↑1,604	(400-1200)

Urinalysis 14 days post surgery

Voided urine is yellow and clear
Specific Gravity: 1.012
Protein, glucose, heme, ketones: Negative
Bilirubin: 2+
Sediment: Other than a small amount of debris, sediment is inactive

Low BUN: Fluid therapy and diuresis can lower the BUN. The BUN will also decrease because of impaired production in liver failure. Severe liver dysfunction can impair hepatic gluconeogenesis with resultant hypoglycemia and can impair production of albumin (which is low here) and cholesterol (which eventually increases). Because the liver enzymes indicate some type of liver disease, liver function tests such as blood ammonia or serum bile acids may be indicated.

Bilirubin, ALP and GGT: These values are normalizing over time, supporting resolution of the cholestasis after surgery.

ALT and AST: Both are following the trends observed in the cholestatic indicators. Because the hepatocellular damage in this patient was suspected to be occurring secondary to cholestasis, decrements in these values are expected with relief of the cholestatic process. Increases in serum ALT occur within 12 hours of liver damage, generally peak by day 5 after an acute insult, and then fall over the next one or two weeks. In acute liver disease, a 50% decrease in serum ALT levels over 24-48 hours is considered a positive prognostic indicator. Although serum ALT has a longer half life than serum AST in dogs (2.5 days vs. 5-12 hours), Nutmeg's ALT is falling faster than the AST. This may be because extrahepatic tissue damage is contributing to the serum AST activity or because there is ongoing, low level release from hepatocytes. AST can be a more sensitive, albeit less specific, indicator of hepatocellular damage.

Hypoalbuminemia with no change in globulin: Considerations for hypoalbuminia with normal globulin generally include loss, impaired liver function, and starvation. Impaired liver function is possible as discussed above, and in some cases albumin production in the liver is physiologically limited because albumin is a negative acute phase reactant. Renal loss of albumin is not supported by the urinalysis data, although the urine is dilute and a urinary protein:creatinine ratio could be performed as a more sensitive test for glomerular loss of protein. Patients should be evaluated for clinical evidence of loss into the third space, gastrointestinal tract or via cutaneous lesions. Acute anorexia alone is not sufficient to cause hypoalbuminemia, although because albumin is a protein reservoir for the body, anorexia combined with surgery, fever, acidosis, or other causes of increased demands on the protein pool could lower albumin.

Hypercholesterolemia: Hypercholesterolemia is commonly associated with cholestasis, possibly secondary to upregulation of cholesterol synthesis and decreased biliary excretion of cholesterol. Endocrinopathies such as hyperadrenocorticism, hypothyroidism, and diabetes mellitus can increase serum cholesterol as well.

Hypomagnesemia: Disorders of magnesium are less well characterized than for most other analytes. Hypomagnesemia is commonly observed in critical care patients and may be related to a combination of decreased intake and possibly increased renal elimination or cellular translocation. Magnesium is a critical ion for the function of numerous enzyme systems and influences calcium metabolism, therefore correction of hypomagnesemia is usually recommended.

Urinalysis: Urine specific gravity in dogs can vary widely and a single isosthenuric sample does not necessarily signify renal disease. In the absence of azotemia or clinical evidence of dehydration, isothenuria in Nutmeg may not be abnormal or may be in response to fluid therapy. Based on her serum biochemistry panel, polyuria secondary to liver disease is possible. Suggested mechanisms include decreased urea production and/or hypokalemia with medullary washout, decreased metabolism of diuretic hormones such as cortisol, and psychogenic polydipsia. The bilirubinuria is expected because of renal elimination of the excess bilirubin in the blood. Mild bilirubinuria may occur in normal dogs because of production of bilirubin by renal tubular epithelial cells and a low renal threshold for elimination. In this case, the 2+ bilirubin in relatively dilute urine combined with the hyper-bilirubinemia and elevated liver enzymes is compatible with hepatic disease.

As seen with Nutmeg, pancreatic and liver pathology often coexist; some of the liver changes may have been related to increased endogenous corticosteroid levels. It is tempting to speculate in Nutmeg's case that chronic pancreatic disease led to occlusion of flow through the bile duct with subsequent cholestasis and secondary hepatocellular damage. In contrast, Quasi's (Case 15) liver enzyme elevations were of a more modest degree and there was no histologic evidence of hepatic pathology; the liver enzyme elevations may have been related to induction by anticonvulsant therapy. Quasi had much more significant lipid changes compared to Nutmeg despite the likely absence of significant liver disease. This may be due to a more acute severe pancreatitis compared to Nutmeg, who seemed to have a rather low grade pancreatic inflammation not associated with effusion or significant peripancreatic steatitis. In many cases, it can be difficult to be sure of the exact pathophysiologic relationships and causative factors in patients with multiple inter-related conditions. In Nutmeg's case, ultrasound findings were supportive of a lesion amenable to surgical correction. Laboratory work alone is not typically adequate for this type of medical decision making.

GI Case 17 – Level 2

"Flame" is a 26-year-old Quarter Horse mare presenting for a six day history of decreased feed intake, colic episodes, right forelimb lameness (previously diagnosed as rotation of the coffin bone in that limb), and possible neurologic abnormalities. She had been seen rolling and laying on her side in her stall along with aggressive pawing at the ground. She was treated with Banamine®. She had been vaccinated for West Nile Virus. On presentation, Flame was very lame on her right forelimb with sensitivity to pressure with hoof testers. She was sweating and dehydrated with a normal body temperature. She had good appetite when offered food, however gut sounds were not noted on either side.

White blood cell count:	↓ 4.3 x 10⁹/L	(5.9-11.2)
Segmented neutrophils:	2.8 x 10⁹/L	(2.3-9.1)
Band neutrophils:	0.1	(0-0.3)
Lymphocytes:	↓ 1.2 x 10⁹/L	(1.6-5.2)
Monocytes:	0.2 x 10⁹/L	(0-1.0)
WBC morphology: Slightly toxic neutrophils		

Hematocrit:	41 %	(30-51)
Red blood cell count:	8.01 x 10¹²/L	(6.5-12.8)
Hemoglobin:	15.2 g/dl	(10.9-18.1)
MCV:	51.7 fl	(35.0-53.0)
MCHC:	37.1 g/dl	(34.6-38.0)
RBC morphology: Normal		
Platelets: Adequate		
Fibrinogen:	200 mg/dl	(100-400)

Glucose:	↑ 278 mg/dl	(6.0-128.0)
BUN:	18 mg/dl	(11-26)
Creatinine:	1.1 mg/dl	(0.9-1.9)
Phosphorus:	2.3 mg/dl	(1.9-6.0)
Calcium:	↓ 9.7 mg/dl	(11.0-13.5)
Magnesium:	↓ 1.0 mEq/L	(1.7-2.4)
Total Protein:	6.9 g/dl	(5.6-7.0)
Albumin:	2.5 g/dl	(2.4-3.8)
Globulin:	4.4 g/dl	(2.5-4.9)
Sodium:	↓ 123 mEq/L	(130-145)
Chloride:	↓ 81 mEq/L	(99-105)
Potassium:	3.2 mEq/L	(3.0-5.0)

HCO3:	30 mEq/L	(25-31)
Anion Gap:	↑ 15.2 mEq/L	(10-14)
Total Bili:	2.2 mg/dl	(0.30-3.0)
Direct bili:	0.20 mg/dl	(0.0-0.5)
Indirect bili:	2.00 mg/dl	(0.2-3.0)
ALP:	229 IU/L	(109-352)
GGT:	↑ 39 IU/L	(5-23)
AST:	↑ 793 IU/L	(190-380)
CK:	212 IU/L	(80-446)
Triglycerides:	↑ 1340 mg/dl	(9-52)

Interpretation
CBC
Leukogram: Flame has a mild leucopenia with lymphopenia. Causes of lymphopenia are numerous, but some possibilities in this case include acute viral disease, endotoxemia, rickettsial diseases and corticosteroid effects. Neutrophil numbers are approaching the lower end of the reference interval and should be monitored. Endotoxemia and rickettsial diseases may suppress neutrophil numbers and cause toxic change, while corticosteroids should result in mild mature neutrophilia with no morphologic abnormalities. The fibrinogen is not supportive of inflammation. The remainder of the CBC was unremarkable.

Serum Biochemical Profile
Hyperglycemia: Elevations in serum glucose in the horse are most often caused by excitement or stress with release of endogenous catecholamines and glucocorticoids, respectively. In this case, this may be the result of pain from episodes of colic, described in the patient's history. A corticosteroid effect is supported by the concurrent lymphopenia. Transient hyperglycemia can also be observed in the very acute phase of endotoxemia prior to hypoglycemia. In an older horse like Flame, insulin resistance associated with hyperplasia or tumor of the pituitary pars intermedia (Equine Cushing's syndrome) can cause hyperglycemia. Insulin-responsive diabetes mellitus is rare in domestic large animal species.

Hypocalcemia: Because a significant fraction of calcium in the blood is complexed to protein, low serum albumin can result in low total serum calcium measurements. In this case, the albumin is low, but not outside of the reference range. Total hypocalcemia associated with hypoalbuminemia does not affect the biologically active ionized fraction, and so is not associated with clinical signs. A recent study of 64 horses with enterocolitis showed that 75% had low total serum calcium and 80% had low ionized calcium (Toribio). The mechanism was unclear, but did not appear to be due to renal wasting as fractional excretion of calcium was significantly lower in horses with colitis than healthy control horses. Serum intact parathyroid concentrations (PTH) were normal to increased, suggesting a variable physiological response to hypocalcemia. Studies in humans and laboratory animals indicate that sepsis and inflammatory hormones can influence hormonal regulation of calcium by calcitonin and PTH. In turn, hypomagnesemia can interfere with PTH secretion and alter the responsiveness of target tissues to PTH stimulation. Primary hypoparathyroidism could cause hypocalcemia, but is rare in horses. More likely, anorexia may also contribute to hypocalcemia in horses.

Hypomagnesemia:
Hypomagnesemia could be due to dietary deficiency, impaired gut absorption or increased renal excretion. Because of the role of magnesium in calcium regulation, correction of low serum magnesium levels may be sufficient to correct hypocalcemia.

Hyponatremia and hypochloremia with mildly increased anion gap: Because of the high concentrations of triglycerides, measurement of electrolytes by ion specific electrode (ISE) should be confirmed. Titrimetric methods will underestimate electrolytes in lipemic samples, while colorimetric methods may overestimate them. Even ISE measurement can have methodologic problems, if there is substantial dilution of lipemic samples with aqueous diluent as part of the analytical procedure. Low serum sodium and chloride in this case are attributable to increased gastrointestinal losses associated with colic, although significant losses from sweating are also likely. When changes in serum chloride are proportional to sodium, no further analysis is required. When the relative decrease in chloride appears to be greater than sodium, considerations include pure gastric vomiting (not seen in horses), sequestration of chloride containing fluids (more common in ruminants), or a compensatory change in response to a primary respiratory acidosis. Because bicarbonate and chloride are both anions, they tend to vary inversely, therefore hypochloremia is usually associated with alkalemia. In this case the HCO3 is within the reference interval despite the hypochloremia, consistent with a mixed acid/base disorder. Increased anion gap is most often associated with elevations in unmeasured anions, many of which are acids.

Increased GGT: In an adult horse, increased GGT is evidence for liver damage and cholestasis. This change is often associated with hyperbilirubinemia, although bilirubin can be efficiently eliminated in the urine. ALP is less liver specific than GGT and may be less sensitive in the horse.

Increased AST: This enzyme is present in multiple tissues and elevations can be difficult to interpret. In Flame, the concurrent increase in GGT and the normal CK supports hepatic rather than muscle origin for the increase in AST, although the shorter half life of CK could influence interpretation.

Hypertriglyceridemia: Fasted horses with hypertriglyceridemia should be evaluated for hyperlipemia/hyperlipidemia syndrome, which is often triggered by feed restriction or anorexia during colic episodes (Mogg). The syndrome is caused by decreased feed intake with subsequent fat mobilization and accumulation in the plasma and liver. Flame is more appropriately categorized as hyperlipidemic because her plasma is clear despite the high triglyceride concentration. Hyperlipemia is a more serious condition accompanied by lactescent plasma, impaired hepatic function and the production of abnormal very low density lipoproteins that have less apolipoprotein B-100 and more apolipoprotein B-48. This substitution may allow greater triglyceride content (Pearson). Although the triglyceride levels in this patient exceeded the 1,200 mg/dl associated with a poor prognosis in the paper originally describing this condition (Mogg), absence of any clinical or laboratory evidence of significant liver dysfunction associated with the hyperlipidemia improves the prognosis.

Case Summary and Outcome

Flame was extremely painful on her right front limb and was very sensitive to pressure from hoof testers. Relief of pain with an abaxial nerve block resulted in improved appetite, which corrected the hyperlipidemia. Flame responded well to intravenous fluids and calcium gluconate to correct the mineral and electrolyte imbalances from the colic. The neurologic abnormalities noted on the history were not confirmed at presentation. Had they been present they would have been an indication for blood ammonia or serum bile acid testing because of the potential for equine hyperlipemia to impair liver function.

The lymphopenia and hyperglycemia may persist if there is pituitary pars intermedia dysfunction, although blood work is often normal in these patients and diagnosis is based on appropriate clinical signs (hirstuism, chronic or recurrent laminitis, polyuria and polydipsia, sweating, and muscle wasting) and elevated endogenous plasma adrenocorticotropin (ACTH) levels (Couetil).

Couetil L, Paradis MR, Knoll J. Plasma adrenocorticotropin concentration in healthy horses and in horses with clinical signs of hyperadrenocorticism. J Vet Int Med 1996;10:1-6.

Mogg TD, Palmer JE. Hyperlipidemia, hyperlipemia, and hepatic lipidosis in American Miniature Horses: 23 cases (1990-1994). J Am Med Assoc 1995;207:604-607.

Pearson EG, Maas J. Hepatic lipidosis. In: Large Animal Internal Medicine, 3rd ed. Ed P Smith. Mosby, Inc. St. Louis, MO. 2002, pp 810-817.

Toribio RE, Kohn CW, Chew DJ, Sams RA, Rosol TJ. Comparison of serum parathyroid hormone and ionized calcium and magnesium concentrations and fractional urinary clearance of calcium and phosphorus in healthy horses and horses with enterocolitis. Am J Vet Res. 2001;62:938-947.

GI Case 18 – Level 2

"Marion" is a 13-year-old spayed female Beagle presenting with a history of recurrent signs of urinary tract infection that are not responding to antibiotics. Upon questioning, the owner says that Marion has been drinking more than usual too. Although it is difficult to notice because Marion has always had indiscriminate eating habits, she does appear to have an even more voracious appetite than usual lately. On physical examination, Marion is slightly thin, but cheerful.

White blood cell count:	↑ 24.5 x 10^9/L	(6.0-17.0)
Segmented neutrophils:	↑ 19.5 x 10^9/L	(3.0-11.0)
Band neutrophils:	0 x 10^9/L	(0-0.300)
Lymphocytes:	↓ 0.7 x 10^9/L	(1.0-4.8)
Monocytes:	↑ 4.3x 10^9/L	(0.2-1.4)
Eosinophils:	0.0 x 10^9/L	(0-1.3)
WBC morphology: Mild toxic change in neutrophils		
The sample is slightly lipemic		
Hematocrit:	↓ 37%	(39-55)
Red blood cell count:	↓ 5.33 x 10^{12}/L	(5.5-8.5)
Hemoglobin:	↓ 12.9 g/dl	(14.0-19.0)
MCV:	69.7 fl	(60.0-75.0)
MCHC:	34.9 g/dl	(33.0-36.0)
RBC morphology: Appears within normal limits		
Platelets:	370 x 10^9/L	(200-450)
Glucose:	↑ 670 mg/dl	(65.0-135.0)
BUN:	24 mg/dl	(8-33)
Creatinine:	0.6 mg/dl	(0.5-1.5)
Phosphorus:	5.3 mg/dl	(3.0-6.0)
Calcium:	10.4 mg/dl	(8.8-11.0)
Magnesium:	2.7 mEq/L	(1.4-2.7)
Total Protein:	5.8 g/dl	(5.2-7.2)
Albumin:	3.2 g/dl	(3.0-4.2)
Globulin:	2.6 g/dl	(2.0-4.0)
A/G Ratio:	1.2	(0.7-2.1)
Sodium:	↓ 137 mEq/L	(142-163)
Chloride:	↓ 99 mEq/L	(106-126)
Potassium:	↑ 5.8 mEq/L	(3.8-5.4)

HCO3:	23 mEq/L	(16-25)
Anion Gap:	20.8 mEq/L	(10-23)
Total Bili:	0.10 mg/dl	(0.10-0.50)
ALP:	↑ 1079 IU/L	(20-320)
ALT:	↑ 115 IU/L	(18-86)
AST:	35 IU/L	(15-52)
Cholesterol:	↑ 663 mg/dl	(110-314)
Triglycerides:	↑ 406 mg/dl	(30-300)
Amylase:	830 IU/L	(400-1200)

Urinalysis: Cystocentesis

Appearance: Yellow and hazy

Specific gravity:1.033	Sediment:
pH: 5.0	0-5 red blood cells/hpf
Protein: 500 mg/dl	20-30 white blood cells/hpf
Glucose: 4+	Occasional epithelial cells
Ketones: Negative	No crystals seen
Bilirubin: Negative	3+ bacteria
Heme: 1+	

Interpretation

CBC: Marion has a mature neutrophilic leukocytosis with toxic change, leukopenia, and a monocytosis. The toxic changes in the neutrophils are consistent with inflammation, although the other elements of the leukogram are also compatible with a corticosteroid response. The mild normocytic normochromic nonregenerative anemia is most compatible with anemia of chronic disease.

Serum Biochemical Profile

Marked hyperglycemia: The magnitude of the hyperglycemia in combination with glucosuria and the clinical signs is most suggestive of diabetes mellitus. However, other causes of hyperglycemia should be ruled out. This patient has hypercholesterolemia and increased triglycerides in addition to marked hyperglycemia. While post-prandial elevations are possible, this degree of hyperglycemia would be unusual even if blood were collected just after eating. Marion had been fasted over night when this sample was collected. Illness of any kind may cause mild elevations in glucose by interfering with insulin action on peripheral tissues. Increases in both endogenous and exogenous corticosteroids may cause significant increases in serum glucose concentrations. This patient had not been treated with corticosteroids within the previous six months, however elevations of endogenous corticosteroid levels cannot be ruled out at this time. Hyperadrenocorticism may cause polyuria and polydipsia, hyperglycemia, and increases in ALP, cholesterol, and triglycerides. Hyperadrenocorticism and diabetes mellitus can be present concurrently, complicating both the interpretation of laboratory tests and the clinical management of the patient.

Hyponatremia and hypochloremia: In many cases, hyponatremia reflects a relative water excess rather than total body depletion of sodium. In patients like Marion that have marked hyperglycemia, the increase in free water is due to the osmotic force generated by the excess glucose in the extracellular fluid. Serum sodium typically decreases by 1.5 mEq/L for each 100 mg/dl increase in glucose concentration above the upper end of the reference interval. Therefore in this case, we would expect serum sodium to decrease by approximately 7.5 mEq/L, which seems an appropriate degree in this case. Changes in sodium are often accompanied by proportional alterations in chloride, as seen in this case. (Please see Chapter 7 for further discussion).

Hyperkalemia: The regulation of potassium balance is complex and involves total body regulation as well as shifts between intracellular and extracellular compartments. For Marion, the mild hyperkalemia is likely due to insulin deficiency. Insulin causes potassium to enter cells, and inadequate amounts of insulin will impair this process. Acidosis may further increase potassium levels in some diabetic patients, however the bicarbonate levels in this patient are within the reference interval. (Please see Chapter 7 for further discussion). Failure of renal elimination can be important, but this is unlikely to be a major mechanism in this case. Hyperkalemia is rarely due to increased intake, although excessive supplementation of fluids can be an issue.

Mildly increased ALP and ALT: There are many potential causes for increased ALP in the dog, including medications, corticosteroid effects, endocrinopathies and cholestatic disease (please see Chapter 2 for a more complete list of differential diagnoses for increased ALP and ALT). In this case, endocrinopathy is the most likely cause. Because of derangements in glucose homeostasis that are present in diabetes mellitus, lipid accumulates within the hepatocytes. This can lead to mild cholestasis and increased ALP. Similarly, hepatocellular enzymes may also increase with diabetes mellitus. While hepatocellular pathologic changes are usually mild, occasional diabetics will also have increased bile acids, suggesting decreased liver function.

Hypercholesterolemia and hypertriglyceridemia: In poorly controlled insulin dependent diabetes mellitus, there is a rapid mobilization of triglycerides, which increases plasma levels of free fatty acids for use as an energy source by numerous tissues except the brain. Deficiency of insulin leads to decreased activation of lipoprotein lipase, so fatty acids cannot be taken up from the circulation for storage in adipose tissue. In addition, down regulation of low density lipoprotein receptors in the absence of insulin results in hypercholesterolemia. Post-prandial hyperlipidemia, pancreatic or liver disease, and other endocrinopathies such as hyperadreno-corticism or hypothyroidism may also cause abnormalities of cholesterol and triglycerides.

Urinalysis: The urine is somewhat concentrated despite significant glucosuria. Once blood glucose levels exceed the renal tubular maximum for reabsorption (approximately 200 mg/dl in the dog), glucosuria will occur, although glucosuria may be seen in patients that are normoglycemic if there is tubular dysfunction. Glucosuria and proteinuria may falsely increase the urine specific gravity slightly (an increase in specific gravity of 0.001 per 400 mg protein/dl or per 270 mg glucose/dl). Proteinuria is present, and may be the result of urinary tract infection, as indicated by the active sediment and presence of bacteria. It should be noted that not all diabetic patients with urinary tract infection will have active sediment, possibly due to neutrophil function defects that have been described in these patients. Proteinuria may also occur as a result of glomerular damage secondary to diabetes or the hypertension that may accompany diabetes.

Case Summary and Outcome

Marion was diagnosed with diabetes mellitus based on clinical signs and laboratory abnormalities. She was not ketotic at the time of presentation, and responded well to insulin therapy. She also was treated with antibiotics for her urinary tract infection.

In contrast to Marmalade (Case 2), the cat with stress induced hyperglycemia, Marion has marked rather than moderate hyperglycemia, and she clinical signs compatible with diabetes mellitus. Other supportive laboratory abnormalities such as glucosuria, hypercholesterolemia, and hypertriglyceridemia are present in Marion but absent in Marmalade. The classification system of diabetes in people as insulin dependent or non-insulin dependent has been applied to domestic species. Dogs are most often insulin dependent, while cats may be either and can actually fluctuate over time in their requirement for insulin. If the insulin deficiency is sufficiently severe, or if concurrent diseases increase diabetogenic hormones such as catecholamines or corticosteroids, ketoacidosis may develop.

Other differential diagnoses for Marion include hyperadrenocorticism, which shares many clinical and laboratory features with diabetes mellitus. Because screening tests for hyperadrenocortism are often abnormal in patients with newly diagnosed or poorly controlled diabetes, these tests should be reserved for patients with classical clinical signs of hyperadrenocorticism (bilaterally symmetric hair loss, calcinosis cutis, adrenomegaly) and patients who have evidence of insulin resistance. Because Marion was easily regulated and did not have other suggestive clinical signs that could not be explained by diabetes, concurrent hyperadrenocorticism was considered unlikely.

Long term monitoring of diabetic patients is required. Although 24 hour glucose curves were once standard methods of monitoring the progress of diabetic patients, these are expensive and stressful for the patient. Results may be misleading because of stress induced increases in blood glucose levels and the reluctance of some patients to eat in the hospital. This is particularly true for feline patients. An attractive alternative is measurement of serum fructosamine levels, which reflect glycemic control over several weeks and can help differentiate stress induced hyperglycemia from diabetes (see Marmalade). Glycated hemoglobin levels are also helpful, however these species specific assays are less widely available to the practitioner.

Once diagnosed, a variety of approaches for home monitoring of blood glucose and glycemic control have been advocated that vary in reliance on clinical signs and/or direct monitoring of blood glucose or glucosuria (Nelson, Briggs). Hand held point of care instruments are particularly successful in diabetic dogs. With proper supervision by veterinary staff, this allows more frequent and less expensive monitoring of patients (Casella, Reusch). Ultimately, the practitioner must balance the costs and benefits of clinical and laboratory evaluation of diabetic patients in the context of each individual case.

Briggs CE, Nelson RW, Feldman ED, Elliott DA, Neal LA. Reliability of history and physical examination findings for assessing control of glycemia in dogs with diabetes mellitus: 53 cases (1995-1998). J Am Vet Med Assoc 2000;217:48-53.

Casella M, Wess G, Reusch CE. Measurement of capillary blood glucose concentrations by pet owners: a new tool in the management of diabetes mellitus. J Am Anim Hosp Assoc 2002; 38:239-245.

Nelson. R Editorial: Stress hyperglycemia and diabetes mellitus in cats. J Vet Intern Med 2002; 16:121-122.

Reusch CE, Wess G, Casella M. Home monitoring of blood glucose concentration in the management of diabetes mellitus. Compendium 2001;23:544-555.

GI Case 19 – Level 3

Amaryllis is a 7-year-old spayed female Doberman Pinscher mixed breed dog presenting for a 20 pound weight loss over the past year attributed to decreased consumption of table food. Over the past month, Amaryllis has been lethargic and anorexic, associated with intermittent vomiting and diarrhea. Her previous history includes an asymptomatic heart murmur. On physical examination, Amaryllis was thin and depressed but alert and responsive. The presence of a left-sided systolic heart murmur was confirmed. She had a tight, distended abdomen, but she was not painful on abdominal palpation. Abdominal ultrasound showed an enlarged hyperechoic liver, changes in the region of the pancreas compatible with pancreatitis, and mild abdominal effusion. Thoracic radiographs were suggestive of pneumonia.

White blood cell count:	13.1 x 10⁹/L	(4.9-17.0)
Segmented neutrophils:	↑ 11.4 x 10⁹/L	(3.0-11.0)
Band neutrophils:	0.1 x 10⁹/L	(0-0.3)
Lymphocytes:	↓ 0.7 x 10⁹/L	(1.0-4.8)
Monocytes:	0.9 x 10⁹/L	(0.2-1.4)
Eosinophils:	0 x 10⁹/L	(0-1.2)
WBC morphology: Small numbers of mildly toxic neutrophils are seen		
Plasma is icteric.		
Hematocrit:	42%	(37-55)
Red blood cell count:	6.13 x 10¹²/L	(5.5-8.5)
Hemoglobin:	14.9 g/dl	(12.0-18.0)
MCV:	69.3 fl	(60.0-77.0)
MCHC:	34.0	(31.0-34.0)
RBC morphology: Normal		
Platelets:	397.0 x 10⁹/L	(181.0-525.0)
Glucose:	↑ 272 mg/dl	(67.0-135.0)
BUN:	13 mg/dl	(8-29)
Creatinine:	0.6 mg/dl	(0.6-2.0)
Phosphorus:	↓ 2.3 mg/dl	(2.6-7.2)
Calcium:	↓ 9.2 mg/dl	(9.4-11.6)
Magnesium:	2.0 mEq/L	(1.7-2.5)
Total Protein:	↓ 4.7 g/dl	(5.5-7.8)
Albumin:	↓ 2.3 g/dl	(2.8-4.0)
Globulin:	2.4 g/dl	(2.3-4.2)
A/G Ratio:	1.0	(0.7-1.6)
Sodium:	149 mEq/L	(142-163)
Chloride:	118 mEq/L	(111-129)
Potassium:	↓ 3.3 mEq/L	(3.8-5.4)
HCO3:	15 mEq/L	(15-28)
Anion Gap:	19.3 mEq/L	(12-23)
Total Bili:	↑ 8.60 mg/dl	(0.10-0.50)
ALP:	↑ 1752 IU/L	(12-121)
GGT:	↑ 51 IU/L	(2-10)
ALT:	78 IU/L	(18-86)
AST:	↑ 397 IU/L	(16-54)

Cholesterol:	↑ 400 mg/dl	(82-355)
Triglycerides:	↑ 441 mg/dl	(30-321)
Amylase:	↑ 2509 IU/L	(409-1203)

Urinalysis: Cystocentesis

Appearance: Yellow and clear	Sediment:
Specific gravity: 1.024	0-5 RBC/high power field
pH: 6.5	0-5 WBC seen
Protein: trace	No bacteria
Glucose: 2+	Occasional epithelial cells
Ketones: 1+	1+ fat droplets and debris
Bilirubin: 3+	
Heme: 3+	

Interpretation

CBC

Leukogram: Amaryllis has a barely perceptible neutrophilia, which in combination with the toxic change supports mild inflammation. Potential sources include pneumonia, pancreatitis, or a urinary tract infection. Although only small numbers of leukocytes and no bacteria were seen, a culture is recommended as urinary tract infections are common in patients with diabetes and they may be occult (Forrester, McGuire). The lymphopenia is likely associated with endogeneous corticosteroids from a protracted illness.

Erythrogram: The erythrogram of this patient is normal, therefore hemolysis can be ruled out as a cause for the icteric plasma. Elevated liver enzymes are compatible with cholestasis as a cause for the hyperbilirubinemia.

Serum Biochemical Profile

Hyperglycemia: There are numerous possible causes of hyperglycemia. During an initial evaluation, post-prandial effects or the possibility of either transient corticosteroid or epinephrine induced elevations should be ruled out. Given the history of weight loss and the presence of significant amounts of glucose and ketones in the urine, diabetes mellitus should be considered a primary differential diagnosis. Whenever blood glucose levels exceed approximately 200 mg/dl, the renal tubular maximum for glucose reabsorption can be exceeded, resulting in glucosuria, regardless of the cause of the hyperglycemia. Glucosuria itself does not rule out stress-induced hyperglycemia, however ketonuria is strongly suggestive for diabetes. Confirmation of a diagnosis of diabetes by measuring serum fructosamine levels could be considered, but is probably not necessary for Amaryllis. Any cause of insulin resistance such as hyperadrenocorticism must also be considered. Amaryllis has a mild neutrophilic leukocytosis and lymphopenia, compatible with a corticosteroid effect. Pancreatitis can be associated with hyperglycemia, either due to stress secondary to pain or due diabetes mellitus. Pancreatitis-induced diabetes may be transient or permanent, depending on the severity of pancreatic damage.

Mild hypophosphatemia and hypocalcemia: Neither of these values is likely to be physiologically significant. The hypocalcemia may be related to the low serum albumin and is unlikely to be associated with a decrease in biologically active ionized calcium. Hypocalcemia has been described in dogs with acute pancreatitis, but it does not appear to be as common as in humans (Hess 1998). Both total and ionized calcium levels may be low in cats with acute pancreatitis. Possible mechanisms for low ionized calcium in animals with pancreatitis include deposition in saponified tissues, glucagon-mediated increases in calcitonin concentration, and decreased parathyroid hormone activity secondary to hypomagnesemia. Hypophosphatemia can result in lethargy, depression, and diarrhea. Hemolytic anemia can occur if the phosphorus drops below 1 mg/dl. Treatment of diabetic patients with insulin can promote a rapid translocation of phosphorus into cells, associated with a precipitous and potentially dangerous decline in serum phosphorus. Acidemia is associated with a cellular translocation from the intracellular to the extracellular space, therefore correction of acid/base disturbances in ketotic patients can further depress the serum phophorus concentration.

Hypoproteinemia with hypoalbuminemia and low normal globulins: Considerations for hypoalbuminemia include decreased production secondary to starvation, liver failure, or a negative acute phase response. The weight loss in this patient is dramatic, and starvation may be an issue if the body condition score is very low, however transient anorexia does not typically lower serum albumin. Liver enzyme elevations are compatible with liver disease, however other analytes that may decrease with impaired liver function (blood urea nitrogen, glucose, and cholesterol) are normal to increased. None of these values are sensitive or specific tests of liver function, and other more specific tests should be performed to evaluate this possibility. Toxic change in neutrophils indicates some inflammation, however increased production of positive acute phase reactants should induce hyperglobulinemia, which is not present at this time. Increased loss of albumin can also cause hypoalbuminemia. Gastrointestinal, cutaneous, and third space losses should be considered, and the abdominal effusion may be a source of protein loss. Isolated loss of albumin is most likely with glomerular lesions. The urinalysis in this case reveals mild proteinuria; a urine protein:creatinine ratio would be helpful in determining the severity of the proteinuria. Because leukocytes and erythrocytes are present in the urine sediment and diabetic patients are at risk for urinary tract infections, the possibility that proteinuria is due to lower urinary tract disease should be ruled out prior to pursuing a diagnosis of glomerular disease.

Hypokalemia: Anorexia can contribute to hypokalemia because of decreased intake of potassium, however it is usually only clinically significant in combination with increased losses. Amaryllis could be losing potassium through her gastrointestinal tract since there is a history of vomiting and diarrhea, or she may be losing it into the abdominal effusion. Renal potassium wastage is associated with osmotic diuresis from glucosuria and ketonuria. While acidemia is often cited as contributing to hypokalemia by causing a shift of potassium into cells, some authors conclude that these shifts are transient and less significant with organic acidosis like ketoacidosis than for mineral acidosis. Although serum potassium levels are not good indicators of total body potassium stores, the history of polyuria and gastrointestinal signs in this patient puts her at risk for potassium depletion. As discussed above in regards to phosphorus, treatment with insulin is expected to cause translocation of potassium into cells that could further depress serum potassium.

Hyperbilirubinemia with increased ALP and GGT: This combination of data is compatible with cholestasis, especially since the hematocrit is within normal limits, making hemolysis unlikely. Serum ALP activity can increase with a variety of endocrinopathies, including diabetes mellitus, however the concurrent hyperbilirubinemia and increased GGT suggests that diabetes alone is unlikely to be the cause of the elevated ALP. Pancreatitis may be the cause of the cholestasis based on the ultrasound study and hyperamylasemia. Although evidence of sepsis in this patient is weak, extrahepatic bacterial infections can result in hyperbilirubinemia and elevated liver enzymes. This syndrome may occasionally mimic a cholestatic process (Meyer). Because of the steroid leukogram and history of chronic illness, corticosteroid effects on the liver could also contribute to increases in ALP and GGT, as well as AST and ALT (see below).

Increased AST with normal ALT: ALT is more specific for hepatocellular damage than AST, however AST is more sensitive. Many tissues contain AST, limiting the usefulness of this test for the diagnosis of liver disease, however some degree of hepatocellular damage secondary to the toxic effects of bile in cholestatic conditions is common. A normal creatine kinase could help rule out muscle as a source for elevated serum AST. As discussed for Quasi (Case 15-pancreatitis) and Nutmeg (Case 16-pancreatitis and hepatitis), extension of the inflammatory process from the pancreas to the liver can cause hepatocellular enzyme elevations in patients with pancreatitis.

Hypercholesterolemia and hypertriglyceridemia: Once post-prandial effects are ruled out, endocrinopathies (hypothyroidism, hyperadrenocorticism, diabetes mellitus) and liver or pancreatic diseases are common causes of hypercholesterolemia and hypertriglyceridemia. Hyperlipidemia may contribute to the development of pancreatitis or may be a consequence of pancreatitis. In some cases, multiple causes of hyperlipidemia can be present. For example, one study of 221 canine diabetics found that 23% had concurrent hyperadrenocorticism, 13% had acute pancreatitis, and 4% were hypothyroid (Hess 2000). Idiopathic hyperlipidemias are described but much less common than secondary causes. Lipoprotein lipase is an enzyme present on the vascular endothelium which hydrolyzes triglycerides into fatty acids and monoglycerides. Insulin enhances this function, therefore insulin deficiency leads to accumulation of triglycerides in the circulation. Insulin deficiency also leads to enhanced lipolysis, with resultant release of free fatty acids into the circulation which will eventually be processed by the liver into more triglycerides and ketone bodies (Kerl). Typically, ketone bodies are utilized as an energy source as they are produced unless stress hormones such as glucagon, epinephrine or cortisol further promote ketogenesis by hepatic mitochondria. Epinephrine and cortisol will contribute to this process by stimulating muscle protein degradation to supply amino acids for the production of ketone bodies. This is one mechanism by which a stressful event or illness can trigger diabetic ketoacidosis. Increases in serum triglycerides may be greater in magnitude than the hypercholesterolemia in diabetic patients. Even when pathologic processes cause hypercholesterolemia in dogs, there are rarely physiologic consequences because the proportion of low density lipoproteins remain low (Bauer). Occasional ocular abnormalities and rare cases of atherosclerosis have been described.

Hyperamylasemia: The increase in serum amylase in this patient could be explained by decreased glomerular filtration rate, however there is no evidence of azotemia. Both intestinal and pancreatic pathology can elevate serum amylase. Imaging studies or additional tests may be helpful to support a diagnosis of pancreatitis. (See Jimbo-Case 22, Quasi-Case 15).

Urinalysis: The specific gravity may be appropriate depending on the hydration status of the patient since there is no evidence of azotemia. Some amount of osmotic diuresis is expected to accompany the glucosuria and ketonuria. The presence of these osmoles may minimally increase the urine specific gravity if present in very large quantities. It appears that the ketones Amaryllis is generating are being utilized or eliminated in the urine rather than accumulating in the blood since she has a normal HCO3, serum chloride, and anion gap. Urine collected by cystocentesis may have a variable amount of blood contamination, which could introduce small amounts of protein, heme, red blood cells, and white blood cells. Although no bacteria are noted, urine culture is still recommended in diabetic patients with clinical signs compatible with urinary tract infection because of the increased incidence of occult infections (McGuire).

Case Summary and Outcome

Based on the laboratory work, Amaryllis was diagnosed with diabetes mellitus with ketosis (but not yet ketoacidosis). Pancreatitis was also considered likely based on laboratory work and imaging studies. She was treated with intravenous fluids, antibiotics and regular insulin. Over several days, Amaryllis was offered small amounts of bland food and water, but her appetite remained poor. The hyperbilirubinemia improved, suggesting improvement in her pancreatitis, however persistent changes in the region of the pancreas were noted on repeat abdominal ultrasound. Amaryllis was discharged on fluids and insulin with home-monitoring of urine for glucose and ketones. Changes in the liver parameters were interpreted to be secondary to diabetes and pancreatitis, so no liver biopsy was performed.

As alluded to above, there are complex relationships between multiple endocrinopathies, liver disease, pancreatic disease, and hyperlipidemia. The presence of one of the abnormalities certainly does not rule out the presence of another, and in fact, they may occur together with some frequency. Hyperadrenocorticism can cause both a steroid hepatopathy and insulin resistance resembling or exacerbating diabetes mellitus. Acute necrotizing pancreatitis can destroy beta cell islets, causing transient or permanent diabetes mellitus. Conversely, hyperlipidemia may be a predisposing factor for pancreatitis. It may be necessary to prioritize for treatment the most severe problems based on clinical history and laboratory abnormalities (in this case diabetes with ketosis). After these are under control, re-assess the patient to determine if secondary problems resolved with initial treatment or if there are multiple primary problems. Sometimes, this can be a prolonged process. For example, it is necessary to control diabetes mellitus to accurately test for hyperadrenocorticism, however hyperadrenocorticism causes insulin resistance and intereferes with treatment for diabetes. It is useful to compare Amaryllis with Marion (Case 7) who had diabetes without confirmed pancreatic or hepatobiliary disease. Liver enzyme changes were similar in both patients, although Amaryllis has hyperbilirubinemia, making it more likely that her liver enzyme elevations indicate the potential for significant hepatic pathology and may not just be occurring secondary to the diabetes or corticosteroid effects. Quasi (Case 15), the dog with pancreatitis, also had hepatocellular enzyme elevations, however measurement of cholestatic enzymes and bilirubin was not possible due to interference secondary to hemolysis. The dog with histologically confirmed pancreatitis and cholangiohepatitis (Nutmeg-Case 16) had elevations in all liver enzymes and hyperbilirubinemia of a degree similar to Amaryllis. Like Nutmeg, it is possible that once the pancreatitis begins to resolve, secondary cholestasis would be relieved and liver enzyme abnormalities and hyperbilirubinemia would improve in subsequent biochemical panels in Amaryllis.

Bauer JE. Evaluation and dietary consdirations in idiopathic hyperlipidemia in dogs. J Am Vet Med Assoc 1995; 206: 1684-1688.

Forrester SD, Troy GC, Dalton MN, Huffman JW, Holtzman G. Retrospective evaluation of urinary tract infection in 42 dogs with hyperadrenocorticism or diabetes mellitus or both. J Vet Intern Med 1999;13:557-560.

Hess RS, Saudners M, VanWinkle TJ, Shofer FS, Washabau RJ. Clinical, clinicopathologic, radiographic, and ultra-sonographic abnormalities in dogs with fatal acute pancreatitis: 70 cases (1986-1995). J Am Vet Med Assoc; 1998; 213:665-670.

Hess RS, Saunders M, Van Winkle TJ, Ward CR. Concurrent disorders in dogs with diabetes mellitus: 221 cases (1993-1998). J Am Vet Med Assoc; 2000; 217:1166-1173.

Kerl ME. Diabetic Ketoacidosis: Pathophysiology and clinical and laboratory presentation. Compendium 2007;23:220-229.

McGuire NC, Schulman R, Ridgway MD, Bollero G. Detection of occult urinary tract infections in dogs with diabetes mellitus. J Am Anim Hosp Assoc; 2002; 38:541-544.

Meyer DJ, Twedt DC. Effect of Extrahepatic Disease on the Liver. In: Kirk's Current Veterinary Therapy XIII. JD Bonagura, ed. 2000. W.B. Saunders Company. Philadelphia, PA. pp 668-671.

GI Case 20 – Level 3

"Hooligan" is a 17-year old-spayed female domestic short haired cat presenting for increased drinking and decreased appetite for the past 2 days. Hooligan was diagnosed with diabetes mellitus 2 years ago, and is currently taking glipizide. No bloodwork has been performed for one year. She occasionally gets urinary tract infections, which are characterized by frequent urinations and usually resolve with antibiotic therapy. On physical examination, Hooligan is dehydrated with increased skin turgor and tacky mucous membranes. She has moderate dental tartar and hepatomegaly.

Glucose:	↑ 373 mg/dl	(70.0-120.0)
BUN:	↑ 141 mg/dl	(15-32)
Creatinine:	↑ 7.1 mg/dl	(0.9-2.1)
Phosphorus:	↑ 10.6 mg/dl	(3.0-6.0)
Calcium:	10.6 mg/dl	(8.9-11.6)
Total Protein:	↑ 9.0 g/dl	(6.0-8.4)
Albumin:	↑ 4.7 g/dl	(2.4-4.0)
Globulin:	4.3 g/dl	(2.5-5.8)
Sodium:	149 mEq/L	(149-164)
Chloride:	119 mEq/L	(119-134)
Potassium:	4.9 mEq/L	(3.6-5.4)
HCO3:	↓ 11 mEq/L	(13-22)
Total Bili:	0.2 mg/dl	(0.10-0.30)
ALP:	36 IU/L	(10-72)
ALT:	↑ 155 IU/L	(29-145)
AST:	↑ 45 IU/L	(12-42)
Cholesterol:	223 mg/dl	(77-258)
Triglycerides:	96 mg/dl	(25-191)
Amylase:	↑ 2207 IU/L	(496-1874)

Urinalysis: Voided

Appearance: Straw colored and hazy	Sediment:
Specific gravity: 1.020	20-30 RBC/hpf
pH: 6.0	0-5 WBC/hpf
Protein: 100 mg/dl	2-5 granular casts/hpf
Glucose: 4+ Ketones: negative	Occasional squamous and transitional epithelial cells seen
Bilirubin: negative	No bacteria present
Heme: 2+	Trace fat droplets and debris

Interpretation

No CBC data is available on this patient

Hyperglycemia: Given the history, the most likely cause for the hyperglycemia and glucosuria is diabetes mellitus, although stress could exacerbate the hyperglycemia. The clinical signs suggest poor control at this point, however serum fructosamine (See Marmalade-Case 2) could be measured as a longer term indicator of serum glucose levels.

Azotemia:
Azotemia should be categorized as pre-renal, renal, or post-renal. There is no clinical evidence of urinary obstruction in this patient, therefore prerenal and renal components should be considered. Hooligan is clinically dehydrated, so at least a portion of the azotemia is likely pre-renal. Given the degree of dehydration, the urine is less than optimally concentrated and suggests some renal impairment. It can be difficult to adequately gauge renal function in poorly controlled diabetic patients. The glucose in the urine will cause some degree of osmotic diuresis, decreasing urine specific gravity. At the same time, the presence of glucose in the urine will increase the specific gravity by approximately 0.001 for every 270 mg/dl of glucose.

Hyperphosphatemia: The most likely cause of hyperphosphatemia in this patient is decreased glomerular filtration rate (GFR), regardless of whether the decreased GFR is due to primary renal insufficiency or is pre-renal in origin.

Hyperproteinemia with hyperalbuminemia: Because overproduction of albumin does not typically occur, hyperalbuminemia is the result of hemoconcentration. This is compatible with Hooligan's dehydrated state.

Decreased HCO3: The decreased HCO3 indicates acidosis. In this case, lactic acidosis due to decreased tissue perfusion secondary to dehydration and uremic acidosis are potential contributors. The absence of urine ketones suggests that ketoacidosis is not a major cause of metabolic acidosis at this time. (Please see Chapter 7 for more complete discussion). Hooligan is certainly at risk for developing ketoacidosis because of anorexia and concurrent disease (possible urinary tract infection, likely renal failure).

Mild increases in ALT and AST: As noted in Chapter 2 on liver enzymes, there are numerous extrahepatic processes that can elevate serum liver enzymes in the absence of primary hepatic pathology. Several endocrinopathies, including diabetes mellitus, may cause these abnormalities in the cat. Significant liver disease is less likely in this cat, because most causes of primary hepatic disease in cats are characterized by hyperbilirubinemia in addition to increased liver enzyme activities. Hyperthyroidism is another serious consideration in an elderly cat with elevated liver enzymes, hyperglycemia, and weight loss. The presence of diabetes mellitus in this patient in no way rules out hyperthyroidism.

Mild hyperamylasemia: Amylase is a very poor test for pancreatitis in the cat. Although pancreatitis cannot be ruled out in Hooligan's case, decreased glomerular filtration is the probable cause for the hyperamylasemia.

Urinalysis: Glucosuria is expected in any patient whose blood glucose concentration exceeds approximately 200 mg/dl, which is the renal threshold for reabsorption. Other abnormalities such as the active sediment, proteinuria, and 2+ heme could be compatible with urinary tract inflammation, especially considering Hooligan's history of urinary tract infections. Diabetic patients are predisposed to urinary tract infections because glucose can provide a substrate for bacterial growth and because of subtle but relatively consistent immune function defects. Bacterial culture and sensitivity testing is recommended for appropriate therapy of this patient. Because renal disease is suspected, urinalysis should be repeated after improved management of the diabetes and treatment of any urinary tract infections. Persistent proteinuria could reflect glomerular protein loss, and should be followed up by a urine protein:creatinine ratio. The history of repeated urinary tract infections suggests that pyelonephritis could be a potential cause for renal failure, however chronic renal disease is a common problem in geriatric cats with no such history.

Case Summary and Outcome

Intravenous fluid therapy and imaging studies of the urinary tract were strongly recommended, however the owner declined therapy and took Hooligan home. Amoxicillin and subcutaneous fluids were administered at home. The case was lost to follow-up.

Hooligan's case illustrates how multiple concurrent diseases and laboratory abnormalities can complicate interpretation of diagnostic tests. In some cases, the correct interpretation of some laboratory data can only be certain after treatment has begun. For example, the degree of renal versus prerenal azotemia cannot be determined until the patient is appropriately hydrated. Furthermore, the true renal concentrating ability may not be clear until glucosuria and the resultant osmotic diuresis is corrected. Although the previous two cases of diabetes mellitus were not azotemic (Marion-Case 18 and Amaryllis-Case 19), patients with diabetes mellitus can present with prerenal azotemia and impaired urinary concentrating ability due to osmotic diuresis in the absence of irreversible renal failure.

As noted above, primary liver disease is less likely to be the cause of liver enzyme elevations than the diabetes. Liver disease cannot be ruled out, however invasive procedures such as liver biopsy are not recommended until other extrahepatic causes of liver enzyme elevations are assessed. Evaluation of the patient for hyperthyroidism is indicated. Similarly, while pancreatic disease cannot be ruled out as a cause for clinical signs or a possible contributing factor to the liver enzyme elevations, amylase is a poor test for pancreatitis in the cat. A trypsin-like immunoreactivity (TLI) test could be done if pancreatitis remains a concern, but results need to be interpreted with caution in a patient with renal disease or dehydration as the results of this test may also be affected by a low glomerular filtration rate. Serum pancreatic lipase immunoreactivity (cPLI) may also be useful in the diagnosis of feline pancreatitis (Forman).

Forman MA, Marks SL, Cock HE V de, Hergesell EJ, Wisner ER, Baker TW, Kass PH, Steiner JM, Williams DA. Evaluation of serum feline pancreatic lipase immunoreactivity and helical computed tomography versus conventional testing for the diagnosis of feline pancreatitis. J Vet Int Med 2004; 18:807-815

GI Case 21 – Level 3

Kabob is a 9-year-old spayed female miniature poodle. She had been seen one year ago by her referring veterinarian for lethargy and anorexia. Blood work at that time showed elevated liver enzymes with hypoglycemia and hypoalbuminemia. Kabob was treated with antibiotics and showed improvement in clinical signs and liver enzyme values, however the serum biochemistry data did not completely normalize. She did well at home until just prior to this presentation, at which time she was lethargic, anorexic, and vomiting. On physical examination, Kabob is icteric, has cranial organomegaly, and has tacky mucous membranes.

	Day 1	
White blood cell count:	↑ 31.7 x 10⁹/L	(4.9-17.0)
Segmented neutrophils:	↑ 24.4 x 10⁹/L	(3.0-11.0)
Band neutrophils:	↑ 1.3 x 10⁹/L	(0-0.3)
Lymphocytes:	2.5 x 10⁹/L	(1.0-4.8)
Monocytes:	↑ 2.9 x 10⁹/L	(.15-1.4)
Eosinophils:	0.6 x 10⁹/L	(0-1.3)
WBC morphology: Slightly toxic neutrophils		
Plasma is icteric.		
Hematocrit:	↓ 24%	(37-55)
Red blood cell count:	↓ 3.89 x 10¹²/L	(5.5-8.5)
Hemoglobin:	↓ 8.0 g/dl	(12.0-18.0)
MCV:	62.5 fl	(60.0-77.0)
MCHC:	33.3	(31.0-34.0)
RBC morphology: Slight anisocytosis with a few macrocytes		
Platelets:	↓ 12.0 x 10⁹/L	(181.0-525.0)
Glucose:	↓ 42 mg/dl	(67.0-135.0)
BUN:	↓ 7 mg/dl	(8-29)
Creatinine:	↓ 0.3 mg/dl	(0.6-2.0)
Phosphorus:	3.3 mg/dl	(2.6-7.2)
Calcium:	↓ 7.9 mg/dl	(9.4-11.6)
Magnesium:	↓ 1.5 mEq/L	(1.7-2.5)
Total Protein:	↓ 4.6 g/dl	(5.5-7.8)
Albumin:	↓ 1.5 g/dl	(2.8-4.0)
Globulin:	3.1 g/dl	(2.3-4.2)
A/G Ratio:	↓ 0.5	(0.7-1.6)
Sodium:	143 mEq/L	(142-163)
Chloride:	119 mEq/L	(111-129)
Potassium:	↓ 2.3 mEq/L	(3.8-5.4)
HCO3:	16 mEq/L	(15-28)
Anion Gap:	↓ 10.3 mEq/L	(12-23)
Total Bili:	↑ 10.00 mg/dl	(0.10-0.50)
ALP:	↑ 2741 IU/L	(12-121)
GGT:	↑ 55 IU/L	(2-10)
ALT:	↑ 459 IU/L	(18-86)
AST:	189 IU/L	(16-54)
Cholesterol:	88 mg/dl	(82-355)
Triglycerides:	214 mg/dl	(30-321)
Amylase:	↑ 2171 IU/L	(409-1203)

Urinalysis: Cystocentesis

Appearance: Dark yellow and clear	Sediment:
Specific gravity: 1.008	0-5 RBC/high power field
pH: 7.0	0 WBC seen
Protein: Neg	Trace bacteria
Glucose: Negative	Occasional epithelial cells and debris
Ketones: Negative	
Bilirubin: 3+	
Heme: 3+	

Bone marrow aspirate: Multiple smears are hemodiluted, however several contain scattered variably sized hypercellular particles. Megakaryocytes are increased. The M:E ratio is 3.0 (reference interval = 0.75-2.5). The maturation of both cell lines is orderly and goes to completion. Rare lymphocytes are present and plasma cells are noted in focal aggregates in some areas but are less than 5% of the total nucleated cell count. Occasional macrophages contain red blood cell breakdown products, and rare intact erythroblastic islands are seen.

Diagnosis: Myeloid and megakaryocytic hyperplasia. Activity is present in the erythroid line but is less than expected for the degree of anemia.

Coagulation Profile Day 1

PT:	↑ 10.2s	(6.2-9.3)
APTT:	↑ 23.5s	(8.9-16.3)
Fibrinogen:	200 mg/dl	(200-400)
FDPs:	↑ >5, <20 μg/ml	(<5)

Interpretation
CBC
Leukogram: Kabob has an inflammatory leukogram with marked neutrophilic leukocytosis with a left shift, monocytosis and toxic change in the neutrophils.

Erythrogram: Kabob has a normocytic, normochromic anemia. This anemia appears nonregenerative, and there is inadequate response by the bone marrow. Chronic disease or inflammation usually produces a mild non-regenerative anemia as a result of suppression of red blood cell production. In this case, it may not completely explain an anemia of this severity. The red blood cell breakdown products in the bone marrow could suggest increased destruction or apoptosis of red blood cell precursors in the marrow, which may be immune-mediated and non-specifically related to the underlying illness. There is no evidence of a neoplastic process in the bone marrow that could suppress erythropoiesis.

Platelets: Because of the megakaryocytic hyperplasia in the marrow, the thrombocytopenia is interpreted to be due to increased peripheral consumption rather than impaired production. Hemorrhage can cause thrombocytopenia and should be considered with anemia and panhypoproteinemia, however the degree of thrombocytopenia resulting from hemorrhage is generally mild to moderate. The owners should be questioned carefully to determine if there is any evidence of gastrointestinal bleeding. Immune-mediated mechanisms appear likely due to the severity of the thrombocytopenia, which is in the range where there is a risk of spontaneous hemorrhage. Immune-mediated thrombocytopenia can occur secondary to neoplasia, however none has been found at this time. Prolonged coagulation times and increased fibrinogen degradation products combined with the thrombocytopenia suggest the development of disseminated intravascular coagulation. Vaccination can be associated with a mild to moderate but transient thrombocytopenia, as can viral infections. A careful history should be taken on all thrombocytopenic patients to rule out exposure to drugs or toxins.

Serum Biochemical Profile

Hypoglycemia: Any single low blood glucose measurement should be confirmed with a repeat sample because of the possibility of in vitro consumption of glucose by cells in unspun samples. This is especially important in samples with high leukocyte counts as observed in this patient. CBC data are compatible with a severe inflammatory process, and low blood glucose levels may be observed in septic patients. Failure of hepatic gluconeogenesis and hypoglycemia can result from severely impaired liver function. Further support for this is concurrent hypoalbuminemia, low BUN, hyperbilirubinemia and prolonged coagulation times. None of these tests are sensitive or specific for decreased liver function. Another potential cause for hypoglycemia is neoplasia. Insulinoma (See Russell-Case 6) and large intra-cavitary masses that produce abnormal insulin-like growth factors (See Kippy-Case 5) can stimulate glucose uptake by cells. Imaging studies and biopsy may be required to establish a diagnosis of neoplasia and should be considered if liver function tests are normal, although they are indicated as part of further work-up of the liver disease regardless. Both hypoalbuminemia and hypoglycemia can be explained by prolonged starvation, however this is unusual and occurs predominantly in cases with poor body condition scores.

Low BUN and Creatinine: Overhydration can dilute blood urea nitrogen, and polyuria will result in increased urinary losses of BUN. The very low urine specific gravity is compatible with polyuria. It is difficult in this case to assess hydration status using laboratory data because the disease processes are likely to have confounding effects on hematocrit and total protein. Despite the dilute urine, the tacky mucous membranes imply dehydration, suggesting that overhydration is unlikely. Further information about any previous fluid therapy would be helpful. Significantly decreased liver function will impair production of BUN. Significant decrease in muscle mass is the major differential diagnosis for decreased creatinine in the absence of retention of free water. As noted above in the discussion of starvation in relation to hypoalbuminemia and hypoglycemia, the poor body condition should be clinically obvious at the point that laboratory abnormalities can be attributed to starvation. Similarly, negative protein balance can decrease production of blood urea nitrogen.

Hypocalcemia: The hypocalcemia is associated with persistently low serum albumin, therefore it is unlikely that there is truly a low ionized calcium. If there were concurrent abnormalities of phosphorus or any clinical signs compatible with hypocalcemia, then ionized calcium measurement would be recommended.

Minimal hypomagnesemia: This abnormality is commonly noted in critically ill patients and in this case may be attributable to either decreased intake or increased renal losses. Because calcium regulation and many other biochemical processes require magnesium as a critical cofactor, supplementation is recommended. Like calcium, ionized magnesium is the physiologically significant value.

Hypoproteinemia with hypoalbuminemia: The disproportionately low albumin compared to globulin could be compatible with decreased hepatic production of albumin or selective loss of albumin via the glomerulus. Many other sources of increased protein loss such as gastrointestinal tract, skin, and third space encompass losses of both albumin and globulins. As noted above, decreased hepatic production of albumin may occur secondary to decreased intake/starvation, poor liver function in general, or as part of the acute phase response since albumin is a negative acute phase reactant. The negative urinary protein data should be interpreted in the context of the low specific gravity and may not rule out renal protein loss. A urinary protein:creatinine ratio is a more accurate way to assess proteinuria in these cases. At this point, decreased liver function appears to be the most likely cause for low serum albumin, however increased demands on the protein pool such as fever or surgery could further deplete albumin.

Hypokalemia: Kabob is predisposed to the development of hypokalemia because of anorexia and poor dietary intake of potassium. Physiologically significant hypokalemia is most likely to develop in concert with increased losses associated with gastrointestinal losses, renal losses associated with polyuria, or third space losses, all of which are possible here. Iatrogenic hypokalemia can develop if low potassium fluids are given in significant quantities.

Mildly decreased anion gap: This mild abnormality is caused by low albumin. Under normal circumstances, most of the unmeasured anions are negatively charged plasma proteins.

Hyperbilirubinemia: Hemolysis, sepsis, cholestasis, and decreased liver function are all possible causes for the hyperbilirubinemia in this case, and all could potentially contribute to varying degrees. While the anemia may suggest hemolysis as a contributor to the bilirubin levels, hemolytic anemias are typically regenerative and are coupled with red blood cell morphologic changes. The inflammatory leukogram and hypoglycemia could be associated with sepsis, which can impair hepatocellular uptake of bile. The elevated ALP and GGT suggest cholestasis. The potential for decreased liver function has been discussed above, and further testing is required to evaluate this component.

Elevated ALP and GGT: Although extrahepatic causes of enzyme elevation can be important, the concurrent hyperbilirubinemia and hyperbilirubinuria support the presence of a cholestatic process. Although not technically out of range, the cholesterol values seem somewhat low for a patient with cholestatic liver disease; this may be another sign of decreased liver function.

Elevated ALT and AST: Elevations in these enzymes support hepatocellular damage. Because the elevations in the hepatocellular enzymes are milder than those noted in the cholestatic enzymes, hepatocellular damage may be occurring secondary to a primary cholestatic process.

Increased amylase: Increased serum amylase is often used as an indicator of pancreatic disease, however intestinal disease, liver disease, and decreased glomerular filtration rate can all increase serum amylase. Because Kabob's elevation is amylase in mild and is later shown to be transient, a primary pancreatic process appears less likely than the other causes for elevations in this enzyme.

Urinalysis: Despite some clinical evidence for dehydration, the urine specific gravity is dilute. Renal failure appears to be unlikely in the absence of azotemia. Other considerations include medullary washout, or decreased liver function. Given the mild electrolyte changes in the context of the other data, liver failure seems likely. Causes for polyuria and dilute urine in liver failure include overstimulation of adrenocorticotropic hormone and chronic hypercorti-solism and impaired osmotic stimulation of antidiuretic hormone release. In some dogs, nausea may stimulate polydipsia, and low BUN may impair the osmotic concentrating gradient in the kidney (Rothuizen).

Hyperbilirubinuria is expected to reflect renal excretion of bilirubin from the blood. Heme and erythrocytes may be an artifact associated with blood contamination of the sample with subsequent hemolysis of erythrocytes in the dilute urine. The presence of bacteria indicates the need for a bacterial culture, especially with other clinical and laboratory indicators of inflammation and potential sepsis.

Bone marrow aspirate: Inflammation is resulting in the myeloid hyperplasia. Megakaryocytic hyperplasia is in response to the peripheral destruction of platelets. The response to anemia was discussed previously.

Coagulation profile: Prolonged PT and APTT can be explained by markedly impaired liver function due to low levels of production of coagulation factors. Elevated fibrinogen degradation products may be seen with liver failure since the liver is responsible for their clearance. The thrombocytopenia is not expected to occur with uncomplicated poor liver function and in combination with the other changes suggest disseminated intravascular coagulation (DIC). A septic process could trigger DIC. Poor baseline liver function could predispose Kabob to DIC because of the central role of the liver in the regulation of coagulation.

Case Summary and Outcome

Abdominal ultrasound revealed an enlarged gall bladder with a thickened wall and gall stones. Kabob was treated with a unit of platelet rich plasma prior to being sent to surgery on Day 1, where a non-expressible gall bladder and a patent bile duct were observed. A cholecystectomy for removal of gall stones and liver biopsy were performed. The liver culture was negative, however the culture of the gall bladder grew alpha *Streptococcus* and *E. coli*. Examination of biopsy samples revealed suppurative cholecystitis and localized suppurative hepatitis with diffuse extramedullary hematopoiesis. Ascending bacterial infection of the biliary tree was considered to be the cause of the liver disease. Kabob was treated with Actigal® (ursodeoxycholic acid), intravenous fluids, and antibiotics.

	Day 3	Day 7	
White blood cell count:	↑64.0 x 10⁹/L	↑18.4	(4.9-17.0)
Segmented neutrophils:	↑58.8 x 10⁹/L	↑14.9	(3.0-11.0)
Band neutrophils:	↑2.6 x 10⁹/L	0.2	(0-0.3)
Lymphocytes:	1.3 x 10⁹/L	2.2	(1.0-4.8)
Monocytes:	1.3 x 10⁹/L	0.9	(.15-1.4)
Eosinophils:	0 x 10⁹/L	0.2	(0-1.3)
WBC morphology: Slightly toxic neutrophils are seen both days			
Plasma is icteric on all days.			
Hematocrit:	↓25%	↓23	(37-55)
Red blood cell count:	↓3.74 x 10¹²/L	↓3.48	(5.5-8.5)
Hemoglobin:	↓8.4 g/dl	↓7.9	(12.0-18.0)
MCV:	65.8 fl	65.9	(60.0-77.0)
MCHC:	33.6	34.0	(31.0-34.0)
RBC morphology: Slight anisocytosis with a few macrocytes on all days			
Platelets:	24.0 x 10⁹/L	39.0	(181.0-525.0)

	Day 3	Day 7	
Glucose:	↓60 mg/dl	↓36	(67.0-135.0)
BUN:	↓7 mg/dl	↓7	(8-29)
Creatinine:	↓0.3 mg/dl	↓0.2	(0.6-2.0)
Phosphorus:	4.9 mg/dl	4.6	(2.6-7.2)
Calcium:	↓8.2 mg/dl	↓8.5	(9.4-11.6)
Magnesium:	1.7mEq/L	↓1.5	(1.7-2.5)
Total Protein:	↓4.0 g/dl	↓5.3	(5.5-7.8)
Albumin:	↓1.9 g/dl	↓1.9	(2.8-4.0)
Globulin:	↓2.1 g/dl	3.4	(2.3-4.2)
A/G Ratio:	0.9	↓0.6	(0.7-1.6)
Sodium:	142 mEq/L	142	(142-163)
Chloride:	↓109 mEq/L	113	(111-129)
Potassium:	↓2.3 mEq/L	4.0	(3.8-5.4)
HCO3:	27 mEq/L	22	(15-28)
Anion Gap:	↓8.3	↓11	(12-23)
Total Bili:	↑7.2 mg/dl	↑4.2	(0.10-0.50)
ALP:	↑720 IU/L	↑618	(12-121)
GGT:	↑11 IU/L	↑19	(2-10)
ALT:	↑160 IU/L	↑87	(18-86)
AST:	↑146 IU/L	↑71	(16-54)
Cholesterol:	113 mg/dl	154	(82-355)
Triglycerides:	108 mg/dl	88	(30-321)
Amylase:	647 IU/L	605	(409-1203)

Abdominal fluid analysis Day 3

Pre-spin color: red	Post-spin color: yellow
Pre-spin turbidity: cloudy	Post-spin turbidity: clear
Specific gravity: 1.021	Total protein: 3.0 g/dl
Total nucleated cells: 46,600/µl	
Abdominal fluid bilirubin: 3.2 mg/dl	

The fluid contains moderate numbers of erythrocytes; there is a predominance of nondegenerate neutrophils and small numbers of macrophages. No etiologic agent is seen. There is no evidence of bile pigment.

Coagulation Profile:	Day 7	
PT:	8.5s	(6.2-9.3)
APTT:	↑ 16.7s	(8.9-16.3)

CBC

Leukogram: On day 3, Kabob has a more marked neutrophilic leukocytosis compared with day 1, a left shift, monocytosis and toxic changes in the neutrophils. By Day 7 the left shift and monocytosis are no longer apparent and the neutrophilia is minimal. The severity of the inflammation appears to be decreasing by Day 7.

Erythrogram: Kabob has a normocytic, normochromic anemia which changes little over the course of his hospitalization (see above).

Platelets: Platelets are increasing over time in response to therapy.

Serum Biochemical Profile

Hypoglycemia: The observation that the hypoglycemia persists as the inflammatory leukogram resolves is less compatible with sepsis than abnormal liver function as a cause for the hypoglycemia. Because of persistent hypoglycemia, an ACTH stimulation test was performed to rule out hypoadrenocorticism, however the results were normal. Some patients with hypoadrenocorticism can have clinical chemistry abnormalities that mimic decreased liver function, such as hypoglycemia and hypocholesterolemia (See Kazoo-Case 12).

Low BUN and Creatinine: As suggested above, a combination of overhydration, polyuria/polydipsia, liver dysfunction, and poor muscle mass could contribute to the low BUN and creatinine.

Hypocalcemia: This value is increasing towards the reference interval, probably related to the rising albumin levels.

Minimal hypomagnesemia on day 7: Magnesium transiently increases to the lower limit of the reference interval on day 3, but is low again on day 7. See discussion above.

Hypoproteinemia with hypoalbuminemia, transient mild hypoglobulinemia: The protein values may change over time with variation in the hydration status.

Hypokalemia on Day 3 that resolves by Day 7: The potassium status may be improving due to appropriate supplementation of the intravenous fluids, if the patient begins to eat, or if ongoing sources of loss are controlled.

Mildly decreased anion gap on Day 7: This mild abnormality is caused by low albumin.

Hyperbilirubinemia, decreasing over time: The inflammatory leukogram and cholestatic enzyme changes parallel the trend in bilirubin over time, supporting the idea that cholestasis is the cause of hyperbilirubinemia rather than hemolysis.

Elevated ALP and GGT: The ALP and GGT are appropriately decreasing after surgical correction of the cause for the cholestasis.

Elevated ALT and AST: As expected, resolution of the cholestatic process and appropriate medical therapy for any infectious component of the liver disease is leading to a decrease in the ALT and AST. A rapid fall of greater than 50% in ALT over a few days is often noted to be a positive prognostic indicator, although scarcity of viable hepatocytes can also be responsible for this change. Hepatocellular enzyme levels in the blood are nearly normal by Day 7.

Abdominal fluid: Because the fluid analysis is compatible with inflammation, a bacterial culture is recommended although no organisms were noted on cytology. The absence of bile pigment and a fluid bilirubin concentration similar to that of the plasma argues for an intact biliary tree at this time.

Coagulation profile: The coagulopathy appears to be improving along with the resolution of inflammation and decreasing liver enzymes and bilirubin, further substantiating a diagnosis of DIC. Impairment of liver function is generally severe by the time prolonged PT and APTT can be attributed to decreased coagulation factor production by the liver. Improvement in PT and APTT should not be interpreted as evidence of normal liver function.

Even though no specific tests of liver function were performed, Kabob's clinical chemistry profile was very suggestive for decreased liver function along with cholestasis and hepatocellular damage. She was discharged from the hospital 10 days after surgery with continuing medical therapy.

Kabob's blood work should be compared with Yap Yap (Case 7), who had a portosystemic shunt with decreased liver function. Yap Yap also had hypoglycemia, hypoalbuminemia (although globulins were normal, making hemorrhage less of a competing differential diagnosis), and isosthenuria. Yap Yap also had hypocholesterolemia, which is a less consistent feature of severely impaired liver function than some of the other abnormalities. Concurrent cholestasis may have upregulated Kabob's cholesterol production into the normal reference range. Despite decreased liver function, Yap Yap had a normal bilirubin, while Kabob had hyperbilirubinemia which could be attributed to several other factors in addition to poor hepatic function. No coagulation studies were peformed on Yap Yap for comparison. Note that Nutmeg (Case 16) also had liver disease, however there were no indicators of impaired liver function on the clinical chemistry profile. This does not guarantee normal liver function, however liver function is not always abnormal even if there is significant hepatic pathology.

Rothuizen J, Meyer HP. History, physical examination, and signs of liver disease. In: In: Textbook of Veterinary Internal Medicine 5th ed. Ettinger and Feldman eds. 2000. W.B.Saunders Company, Philadelphia, PA. pp 1272-1277.

GI Case 22 – Level 3

"Jimbo" is an 8-month-old male Labrador cross who presented because of pronounced lethargy and depression. The owners report that Jimbo vomited about 5 times over the past 3 days and they discovered several coins in one of the piles of vomitus. Jimbo now has pale, icteric mucous membranes and his abdomen is painful. Jimbo is febrile, and premature ventricular complexes are observed on electrocardiogram. He has a history of seizures for which he currently takes phenobarbital and potassium bromide.

White blood cell count:	↑ 32.6 10⁹/L	(4.9-17.0)
Segmented neutrophils:	↑ 29.3 x 10⁹/L	(3.0-11.5)
Band neutrophils:	0 x 10⁹/L	(0-0.3)
Lymphocytes:	1.3 x 10⁹/L	(1.0-4.8)
Monocytes:	↑ 2.0 x 10⁹/L	(0.2-1.5)
Eosinophils:	0 x 10⁹/L	(0-1.3)
Nucleated RBC/100 WBC:	↑ 20	
Plasma appearance: marked hemolysis		
Hematocrit:	↓ 17%	(39-55)
Red blood cell count:	↓ 2.11 x 10¹²/L	(5.5-8.5)
Hemoglobin:	↓ 5.0 g/dl	(12.0-18.0)
MCV:	↑ 79.0 fl	(60.0-77.0)
MCHC:	↓ 29.4 g/dl	(31.0-34.0)
RBC morphology: Heinz bodies present and confirmed with New Methylene Blue stain. Rare spherocytes are noted. There is mild polychromasia.		
Platelets:	495.0 x 10⁹/L	(181.0-525.0)
Glucose:	↑ 417 mg/dl	(90.0-140.0)
BUN:	↑ 67 mg/dl	(8-33)
Creatinine:	1.3 mg/dl	(0.6-2.0)

Phosphorus:	↑ 8.2 mg/dl	(2.6-7.2)
Calcium:	10.0 mg/dl	(8.8-11.0)
Magnesium:	2.5 mEq/L	(1.7-2.5)
Total Protein:	5.8 g/dl	(4.8-7.2)
Albumin:	↓ 2.6 g/dl	(2.8-4.0)
Globulin:	3.2 g/dl	(2.0-4.0)
Sodium:	143 mEq/L	(140-151)
Chloride:	↓ 102 mEq/L	(105-126)
Potassium:	↓ 3.7 mEq/L	(3.8-5.4)
HCO3:	17 mEq/L	(15-28)
Total Bili:	*Invalid	(0.10-0.50)
ALP:	*Invalid	(20-320)
ALT:	↑ 351 IU/L	(10-95)
AST:	↑ 239 IU/L	(16-54)
Cholesterol:	131 mg/dl	(110-314)
Triglycerides:	36 mg/dl	(30-321)
Amylase:	↑ 2094 IU/L	(400-1200)
Lipase:	143 IU/L	(53-770)

Note: Because the specimen is markedly hemolyzed, total protein and albumin may be falsely elevated; GGT, total bilirubin, and ALP are invalid.

Coagulation		
PT:	↑ 12.0s	(6.2-9.3)
APTT:	↑ 64.9s	(8.9-16.3)
FDP:	↑ >20 µg/ml	(<5)

Interpretation
CBC
Leukogram: Jimbo has a mature neutrophilic leukocytosis and monocytosis suggestive for inflammation. Although the inflammation cannot be precisely localized based on the available data, the history and clinical chemistry profile indicates the gastrointestinal tract, liver, and pancreas are potential sites for initial evaluation.

Erythrogram: Jimbo has a marked macrocytic, hypochromic, likely regenerative anemia with increased numbers of nucleated erythroid precursors released into the circulation as part of the regenerative response. A reticulocyte count could be performed to quantify the response. Heinz bodies indicate oxidative damage to erythrocytes as a cause for the hemolysis. In dogs, exposure to onions (raw or cooked), vitamin K, methylene blue, copper and zinc are all potential causes of oxidative damage and Heinz body formation. Spherocytosis is most often associated with immune-mediated damage to erythrocytes, however some toxicities such as some snake venoms and zinc have been reported to cause spherocytes as well.

Plasma: The plasma is markedly hemolyzed. This may occur artifactually or with intravascular hemolysis. Heinz bodies and spherocytes suggest oxidative damage or immune mediated causes for intravascular hemolysis in this case. The combination of spherocytes and Heinz bodies is compatible with zinc intoxication. Icteric mucous membranes suggest hyperbilirubinemia, although this cannot be confirmed because serum bilirubin is not available. Some component of extravascular hemolysis or processing of the heme released in intravascular hemolysis will elevate serum bilirubin. Elevations in hepatocellular enzymes suggest that there is the potential for decreased liver function or cholestasis, however cholestatic enzymes are not available on this panel, nor have specific tests of liver function such as ammonia or serum bile acids been performed. Because of the affinity of bile pigments for connective tissue, clinical icterus may persist beyond when hyperbilirubinemia can be documented on the serum biochemistry profile.

Serum Biochemical Profile

Hyperglycemia: Corticosteroid or epinephrine effects may promote hyperglycemia, however this degree of hyperglycemia would be unusual for stress alone in the dog. Causes of insulin resistance that might exacerbate the hyperglycemia such as hyperadrenocorticism could be considered. While an ALP may be helpful to evaluate this possibility since most dogs with hyperadrenocorticism have elevated ALP levels, interpretation may be confounded by increased ALP secondary to bone growth in a young dog or induction from endogenous corticosteroids in a sick animal. Repeat measurements or long-term indicators of glycemic control such as fructosamine or glycated hemoglobin may be necessary to determine if this patient has diabetes mellitus. Diabetes mellitus is often associated with hypercholesterolemia and increased serum triglycerides, which are not noted in this profile.

Increased BUN with normal serum creatinine: A concurrent urinalysis is required for definitive interpretation of these values and is not available for this case. Nephropathy may be induced by marked hemoglobinuria in some cases. BUN may also increase prior to creatinine in early pre-renal azotemia because of the relatively greater influence of tubular flow rates on the elimination of urea compared to creatinine. When the BUN is elevated but the serum creatinine is within reference range, extra-renal factors need to be assessed. High protein diet, gastrointestinal hemorrhage, fever, and tissue necrosis are other extra-renal causes of increased BUN that should be ruled out in this case.

Mild hyperphosphatemia with normal calcium: The primary differentials for the mild hyper-phosphatemia in this case are bone growth in a young dog and/or hemolysis. Bone bone growth in young large breed dogs may elevate serum phosphorus as will lytic bone lesions, and the patient should be evaluated for evidence of lameness or bone pain. Serum ALP levels may be helpful in evaluating this possibility, however this data is unavailable due to hemolysis of the sample. Decreased glomerular filtration rate is a common cause of hyper-phosphatemia in adult dogs. Typically, the phosphorus will increase as a patient becomes azotemic, and the high BUN is compatible with decreased glomerular filtration rate. However, both the increased BUN and elevated phosphorus could result from tissue trauma or necrosis. Hemolysis itself can increase serum phosphorus because of the high content of phosphorus in erythrocytes. A similar mechanism involving release of phosphorus from lymphoblasts or myeloblasts has been implicated in the hyperphosphatemia associated with the tumor lysis syndrome, which would be highly unusual in an eight-month-old and is rarely observed in adult dogs. Likewise, vitamin D toxicity and primary hypoparathyroidism are less common causes of hyperphosphatemia and are unlikely in this patient because they are often associated with hypocalcemia. Iatrogenic causes of hyperphosphatemia include administration of intravenous phosphate or phosphate containing enemas, however this is not compatible with the medical history. For a more complete discussion of abnormalities of calcium and phosphorus see Chapter 6.

Hypoalbuminemia: Low serum albumin can result from either decreased production or increased losses. Decreased hepatic production of albumin can occur as part of the acute phase response, which is supported by the inflammatory leukogram. Low albumin production secondary to liver failure is possible, however liver function appears adequate to support gluconeogenesis and cholesterol production (remember that these are not good tests of liver function). Prolonged coagulation times could also be attributed to impaired production of coagulation factors secondary to decreased liver function. A liver function test such as serum bile acids or serum ammonia could be performed. Decreased production may result from starvation, which is not compatible with the clinical history. Increased losses of albumin include third space, cutaneous, interstitial, gastrointestinal, and renal. Examination of the patient for effusions and edema along with urine protein measurements could assist in ruling out various sources of loss. Gastrointestinal losses of protein are more difficult to quantify, however measurement of fecal alpha-1-proteinase inhibitor has been suggested as a potential marker of protein loss into the gut. It is lost into the intestinal lumen with increased mucosal permeability, however unlike many other proteins, alpha-1-proteinase inhibitor resists degradation by gut proteases sufficiently that it may be measured in the feces.

Mild hypochloremia: Hypochloremia with normal serum sodium concentration suggests vomiting of gastric contents, consistent with Jimbo's history. Abnormalities of serum chloride may occur with acid/base abnormalities, however the HCO_3 is within reference range in this profile. In general, the chloride varies inversely with HCO_3, however this relationship is not consistent in mixed acid/base abnormalities. Blood gas analysis is required to fully characterize acid/base status, however this test is not necessary to proceed with treatment in this case. Use of diuretics such a furosemide or thiazides can cause wasting, but again is not present in Jimbo's history.

Mild hypokalemia: Increased gastrointestinal losses and low intake because of anorexia contribute to this electrolyte abnormality. Diuresis caused by diabetes mellitus can lead to renal potassium wasting. Hyperglycemia with hyperinsulinemia can cause intracellular translocation of potassium and may be a factor given Jimbo's serum glucose. Similarly, potassium will enter cells in response to alkalemia. Most potassium in the body is intracellular, and low serum potassium does not always accurately reflect total body potassium status. As with chloride, diuretic use can increase renal potassium loss.

Increased serum ALT and AST: Mild to moderate increases in these enzymes may occur with hepatocellular damage, however AST is less tissue specific and muscle damage as well as hemolysis can increase this value. There are several candidate causes for hepatocellular damage in Jimbo's case: hypoxia or hypoperfusion of hepatocytes secondary to anemia and dehydration, local changes in perfusion or increased exposure to toxins or inflammatory cytokines associated with intestinal disease (vomiting) or pancreatic disease (increased amylase), and exposure to exogeneous toxins or drugs (including phenobarbital or corticosteroids). The potential for hepatocellular damage to occur secondary to cholestasis cannot be evaluated because ALP, GGT and total bilirubin are invalidated by hemolysis. Extrahepatic metabolic processes such as diabetes and hyperadrenocorticism also elevate serum liver enzyme activities. As is often the case, the non-specific nature of liver enzyme activities in the blood of dogs necessitates interpreting the data in the context of other clinical and pathological data; cytology or biopsy may be required for specific diagnosis. Hemolysis may cause release of these enzymes from erythrocytes. Please see Chapter 2 for a more comprehensive discussion of liver enzyme interpretation.

Mild hyperamylasemia with normal lipase: Both of these enzymes are considered to be markers of pancreatic damage, however they are not produced exclusively by that organ. The activities of both enzymes may increase in the blood up to two to four times the upper limit of the reference interval with decreased glomerular filtration rate, which may be a factor here, given the elevated BUN and phosphorus. Vomiting and dehydration could be a cause for pre-renal impairment of glomerular filtration rate, or could be compatible with other pancreatic or intestinal diseases that can elevate serum amylase. Although in theory, changes in amylase and lipase should occur simultaneously in response to pancreatic damage, the reality is that in clinical patients there is often discordance between them. Some authors indicate that lipase is a superior test for pancreatitis (Brobst), however some dogs with confirmed pancreatitis fail to show elevations in serum lipase (Strombeck). Based on a variety of recent studies, various authors have advocated the measurement of canine trypsin-like immunoreactivity, canine pancreatic lipase immunoreactivity (Steiner), and plasma trypsinogen activation peptide concentration (Mansfield) for the diagnosis of pancreatitis in dogs with elevated pancreatic enzymes and clinical signs of gastrointestinal disease. None of these tests appears to have ideal sensitivity and specificity under all conditions, and the diagnosis of pancreatitis continues to rely on identifying a convincing combination of clinical signs, laboratory abnormalities, and imaging data.

Coagulation data: Prolonged PT and APTT suggest abnormalities of secondary hemostasis involving both the intrinsic and extrinsic pathways and/or the common pathway. In combination with evidence of increased fibrinolysis (FDP >20 μg/ml), a mixed hemostatic disorder such as disseminated intravascular coagulation is possible despite the normal platelet count. Decreased liver function could also impair production of clotting factors and slow elimination of fibrin degradation products, however no specific tests of liver function are available at this time.

Case Summary and Outcome
Shortly after admission, Jimbo experienced cardiopulmonary arrest. He was resuscitated and briefly maintained on a ventilator, however he died half an hour later. No necropsy was performed, but based on his laboratory work, the clinical history of having vomited coins, zinc toxicity was the presumptive cause of death.

Animals may be exposed to zinc in batteries, paints, cosmetics, wood preservatives, zippers, board game pieces and hardware in addition to pennies minted 1983 or afterward. While metallic zinc is poorly reactive, solubilization by acid in the stomach leads to absorption and toxicity. Toxic effects include direct irritation to the gastric mucosa (which may be exacerbated by the presence of foreign bodies), altered metabolism because of zinc's interference with other ions such as cadmium, calcium, copper, and iron, and anemia secondary to impaired erythrocyte production and hemolysis. The exact mechanisms for hemolysis are not always clear, however inhibition of red blood cell enzymes (especially those protecting the cell from oxidative damage), membrane damage, and hapten-induced immune destruction have been suggested (Cahill-Morasco). Therefore, both Heinz bodies and spherocytes may be seen in patients with zinc toxicosis. Because of the presence of spherocytes, hemolysis, and a regenerative anemia, immune-mediated hemolytic anemia may be a differential diagnosis. Coombs' testing may be POSITIVE in zinc toxicosis patients in the absence of a primary immune mediated disease because of non-specific adsorption of proteins to red blood cell membranes that have been damaged by the zinc, or because of the presence of zinc on the red blood cell surface.

Zinc may cause hepatocellular and pancreatic damage, leading to elevations in ALP, ALT, AST, amylase and lipase. Toxic damage could be compounded by poor oxygenation of tissues associated with severe anemia and inadequate perfusion from dehydration and low cardiac output resulting from the arrhythmia. Increased BUN and phosphorus, and possible elevated amylase could result from kidney damage associated with heavy metal intoxication or toxic effects of hemoglobin. Pre-renal azotemia from dehydration is also a possibility given the history of vomiting; because the patient is anemic and may have liver disease, the packed cell volume and albumin do not necessarily reflect hydration status and clinical indicators must be used. A urine specific gravity is needed to assess urinary concentrating ability, and the red urine noted in the history is likely to be hemoglobinuria from the hemolysis. Granular casts are occasionally noted in urine samples from zinc toxicosis patients because of renal tubular necrosis. Jimbo is likely to have glucosuria since the renal tubular threshold for glucose reabsorption has been exceeded, however renal tubular dysfunction can lead to glucosuria even in normoglycemic patients (this has been observed in patients with lead poisoning). Glucosuria will occur regardless of the cause of the hyperglycemia and the subsequent osmotic diuresis could interfere with Jimbo's urinary concentrating ability, therefore a finding of isosthenuria should be interpreted with caution.

Prolongations of the PT and APTT have been described with zinc toxicosis; zinc may directly or indirectly interfere with the enzymatic functions of the coagulation proteins.

Brobst DF. Pancreatic Function. In JJ Kaneko, JW Harvey, and ML Bruss (eds): Clinical Biochemistry of Domestic Animals, 5th ed. San Diego, CA. Academic Press, 1997, p 353-366.

Cahil-Morasco R and DePasquale MA. Zinc toxicosis in small animals. Compend Contin Educ Pract Vet 2002;24:712-719.

Mansfield CS, Jones BR. Trypsinogen activation peptide in the diagnosis of canine pancreatitis. J Vet Int Med 2000;14:346

Steiner JM. Broussard J, Mansfield CS, GHumminger SR, Williams, DA. Serum canine pancreatic lipase immunoreactivity (cPLI) concentrations in dogs with spontaneous pancreatitis. J Vet Int Med 2001;15:274.

Steiner JM, Williams DA. Development and validation of a radioimmunoassay for the measurement of canine pancreatic lipase immunoreactivity in serum of dogs. Am J Vet Res 2003;64:1237-1241.

Strombreck DR, Farver T, Kaneko JJ. Serum amylase activities in the diagnosis of pancreatitis in dogs. AM J Vet Res 1981; 42:1966-1970.

Overview

Step 1: Rule out any processing abnormalities that could influence your data, such as prolonged in vitro contact of serum with cells (Case 3).

Step 2: Consider temporary physiological states that may influence an analyte such as a recent meal (hypertriglyceridemia in Case 1), stress (hyperglycemia in Case 2), or dehydration (hyperamylasemia). CBC data may provide supportive data such as a corticosteroid or epinephrine leukogram for stress or polycythemia, or hyperalbuminemia and prerenal azotemia for dehydration.

Step 3: Endocrinopathies are important causes for abnormalities of glucose, cholesterol, and triglyceride. This was also true for abnormalities of liver enzymes. Carefully screen the CBC and biochemical profile data for other abnormalities that would suggest an endocrinopathy such as hypothyroidism (Case 10), hyperthyroidism, hypoadrenocorticism (Case 12), hyperadrenocorticism (Case 17), or diabetes mellitus (Case 18, 19, 20). Additional testing is often required to confirm the presence of an endocrinopathy.

Step 4: Evaluate organs known to influence these analytes for evidence of pathology. Specifically, liver disease can result in abnormalities of glucose, cholesterol, and triglycerides (Case 7, 21). Pancreatic disease can also impact these analytes, in addition to causing elevations in serum amylase and lipase (Case 13, 14, 15). Remember to consider the close relationship between the pancreas and liver as pathology may be present in both organs (Case 16). Renal disease can cause increases in amylase and lipase (Case 20, 21) and can be associated with altered lipid metabolism (see Chapter 5). As seen in step 3, further testing beyond the CBC, serum biochemical profile, and urinalysis are often required to confirm a specific diagnosis.

Step 5: Some types of neoplasia (Case 4, 5, 6, 13, 14), systemic infections (Case 8, 9), or medications and toxins (Case 11, possible Case 21) may influence analytes.

Chapter 4

Serum Proteins

Review of Proteins

Albumin makes up approximately 35-50% of the total serum protein in most domestic animals. It is synthesized in the liver and functions as a storage pool of protein and transporter of amino acids. In addition, albumin acts as a general binding and transport protein that can prevent loss of constituents via the kidneys. Albumin accounts for approximately 75% of the osmotic activity of the plasma because it is small and abundant.

Globulin proteins account for the majority of the non-albumin protein measured in the blood. When separated by electrophoresis, alpha globulins include lipoproteins and some acute phase reactants. Beta globulins include other acute phase reactants and some immunoglobulins, while gamma globulins are predominantly immunoglobulins.

Measurement of Serum Proteins

Several methods are available to the clinician for measurement of serum proteins. A common screening method used in practice is refractometry. This method is based on the refraction of light as it passes through materials of different densities and it really measures TOTAL SOLIDS, which includes total protein (which make up most of the total solids), electrolytes, glucose, urea, and lipids. In health, the total solids are somewhat higher than the total protein of serum or plasma, but conversion factors in the refractometer account for the difference under normal circumstances. These corrections may not be accurate in disease states, and methodologic issues may account for differences between the "total protein" measured using a refractometer and that measured using an automated chemistry analyzer. Therefore, we consider refractometry to be an estimate of the total protein.

Automated chemistry analyzers can usually measure total protein and albumin, and then calculate globulin proteins as the difference between the two. These analyzers measure colored complexes between proteins and reagents. Total protein measurement is typically accomplished by measuring protein-copper complexes, while albumin measurement is determined by measuring albumin binding of dyes such as bromcresol green (BCG). Binding affinities vary by type of protein and species of the patient, and so these measurements are also subject to some methodologic variability, but are more accurate than refractometry and allow fractionation of albumin and globulin proteins.

Serum protein electrophoresis separates various classes of proteins by size and charge and is superior to both refractometry and automated chemistry analyzers for protein determination. The cost and time required for serum protein electrophoresis make it less practical for most purposes, and it is primarily performed to distinguish polyclonal and monoclonal gammopathies in patients who may have lymphoid neoplasms.

Interpretation of Serum Protein Data

Like many analytes, protein measurements reflect the sum of production, loss, and dilution or concentration as a consequence of hydration status. Therefore, when considering abnormalities of protein in a clinical patient, factors influencing production, potential sources of loss, and hydration must all be considered. In some instances, combinations of abnormalities may result in an albumin or globulin value within the reference interval despite marked changes in production, loss and/or hydration status. Albumin and globulins should be considered separately, since different factors may influence their handling by the body.

Hyperalbuminemia: Reflects excessive loss of fluid compared with protein and should be interpreted as evidence of dehydration and hemoconcentration since the liver does not over-produce albumin.

Hypoalbuminemia: Hemodilution in fluid retaining states such as pregnancy, heart failure, or iatrogenic fluid overload.

Decreased production
  Liver failure

  Downregulation of production because albumin is a negative acute phase reactant

  Starvation if chronic or severe and associated with poor body condition (increased use of albumin as a fuel and source of protein also contributes)

Increased losses
  Selective loss of albumin via the glomerulus (globulins may be normal or increased)

  Concurrent loss of albumin and globulin (globulins may be low, normal, or high depending on the presence of any factors that increase production)
    Hemorrhage
    Gastrointestinal loss
    Third space losses into body cavities
    Third space loss into interstitium
    Exudative dermal loss

Increased breakdown/utilization secondary to surgery, trauma, fever, starvation and other catabolic states

Hyperglobulinemia Dehydration (hemoconcentration)

Increased production
  Inflammation can increase production of acute phase reactants and/or immunoglobulins. This is typically a polyclonal increase, however infectious diseases such as feline infectious peritonitis, tick borne diseases, or leishmania rarely can cause a monoclonal gammopathy

  Neoplastic processes such as lymphoma or multiple myeloma can cause the production of excessive amounts of a single immunoglobulin, causing a monoclonal, or less often a biclonal gammpathy.

  Globulin levels may increase just prior to production of colostrum.

Hypoglobulinemia Hemodilution

Decreased production
  Rarely associated with starvation

  Rarely associated with congenital disorders of the immune system

Failure of transfer of passive immunity (This is really decreased "acquisition")

Non-selective protein loss
  Hemorrhage
  Gastrointestinal loss
  Third space losses into body cavities
  Third space loss into interstitium
  Exudative dermal loss

Case 1 – Level 1

"Belinda" is a 6-year-old spayed female German Shepherd dog with a history of unilateral hip replacement for hip dysplasia. Belinda has presented three times within the last year for vomiting and diarrhea related to dietary indiscretion. She presented again today for vomiting associated with getting into the garbage last night. On physical examination, Belinda is quiet and alert. She is very thin with a dull haircoat. No abnormalities or pain are noted on abdominal palpation. Mucous membranes are slightly tacky but pink.

White blood cell count:	9.0 x 10^9/L	(6.0-17.0)
Segmented neutrophils:	6.1 x 10^9/L	(3.0-11.0)
Band neutrophils:	0.0 x 10^9/L	(0-0.3)
Lymphocytes:	2.0 x 10^9/L	(1.0-4.8)
Monocytes:	0.6 x 10^9/L	(0.2-1.4)
Eosinophils:	0.3 x 10^9/L	(0-1.3)
WBC morphology: No abnormalities seen		
Hematocrit:	38%	(37-55)
RBC morphology: Normal		
Platelets:	250.0 x 10^9/L	(200-450)
Glucose:	85 mg/dl	(65.0-120.0)
BUN:	9 mg/dl	(8-33)
Creatinine:	↓ 0.4 mg/dl	(0.5-1.5)
Phosphorus:	5.0 mg/dl	(3.0-6.0)
Calcium:	↓ 8.5 mg/dl	(8.8-11.0)
Magnesium:	1.6 mEq/L	(1.4-2.2)
Total Protein:	6.0 g/dl	(4.7-7.3)
Albumin:	↓ 2.5 g/dl	(3.0-4.2)
Globulin:	3.5 g/dl	(2.0-4.0)
A/G Ratio:	0.7	(0.7-2.1)
Sodium:	150 mEq/L	(140-163)
Chloride:	120 mEq/L	(105-126)
Potassium:	4.0 mEq/L	(3.8-5.4)
HCO3:	26.0 mEq/L	(16-28)
Total Bili:	0.1 mg/dl	(0.10-0.50)
ALP:	103 IU/L	(20-320)
GGT:	5 IU/L	(2-10)
ALT:	51 IU/L	(10-86)
AST:	30 IU/L	(15-52)
Cholesterol:	115 mg/dl	(110-314)
Amylase:	738 IU/L	(400-1200)

Interpretation

CBC: No abnormalities are noted.

Serum Biochemical Profile

Low creatinine: The low creatinine reflects Belinda's poor body condition and decreased muscle mass.

Hypocalcemia: This mild change is likely related to the hypoalbuminemia.

Hypoalbuminemia: Decreased production and increased losses contribute to low serum albumin levels. Decreased production in this case may be related to nutritional factors given Belinda's poor body condition. Decreased liver function is possible and may be specifically evaluated by performing serum bile acid testing; however there are no other serum biochemical abnormalities that would suggest liver disease. Increased losses should also be considered with protein loss through the gut as a possible route given Belinda's history of gastrointestinal issues. No effusions or extensive skin lesions are noted on the physical examination. A urinalysis should be considered to rule out glomerular loss of albumin since globulins are within the normal reference interval.

Case Summary and Outcome

Upon further questioning regarding Belinda's history, it was revealed that her owner severely restricted her food intake based on recommendations made at the time of her hip replacement to "keep her lean." In this case, hypoalbuminemia appears to be related to inadequate nutritional plane, and the repeated episodes of dietary indiscretion were due to Belinda's efforts to get more food. The owner was given a plan to slowly increase Belinda's food intake to an adequate level. Eventually Belinda achieved a healthy body weight with improvement in the quality of her coat and resolution of her laboratory abnormalities. The next year, when Belinda presented to the hospital for heartworm testing and preventive, she was overweight, but she appeared happy and had not eaten garbage in over a year.

Hypoalbuminemia in domestic animals on adequate commercial diets is rarely nutritional in origin. The author has most frequently noted nutritional hypoalbuminemia in cases of animal neglect or abandonment, although other patients with diseases causing severe or prolonged anorexia may develop hypoalbuminemia, particularly if there are concurrent losses or increased demand for protein. In starved animals, hypoalbuminemia may be accompanied by low BUN and/or creatinine, while patients often are able to maintain blood glucose levels if liver function is adequate. Belinda may be compared with Chapter 5, Case 3 (Marsali), in which a neglected horse presented with hypoalbuminemia related to nutritional factors. That horse was also hyperglobulinemic, suggesting that there may have been some downregulation of albumin production in response to inflammation in addition to starvation. Chapter 6, Case 16 (Diva) describes a missing cat who lost approximately half her body weight. Despite this extreme nutritional deprivation, Diva's blood glucose and albumin were within reference intervals at presentation. Her albumin level did drop just slightly below reference range after correction of her marked dehydration.

Case 2 – Level 1

"Dylan" is a 2-year-old neutered male Yorkshire Terrier. About 8 months ago, Dylan began to appear weak and lethargic. He had episodes of vomiting digested and undigested food and diarrhea that appeared to be responsive to antibiotic treatment. Last month, Dylan had surgery for removal of ammonium biurate cystoliths. The owner reports that Dylan is polyuric and polydipsic. Dylan has no abnormalities on physical examination.

White blood cell count:	↑ 14.8 x 10⁹/L	(4.0-13.3)
Segmented neutrophils:	10.2 x 10⁹/L	(2.1-11.2)
Band neutrophils:	0.0 x 10⁹/L	(0-0.3)
Lymphocytes:	3.3 x 10⁹/L	(1.0-4.5)
Monocytes:	0.3 x 10⁹/L	(0.2-1.4)
Eosinophils:	1.0 x 10⁹/L	(0-1.2)
Basophils:	0.0 x 10⁹/L	
WBC morphology: Within normal limits		

Hematocrit:	40%	(37-60)
Red blood cell count:	6.83 x 10¹²/L	(5.5-8.5)
Hemoglobin:	13.0 g/dl	(12.0-18.0)
MCV:	↓ 58.5 fl	(64.0-73.0)
MCHC:	↓ 32.4	(33.6-36.6)
RBC morphology: 2+ anisocytosis, 1+ polychromasia, 3+ target cells		

Platelets:	227 x 10⁹/L	(200-450)

Glucose:	↓ 64 mg/dl	(80.0-125.0)
BUN:	10 mg/dl	(8-33)
Creatinine:	0.7 mg/dl	(0.6-1.5)
Phosphorus:	5.4 mg/dl	(5.0-9.0)
Calcium:	10.3 mg/dl	(8.8-11.0)
Total Protein:	5.1 g/dl	(4.8-7.2)
Albumin:	↓ 2.3 g/dl	(2.5-3.7)
Globulin:	2.8 g/dl	(2.0-4.0)
Sodium:	151 mEq/L	(140-151)
Chloride:	120 mEq/L	(105-120)
Potassium:	4.4 mEq/L	(3.8-5.4)
HCO3:	25 mEq/L	(16-28)
Anion Gap:	10.4 mEq/L	(6-16)
Total Bili:	0.4 mg/dl	(0.10-0.40)
ALP:	91 IU/L	(20-320)
GGT:	7 IU/L	(0-7)
ALT:	↑ 186 IU/L	(10-86)
AST:	↑ 96 IU/L	(16-54)
Cholesterol:	162 mg/dl	(110-314)
Amylase:	502 IU/L	(400-1200)

Interpretation

CBC: The mild leukocytosis is not likely to be clinically significant because individual types of leukocytes all fall within reference intervals and there are no morphologic abnormalities that suggest inflammation or antigenic stimulation. Dylan is not anemic, however his erythrocytes are microcytic and mildly hypochromic. Microcytosis is most often associated with either portosystemic shunts or iron deficiency. A low MCHC may be associated with incomplete hemoglobinization of reticulocytes or low hemoglobin content because iron is not available to produce it. The presence of target cells and absence of red cell fragments or thrombocytosis could be more compatible with liver disease than with iron deficiency, however these are weak associations and further testing may be necessary to determine the cause of the microcytosis and hypochromasia.

Serum Biochemical Profile

Hypoglycemia: In patients with no clinical signs of hypoglycemia, artifactual hypoglycemia due to processing errors should be ruled out by measuring glucose on a freshly collected sample with prompt separation of serum from cells. After processing error, the most likely cause for low blood glucose in this case is decreased liver function, possibly related to a portosystemic shunt. Nutritional factors should not be an issue since Dylan has adequate body condition. Dylan would be unusually young for paraneoplastic hypoglycemia. Sepsis is unlikely in a dog presenting with a normal physical examination and CBC parameters.

Hypoproteinemia with hypoalbuminemia: Hypoalbuminemia can be due to decreased production or increased losses. Because the liver is the site of albumin production, poor liver function, such as occurs with a portosystemic shunt, can cause hypoalbuminemia. Selective loss of albumin could occur with glomerular disease and should be considered because the owners do report polyuria and polydipsia. Again, polyuria and polydipsia may also be related to decreased liver function (See YapYap, Chapter 3, Case 7 for a mechanistic discussion). Urinalysis should detect proteinuria if renal protein loss is occurring, however performing a urine protein:creatinine ratio may be more sensitive if the urine is dilute. Recall that a normal BUN and creatinine are not sensitive indicators of kidney pathology, and protein losing nephropathy may exist with minimal to no elevations in these analytes (see Denver, this chapter, Case 5).

Mild increase in ALT and AST: These changes are mild and indicate hepatocellular damage. Because of close anatomic relationships, intestinal disease can lead to secondary involvement of the liver.

Case Summary and Outcome

The concurrent hypoglycemia, hypoalbuminemia, and ammonium biurate stone formation are compatible with decreased liver function; serum bile acids and imaging studies are indicated to further evaluate the potential for liver disease. Both fasted and fed serum bile acids were elevated. At surgery, a single extrahepatic portocaval shunt was identified and an ameroid constrictor was placed. Biopsy specimens collected at surgery were compatible with the presence of a shunt, but also indicated mild mixed inflammation in the periportal areas, which could contribute to the liver enzyme elevations. Dylan did well in the immediate post-operative period, but re-presented several days after discharge from the hospital for weakness, anorexia, and "twitching". He was slightly dehydrated at presentation. His laboratory work was unremarkable aside from a mild anemia, and his serum bile acids were within reference intervals. Dylan was treated with fluids, antibiotics and medications to control seizures, which occur rarely and for uncertain cause after surgical repair of portocaval shunts. Dylan was discharged and, several weeks after the last presentation, was doing well at home, other than occasional soft stools.

The combination of microcytosis and evidence of liver dysfunction (some combination of low glucose, BUN, albumin, cholesterol, prolonged coagulation times) and mildly elevated liver enzymes in a young dog should prompt consideration of a portosystemic shunt, particularly in a high risk breed. Dylan's case should be compared with other cases of portosystemic shunts to observe variability in laboratory abnormalities that may occur with this condition. Dylan and Pugsley (Chapter 5, Case 12) were microcytic, while YapYap (Chapter 3, Case 7) and Binar (Chapter 2, Case 12, a cat) had normal MCV. While all of these cases were characterized by hypoalbuminemia, only Dylan, YapYap, and Pugsley were hypoglycemic. All except for YapYap had at least one elevated liver enzyme, but serum bilirubin was normal in all cases. Only YapYap was hypocholesterolemic. BUN was low in all of the previous cases, but Dylan's BUN was within reference intervals.

Case 3 – Level 1

"Princess" is a 6-year-old intact female German Shepherd that was hit by a car. She presents in lateral recumbancy with thready pulses. She has at least eight broken ribs and is extremely painful. A quick PCV and total protein are within reference intervals at presentation. After fluid therapy and medication for pain, samples are drawn for CBC and serum biochemical profile.

White blood cell count:	↑ 34.2 x 10⁹/L	(6.0-16.3)
Segmented neutrophils:	↑ 32.1 x 10⁹/L	(3.0-11.0)
Band neutrophils:	0 x 10⁹/L	(0-0.3)
Lymphocytes:	↓ 0.7 x 10⁹/L	(1.0-4.8)
Monocytes:	↑ 1.4 x 10⁹/L	(0.2-1.4)
Eosinophils:	0.0 x 10⁹/L	(0-1.3)
Nucleated RBC/100 WBC: 1		
WBC morphology: Within normal limits		

Hematocrit:	↓ 26%	(37-55)
Red blood cell count:	↓ 3.88 x 10¹²/L	(5.5-8.5)
Hemoglobin:	↓ 8.7 g/dl	(12.0-18.0)
MCV:	66.8 fl	(60.0-77.0)
MCHC:	33.5 g/dl	(31.0-34.0)
RBC morphology: Within normal limits		

Platelets: Moderately decreased

Glucose:	75 mg/dl	(65.0-120.0)
BUN:	26 mg/dl	(8-33)
Creatinine:	1.9 mg/dl	(0.5-2.0)
Phosphorus:	↑ 8.6 mg/dl	(3.0-6.0)
Calcium:	↓ 8.6 mg/dl	(8.8-11.0)
Magnesium:	2.2 mEq/L	(1.4-2.7)
Total Protein:	↓ 3.2 g/dl	(5.5-7.8)
Albumin:	↓ 1.7 g/dl	(2.8-4.0)
Globulin:	↓ 1.5 g/dl	(2.3-4.2)
A/G Ratio:	1.1	(0.7-2.1)
Sodium:	147 mEq/L	(140-151)
Chloride:	109 mEq/L	(105-120)
Potassium:	4.7 mEq/L	(3.8-5.4)
HCO3:	27 mEq/L	(16-28)

Anion Gap:	15.2 mEq/L	(15-25)
Total Bili:	0.2 mg/dl	(0.10-0.30)
ALP:	55 U/L	(20-121)
GGT:	10 IU/L	(2-10)
ALT:	↑ 1943 IU/L	(18-86)
AST:	↑ 2135 IU/L	(15-52)
Cholesterol:	83 mg/dl	(82-355)
Triglycerides:	50 mg/dl	(30-321)
Amylase:	967 IU/L	(400-1200)

Interpretation

CBC: Princess has a moderate mature neutrophilic leukocytosis with lymphopenia and monocytosis. Although inflammation is likely based on the degree of trauma, these findings can be explained by corticosteroid effects alone. There is a normocytic, normochromic anemia that does not appear to be regenerative at this time, however several days should be allowed for the marrow to respond to an acute episode of blood loss. Serial reticulocytes counts would resolve this issue. Thrombocytopenia may be attributable to consumption with hemorrhage.

Serum Biochemical Profile
Hyperphosphatemia and hypocalcemia: Tissue trauma or necrosis is the most likely cause for the increased serum phosphorus (leakage from cells), and is likely also causing some of the increase in AST. The hypocalcemia is most likely related to the hypoalbuminemia. Other differential diagnoses include renal disease (the patient is not currently azotemic) or hypoparathyroidism, which is possible but further diagnostic testing should not be pursued unless the abnormalities are persistent once the current presenting problem is resolved.

Panhypoproteinemia: Decreases in both albumin and globulins are evidence of non-selective protein losses. Of the many potential sites of protein loss, Princess is most likely to be hypoproteinemic secondary to hemorrhage associated with trauma. If the presentation is extremely acute, patients with significant hemorrhage may initially have normal serum total protein values because there has not been sufficient time for fluid shifts to occur that compensate for the hypovolemia. Albumin is also a storage pool protein that may be depleted if increased protein is required for tissue repair after trauma or surgery. With extensive tissue damage or vascular compromise, protein may move from the circulation into the interstitial space, further lowering serum albumin concentration.

Increased ALT and AST: Hepatocellular damage may be related to direct trauma of the liver, however perfusion deficits associated with hemorrhage and shock may contribute. While the increased ALT indicates that a significant amount of the increase in AST may be hepatic, this history of trauma and shock is also likely to result in damage to muscle and other tissues which may contain and release AST. A CK could be measured to assess the muscle component.

Case Summary and Outcome

Over the next few days, Princess began vomiting and developed hyperbilirubinemia and elevations in ALP and GGT, which indicated cholestatic disease in addition to or as the result of the initial hepatocellular damage (See Chapter 2 for further discussion of the relationship of these two processes). A week after presentation, the ALT and AST were almost within reference intervals, however the ALP and GGT remained elevated. At that time, schistocytes were noted on the blood film. Microangiopathic hemolysis was suspected based on the potential for severe tissue trauma and necrosis to result in activation of coagulation or even disseminated intravascular coagulation. Breakdown of extravasated RBCs may have been contributing to the hyperbilirubinemia. The coagulation panel was normal, however Princess was treated with anticoagulants because of the potential for the development of thrombosis. By 10 days after presentation, Princess appeared clinically improved and the bilirubin, ALP, and GGT levels were declining. She was discharged and had an uneventful recovery at home.

Case 4 – Level 1

"Red Molly" is a 12-year-old spayed female Cairn Terrier presenting for weight loss and flatulence. On presentation, Red Molly is well hydrated, with a mild sinus arrhythmia. The abdomen feels slightly doughy, but is non-painful. There is a grade I/IV patellar luxation on the right.

White blood cell count:	7.0 x 10⁹/L	(6.0-17.0)
Segmented neutrophils:	4.1 x 10⁹/L	(3.0-11.0)
Band neutrophils:	0.0 x 10⁹/L	(0-0.3)
Lymphocytes:	2.0 x 10⁹/L	(1.0-4.8)
Monocytes:	0.6 x 10⁹/L	(0.2-1.4)
Eosinophils:	0.3 x 10⁹/L	(0-1.3)
WBC morphology: No abnormalities seen		
Hematocrit:	45.2%	(37-55)
MCV:	70.9 fl	(64.0-73.0)
MCHC:	34.8 g/dl	(33.6-36.6)
RBC morphology: Normal		
Platelets:	450 x 10⁹/L	(200-450)
Glucose:	101 mg/dl	(65.0-120.0)
BUN:	9 mg/dl	(8-33)
Creatinine:	0.6 mg/dl	(0.5-1.5)
Phosphorus:	4.0 mg/dl	(3.0-6.0)
Calcium:	↓ 8.4 mg/dl	(8.8-11.0)
Magnesium:	1.9 mEq/L	(1.4-2.2)
Total Protein:	↓ 3.0 g/dl	(4.7-7.3)
Albumin:	↓ 1.5 g/dl	(3.0-4.2)
Globulin:	↓ 1.5 g/dl	(2.0-4.0)
A/G Ratio:	1.0	(0.7-2.1)
Sodium:	148 mEq/L	(140-163)
Chloride:	115 mEq/L	(105-126)
Potassium:	5.1 mEq/L	(3.8-5.4)
HCO3:	26.0 mEq/L	(16-28)
Anion Gap:	12.1 mEq/L	(10-20)
Total Bili:	0.1 mg/dl	(0.10-0.50)
ALP:	63 IU/L	(20-320)
GGT:	2 IU/L	(2-10)
ALT:	15 IU/L	(10-86)
AST:	25 IU/L	(15-52)
Cholesterol:	↓ 95 mg/dl	(110-314)
Amylase:	873 IU/L	(400-1200)

Urinalysis: Cystocentesis
Apperance: Yellow and clear
Urine specific gravity: 1.013
Negative for bilirubin, glucose, ketones, blood, protein
Sediment: inactive

Interpretation

CBC: No abnormalities

Serum Biochemical Profile

Hypocalcemia with normal phosphorus: The hypocalcemia may be due to the hypoalbuminemia, although low ionized calcium has been described in dogs with malabsorptive intestinal diseases due to the formation of calcium-fatty acid complexes in the intestinal lumen or decreased absorption of Vitamin D (Kull).

Panhypoproteinemia: While both decreased production and increased losses may contribute to low serum total protein, panhypoproteinemia is usually attributable to increased nonselective loss of protein. Red Molly does not have any evidence of hemorrhage, severe skin disease, or body cavity effusions, however she does present for gastrointestinal disease. Liver dysfunction could compound increased losses of albumin, and could also account for the hypocholesterolemia.

Hypocholesterolemia: This abnormalitiy is of limited clinical significance, but can be present with severe protein losing enteropathy, decreased liver function, or malnutrition.

Case Summary and Outcome

To confirm gastrointestinal loss of protein, three fecal samples were submitted for measurement of alpha 1 proteinase inhibitor. This is a protein that is generally not present in the gut of the dog, but when present, it cannot be degraded by intestinal bacteria. Red Molly's fecal alpha 1 proteinase activity levels were consistently high (mean 19.5 µg/g, reference interval 0-5.0), supporting increased intestinal permeability. Unfortunately, this test does not differentiate between the different types of intestinal lesions that can cause protein losing enteropathy. Protein losing enteropathy may occur secondary to congenital or acquired pathology. Acquired cases in dogs are often attributable to inflammation or neoplasia (German). Definitive diagnosis requires invasive procedures such as endoscopy or laparotomy with collection of biopsy samples for histologic examination (Melzer). Even with biopsy, inter-observer variation between pathologists' interpretations of biopsy samples can lead to confusion regarding diagnosis of intestinal disease (Willard), and these patients are at risk for complications including delayed healing due to low protein levels (Melzer). Red Molly's owners elected to try dietary management with hypoallergenic food prior to invasive procedures or medical therapy.

Red Molly is similar to the previous case (Princess), in that non-selective protein loss resulted in decreases in both albumin and globulins. The clinical history provided critical information about the likely sources of non-selective protein loss, which was supported somewhat by other laboratory data (anemia compatible with hemorrhage in Princess and hypocholesterolemia in Red Molly).

German AJ, Hall EJ, Day MJ. Chronic intestinal inflammation and intestinal disease in dogs. J Vet Intern Med 2003;17:8-20.

Kull PA, Hess RS, Craig LE, Saunders HM, Washabau RJ. Clinical, clinicopathologic, radiographic, and ultrasonagraphic characteristics of intestinal lymphangiectasia in dogs: 17 cases (1996-1998). J Am Vet Med Assoc 2001;219:197-202.

Melzer KJ, Sellon RK. Canine intestinal lymphangiectasia. Compend Contin Educ 2002;24:953-960.

Willard MD, Jergens AE, Duncan RB, Leib MS, McCracken MD, DeNovo RC, Helman RG, Slater MR, Harbison JL. Interobserver variation among histopathologic evaluations of intestinal tissues from dogs and cats. J Am Vet Med Assoc 2002;220:1177-1182.

Case 5 – Level 2

"Denver" is a 3-year-old spayed female Golden Retriever that presented for recent onset lameness and fever. On physical examination, Denver is bright and alert, moderately dehydrated, mildly febrile, and has edematous paws and generalized peripheral lymphadenopathy.

White blood cell count:	14.2 x 10⁹/L	(6.0-17.0)
Segmented neutrophils:	11.5 x 10⁹/L	(3.0-11.5)
Band neutrophils:	0 x 10⁹/L	(0-0.3)
Lymphocytes:	2.3 x 10⁹/L	(1.0-4.8)
Monocytes:	0.3 x 10⁹/L	(0.2-1.4)
Eosinophils:	0.1 x 10⁹/L	(0-1.3)
WBC morphology: No abnormalities seen		

Hematocrit:	↓ 30%	(39-55)
Red blood cell count:	↓ 4.48 x 10¹²/L	(5.5-8.5)
Hemoglobin:	↓ 11.1 g/dl	(14.0-19.0)
MCV:	71.3 fl	(60.0-75.0)
MCHC:	36.0 g/dl	(33.0-36.0)
RBC morphology: Normal		

Platelets: Moderately decreased

Plasma appears normal

Glucose:	90 mg/dl	(65.0-135.0)
BUN:	↑ 51 mg/dl	(8-33)
Creatinine:	1.6 mg/dl	(0.6-2.0)
Phosphorus:	7.0 mg/dl	(3.0-6.0)
Calcium:	9.2 mg/dl	(8.8-11.0)
Magnesium:	2.7 mEq/L	(1.4-2.7)
Total Protein:	↓ 4.8 g/dl	(5.2-7.2)
Albumin:	↓ 1.7 g/dl	(3.0-4.2)
Globulin:	3.1 g/dl	(2.0-4.0)
A/G Ratio:	↓ 0.5	(0.7-2.1)
Sodium:	151 mEq/L	(142-163)
Chloride:	119 mEq/L	(106-126)
Potassium:	4.5 mEq/L	(3.8-5.4)
HCO3:	24 mEq/L	(16-25)
Anion Gap:	12.5 mEq/L	(10-20)
Total Bili:	0.1 mg/dl	(0.10-0.50)
ALP:	66 IU/L	(12-121)
GGT:	3 IU/L	(1-10)
ALT:	9 IU/L	(10-95)
AST:	↑ 82 IU/L	(15-52)
Cholesterol:	274 mg/dl	(110-314)
Triglycerides:	72 mg/dl	(30-300)
Amylase:	↑ 1822 IU/L	(400-1200)

Coagulation Profile

PT:	7.1s	(6.2-9.3)
APTT:	↑ 16.7s	(8.9-16.3)

Urinalysis: Cystocentesis

Appearance: Yellow and clear
Urine specific gravity: 1.013
Negative for bilirubin, heme, glucose, ketones
Sediment: inactive
Urine protein: Creatinine ratio: 10.3

Lymph node aspirate (Figure 4-1): Numerous smears are submitted, however only two smears have sufficient numbers of intact cells for interpretation. >80% of cells are small, well differentiated lymphocytes. These are mixed with mature plasma cells, nondegenerate neutrophils, and scattered eosinophils. No etiologic agents are seen.

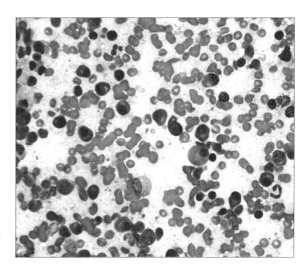

Figure 4-1. Cytology showing plasma cell hyperplasia in a lymph node from a dog.

Interpretation

CBC: Denver has thrombocytopenia and a mild normocytic normochromic nonregenerative anemia. Because Denver is thrombocytopenic, hemorrhage is a possible cause for anemia and the hypoproteinemia. This is less likely since, given sufficient time, blood loss anemias are generally regenerative and there is no history of bleeding. Anemia of chronic disease is likely, although the concurrent thrombocytopenia suggests the possibility of a bone marrow disorder resulting in decreased production of erythrocytes and platelets. Peripheral lymphadenopathy suggests the potential for hematopoietic neoplasia that may involve the marrow, however the results of the lymph node aspirate are more suggestive for a reactive process. Tick borne diseases may cause anemia, thrombocytopenia, and reactive lymphoid hyperplasia, and this patient should be evaluated for these diseases. Tick borne disease may cause thrombocytopenia either by suppressing production of platelets and/or increased destruction associated with vasculitis or immune-mediated processes. Immune-mediated thrombocytopenia (ITP) may be secondary to infectious disease, or it may be a primary idiopathic process. ITP could be considered if the work-up for infectious disease is negative. Peripheral consumption of platelets due to disseminated intravascular coagulation is unlikely because the PT and APTT are essentially normal. The slight increase in APTT is not considered clinically significant.

Serum Biochemical Profile

Mildly increased BUN with normal creatinine: Possible causes for disproportionately increased BUN in this patient include pre-renal azotemia, early renal failure, high protein diet or gastrointestinal hemorrhage. Denver is dehydrated, however he also has poorly concentrated urine, which is compatible with a combination of pre-renal azotemia with possible early renal failure. There does not appear to be any non-renal factors that would interfere with urinary concentrating ability at this time (e.g. osmotic diuresis, medullary washout, liver failure, etc.; see Chapter 5). Anemia, thrombocytopenia, and hypoproteinemia could be compatible with gastrointestinal hemorrhage, so careful evaluation for melena, hematochezia, and hematemesis is recommended.

Hypoproteinemia with hypoalbuminemia and normal globulins: Low serum levels of albumin may occur as a result of decreased production, increased losses, or a combination of the two. Albumin production may be low if there is severe prolonged starvation, if there is severe liver dysfunction, or in the presence of inflammatory disease because albumin is a negative acute phase reactant. Starvation is unlikely based on the physical examination. Liver dysfunction is also unlikely given the normal cholesterol, normal liver enzymes, increased BUN, and normal coagulation times, but specific tests of liver function have not been performed. Reactive lymphoid hyperplasia indicates the potential for antigenic stimulation, which could result in low albumin production and increased globulin production. Protein losses may be selective for albumin (glomerular losses) or non-selective (hemorrhage, gastrointestinal, dermal, third space, interstitial). In this case, the albumin is low and globulins are normal, suggesting selective glomerular protein loss, which is supported by the increased urinary protein:creatinine ratio in the absence of indicators of inflammation in the urinary tract (negative sediment). Non-selective protein losses may also be occurring, which could bring serum globulin levels back into the normal range despite increased production of acute phase reactants and/or immunoglobulins associated with inflammation. The edema noted in Denver's paws could be due to hypoalbuminemia or because vasculitis is increasing capillary permeability, leading to interstitial loss of protein.

Mildly increased AST: In the absence of any other enzyme elevations, the clinical significance of this value is uncertain. The normal ALT makes hepatocellular damage unlikely, so AST may reflect mild hemolysis or muscle damage.

Increased serum amylase: The increased amylase likely reflects decreased glomerular filtration rate. Pancreatitis cannot be ruled out, but clinical signs expected with pancreatitis are not obvious at this time.

Case Summary and Outcome

Denver was treated with intravenous fluids, angiotensin converting enzyme inhibitors, and antibiotics for tick borne diseases, even though serologic evaluation for Lyme disease, Ehrlichia, Rocky Mountain Spotted Fever, heartworm, and leptospirosis were all negative. Unfortunately, his kidney biopsy contained only fragments of medulla and no glomeruli were present to classify the renal disease histologically. Denver was fed a renal diet to help with long term management of kidney disease. Denver's joint pain was evaluated by the orthopedic staff, who felt that it was related to soft tissue swelling outside of the joints, with the exception of a possible partial cruciate tear on the right. Serum antithrombin III (ATIII) levels were also measured, and found to be low (47%, canine reference interval 75-120%). Antithrombin III is an endogeneous anticoagulant protein that is of a similar size as albumin and may be lost via the glomerulus in patients with protein losing nephropathy. Low ATIII predisposes patients to the formation of thrombi, so Denver was also treated with anticoagulants.

Case 6 – Level 2

"Snickers" is a 10-week-old male black Labrador puppy presenting with a 3 day history of anorexia, intermittent vomiting, and bloody diarrhea with mucus. He was adopted three weeks ago along with his sister, who is not sick. According to the owner, he has had one "set" of vaccinations. On physical examination, Snickers is depressed with pale mucous membranes. He has an episode of extremely bloody diarrhea on the examination table.

White blood cell count:	↓ 1.5 x 10⁹/L	(6.0-17.0)
Segmented neutrophils:	↓ 0.4 x 10⁹/L	(3.0-11.0)
Band neutrophils:	0 x 10⁹/L	(0-0.3)
Lymphocytes:	1.1 x 10⁹/L	(1.0-4.8)
Monocytes:	0.0 x 10⁹/L	(0.2-1.4)
Eosinophils:	0.0 x 10⁹/L	(0-1.3)

WBC morphology: No abnormalities seen

Hematocrit:	↓ 31%	(39-55)
Red blood cell count:	↓ 4.6 x 10¹²/L	(5.5-8.5)
Hemoglobin:	↓ 10.2 g/dl	(14.0-19.0)
MCV:	63.6 fl	(60.0-75.0)
MCHC:	33.0 g/dl	(33.0-36.0)

RBC morphology: Slight poikilocytosis

Platelets: Adequate

Plasma appears normal

Glucose:	122 mg/dl	(65.0-135.0)
BUN:	9 mg/dl	(8-33)
Creatinine:	↓ 0.2 mg/dl	(0.5-1.5)
Phosphorus:	↑ 7.2 mg/dl	(3.0-6.0)
Calcium:	9.4 mg/dl	(8.8-11.0)
Magnesium:	1.8 mEq/L	(1.4-2.7)
Total Protein:	↓ 3.7 g/dl	(5.2-7.2)
Albumin:	↓ 2.0 g/dl	(3.0-4.2)
Globulin:	↓ 1.7 g/dl	(2.0-4.0)
A/G Ratio:	1.2	(0.7-2.1)
Sodium:	↓ 136 mEq/L	(142-163)
Chloride:	↓ 100 mEq/L	(106-126)
Potassium:	3.8 mEq/L	(3.8-5.4)
HCO3:	↑ 26 mEq/L	(16-25)
Anion Gap:	13.8 mEq/L	(10-20)
Total Bili:	0.1 mg/dl	(0.10-0.50)
ALP:	↑ 131 IU/L	(12-121)
GGT:	3 IU/L	(1-10)
ALT:	46 IU/L	(10-95)
AST:	16 IU/L	(15-52)
Cholesterol:	181 mg/dl	(110-314)
Triglycerides:	89 mg/dl	(30-300)
Amylase:	378 IU/L	(400-1200)

Interpretation

CBC: Snickers has neutropenia and a mild normocytic normochromic nonregenerative anemia. The anemia is likely due, in part, to acute gastrointestinal hemorrhage. The neutropenia may be attributable to sepsis or severe acute inflammation in the gut, although there is no toxic change or left shift to help substantiate this interpretation. Because a bicytopenia is present, marrow disorders should also be considered. In such a young dog, toxic insults should be ruled out, including medication; however the most common cause of neutropenia in young dogs like Snickers is viral infection such as parvovirus. A parvovirus test is strongly recommended, while a bone marrow evaluation is not indicated at this time.

Serum Biochemical Profile
Low serum creatinine: This value may be related to low muscle mass in puppies.

Panhypoproteinemia: The most obvious cause of the hypoproteinemia in this patient is gastrointestinal loss, which is non-selective. Decreased production of albumin because of starvation or liver dysfunction is possible, however not required to explain the hypoalbuminemia given the severity of the gastrointestinal signs. Globulin levels may be low in juvenile animals because they have been exposed to relatively small numbers of antigens compared to adults.

Hyponatremia and hypochloremia: These electrolyte deficits are attributable to gastrointestinal losses. The potassium is at the low end of the reference interval for the same reasons, and may decrease further with continuing losses compounded by inadequate intake.

Mildly increased HCO3: The mild alkalosis may be secondary to vomiting and loss of gastric acid. Blood gas measurement is needed to fully characterize the acid/base disorder in this patient and is probably not necessary at this time.

Mildly increased ALP and phosphorus: As described in Chapter 2, there are numerous nonspecific causes for increased ALP in dogs. In the context of the normal values for the other liver enzymes, nonspecific induction or increases in the bone isoenzyme related to skeletal growth in a young large breed dog should be considered. Increases in phosphorus may also be seen in young, growing animals; however, decreased perfusion secondary to blood loss could also contribute to this change.

Case Summary and Outcome

Snickers' parvo test was positive, and he was treated with intravenous fluids and antibiotics because of his compromised intestines and neutropenia. His electrolyte values rapidly normalized, and his white blood cell numbers began to increase four days after hospitalization. He was released from the hospital on day 5 and had an uneventful recovery at home. His sister never got sick.

Snicker's case may be compared with Red Molly (Case 4), who also had non-selective protein loss through the gut. This potential feature of gastrointestinal disease may be present with a variety of pathologic processes in the gut, and is not diagnostic for any one disease. As highlighted by comparison of these two cases, loss of protein may or may not be accompanied by concurrent loss of erythrocytes, electrolytes, or fluid (water).

Case 7 – Level 2

"Susannah" is a 2-year-old spayed female domestic short haired cat who was adopted 3 months ago after being held as a stray in a veterinary clinic. Her physical examination and blood work were unremarkable prior to adoption. For the last week, Susannah has had dark stool and a decreased appetite. She has become progressively more lethargic for the past three days, and she may be drinking more than usual lately. On physical examination, Susannah is thin and has an unkempt haircoat. She has lost one pound of body weight, has icteric mucous membranes, and is febrile. Susannah's abdomen is distended and the kidneys feel enlarged on palpation. She is feline leukemia virus negative.

White blood cell count:	↑ 17.3 x 10⁹/L	(4.5-15.7)
Segmented neutrophils:	↑ 15.7 x 10⁹/L	(2.1-13.1)
Bands:	↑ 0.5 x 10⁹/L	(0.0-0.3)
Lymphocytes:	↓ 0.9 x 10⁹/L	(1.5-7.0)
Monocytes:	0.2 x 10⁹/L	(0-0.9)
Eosinophils:	0.0 x 10⁹/L	(0.0-1.9)

WBC morphology: Slightly toxic neutrophils

Hematocrit:	↓ 20%	(28-45)
Red blood cell count:	↓ 4.60 x 10¹²/L	(5.0-10.0)
Hemoglobin:	↓ 6.4 g/dl	(8.0-15.0)
MCV:	42.4 fl	(39.0-55.0)
MCHC:	32.0	(31.0-35.0)
Platelets:	↓ 73 x 10⁹/L	(183-643)

Plasma is icteric

Glucose:	↑ 132 mg/dl	(70.0-120.0)
BUN:	20 mg/dl	(15-32)
Creatinine:	1.0 mg/dl	(0.9-2.1)
Phosphorus:	6.0 mg/dl	(3.0-6.0)
Calcium:	↓ 8.1 mg/dl	(8.9-11.6)
Magnesium:	2.4 mEq/L	(1.9-2.6)
Total Protein:	7.5 g/dl	(6.0-8.4)
Albumin:	↓ 1.8 g/dl	(2.2-3.4)
Globulin:	5.7 g/dl	(2.5-5.8)
Sodium:	154 mEq/L	(149-163)
Chloride:	119 mEq/L	(119-134)
Potassium:	↓ 3.3 mEq/L	(3.6-5.4)
HCO3:	22 mEq/L	(13-22)
Anion Gap:	16.3 mEq/L	(13-27)
Total Bili:	↑ 3.1 mg/dl	(0.10-0.30)
ALP:	59 IU/L	(10-72)
GGT:	<3 IU/L	(0-4)
ALT:	29 IU/L	(29-145)
AST:	↑ 101 IU/L	(12-42)
Cholesterol:	77 mg/dl	(50-150)
Amylase:	1386 IU/L	(362-1410)

Coagulation

PT:	↑ 14.0s	(6.9-12.6)
APTT:	↑ 67.2s	(11.5-25.0)

Urinalysis: Cystocentesis

Appearance: Amber and clear	Sediment:
Specific gravity: 1.021	0 RBC/high power field
pH: 6.5	0-5/high power field
Protein: negative	No casts seen, rare bilirubin crystals
Glucose/ketones: negative	No epithelial cells seen
Bilirubin: 3+	No bacteria
Heme: 1+	Trace fat droplets and debris

Abdominal fluid analysis (Figure 4-2)

Pre spin: dark yellow and hazy
Post-spin: dark yellow and clear
Total protein: 6.7 g/dl
Total nucleated cell count: 2,300/µl
Direct smears contain 75% nondegenerate neutrophils, 14% small lymphocytes, and 11% large mononuclear cells. No etiologic agents are present. The background is thick and eosinophilic, compatible with the high protein content of the fluid.

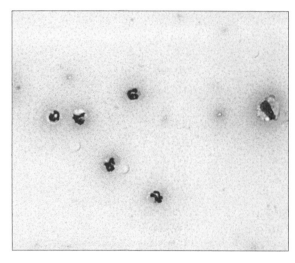

Figure 4-2. Cytology of feline abdominal fluid showing neutrophils and a single large mononuclear cell. The background is compatible with a proteinaceous fluid.

Interpretation

CBC: Susannah has a neutrophilic leukocytosis with a slight left shift and toxic changes, compatible with inflammation. The lymphopenia may be related to corticosteroid effects. She also has a normocytic, normochromic, nonregenerative anemia that is most likely due to inflammatory disease. However, since there is also thrombocytopenia, suppression of production due to a primary bone marrow problem is possible. This seems less likely because of the activity in the myeloid line. Increased consumption of platelets could be immune-mediated or secondary to adhesion to activated or damaged endothelial cells. Hemorrhage could cause both anemia and thrombocytopenia, and the black tarry stool is evidence of melena. In general, blood loss anemias are regenerative, however concurrent inflammatory disease could suppress marrow response. The prolonged coagulation times suggest the potential for abnormal bleeding and/or disseminated intravascular coagulation (DIC) as a cause for increased platelet consumption. Detection of increased fibrin degradation products would further support a diagnosis of DIC. Decreased liver function also may prolong coagulation times.

Serum Biochemical Profile
Hyperglycemia: The increase in serum glucose is mild and likely attributable to stress.

Hypocalcemia with normal phosphorus: Low serum albumin explains the mild decrease in calcium because of a decrease in the protein bound fraction in the blood. This is unlikely to impact the biologically active ionized fraction and therefore should not cause clinical signs. If clinical signs suggestive for hypocalcemia develop, ionized calcium should be measured.

Normal total protein with hypoalbuminemia and high-normal globulins: Hypoalbumiemia could be due to decreased production and/or increased losses. The poor body condition suggests that nutritional factors could impact albumin production in this case. Decreased liver function could also be a contributor. Although no specific tests of liver function were performed, low normal serum cholesterol, poorly concentrated urine, hyperbilirubinemia, and prolonged coagulation times may all be associated with inadequate hepatic function. In addition, albumin production in the liver may be downregulated in response to inflammation (albumin is a negative acute phase reactant) or hyperglobulinemia (to maintain oncotic pressure). Excessive losses of albumin in this patient may be accounted for by high protein effusion in the abdomen and bleeding into the gastrointestinal tract. These two sources of protein loss are non-specific and could lower the globulin concentration back into the reference interval. Inflammation leading to a polyclonal gammopathy is most likely in Susannah because of her age and leukogram data, however monoclonal gammopathies may rarely be associated with inflammatory disease and must be distinguished from paraneoplastic conditions associated with lymphoma or multiple myeloma.

Hypokalemia: Decreased intake associated with a poor nutritional plane and the potential for increased losses via the GI tract or into the abdominal effusion account for the low serum potassium. If Susannah is polyuric and polydipsic, increased renal tubular flow rates may be leading to increased renal wastage of potassium as well.

Hyperbilirubinemia: Sepsis, liver disease, and hemolysis may be factors in causing increased serum bilurubin. Abnormalities in the leukogram combined with fever and coagulation data compatible with DIC could occur as a result of a septic process. The normal ALP and GGT make cholestatic liver disease less likely, however decreased liver function is not always associated with elevated liver enzymes (See Chapter 2). Given the anemia, a hemolytic process is possible, however there are no morphologic abnormalities described such as agglutination, Heinz bodies, spherocytes, schistocytes, etc, that would suggest a cause for hemolysis. Also, given adequate time, hemolytic anemias are usually regenerative, in contrast to the normocytic, normochromic anemia Susannah has at presentation. The increased serum bilirubin explains the bilirubinuria and crystals in the urine.

Increased AST: This mild elevation in the absence of other enzyme elevations suggesting liver disease may indicate mild muscle damage of uncertain cause. Prolonged coagulation times with thrombocytopenia suggest DIC. Liver dysfunction also may contribute to secondary hemostatic defects.

Urinalysis: Since the patient is not azotemic and there is no description of dehydration in the physical examination, the urine specific gravity may be compatible with normal function. The history does indicate increased water consumption, which could be in response to the production of larger volumes of more dilute urine, or conversely, could cause the production of larger volumes of more dilute urine. Urine concentrating ability is usually lost prior to the development of azotemia during the progression of renal disease, although this may not always be true in cats.

Abdominal fluid analysis: The results of this analysis indicate a non-septic exudate. One study of 65 cats with peritoneal effusion showed the following causes in decreasing order of frequency: cardiovascular disease, neoplasia, liver disease, renal disease, feline infectious peritonitis, other peritoneal disease, and urinary tract trauma (Wright). Non-septic exudates are often associated with neoplasia or feline infectious peritonitis.

Case Summary and Outcome

The combination of the neutrophilic leukocytosis with left shift, nonregenerative anemia, and non-septic exudate in the abdomen was suggestive for feline infectious peritonitis (FIP) in this young cat. A diagnosis of FIP may be suggested by the presence of this combination of abnormalities on routine blood testing, however definitive diagnosis is not possible without further work-up (Hartmann). A feline coronavirus titer was positive at 1:1600. Feline coronavirus titers must be interpreted with care, since many cats that never develop FIP have positive titers. Some cats with effusive FIP can have negative or low titers because antibodies are bound in the production of antigen-antibody complexes and are not available for binding with test antigen (Addie). Hyperbilirubinemia in the absence of liver enzyme abnormalities also occurs in cats with FIP and is unlikely in cats with other types of hepatobiliary disease. Because of poor quality of life and questionable prognosis, Susannah was euthanized. At necropsy, she had accumulation of gelatinous fluid in both the abdominal and thoracic cavities. There were multifocal raised yellow nodules covering the liver, intestines and kidneys, compatible with perivascular granuloma formation characteristic of FIP.

Note that multiple processes in this case are influencing Susannah's protein values and that the sum of the abnormalities is resulting in a normal serum total protein value. This is a good illustration of how a "normal" value does not rule out the presence of disease and demonstrates that fractionation of total protein into albumin and globulins can be much more informative than just the total protein value. In previous patients, a "normal" total protein value failed to reflect low serum albumin due to starvation (Belinda, Case 1) and decreased liver function associated with a portosystemic shunt (Dylan, Case 2).

Hartmann K. Feline infectious peritonitis. Vet. Clin North Amer Sm An Prac 2005;35:39-79

Wright KN, Gompf RE, DeNovo RC. Peritoneal effusions in cats: 65 cases (1981-1997). J Am Vet Med Assoc 1999;214:375-381.

Case 8 – Level 2

"Slurpee" is a 9-year-old spayed female Golden Retriever presenting for anorexia, lethargy, and increased urinations. On presentation, she is bright and alert, in good body condition, but slightly dehydrated.

White blood cell count:	↓ 3.3 x 10⁹/L	(6.0-17.0)
Segmented neutrophils:	↓ 2.2 x 10⁹/L	(3.0-11.0)
Band neutrophils:	0 x 10⁹/L	(0-0.3)
Lymphocytes:	1.0 x 10⁹/L	(1.0-4.8)
Monocytes:	↓ 0.1 x 10⁹/L	(0.2-1.4)
Eosinophils:	0.0 x 10⁹/L	(0-1.3)
WBC morphology: Within normal limits		

Hematocrit:	↓ 31%	(39-55)
Red blood cell count:	↓ 4.72 x 10¹²/L	(5.5-8.5)
Hemoglobin:	↓ 11.0 g/dl	(14.0-19.0)
MCV:	71.8 fl	(60.0-75.0)
MCHC:	35.5 g/dl	(33.0-36.0)
RBC morphology: Rouleaux present		

Platelets: Moderately decreased

Plasma appears normal

Glucose:	88 mg/dl	(65.0-135.0)
BUN:	18 mg/dl	(8-33)
Creatinine:	1.1 mg/dl	(0.5-1.5)
Phosphorus:	4.9 mg/dl	(3.0-6.0)
Calcium:	↑ 13.7 mg/dl	(8.8-11.0)
Magnesium:	2.1 mEq/L	(1.4-2.7)
Total Protein:	↑ 12.5 g/dl	(5.2-7.2)
Albumin:	↓ 1.6 g/dl	(3.0-4.2)
Globulin:	↑ 10.9 g/dl	(2.0-4.0)
A/G Ratio:	↓ 0.1	(0.7-2.1)
Sodium:	154 mEq/L	(142-163)
Chloride:	115 mEq/L	(106-126)
Potassium:	4.1 mEq/L	(3.8-5.4)
HCO3:	19 mEq/L	(16-25)
Anion Gap:	24.1 mEq/L	(15-25)
Total Bili:	0.21 mg/dl	(0.10-0.50)
ALP:	↓ 19 IU/L	(20-320)
GGT:	2 IU/L	(1-10)
ALT:	↓ 6 IU/L	(10-95)
AST:	25 IU/L	(15-52)
Cholesterol:	132 mg/dl	(110-314)
Triglycerides:	30 mg/dl	(30-300)
Amylase:	1020 IU/L	(400-1200)

Urinalysis: Voided

Appearance: Yellow and hazy	Sediment:
	occasional red blood cells/hpf
Specific gravity: 1.020	occasional WBC/hpf
pH: 6.0	occasional epithelial cells
Protein: 500 mg/dl	no crystals, casts, or bacteria
Glucose: negative	
Ketones: negative	
Bilirubin: negative	
Heme: trace	

Interpretation

CBC: Slurpee has neutropenia, monocytopenia, a mild normocytic normochromic anemia, and thrombocytopenia. A platelet count is recommended to confirm the thrombocytopenia. Pancytopenia is an indication for bone marrow evaluation if peripheral causes cannot account for the cytopenias. While not typically seen in normal dogs, rouleaux may occur in association with the high globulin levels in this patient.

Serum Biochemical Profile

Hypercalcemia with normal phosphorus: The potential for neoplasia should always be considered in hypercalcemic dogs, especially middle aged to older patients. While hypercalcemia is most often associated with adenocarcinomas of the anal sac, lymphoma, or multiple myeloma, it has been reported with numerous other malignancies in domestic animals. There are no specific abnormalities in the history or physical examination that indicate a potential source for the hypercalcemia, however because of the concurrent pancytopenia, the bone marrow should be evaluated for tumor infiltration. The hyperglobulinemia further suggests the possibility of a lymphoid malignancy as the cause for the hypercalcemia. Hypercalcemia of malignancy is often associated with normal or low phosphorus. Decreased glomerular filtration rate secondary to hypercalcemic nephropathy and/or dehydration may cause the serum phosphorus to be normal to increased.

Hyperproteinemia with hypoalbuminemia and hyperglobulinemia: Despite hypoalbuminemia, the total serum protein level is high because of marked increases in serum globulins. Hypoalbuminemia may be due to decreased production or increased losses, while the hyperglobulinemia indicates increased production. Decreased production of albumin may be related to nutritional status (unlikely here because the patient has good body condition), decreased liver function (cannot be ruled out since blood ammonia or serum bile acids were not measured, however BUN, cholesterol, and bilirubin are within reference intervals), a compensatory change in response to inflammation (albumin is a negative acute phase reactant) or a response to the increased oncotic pressure exerted by the high globulin levels. Increased losses may occur with or without decreased production. Selective loss of albumin is most frequently associated with glomerular lesions, and proteinuria is noted on the urinalysis. This should be further evaluated by measuring a urine protein:creatinine ratio on a urine collected by cystocentesis to avoid potential contamination with protein from the lower urinary tract. A high urine protein:creatinine ratio in the absence of evidence of inflammatory disease is compatible with glomerular protein loss. The test strips used for routine urinalysis are more sensitive for albumin than globulins, and false negatives may occur in the rare case where urine protein is predominantly globulin. Other types of protein loss (GI, dermal, third space, interstitial) are generally non-selective and result in loss of albumin and globulins. Loss of globulin in this case may be masked by the marked hyperglobulinemia. Over production of globulins is most often due to inflammatory disease, in which case both acute phase reactants and immunoglobulins may be produced. The increase in immunoglobulins will generally be polyclonal, however in rare cases inflammatory disease can cause a monoclonal gammopathy. Examples include feline infectious peritonitis, rickettsial diseases, and Leishmaniasis. Over production of globulins can be a paraneoplastic syndrome in which a malignant clone of lymphocytes or plasma cells produces a single globulin protein, resulting in a monoclonal gammopathy. Serum protein electrophoresis can be performed as a diagnostic aid to distinguish polyclonal from monoclonal gammopathy.

Mildly decreased ALP and ALT: Decreases in the serum levels of these enzymes do not have diagnostic significance (See Chapter 2). Specifically, they should not be used as evidence of decreased liver function to explain the hypoalbuminemia.

Urinalysis: The urine is not optimally concentrated for a dehydrated patient, however Slurpee is not azotemic, nor is she yet isosthenuric. Abnormalities of urinary concentrating ability may be related to her hypercalcemia (See Chapter 5, Case 4). The proteinuria should be verified, and a urine protein:creatinine ratio performed (see above). In this case, a urine protein electrophoresis may be indicated to identify light chains that may be present in cases of paraneoplastic gammopathy. The occasional white cells and red cells may be contaminants in the voided sample.

Case Summary and Outcome

Based on the pancytopenia, hypercalcemia, and hyperglobulinemia, a lymphoid malignancy was suspected. Bone marrow aspirate revealed that 75% of the nucleated cells in the bone marrow were plasma cells; both mature and immature cells were present mixed with small numbers of normal hematopoietic precursors (Figure 4-3). A monoclonal gammopathy was documented by serum protein electrophoresis. Survey radiographs to look for lytic lesions and urine protein electrophoresis were not performed because of financial concerns. Treatment was initiated for multiple myeloma based on the existing data.

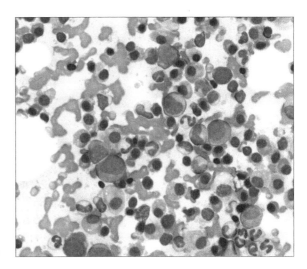

Figure 4-3. Cytology of the bone marrow aspirate showing numerous neoplastic plasma cells.

Slurpee can be compared with Cleopatra (Chapter 6, Case 7), a cat with multiple myeloma. In both cases, concurrent hypercalcemia increased the index of suspicion that hyperglobulinemia could be due to the presence of an immunoglobulin producing malignancy. Neither Slurpee nor Cleopatra had an inflammatory leukogram, in contrast to Susannah (Case 7), who had hypoalbuminemia and high-normal globulins associated with an infectious disease. Serum protein electrophoresis may not be necessary in hyperglobulinemic animals when there is obvious clinical evidence of inflammation and the patient is considered at low risk for neoplasia (Susannah was a young cat). In other cases such as Popcorn (Chapter 5, Case 24), a patient may have inflammatory disease, in this case pyometra, however due to age or concurrent laboratory abnormalities, a more thorough diagnostic work-up is appropriate. In Popcorn's case, hyperglobulinemia was associated with hypercalcemia, therefore a serum protein electrophoresis was performed to help rule out the potential for neoplasia prior to surgical correction of her pyometra.

Case 9 – Level 2

"Salty" is an 11-year-old Quarter Horse stallion presenting for increasingly severe colic of 12 hours duration. On physical examination, Salty is depressed, painful, and attempting to lie down. His coat is drenched with sweat and he has tachycardia. There is dried blood on both nares, possibly related to inadvertent removal of his nasogastric tube during transportation, when he went down several times. He is moderately dehydrated with prolonged capillary refill time and muddy mucous membranes. Salty was immediately treated for pain, however a nasogastric tube could not be passed. Rectal palpation revealed severely distended large bowel. His initial PCV was 60% and total solids were 6.6 g/dl. Further diagnostic evaluation could not be performed because he had to be almost constantly walked to prevent him from going down. As a result, he received several liters of fluids before samples for further laboratory evaluation could be collected.

Hematocrit:	↑ 55%	(30-51)
Glucose:	↑ 226 mg/dl	(6.0-128.0)
BUN:	↑ 46 mg/dl	(11-26)
Creatinine:	↑ 3.6 mg/dl	(0.9-1.9)
Phosphorus:	3.1 mg/dl	(1.9-6.0)
Calcium:	11.9 mg/dl	(11.0-13.5)
Magnesium:	↑ 2.5 mEq/L	(1.4-2.3)
Total Protein:	6.5 g/dl	(5.6-7.0)
Albumin:	↑ 4.0 g/dl	(2.4-3.8)
Globulin:	2.5 g/dl	(2.5-4.9)
Sodium:	136 mEq/L	(130-145)
Chloride:	↓ 93 mEq/L	(97-105)
Potassium:	3.9 mEq/L	(3.0-5.0)
HCO3:	28 mEq/L	(25-31)
Anion Gap:	↑ 18.9 mEq/L	(7-15)
Total Bili:	↑ 2.6 mg/dl	(0.6-1.8)
ALP:	↓ 87 IU/L	(109-352)
GGT:	21 IU/L	(5-23)
AST:	↑ 562 IU/L	(190-380)
CK:	↑ 3640 IU/L	(80-446)

Interpretation

Increased Hematocrit: This is compatible with dehydration or splenic contraction secondary to excitement in the horse.

Serum biochemical profile:

Hyperglycemia: The increased serum glucose is likely related to pain and stress.

Increased BUN and creatinine: Salty is significantly dehydrated and polycythemic at presentation, so there is a pre-renal component to the azotemia. A urine sample could not be obtained, so a urine specific gravity is not available to assess urinary concentrating ability and the potential for renal disease.

Hypermagnesemia: This abnormality is likely associated with decreased glomerular filtration rate secondary to dehydration.

Hyperalbuminemia: Dehydration/hemoconcentration is the cause for increase serum albumin.

Hypochloremia with normal serum sodium: At this time serum sodium is within the reference interval and there is a disproportionate change in chloride, but the significance is unclear in light of the potential effects of fluid therapy initiated prior to sample collection. The low serum chloride could be due to gastrointestinal losses or sweating.

Mildly increased anion gap: Accumulation of unmeasured anions could include increased proteins with hemoconcentration or lactic acidosis associated with poor tissue perfusion. This change is not yet accompanied by a decrease in HCO_3 which often accompanies the accumulation of unmeasured organic acids such as lactic acid. Although Salty is hyperglycemic, ketoacidosis is unlikely given the clinical history. Likewise, although he is azotemic, uremic acidosis is unlikely because pre-renal factors can probably account for the decreased glomerular filtration rate. Ideally, serum glucose, BUN, creatinine, and urine specific gravity should be re-evaluated in subsequent blood work to confirm these impressions.

Hyperbilirubinemia: In horses, anorexia should always be considered as a cause of hyper-bilirubinemia. In this clinical context, sepsis associated with bowel compromise could also contribute. Liver disease is less likely since the GGT is within the reference interval, however hepatic pathology cannot be completely ruled out. Significant intestinal disease can impact the liver secondarily as well.

Increased AST and CK: Elevations in both of these enzymes suggest muscle damage and are compatible with Salty's travel history and episodes of recumbency.

Case Summary and Outcome

During induction of anesthesia in preparation for surgery, Salty suffered respiratory arrest, became non-responsive, and was humanely euthanized. A limited necropsy revealed severely gas-distended large bowel and a 360 degree torsion of the large colon at the base of the cecum. Both arterial and venous supply was compromised, and the mucosa was black, compatible with ischemic necrosis.

Serum albumin levels in horses with intestinal disease may be high, low, or normal. Multiple factors may influence serum albumin in these cases, including fluid and protein loss in the gut or the abdominal cavity, in combination with the effects of fluid therapy. Concurrent electrolyte losses by similar mechanisms may also be present. Sweating can affect electrolyte concentrations and hydration status.

Case 10 – Level 3

"Twister" is a 9-year-old spayed female Brittany Spaniel with a history of histologically confirmed chronic intestinal lymphangiectasia that has been successfully managed with low doses of corticosteroids. At the time of initial diagnosis 2 years ago, Twister had panhypopro-teinemia, mildly elevated ALP (442 IU/L), ALT (174 IU/L), and hypomagnesemia (0.7 mg/dl). Twister is presenting today following a two month history of weight loss. In the last week, she has been anorexic and has vomited twice.

White blood cell count:	10.6 x 10⁹/L	(6.0-17.0)
Segmented neutrophils:	9.8 x 10⁹/L	(3.0-11.0)
Band neutrophils:	0 x 10⁹/L	(0-0.3)
Lymphocytes:	↓ 0.2 x 10⁹/L	(1.0-4.8)
Monocytes:	0.6 x 10⁹/L	(0.2-1.4)
Eosinophils:	0.0 x 10⁹/L	(0-1.3)

WBC morphology: No significant abnormalities

Hematocrit:	54%	(37-55)
Platelets:	450 x 10⁹/L	(200-450)

Plasma is icteric

Glucose:	93 mg/dl	(65.0-120.0)
BUN:	8 mg/dl	(8-33)
Creatinine:	0.6 mg/dl	(0.5-1.5)
Phosphorus:	5.0 mg/dl	(3.0-6.0)
Calcium:	↓ 8.2 mg/dl	(8.8-11.0)
Magnesium:	1.8 mEq/L	(1.4-2.7)
Total Protein:	↓ 4.2 g/dl	(5.2-7.2)
Albumin:	↓ 2.0 g/dl	(3.0-4.2)
Globulin:	↓ 2.2 g/dl	(2.3-4.2)
Sodium:	148 mEq/L	(140-151)
Chloride:	114 mEq/L	(105-120)
Potassium:	5.4 mEq/L	(3.8-5.4)
HCO3:	23 mEq/L	(16-25)
Anion Gap:	16.4 mEq/L	(15-25)
Total Bili:	↑ 2.5 mg/dl	(0.10-0.50)
ALP:	↑ 1044 IU/L	(20-320)
GGT:	↑ 144 IU/L	(3-10)
ALT:	↑ 2088 IU/L	(10-95)
AST:	↑ 195 IU/L	(15-52)
Cholesterol:	264 mg/dl	(110-314)
Triglycerides:	88 mg/dl	(30-300)
Amylase:	778 IU/L	(400-1200)
Lipase:	↑ 8001 IU/L	(53-770)
Fasted bile acids	8 μmol/L	(5-20)

Interpretation

CBC: Lymphopenia may either be due to the effects of treatment with corticosteroids or associated with loss through compromised intestines.

Serum Biochemical Profile

Hypocalcemia with normal phosphorus: Decreased total serum calcium is likely associated with hypoalbuminemia, however decreased ionized calcium has been described in association with malabsorptive intestinal disease (See Case 4, Red Molly). Corticosteroids may also lower calcium.

Panhypoproteinemia: With Twister's clinical history, progression or acute exacerbation of the pre-existing lymphangiectasia is the most obvious cause for the panhypoproteinemia. Nutritional factors can contribute to hypoproteinemia if starvation is severe or prolonged and associated with poor body condition. Decreased liver function could impair Twister's ability to produce sufficient albumin to compensate for ongoing losses. Low-normal BUN and mild hyperbilirubinemia may occur with impaired hepatic function. Her liver enzymes are elevated compared to the earlier values determined at the time of initial diagnosis which could indicate liver pathology. The potential for the enzyme changes to be related to corticosteroid therapy-induced hepatopathy should be considered.

Hyperbilirubinemia: The high-normal hematocrit and relatively normal leukogram indicate that hemolysis and sepsis respectively, are unlikely causes of hyperbilirubinemia. Elevated ALP and GGT suggest cholestasis, but may also be influenced by the presence of corticosteroid hepatopathy. Corticosteroid effects alone are unlikely to explain the hyperbiluribinemia, and causes of cholestasis should be evaluated.

Increased ALP and GGT: As indicated above, both cholestasis and corticosteroid effects may be increasing the amount of these enzymes in the circulation.

Increased ALT and AST: Increases in these enzymes indicate hepatocellular damage, but do not suggest the cause. In some patients with cholestasis, hepatocellular damage may occur secondary to the toxic effects of bile on the hepatocytes (see Chapter 2). Intestinal disease can be associated with increased liver enzymes because the anatomic relationship between the gut and the liver allow greater exposure of hepatocytes to bacteria, toxins, or inflammatory cytokines from compromised bowel. Twister originally presented with elevated ALP and ALT. These values are higher now and may indicate progression of the original disease or additional pathologic processes. Pancreatic disease, suggested by the markedly elevated lipase, can also cause secondary liver damage.

Hyperlipasemia with normal amylase: Both amylase and lipase levels in the blood may increase 3-4 times normal when the glomerular filtration rate is decreased, however this is unlikely in this patient as she is not azotemic. Administration of corticosteroids has been reported to increase serum lipase in dogs up to 3-4 times the upper limit of the reference interval with no significant change in amylase. While this is possible, the increase here exceeds what has been associated with steroid use alone. Hyperlipasemia of 11-93 times the upper limit of the reference range was reported in 6 dogs with tumors of the pancreas or liver (Quigley), which could also account for the other enzyme elevations that are present in this patient.

Case Summary and Outcome

The ultrasound study of Twister's abdomen revealed multiple complex masses in the liver with enlarged mesenteric lymph nodes and a thickened gastrointestinal tract. Aspiration cytology of one of the liver masses was compatible with epithelial neoplasia, likely of biliary origin (Figure 4-4) although no histology was available to confirm this impression. Twister was euthanized because of deteriorating quality of life and poor prognosis.

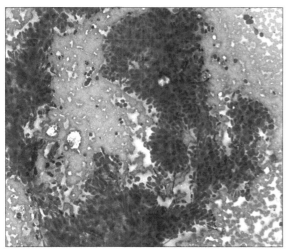

Figure 4-4. Smears from the liver mass contain clusters of cuboidal epithelial cells characterized by scant to moderate basophilic cytoplasm and single round to oval nuclei with coarsely stippled chromatin. Cells occur in branching papillary fronds. Cells appear to have lost polarity and pile up in disorganized masses. These findings were compatible with epithelial neoplasia, likely of bile duct origin.

Twister's data must be interpreted in the context of her previous diagnosis and therapy, both of which could influence her clinical chemistry data. Her data at this second presentation are significantly different from her initial values, which could be related to the effects of the corticosteroids or progression of disease. Unfortunately, the progression or resolution of clinical signs do not always correlate with laboratory parameters. Some patients have good clinical response to therapy with minimal changes in laboratory values, and some have no amelioration of clinical signs despite improvement in laboratory abnormalities. Hence the saying, "treat the patient, not the laboratory work."

For Twister, the hyperbilirubinemia and the dramatic hyperlipasemia with normal amylase were important pieces of information that indicated a new disease process should be considered because they were not readily explicable by the previous disease or treatment. Paradoxically, the normalization of the serum cholesterol may have been the result of increased production secondary to cholestasis rather than decreased gastrointestinal loss following improvement of the lymphangiectasia. This is potentially a patient in which two disease processes working in opposition keep an analyte within the reference range despite significant pathology. This phenomenon can sometimes be an issue in dehydrated hypoalbuminemic patients that initially present with albumin in the normal range, or in hyperglobulinemic patients in which non-selective protein loss drops the globulin value down to within the reference interval.

Twister's case can be compared with Case 4, Red Molly, who also had a protein losing enteropathy with panhypoproteinemia, hypocalcemia, and hypocholesterolemia, however Molly did not have associated liver enzyme elevations as a result of her intestinal disease. Two cases from Chapter 3, have hyperlipasemia associated with pancreatic/hepatic neoplasia like Twister. Shorty the cat (Chapter 3, Case 13) had pancreatic neoplasia with metastases to the liver, however Shorty's liver enzymes were within reference intervals, demonstrating that normal clinical chemistry data cannot be used to rule out hepatic involvement. Muffy the dog (Chapter 3, Case 14) also had a pancreatic carcinoma, but her liver enzymes were elevated. Her liver appeared normal by ultrasonography, however a biopsy was not performed to determine whether the liver enzyme elevations were caused by metastatic disease or another process. Neither Shorty nor Muffy were being treated with medications that commonly result in liver enzyme elevations.

Quigley KA, Jackson ML, Haines DM. Hyperlipasemia in 6 dogs with pancreatic or hepatic neoplasia: evidence for tumor lipase production. Vet Clin Path 2001;30:114-120.

Case 11 – Level 3

"June" is a one-year-old spayed female domestic short haired cat presenting with a history of chronic respiratory and sinus infections. On physical examination, June is thin, quiet, and responsive. She is slightly hypothermic and has pale mucous membranes. While she has obvious dyspnea and tachypnea, her right thorax is quiet on auscultation and 200 ml of purulent fluid is removed. Blood is collected for analysis. She is placed in an oxygen cage and treated with intravenous fluids and antibiotics. June suffers cardiopulmonary arrest during chest tube placement, but is successfully resuscitated.

White blood cell count:	↑ 42.7 x 10⁹/L	(4.5-15.7)
Segmented neutrophils:	↑ 24.3 x 10⁹/L	(2.1-13.1)
Bands:	↑ 7.4 x 10⁹/L	(0.0-0.3)
Metamyelocytes:	↑ 1.3 x 10⁹/L	(0)
Lymphocytes:	↑ 9.5 x 10⁹/L	(1.5-7.0)
Monocytes:	0.2 x 10⁹/L	(0-0.9)
Eosinophils:	0.0 x 10⁹/L	(0.0-1.9)
Nucleated RBC/100 WBC:	15	

WBC morphology: Lymphocytes are mature. Neutrophils often have moderate to marked toxic change characterized by cytoplasmic basophilia and vacuolization. Giant band forms are seen with occasional metamyelocytes. Occasional neutrophils appear to have hyposegmented nuclei despite otherwise mature morphology, compatible with pseudo Pelger-Huet anomaly.

Hematocrit:	↓ 17%	(28-45)
Red blood cell count:	↓ 3.45 x 10¹²/L	(5.0-10.0)
Hemoglobin:	↓ 5.3 g/dl	(8.0-15.0)
MCV:	52.9 fl	(39.0-55.0)
MCHC:	31.2	(31.0-35.0)
Reticulocytes:	1.5% or 51.8 x 10⁹/L	

Platelets: Numbers appear adequate with occasional macroplatelets

Plasma is icteric

Glucose:	↓ 60 mg/dl	(70.0-120.0)
BUN:	↑ 48 mg/dl	(15-32)
Creatinine:	↓ 0.7 mg/dl	(0.9-2.1)
Phosphorus:	↑ 7.8 mg/dl	(3.0-6.0)
Calcium:	↓ 7.2 mg/dl	(8.9-11.6)
Magnesium:	↑ 3.1 mEq/L	(1.9-2.6)
Total Protein:	↓ 5.6 g/dl	(6.0-8.4)
Albumin:	↓ 2.2 g/dl	(2.5-4.0)
Globulin:	3.4 g/dl	(2.5-5.8)
Sodium:	↓ 141 mEq/L	(143-153)
Chloride:	↓ 106 mEq/L	(119-134)
Potassium:	3.8 mEq/L	(3.6-5.4)
HCO3:	17 mEq/L	(13-22)
Anion Gap:	21.8 mEq/L	(13-27)

Total Bili:	↑ 0.95 mg/dl	(0.10-0.30)
ALP:	8 IU/L	(10-72)
GGT:	1 IU/L	(0-4)
ALT:	↑ 190 IU/L	(29-145)
AST:	↑ 557 IU/L	(12-42)
Cholesterol:	105 mg/dl	(50-150)
Amylase:	743 IU/L	(362-1410)

Pleural fluid analysis

Pre spin appearance: yellow and cloudy
Post-spin appearance: yellow and clear
Total protein: 3.4 g/dl
Total nucleated cell count: 63,700/µl
Description: There are massive numbers of degenerate neutrophils with small numbers of macrophages. Large numbers of intracellular and extracellular bacteria are present. While predominantly rod shaped, bacteria are of mixed morphology with long, short, and chaining organisms noted. Both Gram positive and negative organisms are present.

Interpretation

CBC: June has a neutrophilic leukocytosis with an extreme left shift and marked toxic change compatible with severe inflammation; the focus is assumed to be the thoracic cavity based on the gross appearance of the fluid removed via thoracocentesis. The mature lymphocytosis may be attributable to either epinephrine effects or antigenic stimulation, although no reactive cells are described to differentiate between the two mechanisms. June has a normocytic, normochromic, nonregenerative anemia. This is most likely anemia of inflammation, however the hematocrit is slightly lower than is typical for anemia of inflammation. Increased numbers of nucleated red blood cells may be part of a regenerative response to anemia or may reflect increased release secondary to endothelial damage in hematopoietic organs. Endothelial damage is likely given the severity of inflammation and the septic focus in the thorax.

Serum Biochemical Profile

Hypoglycemia: If processing errors are eliminated, the hypoglycemia is explained by sepsis.

Increased BUN with low creatinine: Decreased glomerular filtration or slow renal tubular flow rates increasing available time for reabsorption of urea could explain the increased BUN. No urine specific gravity is available to evaluate renal function because June had a small urinary bladder at presentation and did not produce sufficient urine for collection until after therapy was instituted. Sepsis may also increase the BUN because of intensified protein turnover. The low creatinine may be due to low muscle mass.

Hypocalcemia with hyperphosphatemia and hypermagnesemia: Low serum albumin explains the mild decrease in calcium because of a decrease in the protein bound fraction in the blood. This is unlikely to impact the biologically active ionized fraction and therefore should not cause clinical signs. If clinical signs suggestive for hypocalcemia develop, ionized calcium should be measured. In the context of the clinical presentation and increased BUN, hyperphosphatemia and hypermagnesemia are related to decreased glomerular filtration rate.

Hypoproteinemia with hypoalbuminemia and normal globulins: Hypoalbumiemia could be due to decreased production and/or increased losses. Poor body condition suggests that nutritional factors could impact albumin production in this case. Decreased liver function could also contribute, however no specific tests of liver function were performed to evaluate this possibility. Decreased liver function can result in hypoglycemia and hyperbilirubinemia, however both of these abnormalities can also be explained by sepsis. Albumin production in a healthy liver may be downregulated in response to inflammation because albumin is a negative acute phase reactant. Third space loss of protein into the effusion may be decreasing both albumin and globulin since it is a non-selective site of protein loss. The potential for renal loss of protein cannot be evaluated without a urinalysis. With nonselective protein loss, globulins may be maintained within the normal range by increased production secondary to antigenic stimulation.

Hyponatremia with proportional hypochloremia: These are mild changes of questionable clinical significance, but are likely present because of electrolyte losses into the thoracic effusion.

Hyperbilirubinemia: Sepsis, liver disease, and hemolysis may all be factors in causing June's hyperbilirubinemia. Significant cholestatic liver disease is ruled out based on the normal ALP and GGT. Hemolytic anemias are typically regenerative given sufficient time, and June's anemia is non-regenerative at presentation, making this less likely than sepsis and liver disease as causes for this abnormality.

Increased ALT and AST:
Increased ALT suggests hepatocellular damage, which may be related to hypoxia (anemia and respiratory difficulty), sepsis, or hypoperfusion related to shock. Since the increase in AST is greater than the elevation in ALT, some of the increase in this enzyme may be related to muscle damage from the same causes. No CK is available to confirm this impression.

Pleural fluid analysis (Figure 4-5): Septic suppurative exudate

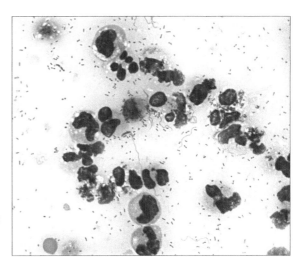

Figure 4-5. Cytology of pyothorax showing degenerate neutrophils and numerous bacteria.

Case Summary and Outcome
Further testing performed while June was hospitalized revealed the presence of feline leukemia virus (FeLV) antigen. She was feline immunodeficiency virus (FIV) negative. Despite June's condition at presentation and FeLV status, she responded well to treatment and was discharged 6 days after presentation on oral antibiotics. She was re-evaluated 6 weeks later. At that time her lungs were clear and she had gained some weight, but had some residual upper airway stridor. All of her laboratory abnormalities were resolved except for a persistent non-regenerative anemia. Bone marrow evaluation demonstrated erythroid hypoplasia, but myeloid and megakaryocytic activity was normal and there was no evidence of dysplasia in the erythroid line. The suppression of red blood cell production was assumed to be related to June's FeLV status.

This case is similar to Susannah (Case 7), in which poor body condition, severe inflammatory disease, and cavity effusion combine to influence serum protein data. In both cases, the globulin levels are within reference intervals despite the expected increases in acute phase reactants and/or immunoglobulins. This may reflect concurrent protein losses, however note that the reference interval is much greater for albumin than globulin, indicating greater biological variability under "normal" circumstances.

Case 12 – Level 3

"Ellis" is an 11-month-old neutered male Labrador Retriever who presented having collapsed acutely after a run. He had profuse diarrhea in the car on the way to the hospital. On physical examination, Ellis is depressed and unresponsive, and his mucous membranes are bright red.

	Day 1	Day 2	
White blood cell count:	↓ 4.8 x 10⁹/L	10.7	(6.0-17.0)
Segmented neutrophils:	↓ 2.1 x 10⁹/L	9.0	(3.0-11.0)
Band neutrophils:	0 x 10⁹/L	↑ 0.4	(0-0.300)
Lymphocytes:	2.5 x 10⁹/L	1.1	(1.0-4.8)
Monocytes:	0.0 x 10⁹/L	0.1	(0.2-1.4)
Eosinophils:	0.2 x 10⁹/L	0.1	(0-1.3)
Nucleaded RBC/100 WBC:	↑ 105	↑ 14	
WBC morphology:	Normal	Slight Toxic change	
Hematocrit:	↑ 60%	↓ 37	(39-55)
Red blood cell count:	↑ 8.53 x 10¹²/L	↓ 4.93	(5.5-8.5)
Hemoglobin:	↑ 21.0 g/dl	↓ 12.2	(14.0-19.0)
MCV:	76.0 fl	↑ 77.8	(60.0-76.0)
MCHC:	35.0 g/dl	33.0	(33.0-36.0)
RBC morphology:	Normal	↑ anisocytosis, polychromasia	
Platelets:	↓ 125 x 10⁹/L	↓ 16	(200-450)
Plasma appearance:	normal	normal	
Glucose:	66 mg/dl	↑ 127	(65.0-120.0)
BUN:	33 mg/dl	27	(8-33)
Creatinine:	2.0 mg/dl	0.9	(0.6-1.5)
Phosphorus:	3.6 mg/dl	6.0	(3.0-6.0)
Calcium:	↑ 12.3 mg/dl	9.4	(8.8-11.0)
Magnesium:	2.1 mEq/L	↓ 1.2	(1.4-2.7)
Total Protein:	↑ 7.7 g/dl	↓ 4.8	(5.2-7.2)
Albumin:	↑ 4.5 g/dl	↓ 2.9	(3.0-4.2)
Globulin:	3.2 g/dl	↓ 1.9	(2.0-4.0)
A/G Ratio:	1.4	1.6	(0.7-2.1)
Sodium:	148 mEq/L	157	(142-163)
Chloride:	111 mEq/L	125	(106-126)
Potassium:	4.7 mEq/L	↓ 3.7	(3.8-5.4)
HCO3:	↓ 12 mEq/L	18	(16-25)
Anion Gap:	↑ 29.7 mEq/L	17.7	(15-25)

Total Bili:	↑ 0.54 mg/dl	0.22	(0.10-0.50)
ALP:	↑ 839 IU/L	↑ 880	(12-121)
GGT:	not available	9	(1-10)
ALT:	↑ 114 IU/L	↑ 2906	(10-95)
AST:	↑ 703 IU/L	↑ 7166	(15-52)
Cholesterol:	↑ 342 mg/dl	217	(110-314)
Triglycerides:	47 mg/dl	53	(30-300)
Amylase:	1008 IU/L	1147	(400-1200)

Coagulation profile Day 1

PT:	6.4s	(6.2-9.3)
APTT:	11.6s	(8.9-16.3)
FDPs:	<5 µg/ml	(<5)

Urinalysis Day 1: catheter

Appearance: Yellow and clear	Sediment:
Urine specific gravity: 1.014	0-5 RBC/hpf
pH: 8.0	5-10 WBC/hpf
Protein: 100 mg/dl	no casts or crystals seen
Glucose: 2+	
Ketones: negative	
Bilirubin: negative	
Heme: 3+	

Interpretation

CBC: On Day 1, Ellis is leukopenic due to neutropenia with no evidence of a left shift or toxic change. This may be due to acute margination of granulocytes, or consumption in an acute, overwhelming inflammatory process. The thrombocytopenia could also be due to increased peripheral consumption associated with vascular pathology or immune mediated destruction. The polycythemia is likely related to dehydration, as supported by the increased serum albumin. Normoblastemia (increased nRBCs) could be compatible with a regenerative response or a primary hematopoietic disorder. There is no evidence of regeneration at this time (no polychromasia). Increased numbers of nucleated erythrocytes can be present in the circulation associated with endothelial damage of any cause, including sepsis, shock, hyperthermia, neoplasia, or any potential cause of hypoxia or hypoglycemia. Given the neutropenia in combination with the thrombocytopenia and metarubricytosis, a marrow disorder leading to depressed production of cells is possible. If peripheral processes cannot account for the hematologic changes, a bone marrow aspirate and biopsy are indicated. Coagulation status appears normal at presentation.

By Day 2, neutrophil numbers have normalized, however there is a minor increase in bands and some toxic change, supporting inflammation. The thrombocytopenia is severe by this time. Ellis is at risk for spontaneous bleeding and should be monitored carefully. The apparent response in the granulocyte line makes a primary bone marrow disorder less likely, and peripheral consumption is suspected. In contrast to the previous polycythemia, Ellis is now mildly anemic with a mild macrocytosis that could be explained by incipient regeneration. Fluid therapy decreased the red cell numbers, however concurrent blood loss is also likely given the anemia and hypoproteinemia.

Serum Biochemical Profile

Glucose: On day 1, the serum glucose is at the lower end of the reference range, which is compatible with sepsis (see leukogram data), however on day 2, there is mild hyperglycemia that could be nonspecifically related to stress, illness, or to administration of glucose containing fluids.

Increased creatinine with high normal BUN: On day 1, the polycythemia and hyperalbuminemia suggest that Ellis is dehydrated, compatible with some degree of pre-renal azotemia. The urine is close to the isosthenuric range despite the dehydration, suggesting compromised renal function. Glucosuria indicates the potential for osmotic diuresis. Glucosuria in association with low normal blood glucose levels is evidence of renal tubular dysfunction if the urine sample does not contain contaminants that could cause a false positive reaction on the test strip. Urinalysis should be repeated to determine if there was transient renal dysfunction related to an acute event or if longer term compromise in renal function is likely.

Hypercalcemia with normal phosphorus: Generally, one of the primary differential diagnoses for hypercalcemia is neoplasia, however Ellis is a young dog and is unlikely to have a malignant process. Growing large breed dogs may have slightly elevated calcium associated with bone growth, however the hypercalcemia in this case is most likely because of increased protein bound calcium associated with hyperproteinemia. This interpretation is supported by normalization of the serum calcium as the albumin in the serum drops by Day 2.

Hypomagnesemia: Hypomagnesemia on Day 2 could be related to gastrointestinal losses associated with the diarrhea or to low serum protein. Like calcium, a proportion of serum magnesium is protein bound.

Hyperproteinemia with increased serum albumin on Day 1, then mild panhypoproteinemia on day 2: Because the liver does not overproduce albumin, increased serum albumin is evidence of dehydration. The dramatic change on the following day reflects correction of fluid deficits as well as some type of non-selective protein loss. The thrombocytopenia indicates risk for hemorrhage, which should be evaluated clinically. Gastrointestinal blood or protein loss is less easily documented than other types, but the presence of diarrhea suggests the potential for gastrointestinal lesions. The thrombocytopenia and metarubricytosis are compatible with endothelial damage, which could increase vascular permeability and allow loss of protein into the interstitial space. Proteinuria is present and can be quantified by measuring a urine protein:creatinine ratio. Because pyuria is also noted on the sediment examination, urinary tract inflammation rather than selective glomerular loss of albumin should be ruled out first. Urine culture is recommended to document any treatable infectious causes for the pyuria and proteinuria.

Acidemia (low HCO3) with increased anion gap: These abnormalities indicate a metabolic acidosis with increased unmeasured anions. Dehydration and collapse suggest the potential for lactic acidosis from decreased perfusion of tissues, while the azotemia could be compatible with uremic acidosis as well. Acid/base status normalizes by Day 2.

Mild hyperbilirubinemia: Potential causes of hyperbilirubinemia in this case include sepsis (neutropenia, low normal blood glucose), decreased liver function (not specifically evaluated by serum bile acid or blood ammonia measurement), cholestasis (increased ALP), or hemolysis (less likely because the bilirubin is high when Ellis is polycythemic, but normal by the time his anemia develops). Whatever the cause, the hyperbilirubinemia is minimal and transient, and unlikely to be clinically significant.

Increased ALP: There are numerous potential hepatic and extrehepatic causes of elevated ALP in the dog. Young large breed dogs may have elevated ALP because of bone growth. A complete medication history should be taken to rule out the influence of medications, particularly anti-convulsants, corticosteroids, or non-steroidal anti-inflammatory drugs. Various endocrinopathies and metabolic disorders can increased ALP, but are uncommon in young dogs. In the context of the clinical history and other elevated liver enzymes, some degree of hepatic damage is likely, and the increased ALP could suggest a cholestatic component.

Increased ALT and AST: These enzyme changes indicate hepatocellular damage, possibly in combination with some muscle damage, however a CK is not available to corroborate that interpretation. Decreased perfusion associated with shock is likely to be a factor in this patient; sepsis is another possibility. The potential for trauma such as being hit by a car should also be evaluated. Primary liver disease cannot be ruled out, but this is less likely in a young dog and secondary causes are suggested by the history. A liver biopsy is not indicated at this time.

Case Summary and Outcome

Ellis was treated with plasma, fluids, and broad spectrum antibiotics. His history, clinical signs, and laboratory data were compatible with heat stroke. The hematologic abnormalities largely reflect thermal endothelial damage compounded by hypovolemia, shock, and possible bacteremia/endotoxemia from translocation of gut organisms through compromised bowel. Changes in the clinical chemistry profile also largely reflect the same processes, however acute renal compromise and liver damage can be the results of hemodynamic instability and thermal injury to renal tubular cells and hepatocytes. This case may be compared with Sally (Chapter 5, Case 14), who suffered from more severe heat stroke. While Ellis responded well to management, Sally progressed to renal failure secondary to her episode.

Ellis is a good example of how rapidly shifts in fluid and protein can occur. At presentation, losses of fluid in excess of protein loss cause hyperproteinemia, but just 24 hours later, fluid therapy and on-going protein loss result in panhypoproteinemia. Similar changes are noted in the hematocrit.

Case 13 – Level 3

"Sara" is a five-hour-old Thoroughbred foal born one month prematurely to a primiparous mare. The pregnancy and delivery were uncomplicated other than the prematurity; however the foal could not stand after delivery.

White blood cell count:	↓ 3.4 x 10⁹/L	(5.9-11.2)
Segmented neutrophils:	2.6 x 10⁹/L	(2.3-9.1)
Band neutrophils:	0.0	(0-0.3)
Lymphocytes:	↓ 0.6 x 10⁹/L	(1.0-4.9)
Monocytes:	0.2 x 10⁹/L	(0-1.0)
Eosinophils:	0.0 x 10⁹/L	(0.0-0.3)
WBC morphology: No abnormalities seen		

Hematocrit:	37%	(30-51)
Red blood cell count:	8.51x 10¹²/L	(6.5-12.8)
Hemoglobin:	13.3 g/dl	(10.9-18.1)
MCV:	43.7 fl	(35.0-53.0)
MCHC:	35.9 g/dl	(34.6-38.0)
RBC morphology: Mild anisocytosis		

Platelets: Adequate

Fibrinogen:	100 mg/dl	(100-400)
Glucose:	↓ 28 mg/dl	(6.0-128.0)
BUN:	18 mg/dl	(11-26)
Creatinine:	↑ 4.4 mg/dl	(0.9-1.9)
Phosphorus:	5.9 mg/dl	(1.9-6.0)
Calcium:	↑ 14.5 mg/dl	(11.0-13.5)
Magnesium:	2.4 mEq/L	(1.7-2.4)
Total Protein:	↓ 3.9 g/dl	(5.6-7.0)
Albumin:	2.4 g/dl	(2.4-3.8)
Globulin:	↓ 1.5 g/dl	(2.5-4.9)
A/G Ratio:	1.5	(0.7-2.1)
Sodium:	137 mEq/L	(130-145)
Chloride:	↓ 88 mEq/L	(97-105)
Potassium:	4.8 mEq/L	(3.0-5.0)
HCO3:	↑ 47 mEq/L	(25-31)
Anion Gap:	↓ 6.8 mEq/L	(7-15)
Total Bili:	↑ 6.1 mg/dl	(0.6-1.8)
ALP:	↑ 2877 IU/L	(109-352)
GGT:	↑ 29 IU/L	(5-23)
AST:	↓ 173 IU/L	(190-380)
CK:	406 IU/L	(80-446)

Interpretation

CBC: The lymphopenia may be related to corticosteroid effects from stress or may be due to an immature immune system.

Serum Biochemical Profile

Hypoglycemia: This foal is predisposed to sepsis due to immaturity and compromised ability to nurse, so sepsis is a potential cause of hypoglycemia. Although starvation rarely results in hypoglycemia in adult animals, neonates may be predisposed to hypoglycemia with decreased food intake because of low fat stores and inadequate hepatic gluconeogenesis.

Normal BUN and increased creatinine: A urine specific gravity measurement would be helpful in assessing the elevated creatinine. This foal could be dehydrated if it is unable to nurse, however renal disease is possible.

Hypercalcemia: Hypercalcemia and high-normal phosphorus may be attributed to age-related skeletal development, however renal failure in horses can be associated with hypercalcemia (See Chapter 5, Case 9).

Hypomagnesemia: Low intake and increased gastrointestinal losses likely combine to cause the hypomagnesemia.

Hypoproteinemia with normal albumin and hypoglobulinemia: Neonatal animals have relatively higher total body water content, which may slightly depress serum protein levels. In addition, young animals have relatively lower globulin levels because they have been exposed to fewer antigens. In this case, the history suggests failure of transfer of passive immunity due to inadequate intake of colostrum. Serum total globulin is not considered a sensitive or specific test for failure of transfer of passive immunity, which should be evaluated by a more specific test than quantitates IgG.

Normal sodium with hypochloremia and increased HCO3: This foal has a hypochloremic metabolic alkalosis, however hypochloremia may also reflect a response to a respiratory acidosis. Various gastrointestinal problems may cause a metabolic alkalosis, as could excessive supplementation with bicarbonate. With the complex history and potential for respiratory compromise, blood gas analysis is strongly recommended to fully characterize the acid/base status.

Low anion gap: Hypoproteinemia can cause a mildly decreased anion gap because proteins are unmeasured anions.

Hyperbilirubinemia: In horses, anorexia should always be considered as a cause of hyper-bilirubinemia. Sepsis is also possible in this case. Neonatal foal referance intervals are higher than adults; this value may be normal for this age foal.

Increased ALP and GGT: The increased ALP is at least in part due to bone development, however the concurrent increase in GGT could be compatible with hepatic pathology.

Case Summary and Outcome

Sara was treated with oxygen, intravenous fluids, and plasma. A nasogastric tube was placed for nutritional support. Although she remained recumbent, Sara appeared to respond well initially. She had a good suckle reflex and would intermittently attempt to rise. Unfortunately, she suffered a cardiac arrest the next day. Necropsy revealed mild atelectasis with a scant amount of intra-alveolar meconium that indicated intrauterine stress or hypoxia. Interestingly, the liver was characterized by moderate multifocal portal bridging with immature fibrous connective tissue, oval cell hyperplasia with histiocytosis, and intrahepatic cholestasis compatible with congenital biliary dysplasia. This is an unusual lesion that accounts for the elevated GGT and possible some of the elevations in ALP and bilirubin, but is unlikely to have contributed to the death of the patient. The etiology of the lesion was unclear.

Case 14 – Level 3

"Cha-Cha" is a 4-year-old Throughbred stallion that presented for surgical correction of left laryngeal hemiplegia by laryngoplasty. Presurgical CBC and serum biochemical profile were unremarkable. The surgery and initial recovery period were uneventful, however Cha-Cha did not eat well during this time. About a week after surgery, Cha-Cha developed distal limb edema. He presented again 2 weeks after surgery and was lethargic and dehydrated with bright red mucous membranes. On physical examination, Cha-Cha has upper airway edema, an elevated heart rate, and a distended abdomen. He has recently had soft manure, but now has profuse watery diarrhea. A tracheostomy was performed to relieve upper airway distress.

White blood cell count:	↓ 3.3 x 10⁹/L	(5.9-11.2)
Segmented neutrophils:	↓ 1.4 x 10⁹/L	(2.3-9.1)
Band neutrophils:	0.0	(0-0.3)
Lymphocytes:	1.7 x 10⁹/L	(1.0-4.9)
Monocytes:	0.2 x 10⁹/L	(0-1.0)
Eosinophils:	0.0 x 10⁹/L	(0.0-0.3)
WBC morphology: Neutrophils are slightly toxic		

Hematocrit:	↑ 58%	(30-51)
Red blood cell count:	↑ 13.61 x 10¹²/L	(6.5-12.8)
Hemoglobin:	↑ 21.6 g/dl	(10.9-18.1)
MCV:	38.2 fl	(35.0-53.0)
MCHC:	37.2 g/dl	(34.6-38.0)
RBC morphology: Normal		

Platelets: Can not estimate due to clumping

Plasma color: Normal

Fibrinogen:	300 mg/dl	(100-400)

Glucose:	107 mg/dl	(6.0-128.0)
BUN:	↑ 27 mg/dl	(11-26)
Creatinine:	1.2 mg/dl	(0.9-1.9)
Phosphorus:	4.2 mg/dl	(1.9-6.0)
Calcium:	↓ 10.0 mg/dl	(11.0-13.5)
Magnesium:	↓ 1.0 mEq/L	(1.7-2.4)
Total Protein:	↓ 4.1 g/dl	(5.6-7.0)
Albumin:	↓ 1.7 g/dl	(2.4-3.8)
Globulin:	↓ 2.4 g/dl	(2.5-4.9)
A/G Ratio:	0.7	(0.7-2.1)
Sodium:	↓ 125 mEq/L	(130-145)
Chloride:	↓ 94 mEq/L	(97-105)
Potassium:	3.5 mEq/L	(3.0-5.0)
HCO3:	28 mEq/L	(25-31)
Anion Gap:	↓ 6.5 mEq/L	(7-15)
Total Bili:	↑ 4.6 mg/dl	(0.6-1.8)
ALP:	↑ 669 IU/L	(109-352)
GGT:	21 IU/L	(5-23)

AST:	↑ 595 IU/L	(190-380)
LDH:	↑ 881 IU/L	(160-500)
CK:	↑ 907 IU/L	(80-446)

Coagulation Profile

PT:	↑ 17.1s	(109-14.5)
APTT:	↑ 96.6s	(54.7-69.9)
Platelets:	↓ 38 x 10⁹/L	(83-271)
FDPs:	>20 µg/ml	(<5)

Abdominal fluid analysis (Figure 4-6):

Appearance: Yellow and hazy

Total protein: <2.0 g/dl

Total nucleated cell count: 640/µl.

Description: Scattered large mononuclear cells and nondegenerate neutrophils are present. No etiologic agents seen.

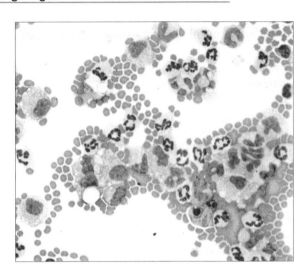

Figure 4-6. Cytocentrifuge preparation of equine abdominal fluid.

Interpretation

CBC: The leucopenia and neutropenia with toxic changes are compatible with severe acute inflammation or endotoxemia. The clinical history of dehydration suggests that the polycythemia is relative and will likely decrease when fluid deficits are corrected. The combination of the neutropenia and thrombocytopenia could be compatible with a primary marrow problem, however since these changes can be explained by sepsis, bone marrow evaluation is not indicated at this time.

Serum Biochemical Profile

Mildly increased BUN: This is compatible with dehydration and pre-renal azotemia, however sepsis may also increase the BUN. A urine specific gravity should be performed to ensure adequate urinary concentrating ability and rule out renal failure.

Hypocalcemia: Low total calcium in this case is attributed to hypoalbuminemia.

Hypomagnesemia: Low intake is the likely cause of the hypomagnesemia.

Panhypoproteinemia: Both globulins and albumin are low, suggesting non-specific protein losses, however the albumin is proportionally lower. This may be because the causes for hypoalbuminemia are more severe or prolonged, or because the globulin protein levels are proportionally increased due to increased production of acute phase reactants or immunoglobulins associated with inflammation. A combination of factors could cause hypoalbuminemia in this horse. While Cha-Cha has not been eating well lately, starvation must be advanced before it causes hypoalbuminemia. Serum albumin is a storage pool of protein, which may be depleted after surgery or trauma. Decreased hepatic production of albumin is possible given the elevated liver enzymes, however these are not adequate liver function tests (See Chapter 2) and the absence of a pre-surgical history of liver enzyme elevations or signs of liver disease makes this less likely. A severe, acute, diffuse liver insult cannot be ruled out though. There may be a physiologic decrease in albumin production by the liver since Cha-Cha has inflammatory disease and albumin is a negative acute phase reactant. Nonspecific protein losses that could result in hypoalbuminemia and hypoglobulinemia include gastrointestinal lesions and interstitial displacement of protein. Both are likely given the history of diarrhea and distal limb edema. Hemorrhage secondary to the coagulopathy is also possible, but is not described in the clinical history and does not appear likely with polycythemia.

Hyponatremia and hypochloremia: These electrolyte changes are proportional and reflect gastrointestinal losses that exceed water losses or volume repletion with hypotonic solutions.

Low anion gap: Hypoalbuminemia can cause a decreased anion gap because is it an unmeasured anion.

Hyperbilirubinemia: In horses, anorexia should always be considered as a cause of hyperbilirubinemia. The concurrently elevated ALP, AST, and LDH indicate that liver disease is another potential contributor to increased serum bilirubin. Hemolysis as a cause of hyperbilirubinemia is unlikely given the polycythemia.

Increased ALP, AST, LDH, and CK: The increased ALP, AST, and LDH are compatible with liver disease, however these enzymes are not liver specific. The CK is also elevated, supporting some contribution by muscle damage. GGT is more liver specific than the ALP in large animals, however it is normal at this time. LDH has a short half-life, and suggests on going tissue damage. Poor perfusion of many tissues secondary to dehydration and sepsis is likely. The coagulation data is compatible with disseminated intravascular coagulation (DIC) and suggests the potential for tissue necrosis secondary to thromboembolic disease. Intestinal disease alone can cause secondary liver pathology as the portal circulation delivers potentially high quantities of bacteria, bacterial toxins, and inflammatory mediators to the liver.

Coagulation profile: The combination of thrombocytopenia and prolonged PT and APTT with increased fibrin degradation products meets the criteria for a mixed hemostatic defect, likely DIC. Sepsis and vasculitis are likely causes for DIC in this patient, although severe liver disease may also trigger DIC or DIC-like changes in coagulation data.

Abdominal fluid analysis: Transudate. This is within normal limits for abdominal fluid in the horse.

Case Summary and Outcome

Cha-Cha's condition continued to deteriorate despite aggressive therapy, and she died after developing profuse nasal bleeding. At necropsy, the cause of death was determined to be extensive pulmonary thromboembolism. Severe necrotizing and ulcerative typhlocolitis and acute neutrophilic periportal hepatitis and hepatocellular necrosis were also present.

This case may be compared to Salty (Case 9), who presented with a similarly severe gastrointestinal lesion in a more acute setting. At Salty's presentation, fluid losses exceeded protein loss so he was hyperalbuminemic. It is likely that had he survived longer, his laboratory data could have eventually become similar to Cha Cha's, in which tissue compromise and sepsis resulted in marked loss of protein from the circulation. Chapter 5, Case 19 (Faith) is another horse presenting with compromised bowel with protein loss into the gut who had a similar negative outcome to Salty and Cha Cha. All of these horses had some evidence of concurrent electrolyte loss assumed to be via the gut. This loss of protein and electrolytes into the GI tract was also observed in Snickers, the puppy with parvoviral enteritis (Case 6).

Overview

Step 1: Remember that total proteins may be misleading and fractionation into albumin and globulin may reveal abnormalities not apparent with only a total protein measurement (Cases 1, 2, 7, 9)

Step 2: Evaluate the patient's hydration status.

Dehydration may cause hyperalbuminemia (Case 9, 12) or may push a hypoalbuminemic patient into the reference interval. Less often, dehydration may cause mild hyperglobulinemia or push a hypoglobulinemic patient into the reference range.

Overhydration may have a dilutional effect.

Step 3: Does the patient have panhypoproteinemia? This suggests non-selective protein loss.

Is the patient bleeding? Case 3
Does the patient have exudative skin lesions?
Does the patient have cavity effusions? Case 3, 7
Does the patient have gastrointestinal disease? Case 4, 6, 9, 12, 14
Does the patient have edema/vasculitis? Case 5, 12

Step 4: If the patient has selective hypoalbuminemia, consider the following.

Evaluate body condition and diet for nutritional influences, which are rare (Case 1).

Consider increased demand for protein if the patient is febrile or has a history of surgery or trauma. This usually causes only mild hypoalbuminemia in the absence of other factors.

Consider physiological downregulation of albumin production if there is evidence of inflammation (albumin is a negative acute phase reactant) or concurrent hyperglobulinemia (to regulate oncotic pressure). Case 7, 8

Evaluate liver function, especially if there is any combination of the following: hypoglycemia, low BUN, hypocholesterolemia, hyperbilirubinemia, prolonged coagulation times. Case 2

Perform a urinalysis. If there is proteinuria in a sample collected by cystocentesis with no evidence of inflammation, glomerular loss of albumin may be occurring. This may be further quantified by performing a urine protein:creatinine ratio. This is also recommended as a more sensitive way to evaluate proteinuria if the urine is dilute (Case 5).

Step 5: If the patient is hyperglobulinemic, evaluate for inflammation/antigenic stimulation vs. neoplasia.

The presence of inflammation can be supported by leukogram data, including the presence of neutrophilia, left shift, toxic change, and lymphocytosis with reactive cells. This is a more common cause of hyperglobulinemia and is usually associated with a polyclonal gammopathy. Rarely a monoclonal gammopathy can occur with some inflammatory diseases (Case 7).

The presence of neoplasia should be considered in older patients, patients with hypercalcemia, mass lesions or organomegaly, lytic bone lesions, or patients with peripheral cytopenias. Lymphadenopathy may occur with either neoplasia or inflammation/antigenic stimulation. Monoclonal gammopathies usually reflect production of a single immunoglobulin by neoplastic lymphocytes or plasma cells (Case 8).

Step 6: Consider the sum of the effects of all clinical factors on the protein values. Additive effects may result in values within the reference range despite significant pathology.

Chapter 5

Tests of Renal Function

The kidney is a central organ in the regulation of electrolyte, acid/base, and fluid balance, in addition to having an important endocrine role in controlling calcium and phosphorus homeostasis and erythropoiesis. This chapter will focus on BUN, creatinine, and urine specific gravity as tests of renal function. Other abnormalities associated with renal disease will be explained as has been the case in previous chapters, however for more detailed discussions of electrolytes and minerals, the reader is referred to appropriate chapters in this text. Urinalysis data will be discussed when available for the cases in this chapter, but a complete review of urinalysis is beyond the scope of the book. The reader is referred to several excellent resources for this information in the begining of this text.

Two sets of definitions should be reviewed prior to discussing tests of renal function. Both will be important for describing and classifying patients with renal disease.

Azotemia: The presence of increased non-protein nitrogenous compounds in the blood. This is routinely assessed by the measurement of blood urea nitrogen (BUN) and creatinine.

Uremia: The loss of a critical amount of renal function resulting in a group of clinical signs that can include lethargy, anorexia, mucosal ulceration, vomiting, diarrhea, weight loss, anemia, altered urine output, and hyperparathyroidism.

In general, as renal disease progresses, urinary concentrating ability is lost first, followed by the development of azotemia. Cats may retain some concentrating ability despite the presence of renal azotemia. By the time clinical signs of uremia develop, the patient is almost always azotemic and isosthenuric. In contrast, patients may be azotemic for some period of time prior to the development of uremia. To further classify the potential causes for azotemia, the condition is described as pre-renal, renal, or post-renal. These three descriptors of azotemia are not mutually exclusive; as will be seen in the cases, any of the three may occur in any combination in a patient.

Pre-renal azotemia: This occurs when there is reduced renal perfusion because of hypovolemia or reduced renal perfusion pressures. For example, uncompensated hypovolemia associated with dehydration or hemorrhage can cause pre-renal azotemia. Renal perfusion may be reduced because of low cardiac output secondary to primary heart disease, or if blood pressure cannot be maintained because of systemic vasodilation that is the result of shock or sepsis. When pre-renal azotemia occurs in patients with normal renal function, the urine is generally concentrated, which helps rule out renal azotemia. In some cases, however, extra-renal factors such as medullary wash-out, osmotic diuresis, or endocrine disorders interfere with the kidney's ability to concentrate urine in the absence of significant renal parenchymal damage.

Renal azotemia: Primary renal parenchymal disease of any cause results in renal azotemia. The presence or degree of confirmed renal azotemia does not distinguish an acute from a chronic process. As will be seen below, BUN and serum creatinine are not sensitive indicators of decreased renal function, and they may be influenced by extra-renal factors.

Post-renal azotemia: Failure of urine to be excreted from the body causes post-renal azotemia, which is generally diagnosed by clinical signs such as minimal to absent urinations and possible abdominal distension as urine accumulates. Physical obstruction of urine flow and uroabdomen are two causes of post-renal azotemia. Please note that some patients with post-renal azotemia may be able to pass small amounts of urine. The obstruction of flow does not need to be complete to cause azotemia.

Although creatinine and BUN are most commonly thought of as indicators of renal function, non-renal variables may influence these analytes.

Creatinine measured in the blood originates from either consumption of animal tissues or from irreversible, non-enzymatic degradation of muscle creatine. Therefore, diet (unlikely to be clinically significant), muscle mass, and muscle damage or breakdown could influence serum creatinine concentrations. Volume expansion could dilute serum creatinine. Most of the creatinine formed in the body is eliminated by the kidney, although small amounts may be lost in sweat, in the gastrointestinal tract, or via biochemical recycling pathways. Creatinine is freely filtered in the glomerulus, with a small amount of active transport into the urine in some species. Decreased glomerular filtration rate (GFR) increases serum creatinine, while increased glomerular filtration can slightly decrease serum creatinine concentrations. In general, creatinine is less influenced by extra-renal factors than BUN, however some creatinine assays lack analytic specificity and will measure substances other than creatinine. This may result in some variation in serum creatinine unrelated to changes in GFR in the normal range of serum creatinine concentrations. These noncreatinine chromagens are present in small, relatively constant quantities in the blood and this interference is unlikely to make a normal animal appear to be azotemic or to significantly impact the degree of azotemia in patients with renal failure.

Small amounts of urea are ingested in the diet, however the majority of blood urea nitrogen is generated from protein derived ammonium by the urea cycle in the liver. Thus, similar to creatinine, protein metabolism can influence BUN. High protein diets or increased muscle catabolism can increase BUN, and there is some evidence that individuals with compromised renal function may have impaired ability to eliminate an acute urea load even though they may not be azotemic in the fasted state. Conversely, low muscle mass, low protein diet, or poor urea cycle activity associated with liver failure may lower BUN. Some urea may be lost in the gastrointestinal tract, and in ruminants, gut bacteria may utilize sufficient quantities to blunt elevations in BUN when the GFR is compromised. Unlike creatinine, urea undergoes some passive reabsorption in the collecting ducts. Higher tubular flow rates decrease the amount of time available for reabsorption, and decrease BUN while low tubular flow rates result in greater urea reabsorption. This means that changes in urine flow can alter BUN with no significant change in total glomerular filtration rate.

As noted above, neither creatinine nor BUN is a sensitive indicator of decreased renal function, and patients may have lost as much as 75% of renal function prior to the development of azotemia. In addition, BUN and creatinine do not change linearly with further decrements in renal function, so a patient whose creatinine doubles may have less than half of the original glomerular filtration rate. The ability of non-renal factors to impact serum creatinine and BUN can also contribute to variation in azotemia unrelated to true changes in renal function. Finally, it should be noted that significant glomerular lesions can occur that result in protein losing nephropathy in the absence of azotemia. Eventually, glomerular lesions will cause tubular and interstitial pathology and nephron loss with resultant azotemia, but this can occur late in the disease in some patients.

Case 1 – Level 1

"Marklar" is a 7-year-old castrated male, domestic shorthair cat that has been missing for 4 days. Marklar normally is an exclusively indoor cat. He returned home with some weight loss, although his body condition is still good. He is obviously hungry and thirsty. His owners request a health check and blood work. Marklar has tacky mucus membranes and a slightly prolonged capillary refill time, but he otherwise appears healthy.

White blood cell count:	15.0 x 10⁹/L	(4.5-15.7)
Segmented neutrophils:	↑ 13.7 x 10⁹/L	(2.1-10.1)
Lymphocytes:	↓ 0.7 x 10⁹/L	(1.5-7.0)
Monocytes:	0.6 x 10⁹/L	(0-0.9)
Eosinophils:	0 x 10⁹/L	(0.0-1.9)
WBC morphology: No significant abnormalities		
Hematocrit:	45%	(28-45)
Platelets: Clumped, but appear adequate		
Glucose:	↑ 142 mg/dl	(70.0-120.0)
BUN:	↑ 75 mg/dl	(15-32)
Creatinine:	↑ 3.5 mg/dl	(0.9-2.1)
Phosphorus:	↑ 7.0 mg/dl	(3.0-6.0)
Calcium:	9.6 mg/dl	(8.9-11.6)
Magnesium:	2.5 mEq/L	(1.9-2.6)
Total Protein:	↑ 9.0 g/dl	(6.0-8.4)
Albumin:	↑ 4.5 g/dl	(2.4-4.0)
Globulin:	4.5 g/dl	(2.5-5.8)
Sodium:	↑ 165 mEq/L	(149-163)
Chloride:	134 mEq/L	(119-134)
Potassium:	4.0 mEq/L	(3.6-5.4)
HCO3:	18 mEq/L	(13-22)
Total Bili:	0.2 mg/dl	(0.10-0.30)
ALP:	48 IU/L	(10-72)
ALT:	71 IU/L	(29-145)
AST:	41 IU/L	(12-42)
Cholesterol:	123 mg/dl	(77-258)
Triglycerides:	56 mg/dl	(25-191)
Amylase:	1,523 IU/L	(496-1874)

Urinalysis: Cystocentesis

Appearance: Yellow and slightly cloudy	Sediment:
Specific gravity: >1.060	0 RBC/high power field
pH: 6.0	No WBC seen
Protein: negative	No casts seen
Glucose/ketones: negative	No epithelial cells seen
Bilirubin: negative	No bacteria
Heme: negative	Trace fat droplets and debris

Interpretation

CBC: Marklar has a mature mild neutrophilia and lymphopenia consistent with a corticosteroid leukogram, probably due to stress from being lost.

Serum Biochemical Profile

Hyperglycemia: The most likely cause for the mild hyperglycemia in this patient is stress, which is supported by the concurrent corticosteroid leukogram. Diabetes mellitus cannot be ruled out, but is unlikely based on the mild elevation of glucose, normal urinalysis, and absence of typical clinical history. Note that despite several days of inadequate food intake, there is no hypoglycemia (see Chapter 3 for further discussion of anorexia and serum glucose values).

Increased BUN and creatinine, hyperphosphatemia: These changes are indicators of decreased glomerular filtration rate. The concentrated urine supports a pre-renal cause of azotemia. Marklar has clinical signs as well as laboratory data (hyperalbuminemia and hypernatremia with a proportionally high normal hyperchloremia) compatible with dehydration.

Hyperproteinemia due to hyperalbuminemia: The liver does not over-produce albumin, therefore this value indicates dehydration.

Hypernatremia: Causes of hypernatremia include increased intake (possible but unlikely) or dehydration with the loss of water exceeding the loss of electrolytes such as when access to water is restricted. This is likely given the cat's history of being lost for several days.

Urinalysis: Highly concentrated urine with no significant abnormalities.

Case Summary and Outcome

Marklar was given a bolus of subcutaneous fluids and sent home with his owners. This is a good example of pre-renal azotemia. Marklar had multiple laboratory abnormalities compatible with dehydration because of a pure water deficit and no concurrent losses of protein or erythrocytes. Many patients will be dehydrated and yet have normal electrolytes, protein, or packed cell volume because losses of these analytes occur simultaneously with loss of fluid or other factors are influencing their concentration in the blood. In addition, the reference intervals for some of these analytes are wide, allowing for considerable change without deviation from "normal" values. In these cases, clinical indicators of dehydration will be more reliable than laboratory data to diagnose poor hydration status. Although Marklar had no evidence of renal failure, in some patients dehydration may impose some degree of pre-renal azotemia on top of renal azotemia. In these cases, isosthenuria does not rule out a pre-renal component.

Case 2 – Level 1

"Sherpa" is a 10-year-old castrated male Collie presenting with a 5 month history of hematuria and stranguria. He now requires 3-5 minutes to urinate and dribbles small amounts. Sherpa was treated with antibiotics last month and 6 months ago. He has a history of seizures which are well controlled by phenobarbital. On physical examination, Sherpa has nuclear sclerosis in both eyes, severe dental tartar and moderate gingivitis. His abdomen is taught and difficult to palpate.

White blood cell count:	5.1 x 10⁹/L	(4.0-13.3)
Segmented neutrophils:	4.3 x 10⁹/L	(2.0-11.2)
Band neutrophils:	0.0 x 10⁹/L	(0-0.3)
Lymphocytes:	↓ 0.2 x 10⁹/L	(1.0-4.5)
Monocytes:	0.2 x 10⁹/L	(0.2-1.4)
Eosinophils:	0.4 x 10⁹/L	(0-1.2)
WBC morphology: Appears within normal limits		

Hematocrit:	43.5%	(37-60)
Red blood cell count:	6.77 x 10¹²/L	(5.5-8.5)
Hemoglobin:	15.5 g/dl	(12.0-18.0)
MCV:	64.2 fl	(60.0-77.0)
MCHC:	35.6 g/dl	(31.0-34.0)

Platelets: Appear adequate

Glucose:	124 mg/dl	(90.0-140.0)
BUN:	↑ 33 mg/dl	(6-24)
Creatinine:	1.2 mg/dl	(0.5-1.5)
Phosphorus:	3.2 mg/dl	(2.2-6.6)
Calcium:	10.6 mg/dl	(9.5-11.5)
Total Protein:	6.2 g/dl	(4.8-7.2)
Albumin:	3.1 g/dl	(2.5-3.7)
Globulin:	3.1 g/dl	(2.0-4.0)
Sodium:	149 mEq/L	(140-151)
Chloride:	118 mEq/L	(105-120)
Potassium:	4.6 mEq/L	(3.6-5.6)
Anion gap:	13.5 mEq/L	(6-16)
HCO3:	22.1 mEq/L	(15-28)
Total Bili:	0.3 mg/dl	(0.10-0.50)
ALP:	↑ 606 IU/L	(20-320)
GGT:	8 IU/L	(2-10)
ALT:	↑ 114 IU/L	(10-95)
AST:	29 IU/L	(10-56)
Cholesterol:	↑ 352 mg/dl	(110-314)
Amylase:	↑ 1348 IU/L	(400-1200)

Urinalysis: Catheter

Appearance: Yellow and cloudy	Sediment:
	5-20 erythrocytes/hpf
Specific gravity: 1.015	0-5 WBC/hpf
pH: 7.5	4-8 epithelial cell/hpf with clumping and atypical cells
Glucose, ketones, bilirubin: negative	
Protein: 2+	
Heme: 2+	

Interpretation

CBC: Sherpa has a mild lymphopenia which is compatible with corticosteroid effects.

Serum Biochemical Profile

Elevated BUN and normal serum creatinine: Early pre-renal azotemia is possible if other extra-renal causes of increased BUN are ruled out. However, the relatively low specific gravity raises concerns about urinary concentrating ability. Reduced tubular flow rates may increase the amount of time for reabsorption of urea and elevate levels in the blood even if there is no decrease in the glomerular filtration rate. No fever, sepsis, gastrointestinal hemorrhage, or trauma are present in the history to suggest these potential causes of increased BUN with normal creatinine.

Increased ALP and ALT: In this case, the most likely cause is induction by treatment with anticonvulsants (see Chapter 2). Enzyme induction by corticosteroids or liver disease cannot be completely ruled out without further testing.

Hypercholesterolemia: Hypercholesterolemia of this magnitude is unlikely to be physiologically significant in the dog, and post-prandial elevations should be ruled out first. Multiple endocrinopathies can be associated with hypercholesterolemia, including diabetes (unlikely with normal serum glucose), hypothyroidism (possible, but no compatible clinical signs reported at this time), hyperadrenocorticism (possible as there is concurrent lymphopenia and increased ALP, but no clinical signs), pancreatic and hepatic disease (possible with increased liver enzymes and amylase, but, again, no compatible clinical signs), and renal disease (possible, with clinical signs referable to the urinary system, but only mild elevation in BUN). Idiopathic hypercholesterolemia may be ruled out by examination of any previously normal serum biochemical data.

Hyperamylasemia: Mild elevations are associated with decreased glomerular filtration rate, which is possible in this case, given the elevated BUN. Pancreatic disease may be considered if appropriate clinical signs develop.

Urinalysis: The proteinuria and presence of erythrocytes and leukocytes suggest inflammation of the urinary tract. Atypical epithelial cells may indicate the presence of reactive epithelial hyperplasia in response to the inflammation. Alternatively, with the history of stranguria, the potential for neoplasia with secondary inflammation should be evaluated by imaging of the urinary tract.

Case Summary and Outcome

Ultrasound evaluation of Sherpa's urinary tract revealed an extensive tumor of the urinary bladder which completely blocked the left ureter and resulted in hydronephrosis. The right kidney was not involved, however there was mild ureteral dilation and hydronephrosis of the right kidney as well. Cytologic examination of cells from the bladder mass showed sheets and clusters of anaplastic transitional epithelial cells characterized by scant to abundant deeply basophilic cytoplasm; occasional cells have cytoplasmic tails characteristic of transitional epithelial cells (Figure 5-1). Rare cells have a single large cytoplasmic inclusion of bright pink hyaline material. Most cells contain a single round to oval nucleus, although scattered binucleated cells with nuclear molding were also present. Some cells contain small but prominent nucleoli. The nuclear to cytoplasmic ratio is high but markedly variable. Anisocytosis and anisokaryosis were marked. The diagnosis was transitional cell carcinoma. Sherpa was treated with chemotherapy.

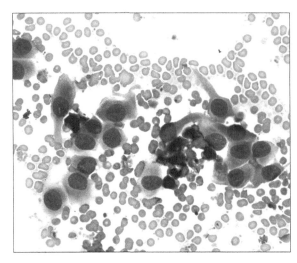

Figure 5-1. Cytology of transitional cell carcinoma from the urinary bladder mass.

Sherpa's case demonstrates how severe urinary tract disease may be present with minimal indication on the serum biochemical profile. What azotemia is present is attributable to the post-renal obstructive effects of the transitional cell carcinoma. Increased pressure in the tubules secondary to outflow obstruction can result in either transient or permanent decreases in tubular function depending on the duration and severity of the pressure. Renal function may increase over time as temporary losses of renal tubular function are regained and as remaining functional nephrons undergo compensatory hypertrophy with enhanced function. Alternatively, there may be ongoing losses of renal function because at a certain point, renal lesions can progress despite correction of the initial cause of injury. Because of these factors, sequential serum biochemical profiles on the patient may show normalization of abnormalities or progressive azotemia with the development of other biochemical abnormalities that accompany renal failure. Chemotherapy may result in temporary relief of obstruction, however the long-term prognosis is poor.

This case should be compared with Case 1, Marklar, in which pre-renal factors caused a more significant increase in BUN and creatinine despite absence of renal disease. Therefore, the degree of azotemia does not always distinguish pre-renal from renal changes or their potential reversibility. Marklar's ability to concentrate his urine was a key indicator of adequate renal function despite the azotemia.

Case 3 – Level 1

"Marsali" is a 10-year-old Paint mare that presents for evaluation after being seized for mistreatment by law enforcement agents. She is extremely thin with a poor hair coat (Figure 5-2A). She appears bright and alert with pale mucous membranes.

Hematocrit:	↓ 26%	(30-51)
Glucose:	↓ 70 mg/dl	(71-106)
BUN:	↓ 9 mg/dl	(13-25)
Creatinine:	↓ 0.8 mg/dl	(0.9-1.9)
Phosphorus:	3.5 mg/dl	(1.9-6.0)
Calcium:	11.4 mg/dl	(10.2-13.0)
Magnesium:	2.2 mEq/L	(1.7-2.4)
Total Protein:	↑ 8.3 g/dl	(5.2-7.1)
Albumin:	↓ 2.1 g/dl	(2.6-3.8)
Globulin:	↑ 6.2 g/dl	(2.5-4.9)
Sodium:	135 mEq/L	(130-145)
Chloride:	99 mEq/L	(97-110)
Potassium:	3.8 mEq/L	(3.0-5.0)
HCO3:	26.4 mEq/L	(25-31)
Total Bili:	0.6 mg/dl	(0.30-3.0)
ALP:	174 IU/L	(109-352)
GGT:	24 IU/L	(4-28)
SDH:	3 IU/L	(1-7)
AST:	313 IU/L	(190-380)
CK:	370 IU/L	(80-446)

Interpretation

CBC: Marsali is anemic. With the limited clinical history, anemia of chronic disease or malnutrition are likely causes, however poor management also suggests the possibility of parasitism. Blood loss is possible with the concurrent hypoalbuminemia, however nutritional factors could influence this analyte as well.

Serum Biochemical Profile
Hypoglycemia: This change is minimal and is unlikely to be clinically significant. Anorexia is an uncommon cause of hypoglycemia but is more likely in cases of advanced starvation like Marsali. Even under these extreme circumstances, blood glucose is often maintained within or just slightly below reference range.

Low BUN and creatinine: Low protein diets and poor muscle mass can result in decreased BUN and creatinine. Increased glomerular filtration rate and water retention associated with pregnancy can decrease creatinine, while polyuria can decrease BUN. Marsali was not pregnant and her urine output appeared to be normal.

Hyperproteinemia characterized by hypoalbuminemia and hyperglobulinemia: Both decreased hepatic production and increased losses can lower serum albumin. Marsali is one of the rare cases in which decreased production may be due to starvation. Because albumin is a negative acute phase reactant, hepatic production may be suppressed with inflammation. This mechanism seems plausible given the hyperglobulinemia, however supporting evidence such as hyperfibrinogenemia and an inflammatory leukogram are not available in this case.

Because albumin is a readily usable protein reserve, hypoalbuminemia can occur with fever, surgery, or other causes of increased catabolism. Selective loss of albumin is characteristic of glomerular lesions, while most other causes of protein loss (gastrointestinal, dermal, or third space loss) include both albumin and globulins. Hyperglobulinemia is due to increased acute phase reactants and/or immunoglobulins. Polyclonal expansions are associated with antigenic stimulation, and infectious disease is likely given the management at Marsali's farm. Hyperglobulinemia due to monoclonal gammopathy is often associated with hematopoietic malignancies such as lymphoma or multiple myeloma, although in small animals, infectious diseases such as feline infectious peritonitis, tick borne pathogens and *Leishmania* rarely can cause monoclonal gammopathy.

Case Summary and Outcome

Marsali was wormed and placed on an appropriate diet. She responded very well, gained 51 pounds while in the hospital, and was transferred to the Minnesota Hooved Animal Rescue Foundation, a local group that rehabilitates abused or neglected livestock, where she completed her recovery (Figure 5-2B).

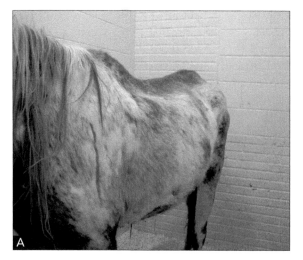

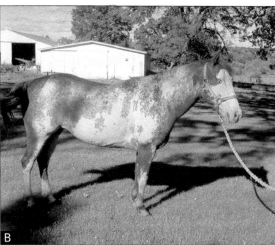

Figure 5-2A & B. Marsali in poor body condition, A. Healthy body condition, B.

Case 4 – Level 1

"Jag" is a 7-year-old castrated male Golden Retriever mixed breed dog presenting with a history of "not doing right." Over the last few days, Jag has begun vomiting and will not eat.

White blood cell count:	9.0 x 10⁹/L	(6.0-17.0)
Segmented neutrophils:	↓ 2.5 x 10⁹/L	(3.0-11.0)
Band neutrophils:	0.0 x 10⁹/L	(0-0.3)
Lymphocytes:	↑ 6.0 x 10⁹/L	(1.0-4.8)
Monocytes:	0.5 x 10⁹/L	(0.2-1.4)
Eosinophils:	0.0 x 10⁹/L	(0-1.3)

WBC morphology: Occasional atypical lymphocytes are seen.

Hematocrit:	39%	(37-55)
MCV:	62.5 fl	(60.0-77.0)
MCHC:	33.1 g/dl	(31.0-34.0)

RBC morphology: Appears within normal limits

Platelets:	↓ 152 x 10⁹/L	(200-450)

Glucose:	103 mg/dl	(65.0-120.0)
BUN:	↑ 63 mg/dl	(8-33)
Creatinine:	↑ 3.8 mg/dl	(0.5-1.5)
Phosphorus:	3.8 mg/dl	(3.0-6.0)
Calcium:	↑ 17.6 mg/dl	(8.8-11.0)
Magnesium:	2.5 mEq/L	(1.4-2.7)
Total Protein:	6.3 g/dl	(5.2-7.2)
Albumin:	3.5 g/dl	(3.0-4.2)
Globulin:	2.8 g/dl	(2.0-4.0)
A/G Ratio:	1.2	(0.7-2.1)
Sodium:	155 mEq/L	(140-163)
Chloride:	114 mEq/L	(105-126)
Potassium:	↓ 3.6 mEq/L	(3.8-5.4)
HCO3:	25 mEq/L	(16-28)
Anion Gap:	19.6 mEq/L	(15-25)
Total Bili:	0.30 mg/dl	(0.10-0.50)
ALP:	184 IU/L	(20-320)
GGT:	9 IU/L	(2-10)
ALT:	47 IU/L	(10-86)
AST:	47 IU/L	(15-52)
Cholesterol:	188 mg/dl	(110-314)
Triglycerides:	85 mg/dl	(30-300)
Amylase:	490 IU/L	(400-1200)

Urinalysis: Cystocentesis

Appearance: Yellow and clear	Sediment: inactive

Specific gravity: 1.007

pH: 7.0

Negative for protein, glucose, ketones, bilirubin, heme

Interpretation

CBC: Jag has a mild neutropenia and thrombocytopenia, while the packed cell volume is still within the normal range. The combination of bicytopenia with the presence of atypical lymphocytes is reason to consider bone marrow evaluation. The concurrent hypercalcemia can be an indication for bone marrow biopsy by itself, and in combination with bicytopenia it is a strong rationale for the procedure if no extramarrow cause for the bicytopenia is apparent.

Serum Biochemical Profile

Azotemia: Classically, the combination of azotemia and isosthenuria is interpreted to be evidence of renal failure. In general, this is true, however in some cases, extra-renal factors may interfere with urinary concentrating ability in the absence of significant structural renal lesions. Examples include diabetes insipidus, medullary washout, or bacterial toxins in pyometra. In this case, the patient is hyposthenuric, which implies some ability of the kidney to modify the filtrate, and therefore some renal function. Hypercalcemia can result in temporary reversible renal dysfunction in the short term, or actual renal damage and subsequent renal failure in the long term. If the azotemia is merely due to the obligatory fluid losses associated with temporary polyuria, the azotemia may be pre-renal. It may not be possible to determine which is more likely from the data available at this time. Imaging studies of the kidney and repeat biochemistry and urinalysis after correction of hypercalcemia are required to categorize the azotemia in these cases. See below for description of the mechanisms for azotemia associated with hypercalcemia.

Hypercalcemia with normal phosphorus: After ruling out laboratory artifact, hypercalcemia of malignancy should be a primary differential diagnosis in this case. Lymphoma is a common cause of hypercalcemia of malignancy, however multiple myeloma, thymoma, anal sac apocrine gland adenocarcinoma, and other carcinomas also may be associated with hypercalcemia. The serum phosphorus is generally normal or decreased in patients with hypercalcemia of malignancy, although concurrent decrements in glomerular filtration rate with the development of renal complications could elevate phosphorus concentrations. Hypercalcemia of malignancy may be confirmed by identifying a causative neoplasm and/or demonstrating increased concentrations of parathyroid hormone related protein (PTHrP) and low to normal parathyroid hormone (PTH). Another consideration for hypercalcemia with normal to low serum phosphorus is primary hyperparathyroidism. In that case, the presence of a parathyroid tumor with an elevated PTH but normal PTHrP would be expected. Renal failure and hypervitaminosis D may also elevate serum calcium, but are typically associated with hyperphosphatemia. Other causes of hypercalcemia such as skeletal lesions and bone growth, granulomatous disease, hemoconcentration, or hypoadrenocorticism are less likely based on the clinical history and the degree of hypercalcemia noted in this patient.

Hypokalemia: A combination of decreased intake with anorexia and increased losses due to polyuria contribute to hypokalemia in this case. Gastrointestinal losses are also possible with the history of vomiting. There is no evidence of acid/base abnormalities that would cause intracellular translocation of potassium.

Case Summary and Outcome

Ultrasound evaluation of the parathyroid gland and abdomen failed to reveal any lesions, however a bone marrow aspirate contained large numbers of immature lymphocytes compatible with a lymphoid neoplasm (Figure 5-3). This was considered sufficient to explain the hypercalcemia, and PTHrP levels were not measured. The pathogenesis of hypercalcemia of malignancy will be discussed in greater detail in Chapter 6, but briefly, PTHrP stimulates osteoclastic bone resorption and renal calcium reabsorption. Dehydration may further compromise renal calcium excretion. Jag underwent chemotherapy for his cancer and the hypercalcemia resolved with therapy. After his calcium levels normalized, Jag began concentrating his urine again with no observable deficit in renal function. Jag should be compared with Marklar in Case 1, who had pre-renal azotemia with concentrated urine, which made it easier to verify adequate renal function. Marklar also had hyperphosphatemia, which generally accompanies decreased GFR, except in cases like Jag, where other factors may be lowering serum phosphorus.

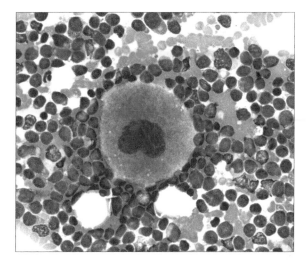

Figure 5-3. Canine bone marrow lymphoma. The very large central cell is a megakaryocyte.

Jag is a good example of a patient with azotemia and a low urine specific gravity that does not have irreversible chronic renal failure, although it was not possible to be sure of this based on only the initial blood work. Hypercalcemia can cause a nephrogenic diabetes insipidus-like syndrome because of decreased tubular reabsorption of sodium and interference with the action of antidiuretic hormone on renal tubules. These responses are mediated by calcium-sensing receptors on renal epithelial cells and are designed to promote excretion of excess calcium. Renal medullary blood flow may increase in hypercalcemic dogs, with resultant medullary washout and impaired concentrating ability. Production of large amounts of dilute urine results in dehydration and pre-renal azotemia.

With chronic and severe hypercalcemia, calcium-mediated vasoconstriction and subsequent ischemia combined with direct toxic effects of calcium on renal tubular cells can cause permanent nephron loss and renal failure. At this point, the patient is typically isosthenuric, and other clinical and laboratory signs of renal failure may become apparent.

Case 5 – Level 1

"Sheba" is a 5-year-old spayed female Labrador Retreiver presenting with a history of decreased appetite and weight loss over the past several months. More recently, Sheba has been experiencing shifting leg lameness. On presentation, Sheba has peripheral lymphadenopathy, and cytologic specimens were collected.

White blood cell count:	7.8 x 10⁹/L	(6.0-17.0)
Segmented neutrophils:	6.0 x 10⁹/L	(3.0-11.0)
Band neutrophils:	0 x 10⁹/L	(0-0.3)
Lymphocytes:	1.3 x 10⁹/L	(1.0-4.8)
Monocytes:	0.2 x 10⁹/L	(0.2-1.4)
Eosinophils:	0.3 x 10⁹/L	(0-1.3)
WBC morphology: Mild toxic changes observed in the neutrophils		

Hematocrit:	↓ 25%	(37-55)
MCV:	73.5 fl	(60.0-77.0)
MCHC:	34.8 g/dl	(31.0-34.0)
RBC morphology: No abnormalities noted		

Platelets:	↓ 40 x 10⁹/L	(181-525)

Glucose:	104 mg/dl	(65.0-120.0)
BUN:	↑ 114 mg/dl	(8-33)
Creatinine:	↑ 5.9 mg/dl	(0.5-1.5)
Phosphorus:	↑ 9.0 mg/dl	(3.0-6.0)
Calcium:	10.2 mg/dl	(8.8-11.0)
Magnesium:	↑ 2.8 mEq/L	(1.4-2.7)
Total Protein:	5.7 g/dl	(5.2-7.2)
Albumin:	↓ 1.9 g/dl	(3.0-4.2)
Globulin:	3.8 g/dl	(2.0-4.0)
Sodium:	147 mEq/L	(140-151)
Chloride:	109 mEq/L	(105-120)
Potassium:	5.4 mEq/L	(3.8-5.4)
HCO3:	25 mEq/L	(16-25)
Anion Gap:	18.4 mEq/L	(15-25)
Total Bili:	0.10 mg/dl	(0.10-0.50)
ALP:	48 IU/L	(20-320)
GGT:	<3 IU/L	(3-10)
ALT:	21 IU/L	(10-95)
AST:	38 IU/L	(15-52)
Cholesterol:	219 mg/dl	(110-314)
Triglycerides:	79 mg/dl	(30-300)
Amylase:	↑ 1894 IU/L	(400-1200)

Urinalysis: Cystocentesis

Appearance: Pale yellow and clear	Sediment: inactive
Specific gravity: 1.010	
pH: 6.0	
Glucose, ketones, bilirubin, heme: negative	
Protein: 2+	

Urine protein:creatinine ratio: 8.1

Lymph node aspirates: Numerous markedly cellular smears consist almost entirely of intact cells. The population of cells is heterogeneous and consists of large numbers of small, mature lymphocytes and well differentiated plasma cells mixed with occasional medium and large cells and scattered Mott cells. A few nondegenerate neutrophils, macrophages and rare heavily granulated mast cells are also present (Figure 5-4).

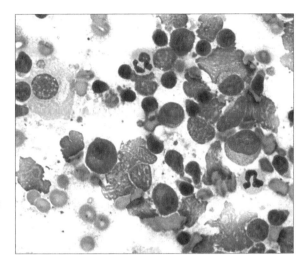

Figure 5-4. Canine reactive lymph node with small, medium, and large lymphocytes and plasma cells.

Interpretation

CBC: Sheba has mild toxic change, which could be compatible with inflammation or marrow insult. Future CBC's should be monitored for additional evidence of inflammation. Sheba also has a normocytic, normochromic anemia and thrombocytopenia. A reticulocyte count should be done to determine if the anemia is nonregenerative. Anemia of chronic disease should always be considered as a potential cause of mild nonregenerative anemia. The isosthenuria and azotemia are evidence of renal damage, which may result in a nonregenerative anemia because of inadequate production of erythropoietin and the toxic effects of uremia on the bone marrow microenvironment. Sheba should also be evaluated for acute blood loss, which could initially cause a nonregenerative anemia and thrombocytopenia. The low normal protein and hypoalbuminemia may be compatible with blood loss. Blood loss is not always obvious to owners, especially if the losses are gastrointestinal and up to a week may be required to see evidence of regeneration on a CBC. If no peripheral causes for the bicytopenia can be found, bone marrow aspirate and biopsy are indicated.

Serum Biochemical Profile
Azotemia and isosthenuria: This combination of laboratory abnormalities in a dehydrated patient is suggestive for renal failure, but there are exceptions when extra-renal factors interfere with renal concentrating ability (See Chapter 5, Case 4). Osmotic diuresis, medullary washout, and liver failure are unlikely based on the fact that all of the abnormalities on the serum biochemical profile can be explained by renal disease alone. Diabetes insipidus is a consideration, but is less likely.

Hyperphosphatemia and hypermagnesemia: The hyperphosphatemia and hypermagnesemia are most likely attributable to decreased glomerular filtration rate.

Hypoalbuminemia: Increased losses of albumin appear most likely in this case, and include the potential for hemorrhage discussed above and the documented excessive protein loss in the urine. The inactive urine sediment makes lower urinary tract disease unlikely, and glomerular loss of protein is suspected as the primary route of protein loss. Causes of decreased production of albumin contributing to the hypoalbuminemia in this case may include starvation, acute phase changes (albumin is a negative acute phase reactant), and liver failure. Depending on her body condition, anorexia/cachexia may be a consideration, but is usually only associated with extreme nutritional deprivation and poor body condition (see Chapter 5, Case 3, Marsali). The toxic change in the neutrophils suggests inflammation that could produce an acute phase response. Liver failure is unlikely given normal glucose, cholesterol, and bilirubin, although these are insensitive indicators of liver function. Serum bile acid or blood ammonia measurement is preferred to confirm poor hepatic function.

Hyperamylasemia: The most likely cause for this change is the decreased GFR, supported by the azotemia and hyperphosphatemia. Clinical signs are vague, and pancreatic disease cannot be completely ruled out.

Case Summary and Outcome

Sheba had hypertension, assumed to be secondary to renal disease, and was treated with antihypertensive medications. Cytologic examination of lymphoid tissue was consistent with reactive hyperplasia and antigenic stimulation; however, there was no evidence of neoplasia. Because of the shifting leg lameness, lymphoid hyperplasia, and thrombocytopenia, samples were collected for serologic titers to Lyme disease, Ehrlichia, Rocky Mountain Spotted Fever, and Leptospirosis. All of the titers were negative except that for Lyme disease, which was positive. Sheba was treated with appropriate antibiotics. During the second day of her hospitalization, Sheba developed petechia on her abdomen and legs. Intravenous fluid therapy was initiated for her renal disease, however she developed severe edema after 24 hours, and the fluids were discontinued. Both the hypoproteinemia and the potential for vasculitis could have potentiated the development of edema. At discharge, Sheba's treatment plan included antibiotics, antihypertensive medications, and subcutaneous fluids.

No kidney biopsy was performed, however hypoalbuminemia with proteinuria and no evidence of lower urinary tract disease or pyelonephritis is strong evidence of glomerular disease. Clinical signs associated with glomerular disease can be varied and non-specific. At least in the early phases of the disease, significant glomerular disease can be present without significant changes in glomerular filtration rate or BUN and creatinine. The degree of azotemia and the progression of disease may depend on the type of glomerular disease. Classification requires biopsy which may not be performed because of the risk of further renal injury and hemorrhage, which is higher in patients with coagulopathy and hypertension. Sheba currently has both of these risk factors. Glomerular damage eventually leads to loss of nephrons and chronic renal failure, however the progression of disease is variable and some patients with glomerular disease may have stable renal function for extended periods of time. In Sheba's case, the history of shifting leg lameness and reactive lymphoid hyperplasia suggest the possibility of antigen:antibody complex deposition as a cause for glomerulopathy. Lyme disease itself can be associated with a rapidly progressive membrano-proliferative glomerulonephritis accompanied by tubular lesions and interstitial inflammation, culminating in renal failure (Dambach). Substantiating a diagnosis of Lyme borreliosis in dogs is complicated by the absence of a pathognomonic signs of infection such as the presence of the erythrema migrans rash in people. In most dogs, measurable antibody production occurs prior to the development of clinical signs (Fritz). Many clinically healthy dogs will test positive for exposure to the Lyme borrelia due to natural exposure or vaccination. Immunoblot band patterns can distinguish antibody production in response to natural exposure from the response to vaccination. Because of a significant rate of false positive tests and the large numbers of dogs in which exposure can be documented, but clinical disease never develops, testing for Lyme disease should be restricted to patients with suggestive history and clinical signs (Fritz).

Dambach DM, Smith CA, Lewis RM, Van Winkle TJ. Morphologic, immunohistochemical, and ultrastructural characterization of a distinctive renal lesion in dogs putatively associated with Borrelia burdorferi infection: 49 cases (1987-1992). Vet Path 1997;34:85-96.

Fritz CL, Kjemtrup AM. Lyme borreliosis. J Am Vet Med Assoc 2003;223:1261-1270.

Case 6 – Level 1

"Gucci" is a 12-year-old spayed female Beagle dog presenting with a one month history of stranguria and leaking urine. She had been eating well up until one day prior to presentation. Abdominal ultrasound revealed an enlarged bladder with echogenic urine and a fimbriated mass in the caudal bladder extending into the urethra. Severe bilateral hydronephrosis and renomegaly with marked hydroureter were noted.

White blood cell count:	14.6 x 10⁹/L	(6.0-17.0)
Segmented neutrophils:	11.7 x 10⁹/L	(3.0-11.9)
Band neutrophils:	0 x 10⁹/L	(0-0.3)
Lymphocytes:	1.2 x 10⁹/L	(1.0-4.8)
Monocytes:	1.6 x 10⁹/L	(0.2-1.8)
Eosinophils:	0.1 x 10⁹/L	(0-1.3)
WBC morphology: Small numbers of reactive lymphocytes are seen.		

Hematocrit:	46%	(37-55)
MCV:	61.6 fl	(60.0-75.0)
MCHC:	35.9 g/dl	(33.0-36.0)
RBC morphology: No abnormalities of erythrocytes		

Platelets: Appear adequate

Glucose:	119 mg/dl	(65.0-120.0)
BUN:	↑ 62 mg/dl	(8-29)
Creatinine:	↑ 2.8 mg/dl	(0.5-1.5)
Phosphorus:	↑ 9.5 mg/dl	(2.6-7.2)
Calcium:	↑ 12.2 mg/dl	(8.8-11.7)
Magnesium:	1.9 mEq/L	(1.4-2.7)
Total Protein:	↑ 7.8 g/dl	(5.2-7.2)
Albumin:	3.3 g/dl	(3.0-4.2)
Globulin:	↑ 4.5 g/dl	(2.0-4.0)
Sodium:	142 mEq/L	(142-163)
Chloride:	↓ 100 mEq/L	(111-129)
Potassium:	4.5 mEq/L	(3.8-5.4)
HCO3:	↓ 14 mEq/L	(15-28)
Anion Gap:	↑ 32.5 mEq/L	(15-25)
Total Bili:	0.20 mg/dl	(0.10-0.50)
ALP:	120 IU/L	(12-121)
GGT:	6 IU/L	(3-10)
ALT:	54 IU/L	(10-95)
AST:	32 IU/L	(15-52)
Cholesterol:	237 mg/dl	(110-314)

Triglycerides:	67 mg/dl	(30-300)
Amylase:	↑ 4400 IU/L	(400-1200)
Lipase:	↑ 5264 IU/L	(53-770)

Urinalysis: Method of collection not indicated

Appearance: Straw and hazy	Sediment: occasional RBC/hpf
Specific gravity: 1.009	0-5 WBC/hpf
pH: 5.0	0-5 transitional epithelial cells
Glucose, ketones, bilirubin: negative	Occasional bilurubin crystals
Heme: 1+	Yeast present (Figure 5-5)
Protein: trace	

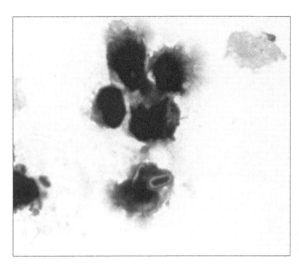

Figure 5-5. Intercellular yeast within a poorly preserved leukocyte in canine urine.

Cytology of bladder mass: Smears are excellent quality with many variably sized clusters of anaplastic epithelial cells mixed with debris, scattered nondegenerate neutrophils, individualized transitional cells with cytoplasmic tails, and broken cells. The cells within clusters are polyhedral with scant to moderate deeply basophilic cytoplasm. The cytoplasm occasionally contains small clear vacuoles and rarely a single large pink inclusion that peripheralizes the nucleus. Nuclei are large and round to oval with coarse chromatin and multiple prominent nucleoli. Occasional cells with two to three nuclei are also present. Anisocytosis and anisokaryosis are moderate to marked. The nuclear to cytoplasmic ratio is high but variable. Occasionall extracellular yeast similar to those seen in the urine are present; rare extracellular rod shaped bacteria are seen.

Interpretation
CBC: Unremarkable

Serum Biochemical Profile
Azotemia and isosthenuria: This combination of laboratory abnormalities is suggestive for renal failure, and the ultrasound findings demonstrate a cause for post-renal obstruction of urine flow with the secondary development of renal lesions resulting in renal failure. If the patient is dehydrated, a pre-renal component may be superimposed on the other causes of azotemia.

Hyperphosphatemia and hypercalcemia: The hyperphosphatemia is the result of decreased glomerular filtration rate, whether due to renal or pre-renal factors. Calcium changes unpredictably in renal failure, and total calcium may be high, low or normal. In older patients, hypercalcemia of malignancy must also be considered. Hypercalcemia has rarely been reported in people with transitional cell carcinoma (Grubb) and may be related to the presence of bone metastases in animals with transitional cell carcinoma (Rosol). Further characterization of the pathophysiology of the hypercalcemia might be possible by measuring ionized calcium (which is most often high in hypercalcemia of malignancy and most often, but not always, low in chronic renal failure), measuring parathyroid hormone related protein (PTHrP), or documenting bone metastases.

Mild increase in total protein and globulin: The increase in total protein is accounted for by an increase in globulins. This may reflect antigenic stimulation and is supported by the presence of reactive lymphocytes in the peripheral blood and inflammation in the urine sediment.

Mild acidemia (decreased HCO3) with increased anion gap: These changes reflect uremic acidosis.

Hypochloremia: This may occur as a result of renal losses secondary to polyuria or may reflect acid/base abnormalities.

Hyperamylasemia and hyperlipasemia: The most likely cause for this change is decreased GFR, supported by the azotemia and hyperphosphatemia. Clinical signs are vague, and pancreatic disease cannot be completely ruled out.

Cytology: Malignant epithelial neoplasia compatible with transitional cell carcinoma; mild suppurative inflammation and opportunistic yeast infection.

Case Summary and Outcome

Thoracic radiographs revealed multiple irregular nodules suggesting metastatic neoplasia. Gucci had surgery to remove the urinary bladder mass and to place a transabdominal Foley catheter. She was treated with chemotherapy for the tumor and antifungal drugs for the yeast infection. Antibiotics were added when her urine culture was positive for bacteria as well. Gucci's azotemia resolved with intervenous fluid therapy. However she remained isosthenuric after discharge from the hospital, and residual renal failure is likely given the changes in the kidneys observed at ultrasound. Gucci was doing well at home several weeks after discharge.

Gucci's data demonstrate the effects of more severe and prolonged urinary tract obstruction than was present in Sherpa, Chapter 5, Case 2, despite an identical underlying cause (transitional cell carcinoma). Sherpa was fortunate in that one kidney was largely spared the effects of obstruction, with the potential for renal function to remain above the threshold of 25% functional renal mass below which azotemia develops. Gucci also has other laboratory data compatible with decreased renal function such as calcium, phosphorus, and acid/base abnormalities. Like Sherpa, Gucci's azotemia is less severe than that observed in the cat with pre-renal azotemia in Chapter 5, Case 1, Marklar, re-emphasizing the limitations of BUN and creatinine in consistently distinguishing pre-renal from renal or post-renal causes of azotemia.

Grubb RL, Collyer WC, Kibel AS. Transitional cell carcinoma of the renal pelvis associated with hypercalcemia in a patient with autosomal dominant polycystic kidney disease. Urology 2004;63:778-780.

Rosol TJ. Parathyroid hormone-related protein (PTHrP): Role in cancer, metastasis, and humoral hypercalcemia of malignancy. Proceedings, 13th Annual European College of Veterinary Internal Medicine Meeting, September 2003, Uppsala, Sweden.

Case 7 – Level 2

"Ringo" is a 3-year-old castrated male, domestic long hair cat presenting with a two to three month history of intermittently urinating next to his litter box. One day prior to presentation, Ringo urinated next to his box, but then did not urinate at all for the next 24 hours. On the morning of presentation, Ringo was found lying near his water bowl. On physical examination, Ringo is hypothermic and has a large, firm urinary bladder which is painful on palpation.

White blood cell count:	↑ 21.1 x 10⁹/L	(4.5-15.7)
Segmented neutrophils:	↑ 17.3 x 10⁹/L	(2.1-13.1)
Lymphocytes:	3.6 x 10⁹/L	(1.5-7.0)
Monocytes:	0.2 x 10⁹/L	(0-0.9)
Eosinophils:	0.0 x 10⁹/L	(0.0-1.9)
WBC morphology: No significant abnormalities seen.		

Hematocrit:	37%	(28-45)
Red blood cell count:	8.53 x 10¹²/L	(5.0-10.0)
Hemoglobin:	13.2 g/dl	(8.0-15.0)
MCV:	43.7 fl	(39.0-55.0)
MCHC:	35.7	(31.0-35.0)
Platelets: Clumped, but appear adequate		

Glucose:	↑ 228 mg/dl	(70.0-120.0)
BUN:	↑ 206 mg/dl	(15-32)
Creatinine:	↑ 12.4 mg/dl	(0.9-2.1)
Phosphorus:	↑ 18.0 mg/dl	(3.0-6.0)
Calcium:	↓ 7.2 mg/dl	(8.9-11.6)
Magnesium:	2.6 mEq/L	(1.9-2.6)
Total Protein:	6.1 g/dl	(5.5-7.6)
Albumin:	3.2 g/dl	(2.2-3.4)
Globulin:	2.9 g/dl	(2.5-5.8)
Sodium:	150 mEq/L	(149-164)
Chloride:	↓ 109 mEq/L	(119-134)
Potassium:	↑ 10.7 mEq/L	(3.9-5.4)
HCO3:	13 mEq/L	(13-22)
Anion Gap	↑ 38.7 mEq/L	(13-27)
Total bili:	0.3 mg/dl	(0.10-0.30)
ALP:	30 IU/L	(10-72)
GGT:	<3 IU/L	(3-10)
ALT:	80 IU/L	(29-145)
AST:	↑ 66 IU/L	(12-42)
Cholesterol:	87 mg/dl	(77-258)
TGA:	73 mg/dl	(25-191)
Amylase:	552 IU/L	(496-1874)

Urinalysis: Catheter

Appearance: Red and cloudy	Sediment:
Specific gravity: 1.018	RBCs too numerous to count/hpf
pH: 6.5	Occasional WBC/high power field
Protein: 500 mg/dl	No casts seen
Glucose: 2+	No epithelial cells are seen
Ketones: negative	No bacteria or crystals present
Bilirubin: negative	Trace fat droplets and debris
Heme: 3+	

Interpretation

CBC: The mild mature neutrophilic leukocytosis is compatible with inflammation.

Serum Biochemical Profile

Hyperglycemia: Given the history, the most likely cause for the hyperglycemia and glucosuria is stress, although supportive changes in the leukogram are not present. Diabetes mellitus should also be considered if the hyperglycemia is persistent or is associated with other suggestive clinical signs such as polyphagia, weight loss, and polyuria/polydipsia. Note that the glucosuria merely reflects hyperglycemia that causes the glomerular filtrate to have a glucose content that exceeds the renal tubular maximum for glucose reabsorption. A single finding of glucosuria does not by itself justify a diagnosis of diabetes mellitus.

Azotemia: Azotemia should be categorized as pre-renal, renal, or post-renal. The minimally concentrated urine supports the possibility of renal dysfunction, however this does not rule out a pre-renal component to the azotemia if there is clinical evidence of dehydration. The presence of a large, firm bladder is suspicious, and this cat may have post-renal azotemia related to urethral blockage.

Hyperphosphatemia and hypocalcemia: The most likely cause of hyperphosphatemia in this patient is decreased glomerular filtration rate, regardless of whether the decreased GFR is due to pre-renal, renal, or post-renal causes. Dogs and cats in renal failure may have high, normal, or low serum calcium levels, and ionized calcium levels may not correlate with total calcium levels as they often do in healthy animals. In a small study of cats with urethral obstruction, 75% had low ionized calcium, and 27% had low total calcium (Drobatz). All cats with low total calcium also had low ionized calcium. While not directly evaluated, formation of calcium-phosphorus complexes and impaired PTH activity were suggested as mechanisms. Renal secondary hyperparathyroidism and primary hypoparathyroidism may also cause hyperphosphatemia and hypocalcemia. PTH levels will be increased in renal secondary hyperparathyroidism as the body attempts to increase serum calcium that has dropped in response to the hyperphosphatemia resulting from the low GFR. In contrast, low PTH levels in primary hypoparathyroidism cannot maintain adequate calcium levels in the blood and fail to promote the excretion of phosphorus into the urine.

Hypochloremia and normal sodium: Loss of chloride in excess of sodium in the gastrointestinal tract can result in disproportionate hypochloremia, but appropriate clinical signs are not described in the history. Chronic respiratory acidosis will trigger increased excretion of chloride by the kidney. Diuretic use can potentiate urinary chloride loss. Because Ringo has hypochloremia and hyperkalemia, hypoadrenocorticism is a possibility, but is rare in cats.

Hyperkalemia and increased anion gap: Hyperkalemia is associated with renal diseases characterized by inability to eliminate urine, whether from urethral blockage, uroabdomen, or oliguric/anuric renal failure. Increased intake or oversupplementation or drug effects are not compatible with the clinical history, and translocation due to acute inorganic acidosis also appears unlikely, although the anion gap suggests a metabolic acidosis (probably uremic). Hypocalcemia may potentiate the effects of hyperkalemia on the heart.

Increased AST: This increase is mild and is not accompanied by an increased ALT. Hemolysis or muscle damage are possible sources of the increased AST.

Urinalysis: The erythrocytes, heme, and protein are compatible with the presence of blood in the urine. The urine is not adequately concentrated for a dehydrated patient, which may be related to tubular dysfunction associated with obstructive nephropathy. This is not necessarily a permanent change and the urine specific gravity should be re-evaluated after treatment.

Case Summary and Outcome

Ringo was found to have a urethral obstruction, and after he was sedated, caseous material was extracted from his urethra. Ringo was treated with intravenous fluids and calcium gluconate following placement of a urethral catheter. The next day Ringo was bright and alert, but continued to pass bloody urine. Two days later his catheter was removed and he continued to pass urine, so he was discharged.

Ringo should be compared with the previous two cases of post-renal azotemia (Chapter 5, Case 2, Sherpa, and Case 6, Gucci). Those two dogs had relatively slowly developing obstructions in which imaging studies revealed renal changes, making it more likely that permanent renal damage occurred with some degree of renal azotemia. Obstructed cats, on the other hand, are more likely to present acutely and have less severe, if any, renal parenchymal lesions. Because Ringo was unable to pass urine for a period of time, he developed hyperkalemia, which was not noted in the two dogs as they were able to continue to pass some urine, albeit with difficulty.

Ringo's relatively dilute urine in combination with the azotemia gives the impression of renal azotemia. Like Gucci (Case 6), temporary tubular dysfunction may be present after relief of the urinary obstruction. The passage of large amounts of relatively dilute urine characterizes a period of post-obstructive diuresis after relief of urethral blockage (Nichols). Osmotic diuresis from elevated urea nitrogen content of the urine may also contribute to post-obstructive diuresis. This process is generally self-limiting, however large amounts of fluid can be lost. The patient must be monitored carefully for electrolyte changes, specifically for hypokalemia as the metabolic acidosis corrects itself and high tubular flow rates result in renal potassium loss. As the pressure is relieved and normal water and electrolyte balance is re-established, urinary concentrating ability generally recovers. This is in contrast to the apparently permanent loss of urinary concentrating ability noted in Gucci (Case 6).

Drobatz KJ, Hughes D. Concentration of ionized calcium in plasma from cats with urethral obstruction. J Am Vet Med Assoc 1997;211: 1392-1395.

Nichols CE. Endocrine and metabolic causes of polyuria and polydipsia. In: Kirk's Current Veterinary Therapy XI, Small Animal Practice. Ed. RW Kirk, JD Bonagura. 1992 W.B. Saunders Company, Philadelphia, PA, pp 293-301.

Case 8 – Level 2

"Riff Raff" is a 4-year-old castrated male Dachshund presenting for abdominal distention. Six days ago, he had had enterotomy at multiple sites for removal of carpet material.

White blood cell count:	↓ 4.7 x 10⁹/L	(6.0-17.0)
Segmented neutrophils:	↓ 1.8 x 10⁹/L	(3.0-11.0)
Band neutrophils:	↑ 2.1 x 10⁹/L	(0-0.3)
Lymphocytes:	↓ 0.6 x 10⁹/L	(1.0-4.8)
Monocytes:	0.1 x 10⁹/L	(0.1-1.4)
Eosinophils:	0.1 x 10⁹/L	(0-1.3)

WBC morphology: Smudged leukocytes are present as well as 3+ toxic change in the neutrophils.

Hematocrit:	↓ 18%	(37-55)
Red blood cell count:	↓ 2.79 x 10¹²/L	(5.5-8.5)
Hemoglobin:	↓ 6.1 g/dl	(12.0-18.0)
MCV:	64.8 fl	(60.0-77.0)
MCHC:	33.7 g/dl	(31.0-34.0)

RBC morphology: Mild anisocytosis

Platelets:	↓ 80 x 10⁹/L	(200-450)

Platelet morphology: Many macroplatelets seen

Glucose:	↓ 70 mg/dl	(80.0-125.0)
BUN:	↑ 27 mg/dl	(6-24))
Creatinine:	0.9 mg/dl	(0.5-1.5)
Phosphorus:	4.2 mg/dl	(3.0-6.0)
Calcium:	9.3 mg/dl	(8.8-11.0)
Magnesium:	2.0 mEq/L	(1.4-2.7)
Total Protein:	5.0 g/dl	(4.7-7.3)
Albumin:	2.8 g/dl	(2.5-4.2)
Globulin:	2.2 g/dl	(2.0-4.0)
A/G Ratio:	1.3	(0.7-2.1)
Sodium:	144 mEq/L	(140-151)
Chloride:	117 mEq/L	(105-120)
Potassium:	↓ 3.6 mEq/L	(3.8-5.4)
HCO3:	19.9 mEq/L	(16-28)
Anion Gap:	10.7 mEq/L	(5-18)
Total Bili:	↑ 3.0 mg/dl	(0.10-0.50)
ALP:	145 IU/L	(20-320)
GGT:	3 IU/L	(2-10)
ALT:	↑ 68 IU/L	(5-65)
AST:	↑ 126 IU/L	(15-52)
Cholesterol:	114 mg/dl	(110-314)
Amylase:	577 IU/L	(400-1200)

Coagulation

PT:	↑ 8.5s	(6.2-7.7)
APTT:	↑ 17.8s	(9.8-14.6)
FDP:	↑ >20 µg/ml	(<5)

Interpretation

CBC: Riff Raff has leucopenia with neutropenia and a degenerative left shift. It is not known if Riff Raff had a left shift prior to the original surgical procedure. However, dogs with a left shift prior to surgery for intestinal anastomoses are at increased risk for anastomotic leakage and should be monitored carefully (Ralphs). Riff Raff also has a normocytic normochromic anemia. The anemia may be nonregenerative, however a reticulocyte count is needed to make this assessment. His anemia is more severe than is typically due to chronic disease or inflammation alone, and blood loss from the previous surgery may have contributed to the decrease in RBC mass. Further blood loss is possible because of Riff Raff's coagulopathy. The thrombocytopenia can be explained by disseminated intravascular coagulation (see coagulation data); however some degree of immune mediated destruction or impaired production cannot be ruled out. The combination of neutropenia, nonregenerative anemia and thrombocytopenia could be compatible with a primary bone marrow problem, however these changes can be accounted for by extramarrow causes and a bone marrow aspirate is not indicated at this time.

Serum Biochemical Profile

Hypoglycemia: Given the leukogram, a septic process is the most likely cause of hypoglycemia, once sample processing errors are ruled out. Inadequate gluconeogenesis as a result of poor liver function is possible. Impaired liver function is compatible with by the albumin and cholesterol which are at the lower limits of the reference ranges, the hyperbilirubinemia, and the prolonged PT and APTT. Serum bile acids could be performed to evaluate this possibility. Small breed dogs may be more likely to develop hypoglycemia with anorexia, however in most cases anorexia must be severe or prolonged to cause low blood glucose. Even then, the decrease in glucose is generally mild (see Marsali, Chapter 5, Case 3 and Chapter 3).

Increased BUN with normal creatinine: Several contributing factors are present to explain increased BUN with normal creatinine. This may represent early pre-renal azotemia, when BUN increases because of slow tubular flow rates and increased time for passive reabsorption of urea. Poor renal perfusion may be the result of dehydration or low blood pressure secondary to septic shock. Hydration status is difficult to assess using laboratory data because of the confounding effects of anemia and the possibility of protein losses from hemorrhage, into the gastrointestinal tract, or into the abdominal effusion. BUN may also increase if there has been bleeding into the gastrointestinal tract, or as a result of protein catabolism associated with fever, sepsis, or surgery. A urinalysis is needed to assess renal concentrating ability.

Hypokalemia: This patient is likely to have been anorexic during the course of his illness, so decreased intake could lower serum potassium concentration. Increased losses via the gastrointestinal tract or into the abdominal effusion are also possible. Hypokalemia is more likely to occur with poor intake if there are concurrent losses of the electrolyte.

Hyperbilirubinemia: Hyperbilirubinemia is often the result of liver disease or hemolysis. Obstructive cholestasis is unlikely given the normal ALP and GGT, however decreased liver function (reference above) can also cause hyperbilirubinemia. Hemolysis is certainly possible given the anemia, however hemolytic anemias are frequently regenerative and no RBC morphologic abnormalities suggesting a cause for hemolysis were noted (i.e. spherocytes, Heinz bodies, etc). Although liver disease and hemolysis cannot be excluded as causes for the hyperbilirubinemia, sepsis can also result in a defect in hepatocellular uptake of bilirubin.

Mildly increased ALT and AST: Elevations in these enzymes suggest hepatocellular damage, however they indicate nothing about the etiology of the damage. Riff Raff has multiple potential sources for liver damage, including sepsis (effects of bacterial toxins and poor perfusion with shock), intestinal disease with increased hepatic exposure to bacteria and bacterial products with inflammatory mediators, trauma during surgery, and hypoxia secondary to anemia. Primary liver disease cannot be ruled out, but is not required to account for these enzyme elevations. The increased AST may refect muscle damage during surgery.

Coagulation profile: Mild prolongation of PT and APTT suggests the development of a secondary hemostatic defect. In combination with the thrombocytopenia and increased fibrin degradation products (indicating increased fibrinolysis), these findings are compatible with disseminated intravascular coagulation, which may occur secondary to sepsis. Decreased liver function can also cause these laboratory changes because of decreased hepatic production of coagulation factors and impaired clearance of fibrin degradation products by the liver. Adherence of platelets to damaged endothelium in the liver can cause thrombocytopenia.

Case Summary and Outcome

Abdominal fluid cytology revealed large numbers of degenerate neutrophils containing intracellular bacteria. Riff Raff was taken to surgery, where it was discovered that two of the four enterotomy sites had dehisced. One was repaired and the other required resection and re-anastomosis. Riff Raff was managed with an open abdomen, fluids, antibiotics, and parenteral nutrition. Unfortunately, 5 days later, Riff Raff suffered cardiopulmonary arrest associated with an episode of vomiting. At necropsy, Riff Raff was noted to have diffuse, fibrous and fibrinous peritonitis. Histologic examination of tissue revealed yeast compatible with *Candida* species attached to the capsular surface of the liver, spleen, and intestine. Yeast were subsequently cultured from these organs.

Although no urine was available to help interpret the increased BUN, multiple extra-renal factors that could potentially influence the BUN were present in the clinical history. It is helpful to compare Riff Raff with Sherpa (Chapter 5, Case 2), who also had a minor elevation of BUN with modest elevations in liver enzymes. Despite these similarities, Riff Raff did not have primary urinary tract disease, while Sherpa's diagnosis was transitional cell carcinoma with hydronephrosis and significant renal pathology due to urinary outflow obstruction. Just as the degree of azotemia cannot always distinguish pre-renal from renal causes, neither can a minor increase in BUN with normal creatinine distinguish renal from extra-renal pathology in all patients.

Ralphs SC, Jessen CR, Lipowitz AJ. Risk factors for leakage following intestinal anastomosis in dogs and cats: 115 cases (1991-2000). J Am Vet Med Assoc 2003;223:73-71.

Case 9 – Level 2

"Margarite" is a 21-year-old Arab mare presenting with a one day history of anorexia and decreased urinations. The owner's had noticed Margarite had been drinking and urinating more than their other horses for about four years. Rectal palpation revealed an enlarged left kidney.

White blood cell count:	10.6×10^9/L	(5.9-11.2)
Segmented neutrophils:	8.7×10^9/L	(2.3-9.1)
Band neutrophils:	0.0×10^9/L	(0-0.3)
Lymphocytes:	1.6×10^9/L	(1.6-5.2)
Monocytes:	0.3×10^9/L	(0-1.0)
WBC morphology: No abnormal findings		

Hematocrit:	34%	(30-51)
Red blood cell count:	6.99×10^{12}/L	(6.5-12.8)
Hemoglobin:	12.6 g/dl	(10.9-18.1)
MCV:	50.3 fl	(35.0-53.0)
MCHC:	37.1 g/dl	(34.6-38.0)
RBC morphology: Appears within normal limits		

Platelets: Clumped but appear adequate

Fibrinogen:	400 mg/dl	(100-400)

Glucose:	↑ 136 mg/dl	(6.0-128.0)
BUN:	↑ 62 mg/dl	(11-26)
Creatinine:	↑ 8.2 mg/dl	(0.9-1.9)
Phosphorus:	↓ 0.6 mg/dl	(1.9-6.0)
Calcium:	↑ 15.7 mg/dl	(11.0-13.5)
Magnesium:	2.4 mEq/L	(1.7-2.4)
Total Protein:	↑ 7.3 g/dl	(5.6-7.0)
Albumin:	3.1 g/dl	(2.4-3.8)
Globulin:	4.2 g/dl	(2.5-4.9)
A/G Ratio:	0.7	(0.7-2.1)
Sodium:	135 mEq/L	(130-145)
Chloride:	↓ 97 mEq/L	(99-105)
Potassium:	↑ 5.1 mEq/L	(3.0-5.0)
HCO3:	31 mEq/L	(25-31)
Anion Gap:	7.0 mEq/L	(5-10)
Total Bili:	0.8 mg/dl	(0.3-3.0)
Direct bili:	0.3 mg/dl	(0.0-0.5)
Indirect bili:	0.5 mg/dl	(0.2-3.0)
ALP:	135 IU/L	(109-352)
GGT:	15 IU/L	(5-23)
AST:	234 IU/L	(190-380)
CK:	174 IU/L	(80-446)

Abdominal fluid analysis

Pre-spin: light red and hazy	
Post-spin: colorless and clear	
Total protein: <2.0 gm/dl	
Total nucleated cell count: 391/µl	

The fluid contains small numbers of erythrocytes and nucleated cells. Nondegenerate neutrophils predominate, with lesser numbers of macrophages and occasional small lymphocytes. No etiologic agents are seen.

Urine specific gravity: 1.011

Interpretation

CBC: No abnormalities noted.

Serum Biochemical Profile

Hyperglycemia: Elevations in serum glucose in the horse are most often caused by excitement or stress with increases in endogenous catecholamines and glucocorticoids. No changes in the CBC are noted to explain the hyperglycemia such as a mature neutrophilia and lymphopenia with corticosteroid effect or a mature neutrophilia and lymphocytosis with epinephrine.

Azotemia: The combination of increased BUN and creatinine with isosthenuria is indicative of renal azotemia in the absence of any extra-renal factors that could interfere with urinary concentrating ability. Isosthenuria alone in a well hydrated patient can be a normal finding.

Hypercalcemia with hypophosphatemia: Because normal equine kidneys excrete large quantities of calcium, decreased glomerular filtration rate can result in hypercalcemia, especially if dietary calcium is high. This is in contrast to the variable calcium measurements that characterize renal failure in the dog and cat. Hypophosphatemia is often described in horses with renal failure and may occur secondary to the hypercalcemia because of mass action. This is in contrast to the hyperphosphatemia that often accompanies decreased GFR in other species. PTH levels in horses with renal disease are reported to be suppressed (Brobstt) or variable (Toribio).

Hyperproteinemia: Given that the serum albumin and globulins are both within reference range, this finding is of questionable clinical significance.

Hypochloremia: The chloride is minimally decreased and is unlikely to be significant at this time. Changes in chloride that are not proportional to sodium can be present if chloride losses exceed sodium, or if there is an acid/base abnormality. In acid/base disturbances, the chloride generally varies inversely with the bicarbonate, which is currently at the upper limit of the reference range. The renal disease in this horse is a risk factor for the development of acid/base abnormalities, so these analytes should be monitored.

Hyperkalemia: When the body cannot eliminate urine, potassium will be retained. This may occur with post-renal azotemia or in the anuric/oliguric phase of renal failure. This is in contrast to the polyuric phase of renal failure, in which increased tubular flow rates promote potassium wasting because of decreased time for reabsorption. As has been noted for other cases with hyponatremia/hypochloremia/hyperkalemia, hypoadrenocorticism is a differential diagnosis and may be evaluated by performing an ACTH stimulation test; however this is unlikely in the horse.

Abdominal fluid analysis: The fluid is a transudate and is considered to be normal.

Case Summary and Outcome

Margarite was treated with intravenous fluids and phosphorus, but she continued to produce only small amounts of urine. The day after presentation, Margarite developed ventral edema, so intravenous fluid administration was reduced and diuretics were administered. The next day she became anuric and began to accumulate fluid in the abdominal cavity and pleural space. Ultrasound of the kidneys showed advanced hydronephrosis in the right kidney and a severely dilated ureter. The left kidney was small and hyperechoic with a dilated renal pelvis. Margarite was euthanized because of anuria, anorexia, and poor long-term prognosis.

Brobst DF, Bayly WM, Reed SM, Howard GA, Torbeck RL. Parathyroid hormone evaluation in normal horses and horses with renal failure. Equine Vet Sci. 1982; 2:150-157.

Toribio RE. Parathyroid gland function and calcium regulation in horses. In: Proceedings 21st Annual American College of Veterinary Internal Medicine Forum. June 4-8, 2003, Charlotte, NC. pp 224-226.

Case 10 – Level 2

"Tramp" is a 14-year-old spayed female Siamese cat with a history of declining appetite over three weeks and lethargy. On physical examination, Tramp is quiet, alert, and responsive. She is estimated to be 10-12% dehydrated and has very poor body condition with no palpable fat deposits. Her mucous membranes are very pale and she is tachycardic.

White blood cell count:	10.3 x 10⁹/L	(4.5-15.7)
Segmented neutrophils:	9.3 x 10⁹/L	(2.1-13.1)
Lymphocytes:	↓ 0.5 x 10⁹/L	(1.5-7.0)
Monocytes:	0.5 x 10⁹/L	(0-0.9)
Eosinophils:	0.0 x 10⁹/L	(0.0-1.9)

WBC morphology: No significant abnormalities noted.

Hematocrit:	↓ 21.6%	(28-45)
Red blood cell count:	↓ 4.65 x 10¹²/L	(5.0-10.0)
Hemoglobin:	↓ 7.0 g/dl	(8.0-15.0)
MCV:	42.9 fl	(39.0-55.0)
MCHC:	35.0	(31.0-35.0)

Platelets: Clumped, but appear adequate

Glucose:	↑ 200 mg/dl	(70.0-120.0)
BUN:	↑ 240 mg/dl	(15-32)
Creatinine:	↑ 13.1 mg/dl	(0.9-2.1)
Phosphorus:	↑ 10.3 mg/dl	(3.0-6.0)
Calcium:	10.0 mg/dl	(8.9-11.6)
Magnesium:	↑ 3.6 mEq/L	(1.9-2.6)
Total Protein:	↑ 8.2 g/dl	(5.5-7.6)
Albumin:	↑ 3.9 g/dl	(2.2-3.4)
Globulin:	4.3 g/dl	(2.5-5.8)
Sodium:	153 mEq/L	(149-164)
Chloride:	126 mEq/L	(119-134)
Potassium:	↓ 2.9 mEq/L	(3.9-6.3)
HCO3:	↓ 9.1 mEq/L	(13-22)
Anion gap:	20.8	(13-27)
Cholesterol:	↑ 300 mg/dl	(77-258)
Amylase:	↑ 1872 IU/L	(362-1410)

Urinalysis: Method of sampling was not indicated

Appearance: Yellow and clear	Sediment:
Specific gravity: 1.011	0 RBC/high power field
pH: 6.5	0 WBC/high power field
Protein: 1+	No casts seen
Glucose: negative	No epithelial cells are seen
Ketones: negative	No bacteria or crystals present
Bilirubin: negative	Trace fat droplets and debris
Heme: trace	

Interpretation

CBC: Lymphopenia could be compatible with stress/corticosteroid effects. Tramp has a normocytic, normochromic anemia which will be somewhat more severe when fluid deficits are corrected. Non-regenerative anemia is common in patients with chronic renal failure because of low renal production of erythropoietin and the effect of uremic toxins on erythropoiesis. Poor nutritional status may also exacerbate these anemias. If leukocyte and platelet numbers are adequate, a bone marrow evaluation is not indicated because a peripheral etiology for the anemia is present.

Serum Biochemical Profile

Azotemia: Azotemia with isosthenuric urine supports renal failure, and there is no evidence of post-renal disease such as fluid in the abdomen, a large, firm bladder, stranguria or failure to urinate. Because the patient is significantly dehydrated, there is likely pre-renal azotemia in addition to renal azotemia.

Hyperphosphatemia and normal calcium: The most likely cause of hyperphosphatemia in this patient is decreased glomerular filtration rate, regardless of whether the decreased glomerular filtration rate is due to pre-renal, renal, or post-renal causes. Small animal patients in renal failure may have high, normal, or low serum calcium levels, and ionized calcium levels may not correlate with total calcium levels. Ionized calcium measurements should be performed if there are clinical signs compatible with hypocalcemia.

Hypermagnesemia: Increased serum magnesium, like hyperphosphatemia, is the result of decreased glomerular filtration rate.

Hyperproteinemia due to hyperalbuminemia: The liver does not over-produce albumin, so this value is interpreted to support the clinical observation of dehydration.

Hypokalemia: Increased renal losses of potassium due to polyuria are compounded by low intake associated with anorexia. Hypokalemia itself can result in renal disease, which may be characterized by renal vasoconstriction and decreased glomerular filtration rate, polydipsia and polyuria because of increased angiotensin II, and refractoriness to vasopressin. Correction of potassium depletion may reverse some of these changes and improve urinary concentrating ability.

Decreased HCO3: This indicates acidemia, which is frequently observed in patients with renal failure. Often this change is associated with increased anion gap due to the presence of uremic acids, which are unmeasured anions. Anion gap is normal in this case. Decreased distal sodium reabsorption in response to potassium depletion will conserve hydrogen and potassium because of the presence of a more positive charge in the tubular luminal fluid, impairing acid excretion and leading to acidemia.

Hypercholesterolemia: Increases in cholesterol have been described in dogs with glomerular nephritis and in dogs with nephrotic syndrome. The mechanism for hypercholesterolemia in nephrotic syndrome may be increased hepatic synthesis, and these patients often have an inverse relationship between albumin and cholesterol, although this is not present in this cat. Abnormal lipoprotein lipase function related to inadequate amounts of its co-factor, heparan sulfate, may also contribute to the hypercholesterolemia in nephrotic syndrome.

Increased amylase: Decreased glomerular filtration rate will increase amylase in the absence of pancreatic disease. Amylase is a poor indicator of pancreatic pathology in cats.

Urinalysis: Small amounts of protein and heme could be compatible with mild blood contamination if the sample was obtained by cytocentesis. A positive reaction for heme may occur with free hemoglobin or the presence of erythrocytes in the urine sediment. However it may not be possible to make this distinction because erythrocytes may lyse in urine with a low specific gravity. Renal failure is associated with variable degrees of proteinuria.

Case Summary and Outcome

Tramp was not hospitalized, but was sent home on management with subcutaneous fluids, a renal failure diet, and potassium supplementation. Chronic renal failure patients may remain stable for unpredictable amounts of time with supportive therapy. Comparison of Tramp with Margarite (Chapter 5, Case 9) illustrates important species differences in calcium and phosphorus responses to renal failure. Horses often present with increased calcium and normal or low phosphorus depending on diet, while dogs and cats often present with variable calcium levels and hyperphosphatemia.

On the other hand, Margarite's hyperkalemia reflects decreased urine production and retention of potassium while Tramp's hypokalemia is characteristic of the polyuric phase of renal failure. These are relatively consistent findings across species.

Case 11 – Level 2

"Joe" is a 9-year-old castrated male Yorkshire Terrier presenting for ingestion of between 4 and 8 200 mg tablets of ibuprofen. His owner came home from work and found multiple piles of vomitus throughout the house. Joe appeared disoriented and was growling. On presentation, Joe's physical examination was unremarkable other than pain on abdominal palpation.

	Day 1	Day 3	Day 4	
PCV	38	↓24	↓18	(38-57)
Glucose:	↑164 mg/dl	97	105	(65.0-120.0)
BUN:	↑35 mg/dl	↑66	↑46	(8-33)
Creatinine:	↑1.7 mg/dl	↑3.1	1.4	(0.5-1.5)
Phosphorus:	5.4 mg/dl	↑6.8	4.8	(3.0-6.0)
Calcium:	↓7.9 mg/dl	↓7.7	↓7.7	(8.8-11.0)
Magnesium:	1.5 mEq/L	1.9	2.4	(1.4-2.7)
Total Protein:	↓5.0 g/dl	↓3.5	↓3.9	(5.5-7.8)
Albumin:	↓2.5 g/dl	↓1.7	↓2.0	(2.8-4.0)
Globulin:	2.5 g/dl	↓1.8	↓1.9	(2.3-4.2)
A/G Ratio:	1.0	0.9	1.1	(0.7-2.1)
Sodium:	141 mEq/L	149	149	(140-151)
Chloride:	115 mEq/L	↑127	↑125	(105-120)
Potassium:	↓3.4 mEq/L	↓3.5	↓3.5	(3.8-5.4)
HCO3:	↓12.2 mEq/L	↓14.9	17.7	(16-28)
Anion Gap:	17.2 mEq/L	↓10.6	↓9.8	(15-25)
Total Bili:	N/A mg/dl	0.3	0.2	(0.10-0.30)
ALP:	N/A IU/L	↑134	40	(20-121)
GGT:	N/A IU/L	5	3	(2-10)
ALT:	N/A IU/L	21	N/A	(18-86)
AST:	N/A IU/L	↑86	51	(15-52)
Cholesterol:	↓114 mg/dl	↓105	↓112	(115-300)
Amylase:	N/A IU/L	568	N/A	(400-1200)

N/A = not available

Urinalysis: Catheter

Appearance: Yellow and clear	Sediment:
Specific gravity: 1.010	2-20 RBC/hpf
Glucose: 1+	no other findings on sediment examination
Ketones: negative	
Bilirubin: negative	
Protein: 2+	
Heme: 2+	

Interpretation

PCV: The patient is not initially anemic, however marked anemia develops over the next several days. While chronic renal disease can be associated with the development of non-regenerative anemia due to failure of erythropoietin production and the impact of uremic toxins on the marrow, this is less likely with acute renal compromise and generally develops more slowly as senescent erythrocytes fail to be replaced by adequate erythropoiesis. Because panhypoproteinemia is developing along with the anemia, blood loss anemia should be considered likely. Non-steroidal anti-inflammatory drugs (NSAIDS) such as ibuprofen may cause gastrointestinal ulceration and hemorrhage. They may also impair platelet function, which could exacerbate bleeding (Tomlinson). Gastrointestinal ulcers and thrombocytopathy also characterize uremia and may contribute to hemorrhage. Indices and reticulocyte counts are not available to assess the erythropoietic response. It is anticipated that it would take 3-5 days before a significant reticulocytosis would be detected in response to hemorrhage. A regenerative response may be blunted due continued loss of iron with external hemorrhage and impaired erythropoietin release by the damaged kidneys.

Serum Biochemical Profile

Hyperglycemia: This change is likely related to stress.

Azotemia: Azotemia with isosthenuria suggests renal disease if there are no other factors such as medullary washout or osmotic diuresis that could impact urinary concentrating ability. The urinalysis on Day 1 indicates glucosuria, which can cause osmotic diuresis. Although the blood glucose level is high, it does not exceed the renal tubular maximum for glucose reabsorption, suggesting that there may be some renal tubular damage or dysfunction. The azotemia worsens despite aggressive fluid therapy on Day 3, however by Day 4 values begin to decline. On Day 4, the BUN remains high despite a normal serum creatinine. This can sometimes occur gastrointestinal hemorrhage, which is strongly suspected given the ibuprofen intoxication and declining PCV and protein values. Other causes of an increased BUN with a normal creatinine include early pre-renal azotemia (unlikely here) or with a high protein diet.

Hyperphosphatemia: On presentation, phosphorus levels are normal. Hyperphosphatemia develops on Day 3 as renal function and glomerular filtration rate decline.

Hypocalcemia: The hypocalcemia may be explained, in part, by the concurrent hypoalbuminemia and would not be expected to result in significant changes in ionized calcium. Hypocalcemia is seen in some patients with renal failure, generally attributed to calcium/phosphorus mass law interactions secondary to elevated phosphorus, although the phosphorus is not markedly elevated in this case. Inadequate calcitriol, leading to skeletal resistance to parathryroid hormone and deficient intestinal absorption of calcium also appears to play a role in the hypocalcemia that may develop with renal failure. These patients usually do not have clinical signs associated with hypocalcemia, although symptoms may be more common in dogs with acute renal failure or ethyelene glycol poisoning. Measurement of ionized calcium should be considered.

Hypoproteinemia: On Day 1 there is mild hypoalbuminemia. Glomerular disease can result in selective loss of albumin in the urine but it seems unlikely that acute intoxication leading to renal damage would cause low serum albumin in a matter of hours. Hemorrhage is a possible cause of the hypoalbuminemia, but the bleeding at this time is not of sufficient duration or severity to lower the PCV or globulins below the lower limit of the reference interval. Comparison with any available historical data to determine if Joe normally has a low normal albumin would be helpful in understanding the clinical significance of this value. By days 3 and 4 there is anemia and panhypoproteinemia characteristic of hemorrhage.

Hyperchloremic acidosis with decreased anion gap: Small bowel diarrhea causes hyperchloremic metabolic acidosis because of the loss of fluid with high bicarbonate content and low chloride concentration. The anion gap often will be normal in these cases. This interpretation is supported by the hypokalemia. Accumulation of uremic acids should increase the anion gap, however this is offset by the developing hypoproteinemia. Negatively charged plasma proteins represent a significant proportion of the unmeasured anions under normal circumstances.

Hypocholesterolemia: Low serum cholesterol is not generally associated with clinical signs, however it may occur in association with protein-losing enteropathy, decreased liver function, or severe malnutrition. The combination of hypoalbuminemia and hypocholesterolemia early in the course of disease could be compatible with a pre-existing liver function problem such as a portocaval shunt, especially in a high risk breed such as the Yorkshire terrier. Serum bile acid measurement should eventually be considered in this patient. Decreased liver function would certainly interfere with Joe's ability to increase albumin synthesis in compensation for increased renal or gastrointestinal losses.

Urinalysis: As noted above, Joe is isosthenuric. The glucosuria could indicate renal tubular dysfunction, or the possibility that the hyperglycemia previously exceeded the tubular maximum for reabsorption of 180-200 mg/dl. The proteinuria may be partially related to the presence of blood in the urine, lower urinary tract disease, or glomerular lesions. Dipstick protein measurements are generally more sensitive to albumin than globulins, and this level of proteinuria is considered significant in dilute urine. A urine protein:creatinine ratio could be performed to quantify the proteinuria, but is only recommended if lower urinary tract sources of protein are ruled out.

Case Summary and Outcome

Joe was admitted to the hospital and activated charcoal was administered to prevent further absorption of any remaining ibuprofen. He also was treated with intravenous fluids, gastroprotectants, antiemetics, total parenteral nutrition, and antibiotics because of the concern that bacterial translocation may occur with compromised intestines. Despite this therapy, Joe vomited blood several times and began to have episodes of diarrhea containing digested blood. A blood transfusion and albumin were given to compensate for his gastrointestinal blood loss. After six days of therapy, he showed signs of fluid overload and was treated with oxygen and diuretics. Despite the propensity for patients with renal disease to develop hypertension, Joe's blood pressure was normal throughout his hospitalization. His azotemia improved over time, and he was discharged from the hospital. While his long term prognosis is unclear, some renal function may be regained over time. Early and aggressive treatment with normalization of BUN and creatinine are encouraging. This case can be compared with ibuprofen toxicity in a ferret (Calvin, Case 20, Chapter 2), where both hepatic and renal abnormalities were present.

Joe's renal disease was acute due to a nephrotoxic drug and was diagnosed early. Many cases of renal failure are diagnosed late in the course of disease (see Chapter 5, Cases 9 and 10), and the initiating causes are never discovered. Differentiation of acute from chronic renal failure can be difficult, and the occurrence of acute exacerbations of more chronic processes can complicate the distinction. Acute presentation, especially with a history of potential ischemia or toxin exposure, implies acute renal failure, however development of clinical signs may be subtle in chronic renal failure, and acute decompensation of chronic renal disease may give the clinical impression of recent onset. Patients with chronic renal failure are more likely to present with poor body condition, or small firm kidneys, versus patients with acute renal failure who may present in good flesh with normal to enlarged kidneys.

Laboratory data are not always helpful in determining whether renal failure is acute or chronic. Patients with acute renal failure may be more likely to present with oliguria/anuria and therefore hyperkalemia (Vaden). However, terminal chronic renal failure can be present with decreased urine production and potassium retention as seen in Margarite (Case 9).

Acute post-renal azotemia can also be associated with hyperkalemia, such as in cats with urinary obstruction (Ringo, Chapter 5, Case 7). Joe's serum potassium was low despite acute renal failure, possibly because of gastrointestinal losses and the maintenance of adequate urine production throughout his hospitalization. The metabolic acidosis may be more severe with acute renal failure because there has been less time for physiologic adaptation to decreased renal function.

The presence of non-regenerative anemia is more common in chronic renal failure, however the above cases illustrate the limitation of this data for prediction of acute versus chronic renal disease. The horse with chronic renal failure (Margarite, Case 9) was not anemic. Ringo, the cat with chronic renal failure was moderately anemic. Joe developed anemia along with his renal failure, because of gastrointestinal hemorrhage associated with non-steroidal anti-inflammatory toxicity. Blood loss anemias are usually regenerative, however Joe's erythropoietic response may have been limited by the presence of renal disease. Indices were not available to judge Joe's response to the blood loss. Often the clinician must rely on the combination of history, clinical signs, and laboratory data to determine the likelihood of acute or chronic renal failure.

Tomlinson J, Blikslager A. Role of nonsteroidal anti-inflammatory drugs in gastrointestinal tract injury and repair. J Am Vet Med Assoc. 2003;222:946-951.

Vaden SL. Differentiation of acute from chronic renal failure. In: Kirk's Current Veterinary Therapy XIII: Small Animal Practice. JD Bonagura Ed. W.B. Saunders Company, Philadelphia, PA. 2000. pp 856-858.

Case 12 – Level 2

"Pugsley" is a 13-month-old castrated male pug presenting for work-up of some abnormalities that were noted on a presurgical serum biochemical profile. No abnormalities were noted on physical examination.

White blood cell count:	↑ 28.7 x 10⁹/L	(4.0-15.5)
Segmented neutrophils:	↑ 23.5 x 10⁹/L	(2.0-10.0)
Band neutrophils:	0.3 x 10⁹/L	(0-0.3)
Lymphocytes:	4.0 x 10⁹/L	(1.0-4.5)
Monocytes:	0.6 x 10⁹/L	(0.2-1.4)
Eosinophils:	0.3 x 10⁹/L	(0-1.2)
Basophils:	0.0 x 10⁹/L	
WBC morphology: Within normal limits		

Hematocrit:	↓ 32%	(37-60)
Red blood cell count:	↓ 5.36 x 10¹²/L	(5.5-8.5)
Hemoglobin:	↓ 10.6 g/dl	(12.0-18.0)
MCV:	↓ 57.5 fl	(60.0-77.0)
MCHC:	33.1 g/dl	(31.0-34.0)
RBC morphology: Occasional target cells seen.		

Platelets:	↓ 173 x 10⁹/L	(200-450)

Glucose:	↓ 65 mg/dl	(70.0-120.0)
BUN:	↓ 6 mg/dl	(8-33)
Creatinine:	↓ 0.4 mg/dl	(0.6-1.5)
Phosphorus:	5.3 mg/dl	(5.0-9.0)
Calcium:	9.8 mg/dl	(8.8-11.0)
Total Protein:	↓ 4.3 g/dl	(4.8-7.2)

Albumin:	↓ 2.1 g/dl	(3.0-4.2)
Globulin:	2.2 g/dl	(2.0-4.0)
Sodium:	142 mEq/L	(140-151)
Chloride:	108 mEq/L	(105-120)
Potassium:	4.6 mEq/L	(3.8-5.4)
HCO3:	28 mEq/L	(16-28)
Anion Gap:	↓ 10.6 mEq/L	(15-25)
Total Bili:	0.10 mg/dl	(0.10-0.50)
ALP:	↑ 409 IU/L	(20-320)
GGT:	<3 IU/L	(4-10)
ALT:	↑ 94 IU/L	(10-86)
AST:	↑ 85 IU/L	(16-54)
Cholesterol:	126 mg/dl	(110-314)
Triglycerides:	119 mg/dl	(30-300)
Amylase:	↓ 386 IU/L	(400-1200)

Urinalysis: Cystocentesis

Appearance: Yellow and clear	Sediment: inactive

Specific gravity: 1.014

pH: 7.0

Protein, glucose, ketones, bilirubin, heme: negative

Interpretation

CBC: Pugsley has a mild neutrophilic leukocytosis which could be compatible with mild inflammation.

There is a mild microcytic, normochromic anemia. Causes of microcytosis in dogs are limited and include breed characteristic (Japanese breeds such as Akitas, Chows or Shar Peis), iron deficiency, and portosystemic vascular anomolies. An iron panel could be performed to clarify Pugsley's iron status, however Pugsley has other data compatible with a portosystemic shunt (hypoglycemia, low BUN, hypoalbuminemia, mild elevations of liver enzymes). If Pugsley is eating a standard commercial dog food, he is unlikely to have a dietary deficiency of iron. No obvious chronic blood loss has been noted by the owner. Pugsley should be checked for evidence of parasites; it would be more cost effective to perform a fecal flotation and to check for fleas and ticks than to run an iron panel at this time. In addition, iron deficiency may be accompanied by hypochromia and schistocytes, which are not seen here, while liver disease can be characterized by the presence of target cells, which were present on this blood film.

The mild thrombocytopenia is of questionable clinical significance at this time. Although no platelet clumping was reported, a repeat CBC should be considered to rule out artifactual thrombocytopenia prior to pursuing any other diagnostics for thrombocytopenia. This degree of thrombocytopenia will not be associated with an increased risk of hemorrhage provided that platelet function and other hemostatic parameters are normal. Because there is evidence of decreased liver function on the serum biochemical profile, a coagulation profile should be run prior to invasive procedures.

Serum Biochemical Profile

Hypoglycemia: In patients with no clinical signs of hypoglycemia, artifactual hypoglycemia due to inappropriate sample processing should be ruled out by measuring glucose on a freshly collected sample with prompt separation of serum from cells. In this case, the hypoglycemia was verified. After processing error, the most likely cause for low blood glucose in this case is decreased liver function, possibly related to a portosystemic shunt. Because of the neutrophilic leukocytosis, sepsis may be considered as a cause for hypoglycemia, however it is unlikely in a dog with no apparent clinical signs. Neoplasia is also unlikely in a young dog, and there is no history of starvation or poor body condition.

Decreased BUN and creatinine: Low BUN may be attributed to poor liver function secondary to the presence of a portosystemic shunt. Given the low urine specific gravity, high tubular flow rates in the kidney with decreased time for reabsorption of urea may contribute to low BUN in this case. Polyuria and polydipsia were not described in the clinical history, but are frequently associated with poor liver function in dogs because of a combination of potential mechanisms including psychogenic polydipsia, alterations in osmoreceptors, stimulation of thirst centers, and/or increased endogenous cortisol levels associated with increased production or decreased degradation of corticosteroids. Low muscle mass in a young, small breed dog could also conceivably contribute to low creatinine. Some patients with portosystemic shunts grow poorly and are small compared to litter mates.

Hypoproteinemia with hypoalbuminemia: Hypoalbuminemia can be due to decreased production or increased losses. Because the liver is the site of albumin production, poor liver function can cause hypoalbuminemia. In some cases, albumin production may be low because of lack of substrate (starvation/malnutrition, unlikely in this case because of lack of supporting clinical data), or because the liver downregulates albumin production as part of the acute phase response (the neutrophilic leukocytosis suggests some degree of inflammation). Most causes of increased protein losses result in the loss of both albumin and globulins (hemorrhage, gastrointestinal losses, dermal or third space protein losses). Because of the microcytic anemia, there is some question of chronic blood loss, however hemorrhage should be associated with loss of both albumin and globulin proteins. Exclusive loss of albumin causing hypoalbuminemia occurs via the glomerulus, however proteinuria was not noted on the urinalysis. Because the urine was relatively dilute, a urine protein:creatinine ratio could be performed as a more sensitive indicator of proteinuria. Based on all of Pugsley's laboratory results, evaluation of liver function by performing fasted and post-prandial bile acids measurements is a better choice to determine the cause of hypoalbuminemia.

Low anion gap: The anion gap is an indicator of unmeasured anions, most of which are negatively charged plasma proteins. As a result, hypoproteinemia causes a decrease in anion gap.

Mild increase in ALP: Increases in ALP are nonspecific in dogs and may be related to a variety of extrahepatic causes, drug or hormone effects, or cholestasis. Significant cholestatic disease is often accompanied by an increase in GGT or bilirubin, which are not seen here. Mild liver enzyme elevations are often described in association with portosystemic shunts and is the most likely cause in this case. Increased ALP is seen with bone formation in young, growing, large breed dogs, but is unlikely in a small dog like Pugsley.

Mild increase in ALT and AST: These changes are mild and indicate hepatocellular damage. As with ALP, many hepatic and extrahepatic causes of liver enzyme elevation are possible, but the preponderance of evidence supports the presence of a portosystemic shunt.

Decreased amylase: This value is not considered clinically significant.

Urinalysis: Pugsley has a low urine specific gravity, but is not azotemic. Interpretation of isosthenuria as physiologic or pathologic depends on clinical information such as hydration status. Because impaired ability to concentrate urine appears prior to azotemia, decreased renal function cannot be ruled out. Liver failure may also interfere with renal concentrating ability in the absence of renal pathology. Polyuria may be seen in animals with portosystemic shunts.

Case Summary and Outcome

Both fasted and post-prandial serum bile acid concentrations were elevated. Ultrasonagraphic evaluation of Pugsley's abdomen showed a small liver and a large extrahepatic portosystemic shunt. The shunt was corrected by cellophane banding. He was discharged and recovered well at home. Pugleys' case demonstrates how a primary liver disease can influence renal variables, including BUN, creatinine, and urine specific gravity. Please see Chapter 2, Case 12 (Binar) and Chapter 3, Case 7 (Yap Yap) for more complete discussions of the pathophysiology of portosytemic shunts.

Case 13 – Level 3

"Opie" is a 5-year-old castrated male domestic short haired cat presenting with a several day history of vomiting and inability to hold down any food. He was taken to another veterinarian last week because the owner thought he was drinking and urinating more than usual, however no blood work was performed at that time. On physical examination, Opie is noted to sneeze occasionally, does not appear to be dehydrated, and has a mass in the area of the left kidney which could be fat. An intermittent II/VI systolic heart murmur is noted on auscultation.

White blood cell count:	11.6 x 10⁹/L	(4.5-15.7)
Segmented neutrophils:	9.9 x 10⁹/L	(2.1-13.1)
Lymphocytes:	1.5 x 10⁹/L	(1.5-7.0)
Monocytes:	0.2 x 10⁹/L	(0-0.9)
Eosinophils:	0.0 x 10⁹/L	(0.0-1.9)

WBC morphology: No significant abnormalities noted.

Hematocrit:	33%	(28-45)
Red blood cell count:	7.44 x 10¹²/L	(5.0-10.0)
Hemoglobin:	11.6 g/dl	(8.0-15.0)
MCV:	44.4 fl	(39.0-55.0)
MCHC:	35.2 g/dl	(31.0-35.0)

Platelets: Clumped, but appear adequate in number.

Glucose:	98 mg/dl	(70.0-120.0)
BUN:	↑ 238 mg/dl	(15-32)
Creatinine:	↑ 13.3 mg/dl	(0.9-2.1)
Phosphorus:	↑ 11.1 mg/dl	(3.0-6.0)
Calcium:	10.8 mg/dl	(8.9-11.6)
Magnesium:	↑ 2.9 mEq/L	(1.9-2.6)
Total Protein:	7.3 g/dl	(5.5-7.6)
Albumin:	2.6 g/dl	(2.2-3.4)
Globulin:	4.7 g/dl	(2.5-5.8)
Sodium:	↓ 146 mEq/L	(149-164)
Chloride:	↓ 97 mEq/L	(119-134)
Potassium:	↑ 7.0 mEq/L	(3.9-5.4)
HCO3:	17 mEq/L	(13-22)
Anion gap:	↑ 39.0 mEq/L	(9.0-21.0)
Total bili:	0.2 mg/dl	(0.10-0.30)
ALP:	17 IU/L	(10-72)

GGT:	3 IU/L	(3-10)
ALT:	↑ 237 IU/L	(29-145)
AST:	↑ 62 IU/L	(12-42)
Cholesterol:	227 mg/dl	(77-258)
TGA:	190 mg/dl	(25-191)
Amylase:	1561 IU/L	(496-1874)

Urinalysis: Catheter

Appearance: Straw and clear	Sediment:
Specific gravity: 1.012	0 RBC/hpf
pH: 6.0	Rare WBC/hpf
Protein: negative	No casts seen
Glucose: negative	No squamous or transitional
Ketones: negative	epithelial cells are seen
Bilirubin: negative	No bacteria or crystals present
Heme: negative	Trace fat droplets and debris

Interpretation

CBC: No abnormalities

Serum Biochemical Profile

Azotemia: Azotemia should be categorized as pre-renal, renal, or post-renal. The isosthenuria supports the possibility of renal failure, however this does not rule out a pre-renal component to the azotemia if there is clinical evidence of dehydration. Other causes for poor urinary concentrating ability should be considered such as medullary washout (hyponatremia and hypochloremia), osmotic diuresis associated with diabetes mellitus (unlikely as there is no hyperglycemia or glucosuria at this time), or diabetes insipidus.

Hyperphosphatemia and hypermagnesemia with normal serum calcium: The most likely cause of hyperphosphatemia and hypermagnesemia in this patient is decreased glomerular filtration rate, regardless of whether the decreased glomerular filtration rate is due to pre-renal, renal, or post-renal causes. Small animal patients in renal failure may have high, normal, or low serum calcium levels, and ionized calcium levels may not correlate with total calcium levels as they often do in healthy animals.

Hyponatremia and hypochloremia: Increased renal losses of electrolytes are possible because patients in renal failure may have abnormalities of renal tubular handling of sodium and chloride. Measurement of urinary fractional excretion of sodium and chloride could be performed to evaluate renal losses of electrolytes. The change in serum chloride is disproportionately greater than that of sodium. This could be attributed to vomiting of gastric contents with high concentrations of chloride, however disproportionate changes in chloride can also occur with acid/base abnormalities. In general, HCO3 and chloride have an inverse relationship. This is not the case here, possibly because alkalemia due to loss of hydrogen and chloride from vomiting is counterbalanced by uremic acidosis. This is compatible with a mixed acid/base disorder. In many cases in which hyponatremia and hypochloremia are due to increased gastrointestinal losses, the potassium is normal or decreased. There exceptions, such as in dogs with salmonella, trichuriasis, or perforated duodenal ulcer, in which volume depletion and decreased distal renal tubular blood flow results in potassium retention. Because Opie has hypochloremia and hyperkalemia, hypoadrenocorticism is a possibility, but is rare in cats. An ACTH stimulation test could be performed to evaluate this possibility.

Hyperkalemia: Hyperkalemia is associated with renal diseases characterized by inability to eliminate urine, whether from urethral blockage, uroabdomen, or oliguric/anuric renal failure. Increased intake, oversupplementation, or drug effects are not compatible with the clinical history, and translocation due to acute inorganic acidosis also appears unlikely, although the anion gap suggests a metabolic acidosis (probably uremic). Translocation from damaged tissue is possible with the concurrent increase in AST and phosphorus.

Increased anion gap: The increased anion gap indicates accumulation of unmeasured anions. Increased serum protein can cause this change, however Opie is not hyperproteinemic. Increased organic acids such as uremic acids, ketoacids, or lactic acid can similarly elevate the anion gap. HCO3 should decrease in response to accumulated acids; this may not occur if there is a mixed acid/base disorder or the decrease may not be proportional to the increased acids if buffers other than bicarbonate are being titrated.

Increased ALT and AST: Small Increases in both of these enzymes are compatible with mild hepatocellular damage. Other tissues, including muscle and erythrocytes also contain AST. The cause for the elevated enzymes is not apparent and cannot be determined based on the available data.

Urinalysis: Other than the isosthenuria discussed above, the urinalysis reveals small numbers of leukocytes. Urine culture is recommended to rule out urinary tract infection, despite the minimal changes in the other parameters.

Case Summary and Outcome

Because of the presence of the mass in the area of the left kidney, an abdominal ultrasound was performed. The imaging study revealed hydronephrosis, hydroureter, and pyelectasia suggestive for pyelonephritis. Two bacterial species were isolated from urine cultures. Note that the urine sediment examination was unremarkable; this may occur in patients with pyelonephritis due to minimal or absent urine flow from the affected kidney. Therefore, normal urine sediment does not completely rule out pyelonephritis. Given the positive urine cultures, mild sepsis is possible and could account for the liver enzyme elevations.

Opie was treated with intravenous fluids and antibiotics with subsequent improvement in his laboratory abnormalities. He was discharged on a treatment plan including antibiotics, subcutaneous fluids, potassium supplementation, and suggestions for a low phosphorus diet. Three weeks after discharge, Opie was doing well at home but had a persistent low grade azotemia, indicating persistent renal dysfunction. The degree to which his remaining functional nephrons may compensate for the previous damage remains to be determined, and chronic renal failure may develop.

Case 14 – Level 3

"Sally" is a 7-year-old Chow mix dog. The day prior to presentation, she collapsed acutely after going for a run with her owner and developed hematemesis and melena. On presentation, she was hypothermic and pulses could not be detected until administration of a 2-liter fluid bolus; after which they were weak but palpable. Petechial hemorrhages were noted on the ventral abdomen.

	Day 1	Day 9	
White blood cell count:	↑ 17.9 x 10⁹/L	12.0	(6.0-17.0)
Segmented neutrophils:	↑ 17.0 x 10⁹/L	11.0	(3.0-11.0)
Band neutrophils:	0.0 x 10⁹/L	0.0	(0-0.3)
Lymphocytes:	↓ 0.4 x 10⁹/L	↓ 0.5	(1.0-4.8)
Monocytes:	0.5 x 10⁹/L	0.0	(0.2-1.4)
Eosinophils:	0.0 x 10⁹/L	0.5	(0-1.3)
WBC morphology: No significant abnormalities noted.			
Hematocrit:	↑ 64%	↓ 24	(37-55)
Red blood cell count:	↑ 9.36 x 10¹²/L	↓ 3.48	(5.5-8.5)
Hemoglobin:	↑ 20.6 g/dl	↓ 8.3	(12.0-18.0)
MCV:	65.0 fl	68.3	(60.0-77.0)
MCHC:	35.0 g/dl	34.6	(31.0-35.0)
RBC morphology: Small numbers of target cells present			
Platelets:	↓ 43 x 10⁹/L	↓ 50	(200-450)
Glucose:	↓ 36 mg/dl	101	(65.0-120.0)
BUN:	↑ 76 mg/dl	↑ 56	(8-33)
Creatinine:	↑ 4.3 mg/dl	↑ 4.2	(0.5-1.5)
Phosphorus:	↑ 11.7 mg/dl	↑ 6.3	(3.0-6.0)
Calcium:	9.1 mg/dl	10.8	(8.8-11.0)
Magnesium:	↑ 3.1 mEq/L	1.7	(1.4-2.7)
Total Protein:	7.0 g/dl	↓ 5.0	(5.2-7.2)
Albumin:	3.4 g/dl	↓ 2.7	(3.0-4.2)
Globulin:	3.6 g/dl	2.3	(2.0-4.0)
A/G Ratio:	0.9	1.2	(0.7-2.1)
Sodium:	↓ 139 mEq/L	151	(140-151)
Chloride:	↓ 92 mEq/L	106	(105-120)
Potassium:	3.8 mEq/L	↓ 3.5	(3.8-5.4)
HCO3:	23 mEq/L	28	(16-28)
Anion Gap:	↑ 27.8 mEq/L	20.5	(15-25)
Total Bili:	0.3 mg/dl	↑ 1.10	(0.10-0.50)
ALP:	270 IU/L	↑ 551	(20-320)
GGT:	6 IU/L	↑ 24	(2-10)
ALT:	↑ 1545 IU/L	↑ 987	(10-86)
AST:	↑ 20958 IU/L	↑ 420	(15-52)
Cholesterol:	↑ 332 mg/dl	233	(110-314)
Amylase:	511 IU/L	854	(400-1200)

Urinalysis Day 1: Collection method not indicated

Appearance: Light red and clear	Sediment:
Specific gravity: 1.010	0-5 erythrocytes/hpf
pH: 8.0	
Protein: 100 mg/dl	
Glucose: 3+	
Ketones: negative	
Bilirubin: 1+	
Heme: 3+	

Coagulation profile Day 1:

PT:	7.8s	(6.2-9.3)
APTT:	12.2	(8.9-16.3)
FDP:	greater than 5 µg/ml, but less than 20	(<5)

Interpretation
CBC
Leukogram: Sally has a mild mature neutrophilic leukocytosis and lymphopenia on Day 1, which is compatible with a stress/corticosteroid leukogram. Mild inflammation cannot be ruled out, however there are no toxic changes or a left shift to corroborate this interpretation. The lymphopenia on Day 9 is also likely attributable to corticosteroid effects; the mature neutrophilia may not be a persistent finding with chronic stress.

Erythrogram: Polycythemia is evident on Day 1. The most common cause of polycythemia is a relative change due to dehydration. An increase in total protein is expected with dehydration, but may be counteracted by blood loss. Splenic contraction may also contribute to a relative increase in circulating red blood cells. Erythrocytosis can occur in patients compensating for cardiopulmonary disease in an attempt to improve oxygenation of tissues. Sally may need to have further diagnostic evalvation to determine if underlying cardiopulmonary disease contributed to her collapse. Alternatively, compressive lesions of the kidney parenchyma (cysts and tumors) can cause renal hypoxia and increased erythropoietin production, and there is evidence of renal azotemia in this case. Much less likely is ectopic production of erythropoietin by an extra-renal tumor or autonomous proliferation of erythroid precursors resulting from polycythemia vera. Evaluation of the patient for cardiopulmonary and renal lesions and measurement of erythropoietin can help distinguish various causes of erythrocytosis if correction of dehydration does not lower the PCV.

By Day 9 Sally has a normocytic, normochromic anemia. The thrombocytopenia and hypoalbuminemia plus the clinical history are suggestive for blood loss anemia. This type of anemia is usually regenerative given sufficient time, however anemia of inflammation/chronic disease and loss of iron with hemorrhage could suppress a marrow response. Renal disease can also impact erythropoiesis via reduced production of erythropoietin and the effect of uremic toxins on erythroid precursors.

Mechanisms for thrombocytopenia include decreased production and increased destruction. The hematemesis and melena suggest hemorrhage and increased consumption of platelets. Hypoxic and ulcerative uremic lesions in the gastrointestinal tract predispose to bleeding even without a coagulopathy. The presence of petechia on the ventral abdomen are compatible with a primary hemostatic defect. Spontaneous bleeding due to thrombocytopenia alone generally occurs at platelet counts of 30×10^9/L or below, however if there is concurrent endothelial cell insult, thrombocytopathy, or a defect in secondary hemostasis, bleeding may occur at higher platelet counts. Defective platelet-endothelial cell interactions occur in uremic patients and contribute to development of a coagulopathy. The normal prothrombin time and activated partial thromboplastic time seem to indicate normal secondary hemostasis on Day 1. However, these tests lack sensitivity and only become prolonged once factor activity is approximately 30% of normal. Enhanced fibrinolysis or decreased degradation by the liver accounts for the increase in fibrin degradation products. If extramarrow causes of the thrombocytopenia and non-regenerative anemia are ruled out, a bone marrow disorder will need to be evaluated.

Serum Biochemical Profile Day 1:
Hypoglycemia: In patients with no clinical signs of hypoglycemia, artifactual hypoglycemia due to processing errors should be ruled out by measuring glucose on a freshly collected sample with prompt separation of serum from cells. In this case, the hypoglycemia was verified and may have contributed to the dog's collapse. Sepsis is a likely cause of hypoglycemia in this case because of the clinical signs indicating breakdown of the intestinal mucosa. However, abnormalities in the leukogram are not consistent with sepsis at this time. Liver failure can impair hepatic gluconeogenesis, however other supportive data are lacking, such as low BUN, hypocholesterolemia, or prolonged coagulation times. Serum bile acids could be performed to assess liver function. Hypoglycemia due to the production of insulin or insulin-like substances by tumors is possible in a middle-aged dog, but is rare.

Azotemia: The azotemia in combination with isosthenuria suggests renal failure, however a pre-renal component is also likely due to dehydration (polycythemia) and poor tissue perfusion (lack of palpable pulses on presentation). Gastrointestinal hemorrhage can further elevate the BUN, as seen with Joe, (Chapter 5, Case 11). Glucosuria in a patient with normal to low blood glucose is compatible with renal tubular dysfunction. Contamination of the sample by oxidants causing false positive results on the urine dipstick should be ruled out.

Hyperphosphatemia with hypermagnesemia: The most likely cause for these elevations is decreased glomerular filtration rate and impaired renal excretion.

Hyponatremia and hypochloremia: Increased losses of sodium and chloride may occur via the gastrointestinal tract and kidneys or via hemorrhage in this case. Dilutional hyponatremia and hypochloremia associated with intravascular accumulation of water is an unlikely mechanism for these changes on day 1, given the polycythemia. The hyponatremia and hypochloremia may be exacerbated if fluid losses are replaced by drinking water or by antidiuretic hormone stimulated free water retention. Sally's hypochloremia is more marked than the hyponatremia, which is mild and of questionable clinical significance. When changes in chloride are greater than changes in sodium, disproportionate losses of chloride such as chronic vomiting or an acid/base imbalance are suspected. Other causes of hyponatremia and hypochloremia such as decreased dietary intake of sodium and chloride are rarely an issue in small animal patients on commercial diets.

Increased anion gap and normal HCO3: Accumulation of unmeasured anions increases the anion gap. Poor tissue perfusion creates the potential for lactic acidosis, and the azotemia suggests uremic acidosis. Hypochloremia is generally associated with alkalosis, but the HCO3 is normal. A mixed acid/base disorder is possible here, and a blood gas analysis would facilitate interpretation of these changes.

Increased ALT and AST: Elevation of AST is severe and could reflect damage to muscle, hepatocytes, and/or erythrocytes. Increases in ALT similarly reflect damage to muscle and hepatocytes. A creatine kinase level could be determined to support a myocyte origin for these elevations given the normal cholestatic enzymes and bilirubin. Since poor tissue perfusion and hypoxia are likely causes for the damage, both liver and muscle could be affected.

Mild hypercholesterolemia: This mild increase in cholesterol is clinically insignificant.

CBC and Serum Biochemical Profile Day 9:
Sally was treated with intravenous fluids, antibiotics, and gastroprotectants for presumptive heat stroke. Many of the differences from day 1 to day 9 reflect the fluid therapy. The PCV, total protein and albumin are now decreased, compatible with restoration of vascular volume in the face of whole blood loss. The continued thrombocytopenia may reflect ongoing consumption through hemorrhage or coagulopathy, and continued monitoring for the development of DIC is warranted.

BUN, creatinine, and phosphorus values have improved but have not normalized, indicating ongoing renal dysfunction. Na and Cl are back within the normal range. K is mildly decreased, and this needs to be monitored so that K depletion secondary to fluid therapy and diuresis does not occur.

On day 9, ALT and AST have decreased, which could indicate some resolution of tissue damage. Because AST has a shorter half life than ALT, this marked fall in AST probably reflects decreased release from muscle. The decrease in ALT is not as dramatic and may also reflect resolving muscle damage. There are indications of ongoing hepatocellular damage. There is now evidence of cholestasis, likely secondary to hepatocellular swelling, as indicated by the increased ALP, GGT and total bilirubin.

Case Summary and Outcome
Sally shows many of the complications that may occur with heat stoke. It is likely that she was hyperthermic the previous day, however some patients with heatstroke may present with hypothermia due to owner's attempts to cool them or if they present in shock (Rozanski). Sally responded well and became brighter with resolution of the vomiting and melena, but her appetite did not recover and she was persistently azotemic. Acute renal failure secondary to heat stroke was suspected, and Sally was discharged from the hospital for continuing management with fluid therapy at home (her owner was a nurse). She presented for acute blindness three days later and was found to have severe hypertension and bilateral retinal detachment. Several factors could have contributed to this development, including hypertension, fluid therapy, and vascular lesions from the heat stroke. She was treated with antihypertensive medications and her fluid rate was reduced. Her azotemia was persistent and fluid therapy was to continue for several more weeks in the hopes that some tubular function would recover.

The presence of glucosuria with normoglycemia suggests tubular dysfunction and is compatible with tubular necrosis. This is more common with acute processes, although laboratory data cannot always distinguish acute from chronic renal failure (see discussion of Joe, Case 11). Sally's clinical history indicates high potential for ischemic insult to the kidney: renal damage in heatstroke is attributed to direct thermal injury to cells, reduced visceral perfusion as blood is shunted peripherally for heat dissipation, or microvascular thrombosis secondary to activation of the coagulation cascade (Bouchama). As with Joe (Case 11) and Opie (Case 13), the ultimate outcome of Sally's renal disease may take time to determine. Her severe complications would suggest that she is more likely than Joe to suffer from continuing health problems related to decreased renal function.

Bouchama A, Knochel JP. Heat Stroke. New Engl J Med 2002;246;1978-1988.
Rozanski EA, Boysen S. Heatstroke. Standards of Care: Emergency and Crit Care Med. 2001;3:4-8.

Case 15 – Level 3

"Elvira" is an 8-year-old spayed female German Shepherd dog presenting with a 7 day history of anorexia and lethargy, during which time she has lost 12 pounds of body weight. The owner had taken Elvira to his parents' farm, where he thinks she may have eaten some garbage. Elvira has been vomiting intermittently, but is drinking water. On physical examination, Elvira was dehydrated and had icteric sclera and mildly enlarged submandibular lymph nodes. Her abdomen was tender on palpation and she had a slightly enlarged spleen.

White blood cell count:	12.2 x 10^9/L	(6.0-17.0)
Segmented neutrophils:	9.0 x 10^9/L	(3.0-11.0)
Band neutrophils:	0.0 x 10^9/L	(0-0.3)
Lymphocytes:	1.7 x 10^9/L	(1.0-4.8)
Monocytes:	1.5 x 10^9/L	(0.2-1.5)
Eosinophils:	0.0 x 10^9/L	(0-1.3)
WBC morphology: Appears within normal limits		

Hematocrit:	50.9%	(37-55)
Red blood cell count:	7.37 x 10^{12}/L	(5.5-8.5)
Hemoglobin:	6.1 g/dl	(12.0-18.0)
RBC morphology: 3+ acanthocytes and rare schistocytes		

Platelets: Appear adequate in number

Glucose:	116 mg/dl	(80.0-125.0)
BUN:	↑ 61 mg/dl	(6-24))
Creatinine:	↑ 3.8 mg/dl	(0.5-1.5)
Phosphorus:	5.4 mg/dl	(3.0-6.0)
Calcium:	10.2 mg/dl	(8.8-11.0)
Magnesium:	2.5 mEq/L	(1.4-2.7)
Total Protein:	↑ 7.5 g/dl	(4.7-7.3)
Albumin:	3.3 g/dl	(2.5-4.2)
Globulin:	↑ 4.2 g/dl	(2.0-4.0)
Sodium:	↓ 135 mEq/L	(140-151)
Chloride:	↓ 102 mEq/L	(105-120)
Potassium:	↓ 2.6 mEq/L	(3.8-5.4)
HCO3:	16.8 mEq/L	(16-28)
Anion Gap:	18.8 mEq/L	(15-25)
Total Bili:	↑ 28.3 mg/dl	(0.10-0.50)
ALP:	↑ 713 IU/L	(20-320)
GGT:	↑ 16 IU/L	(2-10)
ALT:	↑ 226 IU/L	(5-65)
AST:	↑ 60 IU/L	(15-52)
Cholesterol:	120 mg/dl	(110-314)
Amylase:	↑ 1226 IU/L	(400-1200)
Lipase:	↑ 1086 IU/L	(20-189)

Coagulation Profile

PT:	6.5s	(6.2-7.7)
APTT:	12.3s	(9.8-14.6)
FDP:	<5 µg/ml	(<5)

Spleen aspirate: Smears are hemodiluted with proportional numbers of leukocytes. Aggregates of splenic stromal cells are present with scattered myeloid and erythroid precursors and rare megakaryocytes. Rare hemosiderin-laden macrophages are present. There is a heterogeneous population of lymphocytes.

Interpretation

CBC: The numerical data is unremarkable. The presence of acanthocytes can be associated with liver disease, which is supported by the clinical chemistry data. The significance of small numbers of schistocytes is unclear, however they may reflect vascular lesions, including some malignancies such as hemangiosarcoma. This may be a concern in this case because of the splenomegaly and the age and breed of the dog; however there are many other potential causes for enlargement of the spleen.

Serum Biochemical Profile

Azotemia: Urinalysis data is not available, therefore the potential for renal azotemia is difficult to evaluate. Given the dehydration, pre-renal factors certainly contribute to the elevated BUN and creatinine.

Mildly increased total protein and hyperglobulinemia: These changes may be due to dehydration, however they also could be compatible with either antigenic stimulation or increased production of acute phase reactants with inflammatory disease. There is no indication of inflammatory disease on the CBC at this time. Less likely is the potential for a monoclonal gammopathy, signaling possible lymphoid malignancy.

Hyponatremia with proportional hypochloremia: Hyponatremia and hypochloremia are mild and are unlikely to be associated with clinical signs at this time. Decreased intake is rarely a factor contributing to low sodium and chloride. These electrolytes may be diluted if there is excessive retention of free water, however, given the dehydration, this is an unlikely mechanism for the alterations. In this case, increased losses by gastrointestinal or renal routes are most likely. Urinary fractional excretion of sodium and chloride could be performed to quantify renal losses of electrolytes, which should be low under these circumstances if the kidney is functioning. High urinary fractional excretion of these electrolytes would be inappropriate and consistent with renal disease. Hypoadrenocorticism is less likely given the hypokalemia. Third space and cutaneous losses should also be considered if compatible with clinical signs.

Hypokalemia: In contrast to sodium and chloride, low intake can contribute to the development of hypokalemia, especially in combination with increased losses. Potassium could be lost via the same routes as sodium and chloride.

Hyperbilirubinemia: Hyperbilirubinemia is often the result of liver disease or hemolysis. Significant hemolysis is unlikely when the PCV is within the reference range. The elevations in the liver enzymes suggest liver disease; specifically the increased ALP and GGT are compatible with cholestasis. Decreased hepatocellular uptake can also be associated with decreased liver function of any cause, and sepsis can result in diminished hepatocellular uptake of bilirubin. Sepsis is unlikely in this patient and generally can only account for relatively modest elevations in bilirubin.

Increased ALP and GGT: As noted above, increased ALP and GGT with hyperbilirubinemia indicate cholestasis, however there are numerous extrahepatic factors and other liver diseases which can increase ALP and GGT (see Chapter 2 for more details).

Increased ALT and AST: Elevations in these enzymes often indicate hepatocellular damage, however they indicate nothing specific about the etiology of the damage, nor the potential reversibility of the liver disease.

Hyperamylasemia and hyperlipasemia: Decreased glomerular filtration rate can increase both enzymes, however pancreatic disease is also possible. Some patients with pancreatitis can have normal amylase and lipase.

Coagulation profile: Normal

Spleen aspirate: compatible with extramedullary hematopoiesis. The spleen is a large and heterogeneous organ; the presence of this common and benign change does not rule out the potential for other processes, including neoplasia, in the organ.

Case Summary and Outcome

Abdominal ultrasonography revealed a thickened spleen with nodules (see above cytology), however the liver and pancreas were within normal limits. Elvira was treated with fluids and nutritional support, after which the azotemia, hyperbilirubinemia, and liver enzyme elevations improved. Her presumptive diagnosis was pancreatitis with secondary cholestatic liver disease; normal ultrasound findings were thought to be evidence of a resolving process.

One week after discharge from the hospital, Elvira's bilirubin was down to 4.7, however her ALT and ALP were persistently elevated and she was still azotemic. At this time, nephropathy was considered a potential explanation for persistent azotemia and isosthenuria. Four days after that, her bilirubin had halved, but other abnormalities were unchanged. One month after discharge from the hospital, she was still azotemic and mildly hyperbilirubinemic, however her liver enzymes had normalized. At this time, Leptospirosis titers were performed.

L. canicola, hardjo, icterohemorrhagica: negative
L. grippotyphosa: 1:806
L. bratislava: 1:800
L. pomona: 1:6,400

Elvira was treated for Leptospirosis with appropriate antibiotics. Over the next year, she developed clinical signs and laboratory abnormalities characteristic of chronic renal failure, however she had good quality of life at home with daily administration of fluids and other supportive management. Sixteen months after her initial presentation, she presented in oliguric renal failure and was euthanized.

At the time of the first hospitalization, Elvira's azotemia was presumed to be pre-renal and secondary to pancreatic/hepatobiliary disease. This assumption delayed diagnosis of concurrent renal disease and underscores the need for determination of urine specific gravity for appropriate interpretation of BUN and creatinine. Leptospirosis should be a consideration in any dog with the combination of renal azotemia and evidence of liver disease, especially if there is a history of exposure to livestock. This case should be compared with Hilda (Chapter 2, Case 18), another case of leptospirosis with laboratory evidence of renal compromise and liver disease. Diagnosis in Hilda's case was further complicated by her clinical history of eating pastries, cheese cake, and butter, however her laboratory work and her presentation with clinical signs of dehydration and poorly concentrated urine prompted immediate evaluation for causes of renal azotemia. Diagnosis in both of these cases was made using documentation of single markedly elevated titers for *Leptospira spp.* in the presence of compatible clinical signs. Polymerase chain reaction testing of urine is also available. While the negative predictive value of these titers appears to be high, some clinically normal dogs may have positive titers (Harkin, Harkin).

Harkin KR, Roshto YM, Sullivan JT. Clinical application of a polymerase chain reaction assay for diagnosis of leptospirosis in dogs. J Am Vet Med Assoc 2003;222:1224-1229.

Harkin KR, Roshto YM, Sullivan JT, Purvis TJ, Chengappa MM. Comparison of polymerase chain reaction assay, bacteriologic culture, and serologic testing in assessment of prevalence of urinary shedding of leptospires in dogs. J Am Vet Med Assoc 2003;222:1230-1233.

Case 16 – Level 3

"Tinker" is a 12-year-old spayed female domestic short haired cat with a history of weight loss, vomiting, diarrhea, polyuria, and polydipsia. On physical examination, she was thin with an unkempt haircoat. She had tachycardia, however auscultation was difficult because of persistent growling. Her kidneys felt slightly small, but abdominal palpation was otherwise unremarkable.

White blood cell count:	13.0 x 10⁹/L	(5.5-19.5)
Segmented neutrophils:	↑ 12.2 x 10⁹/L	(2.1-10.1)
Lymphocytes:	↓ 0.3 x 10⁹/L	(1.5-7.0)
Monocytes:	0.5 x 10⁹/L	(0-0.9)
Eosinophils:	0 x 10⁹/L	(0.0-1.9)

WBC morphology: No significant abnormalities noted.

Hematocrit:	31%	(28-45)
Hemoglobin:	9.5 g/dl	(8.0-15.0)
MCV:	46.8 fl	(39.0-55.0)
MCHC:	31.0 g/dl	(31.0-35.0)

Platelets: Clumped, but appear adequate

Glucose:	108 mg/dl	(70.0-120.0)
BUN:	↑ 105 mg/dl	(13-35)
Creatinine:	↑ 5.4 mg/dl	(0.6-2.0)
Phosphorus:	↑ 17.7 mg/dl	(3.0-6.0)
Calcium:	↑ 11.8 mg/dl	(8.9-11.0)
Magnesium:	2.5 mEq/L	(1.9-2.6)
Total Protein:	7.6 g/dl	(6.0-8.4)
Albumin:	3.5 g/dl	(2.4-4.0)
Globulin:	4.1 g/dl	(2.5-5.8)
Sodium:	156 mEq/L	(149-163)
Chloride:	117 mEq/L	(108-128)
Potassium:	↓ 2.5 mEq/L	(3.6-5.4)
HCO3:	↓ 11 mEq/L	(13-22)
Anion Gap:	↑ 30.5 mEq/L	(13-27)
Total Bili:	0.49 mg/dl	(0.10-0.50)
ALP:	↑ 108 IU/L	(10-72)
GGT:	1 IU/L	(0-5)
ALT:	↓ 8 IU/L	(10-140)
AST:	↑ 343 IU/L	(12-42)
Cholesterol:	184 mg/dl	(77-258)
Triglycerides:	47 mg/dl	(20-100)
Amylase:	1374 IU/L	(496-1874)

Urinalysis: Cystocentesis

Appearance: Yellow and hazy	Sediment:
Specific gravity: 1.009	0-5 RBC/hpf
pH: 5.0	10-20 WBC/hpf
Protein: 30 mg/dl	No casts seen
Glucose/ketones: negative	No epithelial cells seen
Bilirubin: negative	Bacteria 2+
Heme: negative	Trace fat droplets and debris

Interpretation

CBC: There is a neutrophilia and lymphopenia present, suggestive for a corticosteroid leukogram. However, inflammation cannot be ruled out, especially given the evidence of urinary track infection seen in the urinalysis. The PCV is at the low end of the reference range and should be monitored, especially if Tinker is dehydrated.

Serum Biochemical Profile

Azotemia and hyperphosphatemia: These changes are indicators of decreased glomerular filtration rate. Because the patient is simultaneously isosthenuric, renal azotemia is likely, although a pre-renal component also is probably superimposed given the history of vomiting and diarrhea with increased urine output.

Mild hypercalcemia: While many small animal patients with renal failure present with hypocalcemia, renal disease can be associated with variable changes in serum calcium. Neoplasia is also a common cause of hypercalcemia in small animal patients.

Hypokalemia: Several factors in Tinker's history could contribute to hypokalemia, including decreased intake associated with anorexia, and increased losses due to vomiting and diarrhea or polyuria. While serum electrolyte values may not reflect total body content in many cases, potassium depletion itself can cause metabolic acidosis in cats and dogs (DiBartola) in addition to hypokalemic nephropathy. Potassium depletion results in decreased tubular responsiveness to antidiuretic hormone, leading to polyuria and polydipsia. Renal vasoconstriction depresses glomerular filtration rate. In some cases, hypokalemic nephropathy is reversible with potassium repletion, however in more chronic cases, tubulointerstitial nephritis develops with potentially permanent renal damage.

Decreased HCO3 and increased anion gap: These data indicate acidemia with accumulation of unmeasured anions. The most likely cause here is uremic acidosis, however if dehydration is sufficient to cause poor tissue perfusion, lactic acidosis also may contribute to the acidemia and organic acidosis. The clinical history could be compatible with diabetic ketoacidosis, but this is not supported by the normal serum glucose and absence of glucosuria and ketonuria. Exogenous acids such as ethylene glycol and other toxins can also increase the anion gap.

Increased ALP and AST, low ALT: Increased ALP with normal GGT can be compatible with hepatic lipidosis in cats, which is possible given the history of weight loss, however most cats with hepatic lipidosis are also hyperbilirubinemic (see Squid, Chapter 2, Case 11). Weight loss with tachycardia in an older cat should prompt evaluation of the patient for hyperthyroidism. Elevations in one or more of the liver enzymes is observed in over 90% of cases of hyperthyroidism in cats (Broussard). Liver enzyme elevations are reversible with control of thyroid disease. Further work-up for primary liver disease is not recommended at this time because extra-hepatic factors can account for enzyme changes. Liver enzyme levels below the reference range (ALT) are not considered diagnostically significant and should not be over-interpreted.

Urinalysis: Bacteriuria, pyuria, and proteinuria indicate a urinary tract infection. Bacterial culture and sensitivity should be considered. Pyelonephritis could cause renal failure, and sepsis may also be associated with elevated liver enzymes (see Opie, Chapter 5, Case 13, and Riff Raff, Chapter 5, Case 8) that are also present in this patient.

Case Summary and Outcome

Thyroid hormone testing at a reference laboratory revealed hyperthyroidism (T4 = 7.5 µg/dl, reference interval = 1.2-5.2). In-house ELISA assays for T4 are available, but may correlate poorly with standard radio-immunoassay methods (Lurye). Tinker was also suspected to have some degree of decreased renal function. Azotemia is commonly described in hyperthyroid cats (Broussard), although the mechanisms are not clear. Some cats have concurrent renal disease, while in other patients, the azotemia resolves with successful control of excess thyroid hormone concentration. Increased protein catabolism and pre-renal factors related to dehydration or associated cardiovascular disease also have been suggested as mechanisms underlying the azotemia. Both hyperthyroidism and hypokalemia may have contributed to the polyuria/polydipsia and decreased urine specific gravity seen in Tinker. Excess thyroid hormone has been implicated in the development of dilute urine because of increased renal medullary blood flow and inadequate medullary solute concentration. However, one study of 202 hyperthyroid cats documented low urine specific gravity in only 3% of cases (Broussard).

Identification of concurrent renal disease in hyperthyroid cats is important for several reasons. The presence of non-thyroidal illness can lower thyroid hormone concentrations and interfere with diagnosis of hyperthyroidism (Tomsa, McLoughlin). Potential mechanisms for this include low binding of thyroid hormone to carrier proteins, low concentration or affinity of carrier proteins, and impaired production of T4 (Panciera). In addition, there is some evidence that treatment of hyperthyroidism in older cats may exacerbate underlying renal disease, possibly because of reduction in GFR (DiBartola). Based on this data, it is recommended that reversible medical treatment with methimazole be instituted prior to surgery or radioactive iodide, in order that the effects of treatment on renal function can be determined prior to permanent correction of hyperthyroidism.

Tinker was treated with antibiotics for a urinary tract infection and with methimazole, which works by preventing incorporation of iodine into the tyrosine residues of thyroglobulin. Follow-up blood work sixty days into therapy demonstrated resolution of hyperthyroidism and a normal serum biochemical profile with the exception of a slight elevation in BUN. Tinker was still isosthenuric, however her renal disease did not appear to have progressed after control of the thyroid disease.

Ninety days into her treatment, Tinker presented for lethargy and the following laboratory data were obtained:

	Day 90	
White blood cell count:	↓ 1.3 x 10⁹/L	(5.5-19.5)
Segmented neutrophils:	↓ 0.1 x 10⁹/L	(2.1-10.1)
Lymphocytes:	↓ 1.0 x 10⁹/L	(1.5-7.0)
Monocytes:	0.1 x 10⁹/L	(0-0.9)
Eosinophils:	0.1 x 10⁹/L	(0.0-1.9)
WBC morphology: No significant abnormalities noted.		
Hematocrit:	↓ 12%	(28-45)
Hemoglobin:	↓ 3.9 g/dl	(8.0-15.0)
MCV:	43.2 fl	(39.0-55.0)
MCHC:	32.5 g/dl	(31.0-35.0)
Platelets:	↓ 97 x 10⁹/L	(200-700)

Her CBC revealed pancytopenia. Both agranulocytosis and thrombocytopenia are occasionally reported as a side effect of treatment with methimazole, and they are most often observed within the first ninety days of therapy (Behrend, Retsios). Eosinophilia, leucopenia, and lymphocytosis have been described as potentially transient and do not necessarily warrant drug withdrawal, however the thrombocytopenia is a more serious consequence of treatment which requires discontinuation of therapy (Plumb). The cause of the anemia is less clear, but could be related to the drug, although renal disease may also contribute to the development of non-regenerative anemia due to impaired erythropoietin production.

Tinker's methimazole treatment was withdrawn, and her leukocyte and platelet counts normalized in 2 weeks; there was improvement in her anemia, but it was persistent. During this time, Tinker's azotemia and liver enzyme elevations returned, and she became hyperglycemic, which is common in untreated hyperthyroid cats. Because Tinker did not tolerate methimazole and because her renal disease appeared stable after correction of her hyperthyroidism, treatment with radioactive iodide was planned. Tinker's case may be compared with an uncomplicated case of feline hyperthyroidism (Rover, Chapter 2, Case 6), in which no azotemia was present, nor was there any reaction to methimazole therapy.

Behrend EN. Medical therapy of feline hyperthyroidism. Comp Contin Educ Small Animal. 1999;21:235-244.

Broussard JD, Peterson ME, Fox PR. Changes in clinical and laboratory findings in cats with hyperthyroidism from 1983-1993. J Am Vet Med Assoc. 1995;206:302-305.

DiBartola SP, Broome MR, Stein BS, Nixon M. Effect of treatment of hyperthyroidism on renal function in cats. J Am Vet Med Assoc 1996;208:875-878.

Lurye JC, Behrend EN, Kemppainen RJ. Evaluation of an in-house enzyme-linked immunosorbent assay for quantitative measurement of serum total thyroxine concentration in dogs and cats. J Am Vet Med Assoc. 2002;221:243-249.

McLoughlin MA, DiBartola SP, Birchard SJ, Day DG. Influence of systemic nonthyroidal illness on serum concentration of thyroxine in hyperthyroid cats. J Am Anim Hosp Assoc. 1993;29:227-234.

Panciera DL. Editorial: Thyroid function tests-what do they really tell us? J Vet Intern Med. 2001;15:86-88.

Plumb DC. Veterinary Drug Handbook, 4th ed. Iowa State University Press, Ames, IA. 2002.

Retsios E. Pharm profile: Methimazole. Compend Contin Educ Small Animal. 2001;23:36-41.

Tomsa K, Glaus TM, Kael GM, Pospischil A, Reusch CE. Thyrotropin-releasing hormone stimulation test to assess thyroid function in severely sick cats. J Vet Intern Med 2001;12:89-93.

Case 17 – Level 3

"Ziggy" is a 6-year-old castrated male domestic short haired cat presenting for acute onset of vomiting, lethargy, and anorexia. The owners report that he was not grooming himself and was vocalizing in the basement. Two years ago, Ziggy had a rear limb amputated due to trauma. On physical examination, Ziggy appeared to be approximately 8% dehydrated. Abdominal palpation revealed a small bladder and a small right kidney; the left kidney could not be palpated. Mucous membranes were light pink and tacky. Auscultation was normal.

White blood cell count:	9.9 x 10⁹/L	(4.5-15.7)
Segmented neutrophils:	9.5 x 10⁹/L	(2.1-13.1)
Lymphocytes:	↓ 0.3 x 10⁹/L	(1.5-7.0)
Monocytes:	0.1 x 10⁹/L	(0-0.9)
Eosinophils:	0.0 x 10⁹/L	(0.0-1.9)
WBC morphology: No significant abnormalities noted.		

Hematocrit:	32%	(28-45)
Red blood cell count:	7.32 x 10¹²/L	(5.0-10.0)
Hemoglobin:	11.0 g/dl	(8.0-15.0)
MCV:	42.9 fl	(39.0-55.0)
MCHC:	35.0 g/dl	(31.0-35.0)

Platelets: Clumped, but appear adequate

Glucose:	102 mg/dl	(70.0-120.0)
BUN:	↑ 182 mg/dl	(15-32)
Creatinine:	↑ 8.4 mg/dl	(0.9-2.1)
Phosphorus:	↑ 15.6 mg/dl	(3.0-6.0)
Calcium:	10.3 mg/dl	(8.9-11.6)
Magnesium:	↑ 4.2 mEq/L	(1.9-2.6)
Total Protein:	↑ 8.4 g/dl	(5.5-7.6)
Albumin:	↑ 3.9 g/dl	(2.2-3.4)
Globulin:	4.5 g/dl	(2.5-5.8)
Sodium:	↓ 144 mEq/L	(149-164)
Chloride:	↓ 107 mEq/L	(119-134)
Potassium:	4.1 mEq/L	(3.9-5.4)
HCO3:	13 mEq/L	(13-22)
Anion gap:	↑ 28.1 mEq/L	(13-25)
Cholesterol:	↑ 296 mg/dl	(77-258)
CK:	↑ 426 IU/L	(55-382)

Urinalysis: Catheter

Appearance: Yellow and clear	Sediment:
Specific gravity: 1.015	0 RBC/hpf
pH: 6.5	Occasional WBC/hpf
Protein: 2+	No casts seen
Glucose: negative	No epithelial cells are seen
Ketones negative	No bacteria or crystals present
Bilirubin: negative	Trace fat droplets and debris
Heme: 1+	

Interpretation

CBC: Lymphopenia could be compatible with stress/corticosteroid effects. The PCV is in the normal range, however this patient is significantly dehydrated. This PCV should be re-evaluated once the patient is rehydrated to be sure that the dehydration in not masking a mild anemia.

Serum Biochemical Profile

Azotemia: Azotemia should be categorized as pre-renal, renal, or post-renal. The minimally concentrated urine in the face of severe dehydration supports renal failure. There is no evidence of post-renal disease such as fluid in the abdomen or a large, firm bladder. Because the patient is significantly dehydrated, there is likely pre-renal azotemia in addition to renal azotemia.

Hyperphosphatemia, hypermagnesemia, and normal calcium: The most likely cause of hyperphosphatemia and hypermagnesemia in this patient is decreased glomerular filtration rate, regardless of whether the decreased glomerular filtration rate is due to pre-renal, renal, or post-renal causes. Small animal patients in renal failure may have high, normal, or low serum calcium levels, and ionized calcium levels may not correlate with total calcium levels.

Increased total protein and albumin: Increases these analytes are most likely due to dehydration.

Hyponatremia and hypochloremia: Hyponatremia is rarely due to dietary deficiency of sodium, and dilution because of free water is unlikely given clinical dehydration and hyperalbuminemia. Therefore, excessive loss of sodium is the probable cause for the hyponatremia. While sodium may be lost via multiple routes including gastrointestinal, dermal, third space, and renal, the clinical history is most compatible with renal losses. The diseased kidney may be unable to adequately conserve sodium, and conversely, may be less able to excrete a sodium load. Depending on intake and the relative rates of sodium and water loss, patients with renal disease may have low, normal, or high serum sodium. Chloride often changes in proportion to sodium, however in this case there is a disproportionate decrease in chloride compared to sodium. This may be due to loss in vomitus. However the increased anion gap and low normal HCO3 suggest the possibility of an acid/base disturbance, which could also cause a disproportionate change in chloride.

Increased anion gap: Hyperproteinemia and dehydration can increase the anion gap, as can the presence of increased organic acids in the blood. Ziggy may have increased uremic acids because of his renal disease, and the marked dehydration may cause poor perfusion and lactic acidosis. In general, chloride and HCO3 vary inversely. In this case the combination of hypochloremia and borderline acidosis (low HCO3) suggest the possibility of a mixed acid/base disorder. Vomiting of gastric contents could contribute to alkalemia. Alkalemia itself can increase the anion gap because of loss of protons from plasma proteins resulting in increased negative charge. Alkalemia can also stimulate phosphofructokinase leading to increased production of lactic acid. Complete characterization of the acid/base status of this patient requires blood gas analysis. Correction of the fluid deficits and treatment of the renal disease should improve the acid/base status, regardless of the exact cause.

Hypercholesterolemia: Increases in cholesterol have been described in dogs with glomerular nephritis and dogs with nephrotic syndrome. The mechanism for hypercholesterolemia in nephrotic syndrome may be increased hepatic synthesis, and these patients often have an inverse relationship between albumin and cholesterol (which is not present in this patient). Abnormal lipoprotein lipase function related to inadequate amounts of its co-factor, heparan sulfate, may also contribute to the hypercholesterolemia in nephrotic syndrome.

Increased Creatine kinase: This is evidence for muscle degeneration or necrosis. Muscle breakdown associated with anorexia in cats can elevate serum CK (Fascetti). CK levels normalized in anorexic cats once they were given adequate nutritional support.

Urinalysis: Proteinuria of 2+ in dilute urine with an inactive sediment is compatible with glomerular loss of protein. There is no evidence of blood contamination or lower urinary tract disease in this case to account for the protein in the urine. A urine protein:creatinine ratio is recommended to further evaluate urinary protein losses. It is worthwhile noting that significant glomerular protein loss is not always associated with hypoalbuminemia because of the capacity of a healthy liver for compensatory upregulate of albumin production. Dehydration can also mask hypoproteinemia in some cases.

Case Summary and Outcome

Ziggy was treated with aggressive fluid therapy and potassium supplementation. As his dehydration was corrected, the pre-renal component of his azotemia was eliminated and his other laboratory abnormalities improved but did not normalize. Ziggy was discharged from the hospital with treatment plan including subcutaneous fluids, oral potassium supplementation, and gastroprotectants. His long term prognosis is guarded because the combination of his laboratory work and small kidneys are compatible with chronic renal failure, which is not reversible. This case should be compared with Marklar (Case 1), Jag (Case 4), and Popcorn (Case 24, in this chapter), in which appropriate treatment resulted in complete normalization of laboratory data and restoration of urinary concentrating ability. Note that the degree of azotemia was not predictive of prognosis in these cases, nor did it allow differentiation of renal, pre-renal, or post-renal causes of azotemia.

This case is very similar to Tramp (Chapter 5, Case 10), but Tramp has more severe azotemia and anemia. Tramp's creatinine value is higher than Ziggy's, however this is not conclusive proof that Tramp has worse renal function than Ziggy. First of all, the pre-renal component may be different between the two patients. Second, while serial measurements of BUN and creatinine can be used to monitor renal function in individual patients, the use of BUN and creatinine to compare renal function between patients is questionable because of large interindividual variations in BUN and creatinine values (Braun). The non-specific nature of the Jaffé reaction used to measure creatinine in most veterinary chemistry analyzers leads to variation in creatinine values unrelated to changes in glomerular filtration rate, but this is more likely to cause discrepancies at low creatinine concentrations. In addition, it should be remembered that the relationship between plasma creatinine and glomerular filtration rate is curvilinear. Thus, small changes in the low end of the creatinine range can correspond to large changes in glomerular filtration rate, while at higher creatinine concentrations, relatively large changes in creatinine can be associated with smaller decrements in glomerular filtration rate. Comparison of the two cases illustrates the variable electrolyte findings in chronic renal failure cases. In neither case was the cause for the renal failure determined.

Braun JP, Lefebvre HP, Watson ADJ. Creatinine in the dog: A review. Vet Clin Pathol. 2003;32:162-179.

Fascetti AJ, Mauldin GE, Mauldin GN. Correlation between serum creatinine kinase activities and anorexia in cats. J Vet Intern Med 1997;11:9-13.

Case 18 – Level 3

"Sloop" is a 2-week-old thoroughbred filly with a history of lethargy and decreased nursing for one day. On presentation, the foal was quiet, alert and responsive but had a large, distended abdomen.

White blood cell count:	↑ 11.8 x 10⁹/L	(5.9-11.2)
Segmented neutrophils:	↑ 10.1 x 10⁹/L	(2.3-9.1)
Band neutrophils:	0.0	(0-0.3)
Lymphocytes:	↓ 1.1 x 10⁹/L	(1.6-5.2)
Monocytes:	0.6 x 10⁹/L	(0-1.0)

WBC morphology: A few reactive lymphocytes are seen.

Hematocrit:	38%	(30-51)
Red blood cell count:	9.09 x 10¹²/L	(6.5-12.8)
Hemoglobin:	13.9 g/dl	(10.9-18.1)
MCV:	41.0 fl	(35.0-53.0)
MCHC:	36.6 g/dl	(34.6-38.0)

RBC morphology: No abnormalities seen.

Platelets: Clumped but appear adequate

Fibrinogen:	200 mg/dl	(100-400)

Glucose:	↑ 155 mg/dl	(6.0-128.0)
BUN:	↑ 31 mg/dl	(11-26)
Creatinine:	↑ 3.5 mg/dl	(0.9-1.9)
Phosphorus:	↑ 6.7 mg/dl	(1.9-6.0)
Calcium:	12.7 mg/dl	(11.0-13.5)
Magnesium:	1.9 mEq/L	(1.7-2.4)
Total Protein:	6.9 g/dl	(5.6-7.0)
Albumin:	3.0 g/dl	(2.4-3.8)
Globulin:	3.9 g/dl	(2.5-4.9)
A/G Ratio:	0.8	(0.7-2.1)
Sodium:	↓ 119 mEq/L	(130-145)
Chloride:	↓ 82 mEq/L	(99-105)
Potassium:	↑ 6.1 mEq/L	(3.0-5.0)
HCO3:	26 mEq/L	(25-31)
Anion Gap:	↑ 17.1 mEq/L	(7-15)
Total Bili:	↑ 3.80 mg/dl	(0.30-3.0)
Direct bili:	0.20 mg/dl	(0.0-0.5)
Indirect bili:	↑ 3.40 mg/dl	(0.2-3.0)
ALP:	↑ 1522 IU/L	(109-352)
GGT:	↑ 114 IU/L	(5-23)
AST:	364 IU/L	(190-380)
CK:	336 IU/L	(80-446)

Abdominal fluid analysis

Appearance: Yellow and hazy	
Total protein: <2.0 gm/dl	
Total nucleated cell count: 3.46 x 10³/µl	

Total nucleated cell count: $3.46 \times 10^3/\mu l$

Most of the nucleated cells are nondegenerate neutrophils. No etiologic agents are seen. Scattered large mononuclear cells and rare erythrocytes are also present. The fluid creatinine concentration is 12.6 mg/dl.

Interpretation

CBC

Leukogram: There is a mild mature neutrophilia and lymphopenia, most compatible with corticosteroid effects. The neutrophilia could also be compatible with inflammation, however the normal fibrinogen makes this interpretation less likely because fibrinogen is an acute phase reactant that should increase early in the inflammatory response of horses.

Serum Biochemical Profile

Hyperglycemia: Elevations in serum glucose in the horse are most often caused increases in endogenous catecholamines and glucocorticoids secondary to excitement or stress, respectively. A corticosteroid effect is supported by the concurrent lymphopenia.

Azotemia: With no urine specific gravity to aid interpretation, it is difficult to classify the azotemia. The clinical history, the electrolyte abnormalities, and the high creatinine concentration of the abdominal fluid are compatible with uroabdomen, a cause of post-renal azotemia. Pre-renal factors may also contribute to the azotemia. Accumulation of fluid in the abdomen may cause intravascular volume contraction and lower the glomerular filtration rate. Dehydration because of poor nursing also adds to the pre-renal azotemia.

Hyperphosphatemia: The most likely cause for the hyperphosphatemia in this case is decreased glomerular filtration rate. Serum phosphorus can also be high during skeletal growth and development in young animals.

Hyponatremia and hypochloremia: Because of the abdominal effusion, third space loss of sodium and chloride are likely. In the case of uroabdomen, sodium and chloride diffuse down their concentration gradients into the fluid accumulating in the abdomen. The resulting contraction of the intravascular fluid volume leads to stimulation of the renin-angiotensin system, which will tend to conserve sodium and water. In addition, antidiuretic hormone will stimulate free water retention and thirst, which will have a dilutional effect on the remaining electrolytes in the circulation.

Hyperkalemia: When the body cannot eliminate urine, potassium will be retained. This may occur with post-renal azotemia or in the anuric/oliguric phase of renal failure. This is in contrast to the polyuric phase of renal failure, in which increased tubular flow rates promote potassium wasting, resulting from decreased time for reabsorption. As has been noted for other cases with electrolyte changes of hyponatremia, hypochloremia, and hyperkalemia, hypoadrenocorticism is a differential diagnosis, however this is very unlikely in this patient because of signalment and history.

Hyperbiliruinemia: The most likely cause for the hyperbilirubinemia in this patient is anorexia, Fasted horses typically have increased indirect bilirubin with normal to mildly elevated direct bilirubin. In horses with cholestasis, the reverse pattern of a high direct bilirubin with normal to mildly increased indirect value is usually seen. Mechanisms suggested for fasting-induced hyperbilirubinemia include either increased mobilization of free fatty acids that interfere with bilirubin uptake by hepatocytes, or inadequate availability of glucose for conjugation with bilirubin. Hemolysis is another possible contributor to the hyperbilirubinemia. In this case, the PCV is within the reference range, however some degree of hemolysis cannot be ruled out. In horses, causes of hemolytic anemias include neonatal isoerythrolysis, drug effects, infectious agents (Babesia, Leptospirosis, Equine Infectious Anemia virus), metabolic derangements, or plant intoxication. Microscopic evaluation of erythrocytes did not reveal any morphologic abnormalities such as Heinz bodies, eccentrocytes, or parasites that would suggest that any of the above are likely.

Increased ALP and GGT: While hepatobiliary disease cannot be completely ruled out, these elevations in ALP and GGT are likely to be normal age-related changes. In a young horse, an increased ALP reflects bone growth. GGT activity is normally higher in foals less than one month of age, and can be one and a half to three times the value of adult horses (Patterson). Donkeys and burros may also have higher values. There is no increase in the AST to support hepatic pathology, although an SDH was not measured.

Abdominal fluid analysis: The fluid is a low protein effusion with a creatinine concentration that greatly exceeds the serum creatinine, compatible with the presence of urine in the abdomen. Because of its small size, urea diffuses out of the effusion and is not helpful in the diagnosis of uroabdomen. The slightly increased cell counts and predominance of nondegenerate neutrophils is compatible with a mild chemical peritonitis.

Case Summary and Outcome

Appropriate fluid therapy was initiated, and abdominal radiographs with a contrast study of the bladder indicated bladder rupture. Therapeutic abdominocentesis and therapy to reduce serum potassium were performed to prepare Sloop for surgery, where a four centimeter tear was repaired on the dorsal aspect of her urinary bladder. Recovery was uneventful, and Sloop was able to stand and nurse one hour after surgery. Sloop began to improve steadily and gain weight. She was discharged several days after surgery to complete her recovery at home.

As noted for many of the cases, Sloop's azotemia does not distinguish pre-renal, renal, or post-renal processes. The electrolyte abnormalities can be slightly more helpful, in that hyperkalemia is most often present with urinary outflow obstruction (see Ringo, Case 7) or in the oliguric/anuric phase of chronic renal failure (see Margarite, Case 9).

Patterson WH, Brown CM. Increase of serum gamma glutamyl transferase in neonatal Standardbred foals. Am J Vet Res. 1986;47:2461-2463.

Case 19 – Level 3

"Faith" is a 9-year-old miniature mare presenting with a history of developing laminitis 10 days ago, for which she was treated with a course of oral phenylbutazone. She was referred for signs of colic, and at presentation, she was depressed. On physical examination, Faith had a marked tachycardia, increased respiratory rate with normal lung sounds, and a mild fever. Her mucous membranes were injected and she had an ulcer on her buccal mucosal surface. She has 8/9 body condition score. Nasogastric intubation did not produce reflux. Rectal palpation was not possible due to her small size.

White blood cell count:	↑ 18.9 x 10⁹/L	(5.9-11.2)
Segmented neutrophils:	↑ 14.1 x 10⁹/L	(2.3-9.1)
Band neutrophils:	↑ 2.1 x 10⁹/L	(0-0.3)
Lymphocytes:	2.5 x 10⁹/L	(1.6-5.2)
Monocytes:	0.2 x 10⁹/L	(0-1.0)

WBC morphology: Neutrophils are moderately toxic.

Hematocrit:	31%	(30-51)
Red blood cell count:	7.07 x 10¹²/L	(6.5-12.8)
Hemoglobin:	11.4 g/dl	(10.9-18.1)
MCV:	46.6 fl	(35.0-53.0)
MCHC:	36.8 g/dl	(34.6-38.0)

Platelets: Adequate

RBC morphology: Normal

Fibrinogen:	↑ 600 mg/dl	(100-400)

Glucose:	↑ 318 mg/dl	(60.0-128.0)
BUN:	↑ 39 mg/dl	(11-26)
Creatinine:	↑ 2.2 mg/dl	(0.9-1.9)
Phosphorus:	↑ 11.0 mg/dl	(1.9-6.0)
Calcium:	↓ 10.1 mg/dl	(11.0-13.5)
Magnesium:	↓ 1.3 mEq/L	(1.7-2.4)
Total Protein:	↓ 4.9 g/dl	(5.6-7.0)
Albumin:	↓ 1.9 g/dl	(2.4-3.8)
Globulin:	3.0 g/dl	(2.5-4.9)
A/G Ratio:	0.6	(0.6-2.1)
Sodium:	↓ 121 mEq/L	(130-145)
Chloride:	↓ 81 mEq/L	(99-105)
Potassium:	3.5 mEq/L	(3.0-5.0)
HCO3:	26 mEq/L	(25-31)
Anion Gap:	↑ 17.5 mEq/L	(7-15)
Total Bili:	↑ 6.20 mg/dl	(0.30-3.0)
Direct bili:	0.20 mg/dl	(0.0-0.5)
Indirect bili:	↑ 6.00 mg/dl	(0.2-3.0)
ALP:	↑ 689 IU/L	(109-352)
GGT:	↑ 27 IU/L	(5-23)
AST:	↑ 511 IU/L	(190-380)
CK:	↑ 610 IU/L	(80-446)
Triglycerides:	↑ 906 mg/dl	(80-446)

Moderate lipemia of serum is noted

Urinalysis

Urine specific gravity: 1.030	
Other urinalysis data not available	

Abdominal fluid analysis

Appearance: Gold and hazy	
Total protein: <2.0 gm/dl	
Total nucleated cell count: 483/µl	
Most of the nucleated cells are nondegenerate neutrophils. No etiologic agents are seen. Scattered large mononuclear cells and rare erythrocytes are also present.	

Interpretation

CBC

Leukogram: Faith has a neutrophilic leukocytosis with a regenerative left shift and mild toxic change, all of which support inflammation. The hyperfibrinogenemia corroborates this interpretation.

Erythrogram: Her PCV is at the lower end of the reference interval. Correction of any dehydration may result in mild anemia.

Serum Biochemical Profile

Hyperglycemia: Elevations in serum glucose in the horse are most often caused by endogenous catecholamines and glucocorticoids release secondary to excitement or stress. Leukogram findings are not specific for either of these effects. Diabetes mellitus is rare in domestic large animal species. Hyperadrenocorticism in the horse may predispose to development of hyperglycemia, related to insulin resistance.

Azotemia and Urinalysis: Azotemia in conjunction with concentrated urine indicates pre-renal azotemia. Dehydration secondary to colic will contribute to pre-renal azotemia. Poor tissue perfusion secondary to systemic vasodilation with sepsis can also be a factor. While the urine specific gravity at this time supports pre-renal azotemia, the use of nonsteroidal anti-inflammatories at high doses or in combination with other nephrotoxic drugs or dehydration can cause kidney damage and needs to be monitored (see Joe, Chapter 5, Case 11, and Calvin, Chapter 2, Case 20).

Hyperphosphatemia and hypocalcemia: The most likely cause for the hyperphosphatemia in this case is decreased glomerular filtration rate. The hypocalcemia may reflect the hypoalbuminemia. Colic is often associated with decreases in both total and ionized calcium, though the mechanism is still uncertain. Calcium wasting in the urine did not appear to contribute to the hypocalcemia in horses with colic (Toribio). Acute renal failure in horses also can be characterized by hypocalcemia, possibly due to renal wastage. In contrast, chronic renal failure may be associated with hypercalcemia because the large amounts of calcium that are normally excreted in the urine can no longer be eliminated by this route. Low serum ionized calcium levels can be caused by low magnesium states due to inadequate action of parathyroid hormone. Ionized calcium levels can be performed to further evaluate Faith's calcium status.

Hypomagnesemia: Like calcium, magnesium is protein bound and may decrease secondary to hypoproteinemia. Prolonged anorexia and excess urinary elimination may also be factors. Ionized magnesium may be low in horses with colic (Toribio).

Hypoproteinemia with hypoalbuminemia: Selective hypoalbuminemia is most often the result of either decreased production (inadequate liver function, starvation) or increased losses via glomerular lesions. Most other causes of increased protein loss, such as cutaneous, gastrointestinal, or third space losses, result in a deficit of both globulins and albumin. Based on the clinical history, gastrointestinal losses of protein are most likely in this case. It is likely that Faith actually has increased production of acute phase reactants and/or immunoglobulins secondary to inflammation that is offseting the gastrointestinal losses of protein and keeping the globulin measurement in the reference interval.

Hyponatremia and hypochloremia: Hypertonic fluid losses related to colic are the probable cause of these electrolyte abnormalities. Sweating from pain associated with laminitis or colic is another possible route for loss of sodium and chloride. If isotonic fluid losses are replaced by drinking water, hyponatremia and hypochloremia can result. Lipemia can cause artifactually lower electrolyte values, depending on the methodology used to measure these analytes. If an analyzer employs indirect potentiometry with ion specific electrodes in which the sample is diluted as part of the assay, artifactual lowering of electrolyte concentrations may be observed with severe lipemia. This occurs with analyzers such as the Hitachi 911. With direct potentiometric methods using ion specific electrodes in which there is no sample dilution, lipemic interference with measurement of electrolyte concentrations would not be anticipated. If sodium and chloride are both decreased in an obviously lactescent sample, another methodology should be used to confirm concentrations of these electrolytes.

Increased anion gap: This value reflects an accumulation of unmeasured anions, which could include lactic acid in this patient. Increased anion gap is often associated with a low HCO3 compatible with acidosis, however here the HCO3 is still at the lower end of the reference range.

Hyperbilirubinemia: The most likely cause of hyperbilirubinemia in a sick horse is anorexia. Given the normal PCV, hemolysis is unlikely. Cholestasis is possible given the increased liver enzymes.

Increased ALP and GGT: In an adult horse, increased GGT is evidence for liver damage and cholestasis. This change is often associated with hyperbilirubinemia, although bilirubin can be efficiently eliminated in the urine. ALP is less liver specific than GGT and may be slightly less sensitive in the horse. These enzyme elevations are not specific as to the etiology of the liver insult. The combination of lipemia and elevated liver enzymes in a recently anorexic obese pony suggests the possibility of hyperlipemia and hepatic lipidosis.

Increased AST and CK: AST is present in multiple tissues and elevations can be difficult to interpret. In Faith, the concurrent increase in ALP and GGT supports the potential for hepatic origin, yet the concurrent increase in CK indicates that muscle damage has occurred and may be responsible for some of the increase in AST. Like ALP and GGT, elevations in AST are not specific as to the etiology of the liver damage. Note that none of these enzymes are liver function tests. It is necessary to measure blood ammonia or serum bile acids to confirm liver dysfunction in this case, especially since the hyperbilirubinemia could be explained by decreased feed intake.

Hypertriglyceridemia: Fasting hypertriglyceridemia is considered abnormal, and may be associated with metabolic disorders, liver or pancreatic disease, and endocrinopathies. Fasted horses with hypertriglyceridemia should be evaluated for hyperlipemia/hyperlipidemia syndrome, which can be triggered by feed restriction or anorexia during colic episodes (Mogg). The syndrome is caused by decreased feed intake with subsequent fat mobilization and accumulation in the plasma and liver. Faith is more appropriately categorized as hyperlipemia because her plasma is lipemic and her triglycerides exceed 500 mg/dl. Hyperlipemia is a more serious condition accompanied by lactescent plasma, impaired hepatic function and the production of abnormal very low density lipoproteins that have less apolipoprotein B-100 and more apolipoprotein B-48. This substitution may allow greater triglyceride content.

Abdominal fluid: Normal. There is nothing in the abdominal fluid analysis to suggest peritonitis as the cause of the inflammatory leukogram.

Case Summary and Outcome
Faith was treated with intravenous fluids and dextrose, antibiotics, and analgesics (avoiding nonsteroidal anti-inflammatories). She remained stable overnight, but began to deteriorate, becoming increasingly painful and eventually showing signs of endotoxemia. Ultimately, Faith was euthanized for humane reasons because of her lack of response to therapy. Clinicians felt that the gastrointestinal lesions might have been related to the use of non-steroidal anti-inflammatories used to treat the initial laminitis. Non-steroidal anti-inflammatory drugs are thought to induce injury by direct topical effects and inhibition of prostaglandin synthesis that contributes to maintenance of mucosal barrier in the gastrointestinal system (Tomlinson).

Mogg TD, Palmer JE. Hyperlipidemia, hyperlipemia, and hepatic lipidosis in American miniature horses: 23 cases (1990-1994). J Am Vet Assoc. 1995;207:604-607.

Tomlinson J, Blikslager A. Role of nonsteroidal anti-inflammatory drugs in gastrointestinal tract injury and repair. J Am Vet Med Assoc. 2003;222:946-951.

Toribio RE, Kohn CW, Chew DJ, Sams RA, Rosol, TJ. Comparison of serum parathyroid hormone and ionized calcium and magnesium concentrations and fractional urinary clearance of calcium and phosphorus in healthy horses and horses with enterocolitis. Am J Vet Res 2001;62:938-947.

Case 20 – Level 3
"Forsythia" is a 6.5-year-old female llama presenting for a history of weight loss over 2 years and a one day history of straining to urinate. On physical examination, Forsythia had a fist-sized rectal prolapse and her rectum was stained with diarrhea. She had fetid breath and ptyalism with buccal epithelial sloughing, nasal discharge, and was tachypneic. She was dull and had a 3/9 body condition score.

White blood cell count:	↓ 3.3 x 10⁹/L	(7.5-21.5)
Segmented neutrophils:	↓ 2.6 x 10⁹/L	(4.6-16.0)
Band neutrophils:	0	(0-0.3)
Lymphocytes:	↓ 0.5 x 10⁹/L	(1.0-7.5)
Monocytes:	0.1 x 10⁹/L	(0.1-0.8)
Eosinophils:	0.1 x 10⁹/L	(0.0-3.3)
WBC morphology: Slightly to moderately toxic neutrophils present		

Hematocrit:	↓ 20%	(29-39)
RBC morphology: Normal		
Platelets: Appear adequate		

Fibrinogen:	↑ 500 mg/dl	(100-400)

Glucose:	↑ 206 mg/dl	(90-140.0)
BUN:	↑ 441 mg/dl	(13-32)
Creatinine:	↑ 31.8 mg/dl	(1.5-2.9)
Phosphorus:	7.1 mg/dl	(4.6-9.8)
Calcium:	↓ 7.2 mg/dl	(8.0-10.0)

Magnesium:	↑ 3.3 mEq/L	(1.5-2.5)
Total Protein:	5.8 g/dl	(5.5-7.0)
Albumin:	↓ 2.8 g/dl	(3.5-4.4)
Globulin:	3.0 g/dl	(1.7-3.5)
A/G Ratio:	0.9	(1.4-3.3)
Sodium:	152 mEq/L	(147-158)
Chloride:	↓ 98 mEq/L	(106-118)
Potassium:	↓ 2.8 mEq/L	(4.3-5.8)
Anion gap:	↑ 44.8 mEq/L	(14-29)
HCO3:	↓ 12 mEq/L	(14-28)
Total Bili:	0.1 mg/dl	(0.0-0.1)
ALP:	77 IU/L	(30-780)
GGT:	↑ 51 IU/L	(5-29)
AST:	↑ 1099 IU/L	(110-250)
CK:	↑ 9641 IU/L	(30-400)

Urinalysis: Catheter

Appearance: Straw and clear	Sediment:
Specific gravity: 1.015	0-5 RBC/hpf
pH: 6.0	Occasional WBC/hpf
Protein: 30 mg/dl	Few transitional epithelial cells seen
Glucose: 2+	Trace bacteria and debris
Heme: 3+	
Ketones and bilirubin: negative	

Interpretation

CBC: Forsythia has leucopenia with neutropenia and lymphopenia. Hyperfibrinoginemia and toxic change indicate inflammation, which may be too acute for the development of neutrophilia or a left shift. Sepsis and consumption of neutrophils may contribute to the neutropenia. Alternatively, in combination with the nonregenerative anemia, a primary bone marrow disease could be considered. The clinical history and biochemistry data are compatible with renal disease, which could explain a nonregenerative anemia in the absence of marrow pathology. Lymphopenia may indicate corticosteroid effects, or potentially lysis secondary to a viral infection.

Serum Biochemical Profile
Hyperglycemia: Stress and corticosteroid effects can result in hyperglycemia in llamas, which appear to have poor insulin responses (Cebra). The lymphopenia is also compatible with corticosteroid effects. The combination of hyperglycemia and glucosuria is suggestive for diabetes mellitus, but may also result from transient increases in blood glucose over the transport maximum in the kidney. Persistent hyperglycemia with or without ketonemia is needed for a diagnosis of diabetes.

Severe azotemia: In combination with the isosthenuria and oral lesions, renal disease is the likely cause of the azotemia, although pre-renal factors may exacerbate the increases in BUN and creatinine. The oral lesions are compatible with uremia. Given the history of straining and rectal prolapse, urinary obstruction should be ruled out.

Hypocalcemia: This abnormality may related to the hypoalbuminemia, however a quantitative relationship between the two values cannot be determined. Increased urinary losses of calcium associated with renal disease also could contribute to hypocalcemia. While not present in this patient, decreases in calcium in conjunction with hyperphosphatemia have been described in llamas with decreased glomerular filtration rate secondary to urethral obstruction (Gerros).

Hypermagnesemia: Increased magnesium is associated with decreased glomerular filtration rate.

Hypoalbuminemia: Proteinuria suggests the potential for renal protein loss, however the presence of leukocytes, bacteria, and erythrocytes in the urine indicates that lower urinary tract disease could explain the proteinuria. Urine protein:creatinine ratios should be measured after successful treatment of any urinary tract infection. Although the owners do not report diarrhea, fecal staining of her perineum suggests that gastrointestinal losses of protein are possible. However, one would expect losses of both globulins and albumin in protein losing enteropathy. Globulin loss may be masked by increased production due to inflammation. Forsythia's history of chronic weight loss and poor body condition are compatible with starvation as a cause for hypoalbuminemia.

Hypochloremia with normal serum sodium: Gastrointestinal sequestration and salivary losses of chloride will decrease serum chloride. Acid/base abnormalities are also associated with changes in chloride that are disproportionate to sodium, however chloride usually varies inversely with HCO3, which is not the case in this patient. When chloride and HCO3 change in the same direction, a mixed acid/base disorder is suspected, and arterial blood gases should be evaluated for more complete characterization of the process. Renal losses of chloride can be quantifed by measuring urinary fractional excretion, and normal values are available in the literature (Garry).

Hypokalemia: In this case, the combination of decreased intake and excessive losses via the gastrointestinal or urinary tract explain the low serum potassium. Hypokalemia is most often associated with polyuric renal failure because increased tubular flow rates decrease reabsorption of potassium. Inability to eliminate urine in oliguric/anuric renal failure or with urinary outflow obstruction more often causes retention of potassium and hyperkalemia.

Increased anion gap and low HCO3: These changes suggest acidemia with accumulation of unmeasured anions, such as uremic acids. The hyperglycemia and glucosuria could be compatible with diabetes mellitus, and ketoacids also can increase the anion gap. In this case the urine did not contain ketones, and the hyperglycemia could be attributable to stress.

Increased GGT, AST, and CK: Elevated serum GGT may indicate hepatic necrosis or cholestatic liver disease, though this is unlikely given the normal bilirubin. GGT and AST will increase with hepatic lipidosis which can develop in anorexic camelids. However, lipidosis, usually, occurs when there are increased caloric demands such as with pregnancy or lactation (Tornquist). Both liver and muscle damage can increase AST. Based on the increased CK, at least of portion of the elevation in AST is from muscle. Muscle damage may be related to administration of intramuscular injections or any episodes of recumbency.

Case Summary and Outcome

Based on a poor long-term prognosis, Forsythia was humanely euthanized. At necropsy, only mild lymphoplasmacytic inflammation was noted around larger bile ducts. There was no evidence of liver necrosis or hepatic lipidosis. Erythroid hypoplasia was apparent in the marrow, consistent with chronic renal disease as a cause for the anemia. Proteinaceous casts were found in the renal tubules, some of which contained neutrophils. Glomerular adhesions and sclerosis with diffuse interstitial fibrosis were considered compatible with glomerulonephritis. As is usually the case, the cause of the lesion could not be determined, however the pattern was more consistent with immune complex deposition than nephrotoxicity. The glomerular lesions support protein losing nephropathy as a contributing factor to the hypoalbuminemia.

Immune-complex deposition is a common cause of glomerulonephritis in the horse, and subclinical disease may be present in horses as an incidental finding at necropsy (Slauson). Other times, glomerulonephritis culminates in the development of chronic renal failure, although not all patients with glomerulonephritis are azotemic at presentation (Van Biervliet). It is also possible for patients with glomerulonephritis to present with azotemia and concentrated urine. In the absence of pre-renal azotemia, this may be explained as the result of glomerulo-tubular imbalance in which glomerular filtration decreases to below 75% of normal, but tubular function is maintained (Grant).

Cebra CK, Tornquist SJ, Van Saun RJ, Smith BB. Glucose tolerance testing in llamas and alpacas. Am J Vet Res 62:682-686, 2001

Garry F, Weiser MG, Belknap E. Clinical Pathology of Llamas. Veterinary Clinics of North America: Food Animal Practice. 1994;10:201-209.

Gerros TC. Recognizing and treating urolithiasis in llamas. Vet Med 1998;93:583-590.

Grant DC, Forrester SD. Glomerulonephritis in dogs and cats: Glomerular function, pathophysiology, and clinical signs. Compend Contin Educ Pract Vet 2001;23:739-743.

Slauson DO, Lewis RM. Comparative pathology of glomerulonephritis in animals. Vet Pathol 1979;16:135-164.

Tornquist SJ, Cebra CK, Van Saun RJ, Smith BS, Mattoon JS. Metabolic changes and induction of hepatic lipidosis during feed restriction in llamas. Am J Vet Res 2001;62:1081-1087.

Van Biervliet J, Divers TJ, Poerter B, Huxtable C. Glomerulonephritis in Horses. Compend Cont Educ Pract Vet 2002;24:892-901.

Case 21 – Level 3

"Brianna" is a 1.5-year-old intact female toy poodle presenting with a 2-day history of vomiting bile, lethargy, and anorexia. Her last heat was 2 months ago. Brianna is a show dog with no previous health problems and she is in good body condition. On physical examination, Brianna is 8% dehydrated and hypothermic. Abdominal palpation appears to be painful, especially in the peri-renal area. Owners report that Brianna chews many foreign objects.

White blood cell count:	↑ 14.4 x 10⁹/L	(4.0-13.3)
Segmented neutrophils:	↑ 12.4 x 10⁹/L	(2.0-11.2)
Band neutrophils:	0.1 x 10⁹/L	(0-0.3)
Lymphocytes:	1.2 x 10⁹/L	(1.0-4.5)
Monocytes:	0.7 x 10⁹/L	(0.2-1.4)
Eosinophils:	0.0 x 10⁹/L	(0-1.2)

WBC morphology: Appears within normal limits

Hematocrit:	41%	(37-60)
Red blood cell count:	6.08 x 10¹²/L	(5.5-8.5)
Hemoglobin:	14.6 g/dl	(12.0-18.0)
MCV:	67.5 fl	(60.0-77.0)
MCHC:	35.5 g/dl	(31.0-34.0)

Platelets: Appear adequate

Glucose:	96 mg/dl	(90.0-140.0)
BUN:	↑ 246 mg/dl	(8-33)
Creatinine:	↑ 8.9 mg/dl	(0.5-1.5)
Phosphorus:	↑ 23.8 mg/dl	(5.0-9.0)

Calcium:	↓ 9.0 mg/dl	(9.5-11.5)
Total Protein:	6.3 g/dl	(4.8-7.2)
Albumin:	3.1 g/dl	(2.5-3.7)
Globulin:	3.2 g/dl	(2.0-4.0)
Sodium:	145 mEq/L	(140-151)
Chloride:	↓ 94 mEq/L	(105-120)
Potassium:	↑ 5.8 mEq/L	(3.6-5.6)
Anion gap:	↑ 37.9 mEq/L	(15-25)
HCO3:	18.9 mEq/L	(15-28)
Total Bili:	0.20 mg/dl	(0.10-0.50)
ALP:	67 IU/L	(20-320)
GGT:	9 IU/L	(2-10)
ALT:	63 IU/L	(10-95)
AST:	42 IU/L	(10-56)
Cholesterol:	224 mg/dl	(110-314)
Amylase:	622 IU/L	(400-1200)

Urinalysis: Cystocentesis

Appearance: Yellow and clear	Sediment:
Specific gravity: 1.015	rare erythrocytes
pH: 7.5	
Glucose, ketones, bilirubin: negative	
Protein and heme: trace	

Interpretation

CBC: Brianna has a mild mature neutrophilic leukocytosis which could be compatible with mild inflammation. Correction of the dehydration may lower the PCV and could result in mild anemia.

Serum Biochemical Profile

Azotemia: Azotemia in a dehydrated patient with minimally concentrated urine indicates decreased renal function. In dehydrated patients, pre-renal azotemia may complicate renal azotemia. The potential for congenital renal disease and toxin exposure should be carefully evaluated in young patients with evidence of renal failure.

Hyperphosphatemia and hypocalcemia: Hyperphosphatemia in this case is most likely due to decreased glomerular filtration rate from both renal and pre-renal causes. Calcium levels are variable in renal failure and total values may not correlate with ionized calcium as they often do in patients with normal renal function (see Chapter 6). Hypocalcemia may occur secondary to hyperphosphatemia. Acute renal failure can result in more pronounced hypocalcemia than chronic renal failure because of inadequate time for physiologic compensation. Early effects of ethylene glycol intoxication can include hyperphosphatemia because of the high content of this mineral in the antifreeze fluid. Calcium may be chelated by metabolites of ethylene glycol resulting in hypocalcemia.

Hypochloremia and increased anion gap: Hypochloremia in the absence of hyponatremia may be due to disproportionate loss of chloride with vomiting. Hypochloremia can also be associated with acid/base abnormalities, although the HCO3 in this case is within reference range. Because the elevated anion gap indicates increased unmeasured anions, the normal HCO3 could be compatible with a mixed acid/base disturbance. Candidates for unmeasured anions in this case include uremic acids, lactic acid (poor perfusion and dehydration), or exogenous acids, including metabolites of ethylene glycol.

Hyperkalemia: Hyperkalemia is most often present in renal failure patients with low urine output and reflects inadequate renal elimination of potassium.

Urinalysis: The heme and erythrocytes are probably evidence of mild blood contamination during the cytocentesis procedure.

Case Summary and Outcome

Brianna was treated for acute renal failure with intravenous fluids, diuretics, calcium, antibiotics, and anti-emetics. Some decrease in her azotemia was achieved, however she continued to be anorexic and the vomiting could not be controlled. She developed melena four days into her treatment, and the owners elected euthanasia based on her poor response to therapy and prognosis. On necropsy, Brianna's lungs were edematous and the kidneys were congested and bulged on cut surface. Histologic examination of the kidneys revealed acute tubular necrosis and the presence of light green polarizing crystals, consistent with ethylene glycol intoxication. Examination of other organs did not reveal significant abnormalities.

The presence of calcium oxalate crystals can aid in confirming a diagnosis of ethylene glycol intoxication, however they are not always present, especially several days after exposure to the toxin. Similarly, a commercially available kit can be used (Allelic Biosystems Ethylene Glycol Test Kit, PRN Pharmacal, Inc., Pensacola, FL), however by 24 hours after toxin exposure the test is no longer positive (Gaynor).

This case may be compared with Joe (Case 11), in which acute renal damage was caused by ibuprofen toxicity. Joe appears to have milder disease and an earlier intervention than Brianna, despite the fact that both patients were exposed to nephrotoxic substances. Joe's laboratory work is also complicated by the effects of gastrointestinal hemorrhage. Sally (Case 14) suffered from acute renal damage secondary to heatstroke, and her serum biochemical profile is similar to Brianna's, however the degree of hyperphosphatemia is not as pronounced. Note that the patients presenting with acute renal disease are not anemic, while patients with more chronic renal disease often have non-regenerative anemia (Tramp, Case 10, Ziggy, Case 17, Forsythia, Case 20).

Gaynor AR, Dhupa N. Acute ethylene glycol intoxication. Part II. Diagnosis, treatment, prognosis, and prevention. Compend Contin Educ Pract Vet 1999; 21:1124-1133.

Case 22 – Level 3

"Gerhardt" is a 9-year-old miniature schnauzer who has been treated for diabetes mellitus for the past 2 years. He was brought to the hospital for a glucose tolerance test as part of an evaluation to assess control of his diabetes. The owners noted that for the last 2 weeks, he has had a milky discharge from his right nostril and periodic epistaxis from the left nostril. On physical examination, Gerhardt has bilateral cataracts and severe dental tartar. Lung sounds are normal, but he has an enlarged right submandibular lymph node.

Glucose:	↑ 298 mg/dl	(65.0-120.0)
BUN:	↓ 7 mg/dl	(8-33)
Creatinine:	↓ 0.3 mg/dl	(0.5-1.5)
Phosphorus:	5.3 mg/dl	(3.0-6.0)
Calcium:	10.6 mg/dl	(8.8-11.0)
Magnesium:	2.2 mEq/L	(1.4-2.7)
Total Protein:	6.3 g/dl	(5.2-7.2)
Albumin:	3.0 g/dl	(3.0-4.2)
Globulin:	3.3 g/dl	(2.0-4.0)
Sodium:	↓ 132 mEq/L	(140-151)
Chloride:	↓ 94 mEq/L	(105-120)
Potassium:	↑ 5.6 mEq/L	(3.8-5.4)
HCO3:	21 mEq/L	(16-25)
Anion Gap:	22.6 mEq/L	(15-25)
Total Bili:	0.1 mg/dl	(0.10-0.50)
ALP:	↑ 1022 IU/L	(20-320)
GGT:	5 IU/L	(3-10)
ALT:	↑ 172 IU/L	(10-95)
AST:	↑ 61 IU/L	(15-52)
Cholesterol:	↑ 1092 mg/dl	(110-314)
Triglycerides:	↑ 5565 mg/dl	(30-300)
Amylase:	464 IU/L	(400-1200)
Serum is markedly lipemia and slightly hemolyzed		

Urinalysis: Voided

Appearance: Straw and clear	Sediment:
Specific gravity: 1.012	inactive
pH: 6.0	
Glucose: 2+	
Protein, ketones, bilirubin, heme: negative	

Interpretation

No CBC data are available

Serum Biochemical Profile:

Hyperglycemia: The hyperglycemia is compatible with the history of diabetes mellitus. In Gerhardt's case, a glucose tolerance curve revealed adequate glycemic control. As discussed in Chapter 3, fructosamine could be measured as a longer-term indicator of glucose status.

Low BUN and creatinine: Decreased BUN may be related to inadequate hepatic production of urea, which is unlikely in this case given the normal albumin and hypercholesterolemia.

More sensitive testing of liver function could include measurement of serum bile acids or blood ammonia, but is not necessary in this case unless other clinical signs suggestive for liver failure develop. In this case, osmotic diuresis caused by the glucosuria causes the polyuria and decreased BUN. Polyuria and polydipsia increase renal tubular flow rates, decreasing time for reabsorption of urea. This leads to increased renal losses of urea and lower BUN. Decreased creatinine may reflect muscle wasting that can be associated with diabetes. Decreased creatinine is not clinically significant, and is difficult to confirm because of the effects of non-creatinine chromagens at low creatinine concentrations and because the lower end of the reference range in most species is near the limit of analytical sensitivity of the assay. Glucocorticoid administration has been reported to lower serum creatinine in normal dogs (Braun), but there is no history of glucocorticoid therapy in this patient.

Hyponatremia and hypochloremia: Lipemia can cause artifactually lower electrolyte values, depending on the methodology used to measure these analytes. If an analyzer employs indirect potentiometry with ion specific electrodes in which the sample is diluted as part of the assay, artifactual lowering of electrolyte concentrations may be observed with severe lipemia. With direct potentiometric methods using ion specific electrodes in which there is no sample dilution, lipemic interference with measurement of electrolyte concentrations would not be anticipated. If sodium and chloride are both decreased in an obviously lactescent sample, another methodology should be used to confirm concentrations of these electrolytes. Physiologic causes of decreased sodium and chloride include renal wasting or water retention. Accumulation of free water and dilution of these electrolytes is a potential mechanism in diabetics because of the ability of excessive amounts of glucose to draw water into the circulation via osmosis. Renal losses should also be considered, and can be quantified by performing urinary fractional excretions. Patients with hyponatremia should have low urinary fractional excretion of sodium as the body attempts to conserve the electrolyte. Normal to increased fractional excretion under these circumstances would be abnormal and reflect either renal disease or hypoadrenocorticism (lack of aldosterone to signal the need to conserve sodium in the kidney). Hypoadrenocorticism is a differential diagnosis based on the electrolyte pattern, however the changes can be accounted for by other mechanisms and an ACTH stimulation test is not likely to provide diagnostically useful information. The change in chloride is proportional to the change in sodium and there are no evident acid/base abnormalities (normal HCO3 and anion gap) at this time. Dietary deficiency is rarely the cause of low sodium and chloride in small animal patients on commercial diets.

Hyperkalemia: In this case, a relative or absolute lack of insulin could result in high serum potassium and may explain the mild hyperkalemia seen here. Potassium may accumulate if urine cannot be eliminated from the body, but this explanation is not compatible with the clinical history.

Increased ALP with normal GGT: ALP may increase with cholestasis, however, in the dog, there are numerous extrahepatic causes for elevated ALP (Chapter 2). In this case, the presence of diabetes mellitus is likely to account for some of the liver enzyme elevations, although concurrent endocrinopathies such as hyperadrenocorticism cannot be ruled out.

Increased ALT and AST: Hepatocellular enzymes also may increase with endocrinopathies such as diabetes mellitus or hyperadrenocorticism. Primary liver pathology cannot be ruled out because changes in these enzymes are not specific for the cause.

Hypercholesterolemia and hypertriglyceridemia: Post-prandial effects should be considered, however endocrinopathies such as diabetes are common causes of hypercholesterolemia and hypertriglyceridemia in small animal patients. Hyperadrenocorticism and hypothyroidism are also associated with altered lipid metabolism. Liver and pancreatic disease can elevate these values, and hepatic pathology cannot be completely excluded in this case. Because Gerhardt is a schnauzer, the possibility of a pre-existing primary idiopathic hyperlipidemia should be considered despite its relatively rare occurrence. Examination of any "normal" blood work that may have been performed in the past as part of a routine health screen or prior to elective surgery should be reviewed for evidence of idiopathic hyperlipidemia. Previous episodes of pancreatitis secondary to hyperlipidemia could predispose Gerhardt to the development of diabetes mellitus. Because of the complex relationships between pancreatitis, diabetes mellitus, and hyperlipidemia, it may be difficult to determine which processes are primary and which are secondary.

Case Summary and Outcome

Gerhardt was treated with antibiotics for the nasal discharge. As noted above, his blood glucose curve was acceptable, however he continued to have significant hyperlipidemia, indicating that a fructosamine level should be considered to verify adequate glycemic control. Gerhardt's blood pressure was elevated. Hypertension is associated with diabetes mellitus in people and dogs (Struble), but is not documented in diabetic cats (Sennello). Two months after this presentation, Gerhardt presented for bilateral epistaxis. The owners declined to have this investigated and elected to have Gerhardt euthanized. At necropsy, Gerhardt had good body condition, but the sinuses were cavitated and filled with friable necrotic tissue that contained numerous branched septate hyphae compatible with Aspergillus. The heart showed evidence of atherosclerosis, which is rare in dogs but may be more common in miniature schnauzers (Liu). Atherosclerosis can be associated with hypothyroidism and chronic elevations in plasma lipids. Hypertension may accelerate the development of lesions. Clinical signs associated with atherosclerosis in dogs are rare. There were no significant hepatic lesions despite the enzyme elevations, suggesting that the elevations were secondary to the diabetes mellitus. Histologic examination of the kidneys revealed membranoproliferative glomerulonephritis with mild interstitial fibrosis despite the absence of azotemia at the time of euthanasia.

This and several other cases in this chapter underscore the impact of metabolic derangements unrelated to renal disease on serum BUN and creatinine. Gerhardt had decreases in BUN likely related to osmotic diuresis and polyuria. Decreased BUN and creatinine were noted in Case 3, Marsali, who presented for starvation related to neglect. Pugsley, Case 12, presented with decreased BUN and creatinine related to a portosystemic shunt, while Riff Raff, Case 8, had elevated BUN because of a septic process.

Braun JP, Lefebvre HP, Watson ADJ. Creatinine in the dog: A review. Vet Clin Pathol 2003;32:162-179.

Liu. Clinical and pathologic findings in dogs with atherosclerosis: 21 cases (1970-1983). J Am Vet Med Assoc 1986;189:227.

Sennello KA, Schulman RL, Prosek R, Seigel AM. Systolic blood pressure in cats with diabetes mellitus. J Am Vet Med Assoc 2003;223:198-201.

Struble AL, Feldman ED, Nelson RW, Kass PH. Systemic hypertension and proteinuria in dogs with diabetes mellitus. J Am Vet Med Assoc. 1998;213:822-825.

Case 23 – Level 3

"Miranda" is a 6-year-old spayed female Newfoundland dog presenting for weakness, lethargy, and vomiting. She has become progressively more lethargic and anorexic for the last few days, and the owners also noted shaking. Miranda collapsed on presentation and was reluctant to walk. On physical examination, Miranda's mucous membranes were tacky, and she was bradycardic with weak femoral pulses and prolonged capillary refill time. Because of her episode of collapse, fluids were administered immediately after drawing blood for diagnostic testing.

White blood cell count:	10.6 x 10⁹/L	(6.0-17.0)
Segmented neutrophils:	6.8 x 10⁹/L	(3.0-11.0)
Band neutrophils:	0 x 10⁹/L	(0-0.3)
Lymphocytes:	3.3 x 10⁹/L	(1.0-4.8)
Monocytes:	0.2 x 10⁹/L	(0.2-1.4)
Eosinophils:	0.3 x 10⁹/L	(0-1.3)

WBC morphology: No significant abnormalities noted.

Hematocrit:	↑ 60%	(37-55)
MCV:	71.2 fl	(60.0-77.0)
MCHC:	32.5 g/dl	(31.0-34.0)

Platelets:	214 x 10⁹/L	(200-450)

Glucose:	↓ 41mg/dl	(65.0-120.0)
BUN:	↑ 63 mg/dl	(8-33)
Creatinine:	↑ 5.1 mg/dl	(0.5-1.5)
Phosphorus:	↑ 10.1 mg/dl	(3.0-6.0)
Calcium:	↑ 12.8 mg/dl	(8.8-11.0)
Magnesium:	↑ 3.1 mEq/L	(1.4-2.7)
Total Protein:	↑ 8.2 g/dl	(5.2-7.2)
Albumin:	↑ 4.8 g/dl	(3.0-4.2)
Globulin:	3.4 g/dl	(2.0-4.0)
Sodium:	↓ 135 mEq/L	(140-151)
Chloride:	↓ 100 mEq/L	(105-120)
Potassium:	↑ 8.6 mEq/L	(3.8-5.4)
HCO3:	↓ 8 mEq/L	(16-25)
Anion Gap:	↑ 35.6 mEq/L	(15-25)
Total Bili:	0.2 mg/dl	(0.10-0.50)
ALP:	28 IU/L	(20-320)
GGT:	5 IU/L	(3-10)
ALT:	48 IU/L	(10-95)
AST:	↑ 108 IU/L	(15-52)
Cholesterol:	167 mg/dl	(110-314)
Triglycerides:	45 mg/dl	(30-300)
Amylase:	↑ 1296 IU/L	(400-1200)

Urinalysis: Voided

Appearance: Straw and clear	Sediment:
Specific gravity: 1.020	Occasional WBC
pH: 6.0	2+ bacteria are present
Protein, glucose, ketones, bilirubin, heme: negative	

Interpretation

CBC: Polycythemia is relative and attributable to dehydration. This interpretation is supported by the tacky mucous membranes and hyperproteinemia.

Serum Biochemical Profile

Hypoglycemia: Processing errors should be ruled out in all cases of hypoglycemia, however the episode of collapse and history of shaking suggests that the change may not be artifactual. Although she has been anorexic, hypoglycemia associated with starvation generally requires prolonged food deprivation and poor body condition. Various types of neoplasia can cause low blood glucose levels and are possible in a middle aged large breed dog. Failure of gluconeogenesis because of poor liver function can cause hypoglycemia. This appears unlikely because of the high BUN, high albumin, and normal cholesterol, but specific tests of liver function such as serum bile acids or blood ammonia could be considered to further evaluate this possibility. The shaking and collapse could be related to hepatic encephalopathy. Finally, patients with hypoadrenocorticism may have hypoglycemia due to failure of corticosteroid stimulated gluconeogenesis.

Azotemia: Miranda's poorly concentrated urine in the context of significant dehydration suggests the possibility of a renal cause for the azotemia, although there is certainly a pre-renal component given the dehydration and bradycardia with poor femoral pulses. Low glomerular filtration rate is supported by the hyperphosphatemia and hyperkalemia. Before renal azotemia can be confirmed, other non-renal causes of poor urinary concentrating ability should be considered, including liver failure (unlikely, see above), osmotic diuresis (detectable osmoles such as glucose and ketones are not present in the urine), diuretic usage (none in this history), and medullary washout, which is possible given the hyponatremia and hypochloremia. If medullary washout is the reason for the poorly concentrated urine, appropriate supplementation and fluid therapy should correct the problem.

Hyperphosphatemia and hypercalcemia: Renal failure, vitamin D toxicity, and hypoadreno-corticism can lead to these changes. Both renal failure and hypoadrenocorticism are compatible with the other laboratory data and in both, inadequate glomerular filtration rate for elimination of phosphorus leads to its accumulation in the blood. Hypoadrenocorticism is a cause of hypercalcemia in dogs, but is not associated with increases in ionized calcium and is therefore not expected to cause clinical signs related to hypercalcemia. Diminished renal excretion because of cortisol deficiency and hemoconcentration are potential mechanisms for the hypercalcemia, and the calcium level normalizes quickly after initiation of therapy. The most common cause of hypercalcemia in dogs is hypercalcemia of malignancy, which cannot be ruled out in this case. Hypercalcemia can cause both reversible and irreversible renal dysfunction, predisposing to the development of hyperphosphatemia. Measurement of PTH and PTHrP can help differentiate various causes of hypercalcemia, but is not necessary in this case.

Hypermagnesemia: Decreased glomerular filtration rate is the cause for the high magnesium.

Hyperproteinemia with hyperalbuminemia: Hyperalbuminemia is the result of hemoconcentration. Miranda's tacky mucous membranes are consistent with dehydration, as is the relative polycythemia.

Hyponatremia and hypochloremia: Increased losses are the most likely cause for Miranda's hyponatremia and hypochloremia, which are approximately proportional. Given her history, gastrointestinal losses are possible. The potential for third space and cutaneous losses should be evaluated in the context of the clinical information. Renal losses should also be considered, and can be quantified by performing urinary fractional excretions. Patients with hyponatremia should have low urinary fractional excretion of sodium as the body attempts to conserve the electrolyte; normal to increased fractional excretion under these circumstances would be abnormal and reflect either renal disease or hypoadrenocorticism (lack of aldosterone to signal the need to conserve sodium in the kidney). Dietary deficiency is rarely the cause of low sodium and chloride in small animal patients being fed commercial diets. While accumulation of free water and dilution of these electrolytes is a potential mechanism, evidence of dehydration, including polycythemia and hyperproteinemia, rule it out.

Hyperkalemia: Polyuric renal failure is often associated with hypokalemia because of enhanced urinary potassium loss. It is only when glomerular filtration is markedly limited or when urine cannot be eliminated from the body that hyperkalemia ensues. Miranda has marked dehydration and clinical evidence of poor perfusion (weak femoral pulses and prolonged capillary refill time) that could severely reduce glomerular filtration. Her other laboratory abnormalities are also suggestive for hypoadrenocorticism, which could lead to hyperkalemia because of aldosterone deficiency. Cellular translocation in response to acidosis is also possible, however this appears to be less important with organic acidosis than mineral acidosis.

Low HCO3: The acidemia in this case may be related to either uremic acidosis or lactic acidosis secondary to poor tissue perfusion.

Increased anion gap: As noted above, increased uremic acids or lactic acid could elevate the anion gap. Because most of the anion gap in health is due to negatively charged proteins, the hyperalbuminemia could also contribute to increased anion gap.

Increased AST: This most likely reflects tissue damage secondary to poor perfusion.

Increased amylase: The mild change in this value is most compatible with the decreased glomerular filtration rate, although gastrointestinal disease can also be associated with increased amylase and is compatible with the clinical history. Pancreatic disease cannot be ruled out, but is not required to explain this data.

Urinalysis: The pyuria and bactiuria indicate a urinary tract infection.

Case Summary and Outcome

Miranda's laboratory data normalized after 2 days of appropriate fluid therapy, but unfortunately she developed melena with anemia and hypoproteinemia while in the hospital. Because of the history and laboratory results, an ACTH stimulation test was performed to evaluate Miranda for hypoadrenocorticism. Both pre and post stimulation cortisol levels were less than 1.0 µg/dl, consistent with hypoadrenocorticism. Melena and hypoproteinemia are described in dogs with hypoadrenocorticism. This is the result of hypoperfusion of the gut due to circulatory collapse and because normal glucocorticoid levels are required for maintenance of gastrointestinal mucosa. Miranda was given hormone replacement for her hypoadrenocorticism and was treated with antibiotics for her urinary tract infection. She was also given anthelmintics because of her signs of gastrointestinal disease. Miranda responded to treatment and went home.

These clinical signs are common with hypoadrenocorticism, however some types of gastrointestinal parasites can also cause laboratory abnormalities similar to hypoadrenocorticism (see Chapter 7 for more details). Patients with hypoadrenocorticism may present with laboratory data suggestive for renal failure (dehydration, azotemia, and inadequately concentrated urine). Correction of fluid and electrolyte deficits allows the patient to regain urinary concentrating ability shortly after initiation of therapy, which would be unlikely in a case of primary renal failure. Such response to treatment should prompt consideration of an ACTH stimulation test to evaluate adrenal gland function. This case should be compared with Jag, Case 4, in which hypercalcemia of malignancy also resulted in temporary loss of urinary concentrating ability that may be unrelated to primary renal pathology, although renal lesions may eventually develop with hypercalcemia. Liver disease may also interfere with the production of concentrated urine (See Pugsley, Case 12), although BUN or creatinine may be low rather than high in these cases.

Case 24 – Level 3

"Popcorn" is a 12-year-old intact female Yorkshire Terrier presenting with polyuria and polydipsia. On physical examination, Popcorn is depressed, has a vaginal discharge, and bilateral cataracts. She has tacky mucous membranes and is slightly pale. Because of Popcorn's age, the owner requested a thorough workup to rule out neoplasia prior to any surgical interventions. As a result, a bone marrow and serum protein electrophoresis was done in addition to routine blood work.

White blood cell count:	↑ 48.0 x 10⁹/L	(6.0-17.0)
Segmented neutrophils:	↑ 40.7 x 10⁹/L	(3.0-11.0)
Band neutrophils:	0 x 10⁹/L	(0-0.3)
Lymphocytes:	2.4 x 10⁹/L	(1.0-4.8)
Monocytes:	↑ 4.8 x 10⁹/L	(0.2-1.4)
Eosinophils:	0.1 x 10⁹/L	(0-1.3)

WBC morphology: Small numbers of reactive lymphocytes are seen.

Hematocrit:	↓ 34%	(37-55)
MCV:	68.7 fl	(60.0-75.0)
MCHC:	33.8 g/dl	(33.0-36.0)

RBC morphology: No abnormalities of erythrocytes

Platelets: Appear adequate

Glucose:	↓ 62 mg/dl	(65.0-120.0)
BUN:	↑ 77 mg/dl	(8-29)
Creatinine:	↑ 2.6 mg/dl	(0.5-1.5)
Phosphorus:	↑ 8.8 mg/dl	(2.6-7.2)
Calcium:	↑ 11.7 mg/dl	(8.8-11.0)
Magnesium:	2.4 mEq/L	(1.4-2.7)
Total Protein:	↑ 9.3 g/dl	(5.2-7.2)
Albumin:	↓ 2.2 g/dl	(3.0-4.2)
Globulin:	↑ 7.1 g/dl	(2.0-4.0)
Sodium:	142 mEq/L	(140-151)
Chloride:	105 mEq/L	(105-120)
Potassium:	4.2 mEq/L	(3.8-5.4)
HCO3:	↓ 15 mEq/L	(16-25)
Anion Gap:	↑ 26.2	(15-25)
Total Bili:	0.21 mg/dl	(0.10-0.50)
ALP:	296 IU/L	(20-320)
GGT:	4 IU/L	(3-10)

ALT:	16 IU/L	(10-95)
AST:	48 IU/L	(15-52)
Cholesterol:	285 mg/dl	(110-314)
Triglycerides:	80 mg/dl	(30-300)
Amylase:	↑ 2045 IU/L	(400-1200)

Urinalysis: Cystocentesis

Appearance: Pale yellow and clear	Sediment:
Specific gravity: 1.010	3-5 RBC/hpf
pH: 5.0	Occasional WBC
Protein, glucose, ketones, bilirubin: negative	
Heme: 3+	

Bone marrow evaluation: Scattered hypercellular particles are present, and occasional megakaryocytes are seen. The myeloid to erythroid ratio is markedly increased, but the maturation of both lines is orderly and goes to completion. Rare mature plasma cells and lymphocytes are present.

Interpretation

CBC: Popcorn has a marked neutrophilic leukocytosis with toxic change and monocytosis, indicating severe inflammation. There is also a mild normocytic, normochromic anemia, which is likely nonregenerative, but a reticulocyte count would be needed to confirm this. Anemia of inflammatory disease is the likely cause of this anemia, however the isosthenuria and azotemia indicates that renal disease could also be a factor in the development of this anemia.

Serum Biochemical Profile

Hypoglycemia: If processing errors have been excluded, the leukogram suggests the possibility of sepsis as a cause of the hypoglycemia. Liver failure and various types of neoplasia are also possible causes of hypoglycemia in a patient of this age. Starvation can cause hypoglycemia, particularly in small or very young animals. Hypoalbuminemia could also be associated with inadequate nutrition, but poor body condition should be observed clinically, which is not described here.

Azotemia and isosthenuria: This combination of azotemia and an isosthenuric urine in a dehydrated patient is suggestive for renal failure, but there are exceptions when extra-renal factors interfere with renal concentrating ability. Neither osmotic diuresis nor medullary washout appears probable. Liver failure is a consideration given the hypoglycemia and hypoalbuminemia, however the biliburin and cholesterol are within reference range. While liver enzymes may be normal in hepatic failure, the normal values in this patient suggest that liver failure is unlikely. Diabetes insipidus is a potential consideration. Given the clinical history, Popcorn should be evaluated for a pyometra. Infection of the uterus by *E. coli* results in the elaboration of toxins which may cause polyuria by interfering with sodium and chloride resorption in the loop of Henle and by causing a reversible insensitivity of the tubules to antidiuretic hormone. In this case renal function should be re-evaluated once the pyometra has been successfully treated. The azotemia in this case may be entirely reversible if pyometra is the underlying cause. In any case, the dehydration suggests that there is at least a pre-renal component to the increased BUN and creatinine.

Hyperphosphatemia and hypercalcemia: The hyperphosphatemia is most likely the result of decreased glomerular filtration rate, whether due to renal or pre-renal factors. Calcium changes unpredictably in small animal patients with renal failure, and total calcium may be high, low or normal. In older patients, hypercalcemia of malignancy must also be considered due to its high frequency. Hypercalcemia of malignancy is often associated with increases in parathyroid hormone related protein (PTHrP), which can be measured. Most often, the patient is evaluated for lymphadenopathy, organomegaly, and mass lesions in an attempt to diagnose malignant neoplasia. In this case, the combination of non-regenerative anemia, hypercalcemia, and hyperglobulinemia prompted evaluation of the marrow for the presence of lymphoid malignancy.

Hyperproteinemia with hypoalbuminemia and hyperglobulinemia: In patients with evidence of inflammatory or infectious disease, hyperglobulinemia is most often polyclonal and due to increased production of acute phase reactants or immunoglobulins. In these cases, albumin may be low because of downregulation of production in the liver since albumin is a negative acute phase reactant. Very rarely, infectious diseases such as feline infectious peritonitis, Leishmania, or tick borne diseases may cause a monoclonal gammopathy, which must be distinguished from monoclonal gammopathies produced by neoplastic lymphocytes. In this case, hypoalbuminemia could be exacerbated by losses into the uterus.

Mild acidemia (decreased HCO3) with increased anion gap: These changes may be related to uremic acidosis. Poor tissue perfusion associated with sepsis could create lactic acidosis as well. Abnormally low albumin (an anionic protein) and high immunoglobulins (cationic proteins) generally lower the anion gap.

Hyperamylasemia: The most likely cause for this change is the decreased glomerular filtration rate, supported by the azotemia and hyperphosphatemia. Clinical signs are vague, and pancreatic disease cannot be completely ruled out.

Bone marrow evaluation: Erythroid hypoplasia and myeloid hyperplasia are evident on the marrow aspirate and are compatible with the interpretation of the CBC above. The small numbers of mature plasma cells and lymphocytes are considered normal and there is no evidence of lymphoid malignancy on the smears.

Case Summary and Outcome

Popcorn was treated with intravenous fluids and antibiotics and had an ovariohysterectomy. A serum protein electrophoresis confirmed the presence of a polyclonal gammopathy. Repeat CBC, serum biochemical profile, and urinalysis were normal eight weeks after surgery, and urinary concentrating ability had recovered.

This combination of laboratory abnormalities suggested the possibility of several disease processes. Hyperglobulinemia and hypercalcemia could be compatible with lymphoid malignancy, and secondary hypercalcemic nephropathy could have explained the azotemia and isosthenuria (See Case 4, Jag). Most of the laboratory abnormalities could have been compatible with renal failure alone, especially if the renal failure was related to an inflammatory process such as pyelonephritis (See Opie, Case 13). In this case, the clinical history and physical examination were instrumental in prioritizing pyometra as a differential diagnosis. However, because of the age of the patient, a more intensive evaluation for neoplasia (bone marrow cytology and serum protein electrophoresis) was conducted prior to surgery because the owner did not wish to pursue treatment for the pyometra if Popcorn also had neoplasia. As was noted in other cases in which extra-renal disease influenced BUN, creatinine, or urine specific gravity (Case 8: sepsis, Case 12: portosystemic shunt, Case 16: hyperthyroidism, Case 22: diabetes mellitus, Case 23: hypoadrenocorticism), treatment Popcorn's underlying disease was successful in restoring urinary concentrating ability and BUN/serum creatinine values to normal.

Case 25 – Level 3

"Lucinda" is a 3-year-old LaMancha doe goat who is part of a milking herd of 30 goats. She developed diarrhea 10 days prior to presentation and was treated with gentomycin and Banamine® at unknown doses. She maintained normal appetite and continued to drink water until she was found recumbent and unable to rise on the day of presentation. Physical and neurologic examination was within normal limits.

White blood cell count:	10.7 x 10⁹/L	(4.0-13.0)
Segmented neutrophils:	4.8 x 10⁹/L	(1.2-7.2)
Band neutrophils:	0.0	(0-0.3)
Lymphocytes:	5.8 x 10⁹/L	(2.0-9.0)
Monocytes:	0.1 x 10⁹/L	(0-0.6)
WBC morphology: No significant abnormalities noted.		

Hematocrit:	38%	(22-38)
Red blood cell count:	13.11 x 10¹²/L	(8.0-18.00)
Hemoglobin:	↑ 13.7 g/dl	(8-12)
MCV:	23.3 fl	(16.0-25.0)
MCHC:	↑ 36.1 g/dl	(28.0-34.0)
RBC morphology: No abnormalties noted		
Platelets: Appear adequate		

Fibrinogen:	↑ 700 mg/dl	(100-400)

Glucose:	↑ 162 mg/dl	(6.0-128.0)
BUN:	↑ 216 mg/dl	(17-30)
Creatinine:	↑ 12.8 mg/dl	(0.6-1.3)
Phosphorus:	↑ 23.5 mg/dl	(4.1-8.7)
Calcium:	↓ 5.5 mg/dl	(8.0-10.7)
Magnesium:	2.9 mEq/L	(2.8-3.6)
Total Protein:	6.3 g/dl	(6.1-8.3)
Albumin:	↓ 2.4 g/dl	(3.1-4.4)
Globulin:	3.9 g/dl	(2.2-4.3)
A/G Ratio:	↓ 0.6	(0.7-2.1)
Sodium:	↓ 126 mEq/L	(140-157)
Chloride:	↓ 94 mEq/L	(102-118)
Potassium:	↓ 3.0 mEq/L	(3.5-5.6)
HCO3:	↓ 6 mEq/L	(22-32)
AnionGap:	↑ 29 mEq/L	(6-15)
Total Bili:	0.1 mg/dl	(0.10-0.2)
ALP:	107 IU/L	(40-392)
GGT:	49 IU/L	(28-70)
AST:	↑ 273 IU/L	(40-222)
CK:	↑ 4267 IU/L	(74-452)

Urine: Catheter

Appearance: Pink and cloudy	Sediment:
Specific gravity: 1.018	Numerous erythrocytes
pH: 6	Small numbers of leukocytes
Glucose 1+	No bacteria, crystals or casts
Ketones, bilirubin: negative	
Protein: 3+	
Heme: 4+	

Interpretation

CBC

Leukogram: Although there were no parameters outside the reference intervals in the leukogram, the increased fibrinogen indicates an acute phase response and inflammation. In large animal species, fibrinogen is a more sensitive indicator of inflammation than changes in the leukogram.

Erythrogram: The increased hemoglobin and MCHC are artifactual, since the body does not produce hyperchromatic erythrocytes. Hemolysis, either in vitro or in vivo, can account for these changes. Because the goat is not anemic, in vitro artifact is more likely than intravascular hemolysis. In fact, the PCV is at the high end of the reference interval, suggesting the potential for mild hemoconcentration.

Serum Biochemical Profile

Hyperglycemia: Stress is the most likely reason for this hyperglycemia, although neither corticosteroid effects (mature neutrophilia and lymphopenia) nor epinephrine effects (mature neutrophilia, lymphocytosis) are evident in the leukogram. Both of these hormones elevate serum glucose by inducing gluconeogenesis and/or interfering with insulin action. The glucosuria reflects the fact that the renal tubular maximum for reabsorption of 100 mg/dl in the goat has been exceeded (Belknap), but by itself does not justify a diagnosis of diabetes mellitus, which is very rare in small ruminants. Renal tubular dysfunction can result in glucosuria in the absence of hyperglycemia.

Azotemia: Azotemia should be categorized as pre-renal, renal, or post-renal. The physical examination does not provide evidence for post-renal causes of azotemia (large distended or firm bladder, accumulation of fluid in the abdomen). Renal azotemia appears likely given the isosthenuric urine, however extra-renal causes of poor urinary concentrating ability should be ruled out. Medullary washout could interfere with the kidney's ability to optimally concentrate urine (hyponatremia, hypochloremia, hypokalemia). The glucosuria could contribute to osmotic diuresis. Poor liver function can be associated with polyuria/polydipsia because of failure of urea production to generate a concentration gradient. Other possibilities include psychogenic polydipsia as a component of hepatic encephalopathy, increased central threshold of antidiuretic hormone release, and hypercortisolism from either impaired hepatic degradation or stimulation of ACTH production by abnormal neurotransmitters. Evidence for impaired liver function in this case is weak, however hypoalbuminemia is present and the increased AST could indicate hepatocellular damage. The concurrent elevation in CK supports muscle damage as a source for the AST. The normal neurologic examination argues against hepatic encephalopathy, although signs may be intermittent.

Pre-renal azotemia can exacerbate renal azotemia and pre-renal and renal azotemia often occur together because of ongoing fluid loss via the poorly functioning kidneys. The high-normal PCV is compatible with hemoconcentration.

Clinical indicators of hydration status such as body weight and tacky mucous membranes should be used to support evaluation of hydration status. Hyperproteinemia and hyperalbuminemia are good indicators of dehydration, but are less reliable when protein loss is part of the disease process. Appropriate fluid therapy should reduce the pre-renal component of the azotemia. Increasing tubular flow rates will decrease the amount of time for passive tubular reabsorption of urea, so the BUN may fall to a proportionally greater degree than creatinine with no change in total glomerular filtration rate.

Because of fewer non-renal influences, creatinine is preferred to BUN to assess renal function. This is especially true in ruminants, because ruminal flora may recycle nitrogen, leading to a slower increase in BUN with low glomerular filtration rate than in non-ruminant species.

Hyperphosphatemia and hypocalcemia: The most likely cause for hyperphosphatemia in any azotemic patient is decreased urinary excretion of phosphorus. Reduced phosphorus excretion in the saliva of anorexic ruminants also can result in hyperphosphatemia with any illness associated with poor food intake. Mass law interactions in hyperphosphatemic patients can cause hypocalcemia, and associated deficits of calcitriol can reduce intestinal calcium absorption and increase skeletal resistance to parathyroid hormone. Hypoalbuminemia can lower total serum calcium without affecting ionized calcium. Correction factors for hypoalbuminemia-induced hypocalcemia have not been developed for ruminants and the use of formulas derived for dogs is probably not valid in small animals either. Specific information on the reproductive status of this doe is not available, however dairy goats are susceptible to periparturient hypocalcemia. In cases of periparturient hypocalcemia, magnesium may be increased or decreased, but the serum phosphorus is usually low, making this an unlikely diagnosis in Lucinda's case (Rankins). Increased demand for calcium and phosphorus for gestation and lactation combined with suppressed parathyroid hormone and 1,25-dihydroxy-cholecalciferol production associated with inappropriate diet interferes with the ability to mobilize the required minerals from skeletal reserves and contributes to poor intestinal absorption. Grass tetany is another potential cause of hypocalcemia in ruminants. Hypomagnesemia occurs in grass tetany and can lead to hypocalcemia secondary to a blunted parathyroid hormone response. In Lucinda, magnesium levels are within the reference interval, making this diagnosis unlikely at this time. Alkalosis, which is common in sick ruminants, can predispose to hypocalcemia (Goff), however this patient is acidemic.

Hypoalbuminemia: Increased losses and decreased production can cause hypoalbuminemia. Albumin is a negative acute phase reactant and given the high fibrinogen, hepatic downregulation of production is likely. Other causes of decreased albumin production such as poor liver function or starvation are not supported by other evidence in this case.

Increased losses of albumin are likely in Lucinda. With the azotemia and proteinuria, urinary losses must be considered. The presence of a significant amount of blood suggests that the proteinuria could be due to blood contamination or lower urinary tract disease. Clinically significant glomerulonephritis is uncommon in goats (Smith) but is a possible source of protein loss in this patient because it results in selective loss of albumin. Repeat measure of urine protein on an atraumatically collected urine sample after any lower urinary tract disease has been ruled out or treated could clarify the potential for glomerular protein loss; urinary protein:creatinine ratio may be indicated.

Gastrointestinal losses are possible with her history of diarrhea, but losses generally include both albumin and globulins. Normal serum globulin does not rule out intestinal loss, especially if there may be increased production of globulins associated with an acute phase response or immune stimulation. Gastrointestinal protein loss can be difficult to confirm or quantitate, however measurement of fecal α1-proteinase inhibitor has been used as an indicator of intestinal protein loss in people and dogs (Murphy). Gastrointestinal parasitism is an important cause of hypoproteinemia and should be ruled out by examination of fecal material and herd worming history. Other sources of loss less compatible with the clinical history include dermal and third space losses.

Hypoalbuminemia due to a dilutional effect with overhydration can occur in association with pregnancy, congestive heart failure, or other causes of fluid retention or overload. Physical examination findings are not suggestive for any of these causes.

Hyponatremia with proportional hypochloremia: As described for albumin, relative water excess can result in a dilutional effect on these electrolytes. This is not likely given the high-normal PCV. Hyperglycemia can exert an osmotic effect and result in hyponatremia and hypochloremia by this mechanism, but is not of sufficient magnitude to be an issue in this case. Dietary deficiency is rarely a cause but is possible. Increased loss is most likely and may include mechanisms such as loss into milk with mastitis, sweating (more important for horses), hypertonic fluid loss in the gastrointestinal tract or isotonic loss with replacement by free water. Gastrointestinal stasis may predispose to sequestration of chloride.

Excessive loss via the kidney can also cause hyponatremia and hypochloremia. Given the other evidence for renal disease, this is most likely. Inappropriate renal losses of electrolytes in the context of low serum levels can be quantified by measuring urinary fractional excretion. In this case, urinary fractional excretion of sodium and chloride should be low in response to hyponatremia and hypochloremia. High or normal urinary excretion of these electrolytes would indicate excessive urinary losses. These losses could also reflect hypoad-renocorticism because of failure of endocrine regulation of renal handling of electrolytes, but this is rare in small ruminants and generally would be associated with hyperkalemia rather than hypokalemia. ACTH stimulation test could be run to rule out this possibility.

Hypokalemia: Low intake of potassium is a more likely factor for this electrolyte than for sodium and chloride. Clinically significant hypokalemia is more likely if combined with increased losses. Mechanisms for increased loss are similar to those described for NaCl and include losses through the gastrointestinal tract, into third spaces and through the kidney. Polyuric renal failure is often associated with hypokalemia as increased tubular flow rates decrease the time available for potassium reabsorption. Treatment with insulin for hyperglycemia or with sodium bicarbonate for acid/base abnormalities can cause translocation of potassium into cells and result in hypokalemia. It should be noted that serum levels of sodium, chloride, and potassium do not generally reflect total body stores.

Decreased HCO3 and increased anion gap: These findings indicate acidemia with increased unmeasured anions. In this case, potential unmeasured anions include uremic acids and lactic acids if there is decreased tissue perfusion. Exogeneous acids such as salicylates, paraldehyde, and ethylene glycol can also increase the anion gap. Loss of bicarbonate rich fluids such as saliva or in diarrhea is possible, and renal disease may compromise the kidney's ability to compensate for challenges to acid/base balance. Urine pH in ruminants is generally alkaline, however the acid pH in this case is expected based on the decreased HCO3.

Increased AST and CK: The combination of these changes indicates muscle damage and is compatible with the history of recumbency in this patient.

Case Summary and Outcome

Based on all of the data, renal failure is the most likely diagnosis. Lucinda was initially anuric, but a small amount of urine was eventually produced after treatment with furosemide and dopamine. After one day of hospitalization, Lucinda suffered cardiac and respiratory arrest. Clinical manifestations of renal failure are poorly documented in goats (Belknap), and even in better studied species, clinical signs and laboratory abnormalities can vary markedly between individuals in different stages of disease. The specific cause of renal failure can be impossible to document based only on clinical pathology data or even with histology.

As with other species, a variety of toxins and infectious agents can cause renal failure. Goats have indiscriminate eating habits and zinc toxicity and ingestion of oxalate containing plants can cause renal damage. Although ruminants may be more resistant to ethylene glycol toxicity than monogastric species because they can degrade oxalates, this toxicity has been reported in the goat (Boermans). In this case, treatment with a nephrotoxic antibiotic and a non-steroidal anti-inflammatory is likely to have caused or contributed to renal disease. The toxicity of both of these drugs is exacerbated by dehydration, which is compatible with a history of diarrhea and the high-normal PCV. Non-steroidal anti-inflammatory drugs interfere with prostaglandin synthesis and result in impaired renal autoregulation of blood flow, causing ischemic damage. Urinary GGT activity can be measured to support a diagnosis of tubular damage.

Lucinda may be compared with several other patients of various species presenting with renal failure (horse-Case 9, cat-Cases 10, 13, 17, dog-Cases 11, 14, 15, llama-Case 20). As noted above, there is a great deal of individual variation in laboratory data between different patients with renal failure. Some of this variation is species dependent, but much of which is not. Length and severity of renal failure, concurrent disease processes, and treatment may influence laboratory results.

Belknap EB, Pugh DG. Diseases of the Urinary System. In: Sheep and Goat Medicine. DG Pugh ed. 2002. W.B.Saunders Company, Philadelphia, PA. pp 255-266.

Boermans HJ, Ruegg PL, Leach M. Ethylene glycol toxicosis in a pygmy goat. J Am Vet Med Assoc 1988;193: 694-696.

Goff JP. Pathophysiology of calcium and phosphorus disorders. The Veterinary Clinics of North America, Food Animal Practice. 2000;16:319-335.

Murphy KF, German AJ, Ruaux CG, Steiner JM, Hall EJ. Fecal α_1-proteinase inhibitor concentration in dogs receiving long-term nonsteroidal anti-inflammatory drug therapy. Vet Clin Path 2003;32:136-139.

Rankins DL, Ruffin DC, Pugh DG. Feeding and Nutrition. In: Sheep and Goat Medicine. DG Pugh ed. 2002. W.B.Saunders Company, Philadelphia, PA. pp 19-60.

Smith MC, Sherman DM. Urinary System. In: Goat Medicine, MC Smith and DM Sherman. eds Lea and Febiger, Malvern, PA. 1994. pp 387-405.

Overview

Step 1: Is the patient azotemic?

Step 2: Determine if the patient has pre-renal, renal, or post-renal azotemia or a combination of causes.

> If the patient is azotemic with concentrated urine, pre-renal azotemia is likely (Case 1, 19).

> If the patient is azotemic with isosthenuria, renal azotemia is possible (Case 9, 10, 11, 13, 14, 15, 17, 20, 21, 25). Pre-renal factors may exacerbate renal azotemia.

> If there is evidence of fluid accumulation in the abdomen, an enlarged, firm bladder, or urethral blockage, post-renal azotemia is possible (Case 2, 6, 7, 18).

Step 3: Determine if there are extra-renal influences on BUN, serum creatinine or urine specific gravity that could complicate interpretation.

> Nutritional factors (starvation, Case 3)

> Hypercalcemia (lymphoma, Case 4)

> Sepsis (septic abdomen, Case 8, pyometra, Case 24)

> Liver disease (portosystemic shunt, Case 12)

> Osmotic diuresis (diabetes mellitus, Case 22)

> Medullary washout (hypoadrenocorticism, Case 23)

Step 4: Is there evidence of renal protein loss that could suggest glomerular disease (Cases 5 and 20)? Remember to rule out extra-glomerular protein loss in the urinary tract related to inflammatory or neoplastic conditions (examine urine sediment).

Chapter 6

Abnormalities of Calcium, Phosphorus, and Magnesium

Measurement of Calcium and Phosphorus

The calcium reported in the standard veterinary serum biochemical profile is the total calcium, which is made up of biologically active ionized calcium (approximately 50% of the total under normal circumstances), calcium complexed to anions such as citrate, bicarbonate, lactate, or phosphate (approximately 5%), and protein-bound calcium that is associated primarily with albumin and to a lesser extent, globulins (approximately 45%) (Rosol). Various physiological parameters such as serum protein concentration and pH may influence the proportions of the different fractions, and proportions may be unpredictable in some conditions such as renal failure (Schenck). Some disease conditions may alter total serum calcium, but not impact the biologically active fraction, whereas other conditions may be characterized by normal total serum calcium but changes in the ionized fraction. Therefore, it may be informative to measure ionized calcium in some patients. This requires specialized sample handling and instrumentation (ion specific electrode).

Phosphorus is present in the serum and plasma in organic and inorganic forms, however clinical assays reflect only the inorganic component. Like calcium, inorganic phosphorus exists either free (55%), protein-bound (10%), or complexed to non-protein cations (35%) (Stockham).

Much of the total body magnesium is stored in bone, and most of the remainder is intracellular; approximately 1% is present in extracellular fluid and can be measured. Like calcium, a proportion of the total serum magnesium is bound to albumin or globulins, some forms complexes with anions, and the biologically active ionized fraction predominates. Also similar to calcium, the measurement of the ionized fraction is preferred under some circumstances because the proportions of protein-bound, complexed and ionized magnesium are not constant. Because specialized equipment is required, clinicians must often rely on measurements of total magnesium.

Regulation of Calcium and Phosphorus

A complete discussion of the complex regulation of these minerals is beyond the scope of this chapter, and the reader is referred to textbooks for more detail (Rosol, Stockham). Very briefly, serum calcium and phosphorus levels reflect the balance of intake, absorption from the gut or bone, excretion via the kidney, and cellular translocation. The regulation of magnesium is less clear, however gastrointestinal disease and changes in renal function impact intake and losses.

Parathyroid Hormone (PTH)

Parathyroid hormone secretion from the parathyroid gland is stimulated by low ionized calcium levels in the blood. This hormone stimulates calcium reabsorption from bone and increases absorption of dietary calcium from the intestines. In the kidney, PTH promotes reabsorption of calcium, excretion of phosphorus, and formation of the active form of vitamin D (Calcitriol).

Calcitonin

Calcitonin secretion from the thyroid C cells is continuous under normal circumstances, however secretion will be increased in response to hypercalcemia. Calcitonin decreases reabsorption of calcium from bone, and inhibits renal production of the active form of vitamin D to reduce serum calcium concentrations. Renal losses of calcium and phosphorus increase in response to calcitonin.

Vitamin D

Vitamin D that is activated in the kidney increases serum calcium and phosphorus by increasing intestinal absorption of both minerals and by working with PTH to promote bone resorption. Macrophages in non-malignant granulomatous diseases may produce calcitriol, which can cause hypercalcemia (Vasilopulos).

Parathyroid Hormone-related Protein (PTHrP)

PTHrP does not play an important role in normal calcium and phosphorus homeostasis in adult animals, however it does contribute to hypercalcemia of malignancy, one of the most common causes of hypercalcemia in domestic animals. It is present in multiple tissues at very low levels in normal animals, but it can be produced in large quantities by some tumors. In these patients, PTHrP stimulates PTH receptors and can result in severe hypercalcemia, which will resolve with successful treatment of the malignancy.

Evaluation of Calcium and Phosphorus

Because of shared regulatory pathways, calcium and phosphorus are often evaluated together, and causes of abnormalities may be categorized by the relationship between the two analytes. For a given disease process, abnormalities of calcium tend to be slightly more consistent than changes in phosphorus. As always, laboratory artifacts and processing errors should be considered as potential causes of changes in calcium and phosphorus. Repeated measurement on a fresh, properly collected sample is recommended prior to expensive or invasive diagnostic work up of any laboratory abnormality in the absence of clinical signs compatible with the abnormality. Also, as for any analyte, remember to consider the influence of physiologic variables such as breed, age, or reproductive status on calcium and phosphorus metabolism. Ancillary information from the clinical history, physical examination, imaging studies and other clinical laboratory testing will often help determine the cause of changes in calcium and phosphorus.

Many patients present with serum magnesium values outside the reference range, but are not considered to have clinical signs specifically referable to hypo- or hypermagnesemia. The clinical significance of these abnormalities is unclear because little data is available for domestic animal species. Interest in evaluation of serum magnesium has been stimulated by data in human patients suggesting that hypomagnesemia is a negative prognostic indicator in critical care patients (Rubeiz). There is some data to suggest this may be true in cats (Toll). In one study of horses with surgical colic, low ionized magnesium in the perioperative period appeared to correlate with poor outcome (Garcia-Lopez). Total magnesium measurements were not predictive in this study, and another study examining total serum magnesium in hospitalized horses found that a low serum magnesium level was a positive predictor of survival (Johansson).

Hypocalcemia with Normal Phosphorus

Step 1: Is there hypoalbuminemia? This is a common cause of low serum total calcium because a significant portion of total calcium is bound to plasma protein. Hypocalcemia attributable to low protein is unlikely to cause clinical signs because biologically active ionized calcium is usually normal. (See Chapter 4 for causes of hypoalbuminemia)

Step 2: Is the patient periparturient or lactating? Additional demands for calcium during pregnancy or lactation can lower both total and ionized calcium and may or may not be associated with clinical signs in a variety of species (Fascetti).

Step 3: Is there evidence of pancreatic or gastrointestinal disease? Severe acute pancreatitis has been associated with hypocalcemia in dogs. Hypocalcemia has been reported in a high percentage of horses with enterocolitis.

Step 4: What is the nutritional status? Grass tetany in cattle may cause hypocalcemia, as can blister beetle toxicosis in horses. Anorexia from any cause in ruminants can result in hypocalcemia because of inadequate intake of calcium.

Step 5: Is the patient taking any medications? Some medications such as glucocorticoids, some anticonvulsants, and chelating compounds can lower serum calcium. Check the potential effects of any drugs or toxins that could impact calcium homeostasis. Performing a serum biochemical profile on blood anticoagulated with chelators such as EDTA will cause an artifactual and dramatic decrease in the measured calcium value.

Hypocalcemia with Hyperphosphatemia

Step 1: Is there evidence of renal disease? As noted in Chapter 5, calcium status is unpredictable in many cases of renal disease in small animals, however phosphorus is generally increased because of low glomerular filtration rate. Patients with protein losing nephropathy may be hypocalcemic due to the selective loss of albumin in the urine. Hypocalcemia may be noted in patients with renal failure due to ethylene glycol intoxication because of chelation of calcium with oxalate, and hyperphosphatemia may be exacerbated by the presence of phosphates in anti-freeze (see Chapter 5, Case 21). Renal secondary hyperparathyroidism is characterized by low calcium and hyperphosphatemia. Acute renal failure in horses may be associated with hypocalcemia and hyperphosphatemia (Carlson), however chronic renal failure in the horse is frequently characterized by hypercalcemia and hypophosphatemia (see Chapter 5, Case 9).

Step 2: Could the patient have hypoparathyroidism? In some patients, poor parathyroid function may be related to hypomagnesemia, while in other cases it may be idiopathic (Beyer) or related to immune-mediated destruction or surgical removal of the parathyroid glands.

Hypocalcemia with Hypophosphatemia

Step 1: Is the patient periparturient or lactating? In some cases these patients may have normal phosphorus, however many cows with parturient paresis are also hypophosphatemic. Clinical signs of hypocalcemia may vary with species (tetany in dogs and horses, paresis in cattle). The presence of clinical signs may depend on other physiologic variables, such as acid/base status, which may determine how much of the total calcium is in the biologically active ionized form.

Step 2: Is the diet adequate, or is there evidence of poor intestinal absorption? Malabsorption syndromes or anorexia could contribute to low serum calcium and phosphorus, as can diets with inappropriate calcium:phosphorus ratios.

Hypercalcemia with Normal to Low Phosphorus

Step 1: Is there neoplasia unrelated to the parathyroid gland? Hypercalcemia of malignancy is most frequently associated with hematopoietic neoplasia, however it is also common in patients with anal sac apocrine gland adenocarcinomas, squamous cell carcinomas, and a variety of other tumors (Williams, Vasilopulos). Serum phosphorus is generally low because PTHrP promotes phosphorus excretion in the kidney similar to PTH. However, if renal failure develops secondary to the hypercalcemia, serum phosphorus levels may increase. PTHrP measurements are often high, while PTH will be suppressed.

Step 2: Is there a tumor in the parathyroid gland? Parathyroid tumors may produce an excessive amount of PTH, which increases serum calcium and suppresses serum phosphorus.

Hypercalcemia with Hyperphosphatemia

Step 1: Is there evidence of renal disease? As noted above, serum calcium values can be unpredictable in renal failure, however phosphorus is often high because of decreased renal clearance. In some patients with hypercalcemia of malignancy, the high ionized calcium levels cause nephropathy, which results in elevated serum phosphorus.

Step 2: Has the patient been exposed to excessive amounts of Vitamin D (often found in rodenticides or some toxic plants)? Excessive vitamin D will promote increased absorption of both calcium and phosphorus. Renal damage may ensue, potentially causing further increases in calcium and phosphorus. Rarely, granulomatous disease may result in excessive production of Vitamin D.

Step 3: Does the patient have clinical signs or laboratory abnormalities compatible with hypoadrenocorticism? Glucocorticoid deficiency may increase absorption of calcium in the gut and kidneys. Most of this calcium is protein bound, and the increase is often mild, so clinical consequences of hypercalcemia in these patients are minimal. Phosphorus increases because of pre-renal decrements in glomerular filtration rate relative to hypovolemia.

Step 4: Does the patient have active bone formation or remodeling? Rapid bone growth in young, large breed dogs or large animals can increase serum calcium and phosphorus (see Chapter 2, Case 1). Bone remodeling associated with primary or metastatic tumors or osteomyelitis may also alter mineral homeostasis, however not all patients with radiographic evidence of bone lysis have alterations in serum calcium and phosphorus (see Chapter 2, Case 3).

Normal Calcium with Hyperphosphatemia

Step 1: Does the patient have an identifiable cause for tissue destruction? Phosphate is a major intracellular anion, and cell lysis associated with tissue trauma or muscle damage, hemolysis, and rarely, treatment of hematopoietic tumors (tumor lysis syndrome) can release large amount of phosphorus into the blood.

Step 2: Is the patient hyperthyroid? Feline hyperthyroidism may be associated with increased serum phosphorus, possibly due to decreased losses.

Hypomagnesemia

Step 1: Is the patient hypoproteinemic? Because a significant proportion of serum magnesium is bound to protein, low serum protein levels may cause total magnesium to be low but ionized magnesium is likely normal.

Step 2: Does the patient have gastrointestinal disease? Low serum magnesium may be associated with gastrointestinal disease in both small and large animal species, possibly due to decreased absorption or increased losses (Johansson, Toll).

Step 3: Does the diet have adequate mineral content? This is rarely an issue in small animal species on commercial diets, however sheep and cattle on all milk or other diets deficient in minerals can lead to low serum magnesium. In some situations such as grass tetany, the diet may be replete, however the magnesium does not appear to be adequately absorbed (Rosol).

Hypermagnesemia

Step 1: Evaluate renal function. The most likely cause of hypermagnesemia is decreased glomerular filtration rate, although cows with parturient paresis may also have increased magnesium. Excessive intake is possible.

Beyer MJ, Freestone JF, Reimer JM, Bernard WV, Rueve ER. Idiopathic hypocalcemia in foals. J Vet Intern Med 1997;11:356-360.

Carlson GP. Clinical chemistry tests. In: Large Animal Internal Medicine, 3rd ed. Bradford Smith, ed. Mosby, Inc., St. Louis, MO. 2002. pp 389-412.

Fascetti AJ, Hickman MA. Preparturient hypocalcemia in four cats. J Am Vet Med Assoc 1999;215:1127-1130.

Garcia-Lopez JM, Provost PJ, Rush JE, Zicker SC, Burmaster H, Freeman LM. Prevalence and prognostic importance of hypomagnesemia and hypocalcemia in horses that have colic surgery. Am J Vet Res 2001;62:7-11.

Johansson AM, Gardner SY, Jones SL, Fuquay LR, Reagan VH, Levine JF. Hypomagnesemia in hospitalized horses. J Vet Intern Med 2003;17:860-867.

Rosol TJ, Capen CC. Calcium-regulating hormones and diseases of abnormal mineral (calcium, phosphorus, magnesium) metabolism. In: Clinical Biochemistry of Domestic Animals, 5th ed. Kaneko JJ, Harvey JW, Bruss ML, eds. Academic Press, San Diego, CA. 1997. pp 619-702.

Rubeiz GJ, Thill-Baharozian M, Hardie D, Carlson RW. Association of hypomagnesemia and mortality in acutely ill medical patients. Crit Care Med 1993;12:203-209.

Schenck PA, Chew DJ. Determination of calcium fractionation in dogs with chronic renal failure. Am J Vet Res 2003;64:1181-1184.

Toll J, Erb H, Birnbaum N, Schermerhorn T. Prevalence and incidence of serum magnesium abnormalities in hospitalized cats. J Vet Intern Med 2002;16:217-221.

Vasilopulos RJ, Mackin A. Humoral hypercalcemia of malignancy: Pathophysiology and clinical signs. Compend Contin Educ Pract Vet 2003;25:122-135.

Williams LE, Gliatto JM, Dodge RK, Johnson JL, Gamblin RM, Thamm DH, Lana SE, Szymkowski M, Moore AS. Carcinoma of the apocrine glands of the anal sac in dogs: 113 cases (1985-1995). J Am Vet Med Assoc 2003;223:825-831.

Case 1 – Level 1

"Felix" is an adult castrated male mixed breed dog presenting for extraction of a fractured tooth. He is not currently taking any medications and is healthy. His physical examination is normal except for the tooth.

White blood cell count:	7.5 x 10⁹/L	(6.0-16.3)
Segmented neutrophils:	4.7 x 10⁹/L	(3.0-11.0)
Band neutrophils:	0 x 10⁹/L	(0-0.3)
Lymphocytes:	1.9 x 10⁹/L	(1.0-4.8)
Monocytes:	0.5 x 10⁹/L	(0.2-1.4)
Eosinophils:	0.4 x 10⁹/L	(0-1.3)

WBC morphology: Within normal limits

Hematocrit:	41%	(37-55)
Red blood cell count:	6.04 x 10¹²/L	(5.5-8.5)
Hemoglobin:	14.4 g/dl	(12.0-18.0)
MCV:	68.1 fl	(60.0-77.0)
MCHC:	35.1 g/dl	(31.0-34.0)

Platelets: Appear adequate in number

Glucose:	98 mg/dl	(65.0-120.0)
BUN:	16 mg/dl	(8-33)
Creatinine:	0.7 mg/dl	(0.5-1.5)
Phosphorus:	4.0 mg/dl	(3.0-6.0)
Calcium:	↓ 1.7 mg/dl	(8.8-11.0)
Magnesium:	↓ 0.7 mEq/L	(1.4-2.7)
Total Protein:	5.9 g/dl	(5.5-7.8)
Albumin:	3.4 g/dl	(2.8-4.0)
Globulin:	2.5 g/dl	(2.3-4.2)

A/G ratio:	1.4	(0.7-2.1)
Sodium:	146 mEq/L	(140-151)
Chloride:	109 mEq/L	(105-120)
Potassium:	↑ 11.3 mEq/L	(3.8-5.4)
HCO3:	26 mEq/L	(16-28)
Anion Gap:	22.3 mEq/L	(15-25)
Total Bili:	0.1 mg/dl	(0.10-0.30)
ALP:	26 IU/L	(20-121)
GGT:	3 IU/L	(2-10)
ALT:	29 IU/L	(18-86)
AST:	26 IU/L	(15-52)
Cholesterol:	312 mg/dl	(82-355)
Triglycerides:	57 mg/dl	(30-321)
Amylase:	538 IU/L	(400-1200)

Interpretation

CBC: There are no abnormalities in the CBC

Serum Biochemical Profile
Severe hypocalcemia: The complete absence of clinical signs makes it very unlikely that this is a true value. Processing error or artifact are likely.

Hyperkalemia: As for calcium, this value would be expected to be associated with clinical signs if it were accurate. Recommend repeat analysis.

Hypomagnesemia: In the absence of clinical signs, the significance of this value is unclear.

Case Summary and Outcome

The combination of abnormalities in this sample is compatible with the effects of EDTA anticoagulant, which contains potassium and chelates calcium and magnesium. It would appear that a plasma sample had been used for the chemistry panel. A new sample was collected in a red topped (serum) tube, and all values were within reference intervals.

Case 2 – Level 1

"Daisy" is a 5-year-old Holstein cow in her third lactation. She has a history of uneventful calvings, including twins last year. A fetotomy was performed two nights ago, and the placenta was subsequently delivered normally. However, Daisy was unable to rise after calving.

Glucose:	↑ 98 mg/dl	(55.0-81.0)
BUN:	22 mg/dl	(8-29)
Creatinine:	1.4 mg/dl	(0.6-1.6)
Phosphorus:	↓ 3.6 mg/dl	(3.8-7.7)
Calcium:	↓ 7.3 mg/dl	(8.6-10.0)
Albumin:	3.4 g/dl	(2.8-4.0)
Globulin:	3.0 g/dl	(2.3-4.2)
A/G Ratio:	1.1	(0.7-2.1)
Sodium:	149 mEq/L	(133-149)
Chloride:	108 mEq/L	(98-108)
Potassium:	4.1 mEq/L	(3.9-4.2)
HCO3:	26 mEq/L	(18-30)
Anion Gap:	19.1 mEq/L	(14-21)
ALP:	73 IU/L	(20-80)
GGT:	19 IU/L	(12-39)
AST:	↑ 491 IU/L	(50-120)

Interpretation

Serum Biochemical Profile

Hyperglycemia: The most likely cause for this relatively mild abnormality is stress, or possibly early sepsis. CBC data or fibrinogen concentration would be helpful to further assess the potential for an inflammatory condition. Diabetes mellitus is rare in large animal species.

Hypocalcemia and hypophosphatemia: Recumbancy in a periparturient, high-producing dairy cow should prompt evaluation for bovine parturient paresis (milk fever). The hypocalcemia and hypophosphatemia noted here are compatible with that diagnosis. When measured, serum magnesium is often elevated. Hypocalcemia occurs because of the acute and extreme demand for calcium associated with onset of colostrum and milk production. It is difficult for the body to compensate for such an increase in demand after the dry period, when demand is low and intestinal absorption and bone resorption are likely to be low. As noted in the introduction to the chapter, the ionized fraction of calcium is the biologically active fraction, however only total calcium measurements are usually available under most circumstances, so the appearance and severity of clinical signs may not vary directly with total serum calcium measurements. Because of protein binding of calcium, serum albumin and globulins influence total calcium measurements. Acid/base abnormalities that may occur with concurrent gastrointestinal disease (such as stasis or obstruction) can also influence ionized calcium levels and therefore the severity of clinical signs at a given total calcium concentration. Serum phosphorus levels may be low because of decreased feed intake near parturition and salivary losses of phosphorus. Low bone resorption can impair the ability to maintain serum phosphorus levels in the normal range when there are acute increases in demand at parturition.

Increased AST: Increased AST in a recumbent cow is likely due to muscle damage, which is common in parturient paresis. This impression can be supported by measuring creatine kinase, which is also often elevated in parturient paresis cases.

Case Summary and Outcome

Daisy responded rapidly to treatment with intravenous calcium, which is often the case in uncomplicated parturient paresis patients. Often, milk fever is diagnosed on the basis of clinical signs and the characteristic rapid response to therapy, however collection of pretreatment blood samples can be helpful in case the patient does not respond to appropriate therapy within a reasonable amount of time. Other conditions associated with hypocalcemia in cows include uterine prolapse, dystocia, retained fetal membranes, abomasal displacement, mastitis, renal disease, and metritis (Hunt).

Hunt E, Blackwelder JT. Disorders of calcium metabolism. In: Large Animal Internal Medicine, 3rd ed. P Smith, ed. Mosby, Inc. St. Louis, MO. 2002. pp.1248-1254.

Case 3 – Level 1

"Bear" is a 7-year-old male Cocker Spaniel presenting with a history of chronic vomiting, diarrhea, and muscle tremors.

Glucose:	104 mg/dl	(65.0-120.0)
BUN:	↓ 4 mg/dl	(6-24)
Creatinine:	0.7 mg/dl	(0.5-1.5)
Phosphorus:	5.6 mg/dl	(3.0-6.0)
Calcium:	↓ 4.4 mg/dl	(8.8-11.0)
Magnesium:	1.5 mEq/L	(1.4-2.7)
Total Protein:	6.2 g/dl	(5.2-7.2)
Albumin:	↓ 2.5 g/dl	(3.0-4.2)
Globulin:	3.7 g/dl	(2.0-4.0)
Sodium:	143 mEq/L	(140-151)
Chloride:	109 mEq/L	(105-120)
Potassium:	4.6 mEq/L	(3.8-5.4)
HCO3:	18 mEq/L	(16-25)
Anion Gap:	20.6 mEq/L	(15-25)
Cholesterol:	162 mg/dl	(110-314)
Creatine kinase:	186 IU/L	(55-309)
Ionized calcium:	↓ 2.10 mg/dl	(4.93-5.65)

Interpretation

No CBC data is available.

Serum Biochemical Profile

Low BUN with normal creatinine: Low protein diets, polyuria/polydipsia, and poor liver function may all cause low BUN with normal creatinine. In the absence of clinical signs or other laboratory data supporting these causes, the low BUN in this case is of questionable clinical significance.

Hypocalcemia (both total and ionized) with normal phosphorus: In this case, mild hypoalbuminemia may account for part, but not all of the low total calcium. In addition, ionized calcium usually is normal in cases of hypocalcemia secondary to low albumin. The muscle tremors strongly suggested ionized hypocalcemia, which was confirmed by laboratory measurement. Eclampsia is a potential cause for low ionized calcium in periparturient female dogs, but is not a consideration for Bear. With a history of vomiting and diarrhea, pancreatitis is a differential diagnosis, however the hypocalcemia in these patients is generally mild and does not produce clinical signs. Renal disease can be associated with hypocalcemia, however, Bear is not azotemic. A urine specific gravity is needed to help assess renal function. Hypoparathyroidism is rare in dogs and cats, but is compatible with the clinical signs and relative absence of other serum biochemical abnormalities seen in Bear. In many cases of hypoparathyroidism, the serum phosphorus is increased because low levels of PTH lead to phosphorus retention by the kidney. Serum phosphorus may remain within the reference interval in some cases because of relatively wide reference ranges or because of concurrent phosphate depletion associated with anorexia. Serum PTH levels should be low in cases of hypoparathyroidism. Hypomagnesemia can cause hypocalcemia by interfereing with PTH secretion or function, however the serum magnesium is normal in this case. Keep in mind that, like calcium, this is a total magnesium concentration and the ionized magnesium is the biologically active form, which could be measured if necessary.

Case Summary and Outcome

Bear was treated with calcium and Vitamin D supplementation, which increased his ionized calcium levels and improved his clinical signs. His PTH levels were low at 1.5 pmol/L (reference interval = 2-13), supporting the diagnosis of hypoparathyroidism. Hypoparathyroidism may follow injury of the parathyroid glands during surgical procedures in the neck or may be secondary to immune-mediated destruction of the gland.

Case 4 – Level 1

"Lolita" is a 2-year-old Standardbred mare. During exercise the day before, she broke away from the trainer. After exercise this morning, she began to show signs of tying up including pain, colic, stiffness, a shuffling hindlimb gait, and sweating. She continued to sweat profusely and by 1.5 hr post exercise, she had dark urine (Figure 6-1). The referring veterinarian gave her banamine and xylazine for the trip to the referral hospital. Lolita presented with profuse sweating, synchronous diaphragmatic flutter, and dark urine. She had a history of a similar episode of tying up last year.

	Day 1	Day 3	
White blood cell count:	8.5 x 10⁹/L	9.1	(5.9-11.2)
Segmented neutrophils:	7.1 x 10⁹/L	7.7	(2.3-9.1)
Band neutrophils:	0.0 x 10⁹/L	0.0	(0-0.3)
Lymphocytes:	1.2 x 10⁹/L	1.3	(1.0-4.9)
Monocytes:	0.1 x 10⁹/L	0.0	(0-1.0)
Eosinophils:	0.1 x 10⁹/L	0.1	(0-0.3)
WBC morphology: No abnormalities noted on either Day 1 or Day 3.			

Hematocrit:	47%	34	(30-51)
Red blood cell count:	9.09 x 10¹²/L	7.60	(6.5-12.8)
Hemoglobin:	16.9 g/dl	12.4	(10.9-18.1)
MCV:	44.0 fl	45.0	(35.0-53.0)
MCHC:	36.2 g/dl	36.4	(34.6-38.0)
RBC morphology: No abnormalities noted on either Day 1 or Day 3.			
Platelets: Clumped but appear adequate in number on both Day 1 and Day 3.			
Plasma color:	normal	normal	
Fibrinogen:	245 mg/dl		(100-400)

Glucose:	106 mg/dl	104	(60.0-128.0)
BUN:	14 mg/dl	13	(11-26)
Creatinine:	1.4 mg/dl	1.1	(0.9-1.9)
Phosphorus:	↑ 5.7 mg/dl	2.8	(2.8-5.1)
Calcium:	11.1 mg/dl	11.6	(11.0-13.5)
Total Protein:	6.4 g/dl	↓ 5.5	(5.6-7.0)
Albumin:	3.4 g/dl	2.9	(2.4-3.8)
Globulin:	3.0 g/dl	2.6	(2.5-4.9)
A/G Ratio:	1.1	1.1	(0.7-2.1)
Sodium:	140 mEq/L	138	(130-145)
Chloride:	98 mEq/L	101	(97-105)
Potassium:	3.6 mEq/L	4.2	(3.0-5.0)
HCO3:	↑ 36 mEq/L	↓ 23	(25-31)
Anion Gap:	9.6 mEq/L	↑ 18.0	(7-15)
Total Bili:	↑ 2.5 mg/dl	↑ 2.4	(0.6-1.8)
ALP:	129 IU/L	120	(109-352)
GGT:	↑ 41 IU/L	↑ 30	(5-23)
AST:	↑ 13,030 IU/L	↑ 14,930	(190-380)
CK:	↑ 500,040 IU/L	↑ 15,742	(80-446)

Urinalysis: Free catch

	Day 1	Day 3:
Color:	Dark brown	Yellow
Specific gravity:	1.042	1.023
pH:	Not available	8.5
Protein:	4+	3-4+
Glucose/ketones:	Negative	Negative
Bilirubin:	3+	1+
Heme:	4+	3+
Sediment:	Casts seen	Not available

Ionized Calcium:	↓ 5.7 mg/dl	(6.0-7.2)
Ionized Magnesium:	↓ 0.44 mmol/dl	(0.46-0.66)

Venous blood gas (Day 1):

pH:	7.429	(7.32-7.45)
PO2:	40.1 mmHg	(24-40)
PCO2:	45.3 mmHg	(34-53)
HCO3:	29.5 mmol/L	(23-31)
TCO2:	30.9 mmol/L	(24-32)
Base Excess:	4.8 mmol/L	(-1.0-5.0)

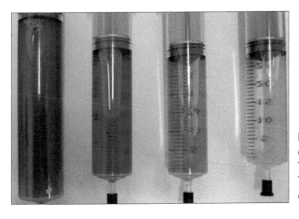

Figure 6-1. Equine urines discolored due to myoglobinuria. The urine on the left is from Day 1. The urine on the right is from the day of discharge and is normal.

Interpretation
CBC: No abnormalities

Serum Biochemical Profile
Hyperphosphatemia: Acute rhabdomyolysis is associated with hyperphosphatemia. The marked elevations in AST and CK and the discolored urine (probably myoglobin) support muscle damage and translocation of phosphorus outside of cells as the most likely cause for the increased phosphorus. Other common causes of increased serum phosphorus include skeletal growth in immature horses, endurance exercise, and renal failure, none of which are consistent with the clinical history or other laboratory data (the patient has concentrated urine and is not azotemic). Less commonly, Vitamin D toxicity will result in hyperphosphatemia.

Normal total calcium with slightly low ionized calcium: Hyperphosphatemia leads to a compensatory decrease in ionized calcium because of mass law interactions and because of decreased active Vitamin D synthesis by the kidney. As has been described in other cases, a discrepancy between total calcium and ionized calcium is present in this case and illustrates the rationale for measurement of the biologically active fraction of the mineral in some situations.

Low ionized magnesium: The serum ionized magnesium concentration in this patient is minimally depressed and may not be clinically significant at this time. The history of sweating indicates potential route for loss of magnesium via the skin, although decreased gastrointestinal absorption, increased gastrointestinal losses or renal wasting are possible.

Increased HCO3: In general, this value is interpreted as evidence of alkalosis, however the normal blood gas results make this unlikely. Artfactual elevations of HCO3 have been reported in two horses and a calf with severe muscle disease (Collins) as a result of interference with the enzymatic method for detection of bicarbonate by LDH released from the injured muscle. The original report also described increased anion gaps, which was not noted in Lolita. LDH was not reported in Lolita, however her serum sample was run on a Hitachi analyzer similar to the chemistry analyzer in the report by Collins et al. By day 3, Lolita has a mild acidemia with elevated anion gap, which could be the result of lactic acidosis or accumulation of another unmeasured anion.

Hyperbilirubinemia: In horses, anorexia should always be considered as a cause of hyperbilirubinemia. The concurrently elevated GGT indicates that cholestasis is another potential contributor to increased serum bilirubin. Hemolysis may also cause hyperbilirubinemia, however Lolita is not initially anemic when she presents with elevated bilirubin. Her PCV does drop significantly over 2 days (although it remains within the reference interval) with no additional change in serum bilirubin. Some of this decrement in packed cell volume may be attributable to rehydration/fluid therapy. It is also possible that her initial PCV was increased due to splenic contraction secondary to excitement of transport and pain.

Increased GGT: Elevations in GGT are compatible with cholestasis, which may be primary or secondary to hypoxia, gastrointestinal disease, sepsis, or other processes. Enzyme elevations are not specific as to etiology, however the trend back towards the upper limit of the reference interval indicates that a complete work up for primary liver disease does not need to be pursued unless other clinical signs or laboratory abnormalities indicative of liver disease appear.

Marked increases in AST and CK: The combination of these abnormalities is supportive of rhabdomyolysis, consistent with the clinical impression of tying up. As with liver enzymes, elevations in muscle enzymes are not specific as to etiology, and many patients with a history of trauma, strenuous exercise, trembling, or intramuscular injections may have increased CK. Conversely, some types of muscle disease do not cause increased CK or AST. The short half-life of creatine kinase explains the precipitous drop in CK by Day 3 while AST levels remain increased.

Urinalysis: The dark brown urine collected on Day 1 is consistent with the presence of either blood, hemoglobin, myoglobin, or bilirubin. Although the information is not available for this patient, examination of the urine for the presence of erythrocytes will rule in or out hematuria as a cause for the discoloration. The normal plasma color with dark urine is suggests myoglobinuria because myoglobin is not significantly protein bound in the plasma and is therefore rapidly cleared in the kidney. Hemoglobinuria is generally associated with hemoglobinemia, which will cause pink to red discoloration of the plasma. Occasionally erythrocytes will lyse in urine, leading to a negative sediment examination and the impression of hemoglobinuria instead of hematuria. An ammonium sulfate test or protein electrophoresis will confirm the presence of myoglobin. Myoglobin will cause protein, bilirubin, and heme test strips to be positive.

On presentation, the urine appears adequately concentrated and fluid therapy is likely causing the production of more dilute urine on day 3. Pigments such as hemoglobin and myoglobin may have toxic effects on the kidney, so the patient should be monitored for isosthenuria and azotemia as signs of nephropathy. This is especially true in this patient because of the presence of casts, which can be a sign of renal damage. Unfortunately, the type and number of casts were not described. Small numbers of hyaline casts may merely reflect diuresis and correction of dehydration, while large numbers of cellular casts can indicate renal tubular cell degeneration and necrosis. The absence of casts in the second sample does not rule out kidney damage.

Case Summary and Outcome

For 4 days, Lolita was treated with lactated ringers supplemented with calcium and magnesium, banamine®, and vitamin E. She was sent home with instructions to hand walk her for 2 weeks, followed by light exercise. Dietary changes also were recommended. A muscle biopsy was suggested as a follow up to assess the potential for polysaccharide storage myopathy, which is documented in Quarter horses and is compatible with her clinical signs and laboratory data.

Collins ND, LeRoy BE, Vap L. Artifactually increased serum bicarbonate values in two horses and a calf with severe rhabdomyolysis. Vet Clin Pathol. 1998;27(3):85-90.

Case 5 – Level 2

"Carley" is a 14-year-old spayed female Border Terrier presenting with a history of vomiting and anorexia. She has previously had several mammary adenomas and carcinomas, that were completely excised based on biopsy evaluation. She also is being treated with low doses of corticosteroids for a previous diagnosis of inflammatory bowel disease.

White blood cell count:	11.1 x 10⁹/L	(4.9-16.8)
Segmented neutrophils:	10.5 x 10⁹/L	(2.8-11.5)
Band neutrophils:	0.0	(0-0.3)
Lymphocytes:	↓ 0.1 x 10⁹/L	(1.0-4.8)
Monocytes:	0.4 x 10⁹/L	(0.1-1.5)
Eosinophils:	0.1 x 10⁹/L	(0-1.4)
WBC morphology: No abnormalities noted.		

Hematocrit:	49%	(39-55)
Red blood cell count:	7.07 x 10¹²/L	(5.8-8.5)
Hemoglobin:	16.4 g/dl	(14.0-19.1)
MCV:	67.7 fl	(60.0-75.0)
MCHC:	33.5 g/dl	(33.0-36.0)
Platelets:	475 x 10⁹/L	(181-525)

Glucose:	93 mg/dl	(65.0-120.0)
BUN:	11 mg/dl	(6-24)
Creatinine:	0.7 mg/dl	(0.5-1.5)
Phosphorus:	3.0 mg/dl	(3.0-6.0)
Calcium:	↑ 12.8 mg/dl	(8.8-11.0)
Magnesium:	2.4 mEq/L	(1.4-2.7)
Total Protein:	6.6 g/dl	(5.2-7.2)
Albumin:	3.4 g/dl	(3.0-4.2)
Globulin:	3.2 g/dl	(2.0-4.0)
Sodium:	144 mEq/L	(140-151)
Chloride:	105 mEq/L	(105-120)
Potassium:	4.1 mEq/L	(3.8-5.4)
HCO3:	23 mEq/L	(16-25)
Anion Gap:	20.1 mEq/L	(15-25)
Total Bili:	↑ 1.4 mg/dl	(0.10-0.50)
ALP:	↑ 996 IU/L	(20-320)
GGT:	↑ 82 IU/L	(3-10)
ALT:	↑ 566 IU/L	(10-95)
AST:	↑ 939 IU/L	(15-52)
Cholesterol:	↑ 371 mg/dl	(110-314)
Triglycerides:	44 mg/dl	(30-300)
Amylase:	439 IU/L	(400-1200)

Urinalysis: Cystocentesis

Appearance: Yellow and clear
Specific gravity: 1.006
pH: 7.5
Protein: trace
Glucose, ketones, bilirubin, heme: negative
Sediment examination: occasional erythrocytes and leukocytes

Interpretation
CBC: The mild lymphopenia is compatible with the history of corticosteroid administration.

Serum Biochemical Profile
Hypercalcemia with low normal phosphorus: In an older patient, a primary consideration for the combination of high serum calcium with normal to low phosphorus is neoplasia. Although many tumors have been documented to cause hypercalcemia of malignancy in small animal patients, hematopoietic neoplasia, anal sac apocrine gland adenocarcinoma, and parathyroid tumors should be primary differential diagnoses. Further diagnostic procedures may include imaging studies to detect masses or enlarged organs, cytologic or histologic examination of affected tissues, and/or measurement of PTH and PTHrP. In this case, the liver should be evaluated because of the enzyme elevations. Hypoadrenocorticism can also mildly elevate serum calcium. However this condition is less likely given Carley's history of steroid treatment, lack of appropriate clinical signs, and lack of significant electrolyte abnormalities.

Hyperbilirubinemia with increased ALP, GGT, and cholesterol: The elevated ALP, GGT, and cholesterol are compatible with the presence of cholestasis as a cause for elevated serum bilirubin. Hemolysis can also contribute to hyperbilirubinemia, however Carley is not anemic, nor does she have any morphologic abnormalities of erythrocytes that would suggest increased red blood cell destruction. Decreased liver function or sepsis can also contribute to mild elevations in serum bilirubin. Sepsis is unlikely with a normal leukogram. Liver enzyme values do not predict liver function, and liver function is best evaluated by measuring serum bile acids or blood ammonia. Other evidence of severe liver dysfunction, such as hypoalbuminemia, low BUN, and hypocholesterolemia are absent in this profile. Therapy with corticosteroids can induce ALP and GGT and, in some cases, can produce a steroid hepatopathy. A variety of endocrinopathies and metabolic derangements also can increase ALP, GGT, and cholesterol, however they appear less likely than the problems described above.

Increased ALT and AST: Elevations in these enzymes support the presence of damage to hepatocytes, but do not specify cause. Potential causes for hepatocellular damage in this patient include cholestasis and steroid hepatopathy, although the hypercalcemia indicates that neoplasia should evaluated as a cause of liver injury.

Urinalysis: The significance of the low urine specific gravity is uncertain in a patient that is not azotemic or dehydrated. Normal urine specific gravity can vary considerably in healthy patients, however hypercalcemia can interfere with urinary concentrating ability via several different mechanisms and may be an issue here (See Chapter 5, Case 4). Pre-renal azotemia may develop if water intake cannot compensate for ongoing losses and laboratory work may be indistinguishable from renal failure. In addition, liver disease may also be associated with polyuria and polydipsia (See Chapter 5, Case 12). Treatment with corticosteroids may contribute to poor urinary concentrating ability.

Case Summary and Outcome
Abdominal ultrasound revealed a markedly enlarged gall bladder compatible with a mucocele, so Carley went to surgery for gall bladder removal and examination of the abdomen for evidence of neoplasia. At surgery, biopsy material was collected from the liver and duodenum, however all other structures appeared grossly normal and were not sampled. Histologically, the liver had evidence of steroid hepatopathy, the gall bladder showed glandular hyperplasia with hypersecretion of mucus, and the duodenum had congestion and lymphoplasmacytic enteritis. There was no evidence of neoplasia in any of the biopsy sections.

Carley recovered well from surgery, and her serum biochemical abnormalities normalized, with the exception of the hypercalcemia, which was persistent over the next several weeks and remained in the range of 12-13 mg/dl. In addition, the phosphorus level dropped to 1.3 mg/dl (2.6-7.2). At this point, ultrasound examination of the neck revealed a small mass in the region of the right parathyroid gland. Carley had another surgery to remove the mass, which was an expansive but non-invasive parathyroid adenoma characterized by uniform cells with low mitotic activity and proliferating in solid sheets. PTH and PTHrP levels were not measured since a parathyroid mass was located using ultrasound.

Case 6 – Level 2

"Picasso" is a 12-year-old intact male Weimeraner presenting for non-painful lumps on his head that the owners noticed two months ago. On physical examination, Picasso's teeth are movable but do not appear painful. Skull radiographs reveal severe bone demineralization in the maxilla and mandible (Figure 6-2A and B).

White blood cell count:	7.0 x 10⁹/L	(4.1-13.3)
Hematocrit:	↓ 36%	(39-55)
Platelets:	Appear adequate in number	
Glucose:	111 mg/dl	(65.0-120.0)
BUN:	↑ 55 mg/dl	(6-24)
Creatinine:	↑ 3.1 mg/dl	(0.5-1.5)
Phosphorus:	↑ 8.0 mg/dl	(3.0-6.0)
Calcium:	↑ 13.7 mg/dl	(8.8-11.0)
Magnesium:	2.1 mEq/L	(1.4-2.2)
Total Protein:	5.5 g/dl	(5.2-7.2)
Albumin:	2.6 g/dl	(2.5-3.7)
Globulin:	2.9 g/dl	(2.0-4.0)
Sodium:	148 mEq/L	(140-151)
Chloride:	121 mEq/L	(108-121)
Potassium:	4.6 mEq/L	(3.8-5.4)
HCO3:	19.2 mEq/L	(16-25)
Anion Gap:	12.4 mEq/L	(15-25)
Total Bili:	0.3 mg/dl	(0.10-0.50)
ALP:	↑ 656 IU/L	(20-320)
GGT:	7 IU/L	(3-10)
ALT:	52 IU/L	(10-95)
AST:	33 IU/L	(15-52)
Cholesterol:	263 mg/dl	(110-314)
Amylase:	1048 IU/L	(400-1200)

Urinalysis: Catheter
Appearance: Yellow and slightly cloudy
Specific gravity: 1.011
pH: 6.0
Protein: 3+
Glucose, ketones, bilirubin, heme: negative
Sediment examination: Occasional erythrocytes and epithelial cells
Protein:creatinine ratio: 2.28 (<1.0)

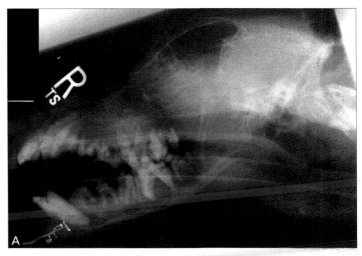

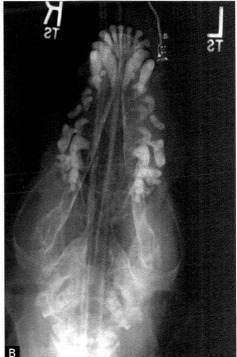

Figure 6-2A & B. Canine skull radiographs showing skeletal mineral depletion.

Interpretation

CBC: Only limited data are available. There is an anemia that cannot be adequately characterized as regenerative or non-regenerative without erythrocyte indices or a microscopic evaluation of anisocytosis and polychromasia and reticulocyte count. A nonregenerative anemia in association with azotemia, isosthenuria, and abnormalities of calcium and phosphorus is compatible with renal failure. Hypercalcemia of malignancy with secondary effects on the kidney can result in similar laboratory abnormalities. Anemia of chronic disease is a common cause of mild, nonregenerative anemia in small animal patients and is likely a factor in the development of Picasso's anemia. Alternatively, hematopoietic malignancies replacing bone marrow can result in a non-regenerative anemia.

Serum Biochemical Profile
Azotemia with isosthenuria: These findings indicate renal azotemia, however if Picasso is dehydrated, there may be a concurrent pre-renal component. A consideration here is the

ability of hypercalcemia to interfere with urinary concentrating ability. If diagnosed sufficiently early in the process, the effects of hypercalcemia on the kidney may be reversible; in other cases, irreversible damage occurs. The BUN, creatinine, and urine specific gravity should be re-evaluated once the hypercalcemia is corrected to re-assess renal function.

Hypercalcemia with hyperphosphatemia: Hypercalcemia should be associated with hypophosphatemia due to mass law interactions unless there is another process elevating phosphorus. Vitamin D toxicity causes elevations in both calcium and phosphorus and should be ruled out here, although it is less common than the following differential diagnoses. Azotemia with isosthenuria implicates renal failure as a cause for hyperphosphatemia due to decreased glomerular filtration rate. Total serum calcium can be high, low, or normal in renal failure patients, and may not correlate with ionized calcium. In renal failure, hyperphosphatemia inhibits renal 1α-hydroxylase, which decreases production of calcitriol and reduces intestinal calcium absorption and decreases ionized calcium concentration. In response, PTH secretion is stimulated, which promotes renal excretion of phosphorus and bone demineralization. In many renal failure patients with high total calcium, ionized calcium may be normal to low. The discrepancy may be due to increased amounts of calcium complexed to anions such as lactate, sulfate, or phosphate. On the other hand, hypercalcemia associated with hyperparathyroidism or paraneoplastic hypercalcemia may damage kidneys and precipitate renal failure. Measurement of ionized calcium, PTH, and PTHrP may help distinguish between these various pathophysiologic scenarios.

Increased ALP: There are numerous potential causes for increased ALP in dogs, including enzyme induction by hormones or drugs, metabolic alterations, and liver disease. As an isolated abnormality, its clinical significance is unclear, particularly if the patient is not taking any medications that could elevate ALP. Re-evaluation of liver enzymes in 2-4 weeks may reveal whether the abnormality is persistent and should be investigated further (See Chapter 2).

Urinalysis: The significance of the isosthenuria is discussed above. The urine sediment is inactive and there is no evidence of inflammation or other lower urinary tract pathology. Thus, the elevated protein:creatinine ratio can be interpreted as compatible with glomerular loss of protein.

Case Summary and Outcome

Further investigation of Picasso's disease revealed increased ionized calcium of 1.85 mmol/L (reference interval = 1.25-1.45). Intact PTH was increased while PTHrP was within reference intervals. The combination of high PTH and increased ionized calcium is compatible with primary hyperparathyroidism with secondary renal damage. Renal secondary hyperparathyroidism may be associated with either high, low, or normal total calcium, but ionized calcium is generally low. Because ionized calcium can be high in dogs with renal failure (Schenck), ultrasound examination of the neck and parathyroid glands was recommended. The owners did not elect to pursue this option so the diagnosis could not be confirmed.

This case should be compared with Carley (Case 5), in which primary hyperparathyroidism was confirmed by identification of a parathyroid adenoma. Her case was complicated with concurrent hepatobiliary disease, however her renal function appeared to be better than Picasso's based on the normal BUN, creatinine, and normal to low phosphorus. Like Picasso, Carley's urine was not concentrated, probably related to the effects of high ionized calcium on the renal tubules.

Schenck PA, Chew DJ. Determination of calcium fractionation in dogs with chronic renal failure. Am J Vet Res 2003;64:1181-1184.

Case 7 – Level 2

"Cleopatra" is a 12-year-old domestic short haired cat presenting with a two month history of reluctance to jump. Her physical examination is within normal limits except for pain in her lumbar spine. Her neurologic examination is normal.

White blood cell count:	7.0 x 10⁹/L	(6.0-17.0)
Segmented neutrophils:	5.8 x 10⁹/L	(3.0-11.0)
Band neutrophils:	0 x 10⁹/L	(0-0.3)
Lymphocytes:	↓ 0.6 x 10⁹/L	(1.1-4.8)
Monocytes:	0.5 x 10⁹/L	(0.2-1.4)
Basophils:	0.1 x 10⁹/L	(0-1.3)

WBC morphology: No significant abnormalities noted.

Hematocrit:	37%	(31-46)
MCV:	51.6 fl	(39.0-56.0)
MCHC:	32.5 g/dl	(30.5-36.0)

Platelets: Present but clumped, cannot estimate number.

Glucose:	106 mg/dl	(70.0-120.0)
BUN:	↑ 35 mg/dl	(8-33)
Creatinine:	1.6 mg/dl	(0.9-2.1)
Phosphorus:	3.4 mg/dl	(3.0-6.3)
Calcium:	↑ 14.2 mg/dl	(8.8-11.5)
Magnesium:	2.6 mEq/L	(1.4-2.6)
Total Protein:	↑ 9.7 g/dl	(5.2-7.2)
Albumin:	3.1 g/dl	(3.0-4.2)
Globulin:	↑ 6.6 g/dl	(2.0-4.0)
Sodium:	149 mEq/L	(149-164)
Chloride:	↓ 115 mEq/L	(119-134)
Potassium:	4.3 mEq/L	(3.6-5.4)
HCO3:	24 mEq/L	(16-25)
Anion Gap:	14.3 mEq/L	(13-27)
Total Bili:	0.1 mg/dl	(0.10-0.50)
ALP:	17 IU/L	(10-72)
GGT:	<3 IU/L	(0-5)
ALT:	30 IU/L	(29-145)
AST:	25 IU/L	(12-42)
Cholesterol:	93 mg/dl	(77-258)
Triglycerides:	108 mg/dl	(30-300)
Amylase:	↑ 2014 IU/L	(400-1200)

Interpretation

CBC: Mild lymphopenia could be compatible with stress/corticosteroid effects

Serum Biochemical Profile
Mild increase in BUN with normal creatinine: The elevated BUN could be attributable to a high protein diet or gastrointestinal bleeding. Mildly decreased renal tubular flow rates, which increase the time available for renal reabsorption of urea may also increase BUN. Early pre-renal or renal azotemia may first manifest itself as increased BUN if extra-renal causes of

increased BUN are ruled out. Sepsis is unlikely given the clinical history and relatively normal leukogram. Hypercalcemia can lead to production of dilute urine, polyuria/polydipsia, dehydration, or ultimately renal failure in some cases. A urine specific gravity should be obtained to help interpret the increased BUN. The high normal magnesium and increased amylase could be compatible with low glomerular filtration rate from renal or pre-renal causes.

Hypercalcemia with normal phosphorus: If the presence of hypercalcemia is verified by repeat measure, then neoplasia, renal disease, bone lesions or some infectious/inflammatory diseases should be considered. Primary hyperparathyroidism is much less common than humoral hypercalcemia of malignancy with increased PTHrP. Measurement of PTH and PTHrP can help distinguish these processes if a malignancy is difficult to identify clinically. However, not all neoplasms that cause hypercalcemia produce PTHrP. Renal disease is a possibility here with elevations in BUN and amylase that could indicate low glomerular filtration rate. Measurement of ionized calcium could be helpful because hypercalcemia of malignancy is generally associated with increased ionized calcium. In contrast, most patients with renal failure have low ionized calcium regardless of total serum calcium values. There are exceptions, and increased ionized calcium does not rule out renal failure. Distinguishing between hypercalcemia of malignancy and renal disease is further complicated by the ability of hypercalcemia of malignancy to cause renal dysfunction (See Jag Chapter 5, case 4). The combination of hypercalcemia, possible bone pain, and hyperglobulinemia suggests multiple myeloma, although bone remodeling unrelated to neoplasia may also increase serum calcium. Radiographic evaluation of the skeleton is indicated. Occasionally, inflammatory diseases such as blastomycosis and schistosomiasis can cause hypercalcemia, and the presence of these organisms could stimulate polyclonal hyperglobulinemia associated with an immune response.

Mild hypochloremia: The cause for the mild hypochloremia is not clear in this case. There is no history of vomiting or any apparent acid/base disorders, however the HCO3 is at the higher end of the reference interval. Treatment with diuretics can be ruled out by the history. Further monitoring is recommended to determine if acid/base abnormalities are developing or if the chloride value normalizes. Because of the way reference ranges are constructed (see Chapter 1), healthy animals may have results that fall slightly outside of the reference range, but are normal due to biological variation.

Hyperproteinemia with hyperglobulinemia: Hyperglobulinemia can be due to numerous causes and can be classified as polyclonal or monoclonal using serum protein electrophoresis. Polyclonal gammopathies are associated with inflammation/antigenic stimulation with increased production of acute phase reactant proteins and several types of immunoglobulins. Monoclonal gammopathies indicate production of a single type of immunoglobulin and are usually associated with neoplastic proliferation of a single clone of lymphocytes or plasma cells. Rarely, infectious diseases such as *Leishmania, Ehrlichia*, or feline infectious peritonitis can result in monoclonal gammopathy.

Increased amylase: The mild change in this value is most compatible with the decreased glomerular filtration rate. Gastrointestinal disease can also be associated with increased amylase and is compatible with the clinical history. Pancreatic disease cannot be ruled out, but is not required to explain this value. Amylase is a poor indicator of pancreatitis in the cat.

Case Summary and Outcome

Radiographic evaluation of the lumbar spine revealed lysis of the vertebral body of L4 and kidneys at the lower limit of normal size. A needle aspirate of the lesion consisted of round cells containing eccentric nuclei with tightly condensed chromatin and a moderate amount of basophilic cytoplasm, compatible with plasma cells. A serum protein electrophoresis documented a monoclonal gammopathy. Cleopatra was diagnosed with multiple myeloma. She was treated with chemotherapy and responded well, with resolution of her serum biochemical abnormalities.

Multiple myeloma is rare in dogs, and only scattered reports describing the condition in cats are available. These suggest that hypercalcemia and osteolytic lesions with accompanying bone pain may be less common in cats than dogs, but data on cats are sparse (Hickford, Sheafor, Weber). The hypercalcemia that can accompany multiple myeloma may be caused by several different mechanisms, including the production of PTHrP, direct osteolysis, or binding of calcium to myeloma proteins. This will increase the total serum calcium but ionized calcium should be unaffected. With multiple myeloma, the production of inhibitors of osteoblast differentiation may help explain why bone lysis is not followed by bone formation as it is during normal bone remodeling (Glass). Renal disease is frequently a complication of multiple myeloma in people (Bataille), and has been described in dogs and cats. Renal insufficiency may be related to concurrent hypercalcemia, neoplastic infiltration of the kidney, protein precipitation in the kidney, or amyloidosis or glomerulonephritis (Sheafor). As noted above, renal disease can cause an increase in total serum calcium and contribute to the hypercalcemia seen with malignancy.

Bataille R, Harousseau JL. Multiple myeloma. N Eng J Med 1997;336:1657-1661.

Glass DA, Patel MS, Karsenty G. A new insight into the formation of osteolytic lesions in multiple myeloma. N Eng J Med 2003;349:2479-2480.

Hickford FH, Stokol T, vanGessel YA, Randolph JF, Schermerhorn T. Monoclonal immunoglobulin G cryoglobulinemia and multiple myeloma in a domestic shorthair cat. J Am Vet Med Assoc. 2000;217:1029-1033.

Sheafor SE, Gamblin RM, Couto CG. Hypercalcemia in cats with multiple myeloma. J Am An Hosp Assoc 1996;32:503-508.

Weber NA, Tebeau CS. An unusual presentation of multiple myeloma in two cats. J Am An Hosp Assoc 1998;34:477-483.

Case 8 – Level 2

"General" is a 1-day-old male Thoroughbred foal. The owners report that the birth was "difficult". His dam was colicky before and after delivery. She died several hours after delivery despite medical therapy for colic. The foal appeared to nurse well after birth despite the poor condition of the mother, and the owners feel that he likely got adequate colostrum. On presentation, the foal is bright, alert, and responsive, but appears weak in the hindlimbs and occasionally drags the right hind limb. All joints appear to be of normal size with no excessive heat, swelling, or pain on palpation. He passed feces, but appears mildly colicky.

All reference intervals were generated for adult horses.

White blood cell count:	9.0 x 10⁹/L	(5.9-11.2)
Segmented neutrophils:	7.0 x 10⁹/L	(2.3-9.1)
Band neutrophils:	0.0	(0-0.3)
Lymphocytes:	1.5 x 10⁹/L	(1.0-4.9)
Monocytes:	0.5 x 10⁹/L	(0-1.0)
Eosinophils:	0.0 x 10⁹/L	(0.0-0.3)

WBC morphology: No abnormalities seen

Hematocrit:	35%	(30-51)
Red blood cell count:	9.15x 10¹²/L	(6.5-12.8)
Hemoglobin:	13.0 g/dl	(10.9-18.1)
MCV:	38.3 fl	(35.0-53.0)
MCHC:	37.0 g/dl	(34.6-38.0)

RBC morphology: No abnormalities seen.

Platelets: Clumped but appear adequate

Fibrinogen:	200 mg/dl	(100-400)

Glucose:	↑ 123 mg/dl	(71-106)
BUN:	↑ 54 mg/dl	(13-25)
Creatinine:	↑ 3.6 mg/dl	(0.9-1.7)
Phosphorus:	↑ 5.6 mg/dl	(2.8-5.1)
Calcium:	10.6 mg/dl	(10.2-13.0)
Total Protein:	↓ 4.0 g/dl	(5.2-7.1)
Albumin:	2.8 g/dl	(2.4-3.8)
Globulin:	↓ 1.2 g/dl	(2.6-3.8)
Sodium:	137 mEq/L	(130-145)
Chloride:	97 mEq/L	(97-105)
Potassium:	3.6 mEq/L	(3.0-5.0)
HCO3:	29.9 mEq/L	(25-31)
Total Bili:	↑ 8.3 mg/dl	(0.6-1.8)
ALP:	↑ 1601 IU/L	(109-352)
GGT:	24 IU/L	(4-48)
SDH:	2.0 IU/L	(1-5)
AST:	226 IU/L	(190-380)
CK:	↑ 1626 IU/L	(80-446)

Urinalysis: Free catch
Color: not indicated
Specific gravity: 1.025
pH: 6.0
Protein: trace
Glucose/ketones: negative
Sediment: not done

Interpretation

CBC: No abnormalities

Serum Biochemical Profile

Hyperglycemia: This may be attributable to stress, however neonatal foal serum glucose may be higher than adults, with an average of 135-150 mg/dl (Vaala).

Azotemia and hyperphosphatemia: Common causes of increased serum phosphorus include skeletal growth in immature horses, endurance exercise, and decreases in glomerular filtration rate secondary to acute renal failure or pre-renal causes. The signalment of this foal suggests that at least part of the hyperphosphatemia is age-related. The average phosphorus of a neonatal foal is 5-6 mg/dl. However General is also azotemic. Because of high milk intake, foals generally produce large volumes of dilute urine, and specific gravity readings of 1.018-1.025 are indicative of maximal concentration (Madigan). General's urine specific gravity is somewhat concentrated, so the azotemia is likely pre-renal.

Hypoproteinemia: Low total protein in neonatal animals may reflect the increased total body water content, however albumin is within reference range. The globulins are often lower in young animals because of a relatively naïve immune system. Given the perinatal history, evaluation of passive transfer status using a test such as IgG is recommended.

Hyperbilirubinemia: Neonatal foals have higher serum bilirubin values than adult horses (average 4.3 mg/dl), however this is still elevated even for a foal. In horses, anorexia should always be considered as a cause of hyperbilirubinemia. Hemolysis is another possible cause of hyperbilirubinemia. Although his PCV is normal, this foal should be monitored for evidence of developing neonatal isoerythrolysis.

Increased ALP: This is likely an age-related change due to increased release of the bone isoform of ALP secondary to skeletal growth and development. Bone disease is a consideration because of General's clinical presentation.

Increased CK: Increased CK indicates muscle damage and is compatible with the history of dystocia and lameness. CK may be a more sensitive indicator of muscle damage than AST.

Case Summary and Outcome

General was treated with nutritional supplementation after the death of his mother. Over a few days, his mobility improved and his prognosis was considered good. Repeat blood work 24 hours after presentation showed diminished azotemia and normal CK. His serum phosphorus normalized with a persistently elevated ALP, indicating that the initial hyperphosphatemia was more likely related to the pre-renal azotemia than bone growth. Unless otherwise specifically indicated, reference ranges for domestic animal species are usually generated in adult animals. It is important to consider the potential impact of signalment, including age, on "normal" values for clinical pathology data. This case can be compared with Spunky (Chapter 2, Case 1), a puppy with age related changes in calcium, phosphorus, and ALP. Interpretation of data on analytes that could be influenced by age should be considered in light of clinical signs and other laboratory data. For example, because General had a high risk history and concurrent azotemia, his hyperphosphatemia was considered to potentially be related to decreased glomerular filtration rate, while Spunky had hyperphosphatemia but no other laboratory data suggesting alterations in glomerular filtration rate. In both General and Spunky, the absence of any other liver enzyme elevations to accompany the increased ALP was taken as evidence of an age-related change rather than an indication of liver disease. In General, this interpretation was slightly more difficult because of the concurrent hyperbilirubinemia, which could be compatible with cholestasis/liver disease. Here, species variation plays a role in interpretation, because anorexic horses commonly have hyperbilirubinemia unrelated to hepatic pathology.

Madigan JE. Oliguria and stranguria. In: Large Animal Internal Medicine, 3rd ed. Bradford P. Smith, ed. Mosby, St. Louis, MO. pp. 371-372.

Vaala WE, House JK, Madigan JE. Initial management and physical examination of the neonate. In: Large Animal Internal Medicine, 3rd ed. Bradford P. Smith, ed. Mosby, St. Louis, MO. pp. 277-293.

Case 9 – Level 2

"Nevada" is a 17-year-old Hackney cross gelding. Five days prior to presentation, Nevada had an episode of colic, which was treated with non-steroidal anti-inflammatory medication. After treatment, Nevada's signs of colic improved, however he did not regain his attitude or a normal appetite. He has been polyuric and polydipsic for the past two days. On presentation, Nevada was bright, alert, and responsive. He had increased dental plaque and a soft systolic heart murmur with maximal intensity over the mitral valve.

White blood cell count:	7.8×10^9/L	(5.9-11.2)
Segmented neutrophils:	5.5×10^9/L	(2.3-9.1)
Band neutrophils:	0.0×10^9/L	(0-0.3)
Lymphocytes:	2.1×10^9/L	(1.6-5.2)
Monocytes:	0.2×10^9/L	(0-1.0)
WBC morphology: No morphologic abnormalities seen.		

Hematocrit:	36%	(30-51)
Red blood cell count:	6.98×10^{12}/L	(6.5-12.8)
Hemoglobin:	12.8 g/dl	(10.9-18.1)
MCV:	51.9 fl	(35.0-53.0)
MCHC:	35.6 g/dl	(34.6-38.0)
RBC morphology: Normal		

Platelets: Appear adequate in number.

Fibrinogen:	↑ 500 mg/dl	(100-400)

Glucose:	117 mg/dl	(60.0-128.0)
BUN:	↑ 33 mg/dl	(11-26)
Creatinine:	↑ 2.6 mg/dl	(0.9-1.9)
Phosphorus:	2.4 mg/dl	(1.9-6.0)
Calcium:	↑ 15.4 mg/dl	(11.0-13.5)
Magnesium:	2.1 mg/dl	(1.7-2.4)
Total Protein:	6.4 g/dl	(5.6-7.0)

Albumin:	3.1 g/dl	(2.4-3.8)
Globulin:	3.3 g/dl	(2.5-4.9)
A/G Ratio:	0.9	(0.6-2.1)
Sodium:	132 mEq/L	(130-145)
Chloride:	↓ 98 mEq/L	(99-105)
Potassium:	4.7 mEq/L	(3.0-5.0)
HCO3:	28 mEq/L	(25-31)
Anion Gap:	10.7 mEq/L	(7-15)
Total Bili:	0.7 mg/dl	(0.3-3.0)
Direct bili:	0.2 mg/dl	(0.0-0.5)
Indirect bili:	0.5 mg/dl	(0.2-3.0)
ALP:	155 IU/L	(109-352)
GGT:	↑ 43 IU/L	(5-23)
AST:	↑ 415 IU/L	(190-380)
CK:	↑ 2691 IU/L	(80-446)

Urinalysis: Voided urine

Appearance: straw and clear

Urine specific gravity: 1.011

pH: 6.0

Protein, glucose, ketones, bilirubin: negative

Sediment: Occasional erythrocytes and leukocytes seen. No casts, crystals, or bacteria noted.

Interpretation

CBC

Leukogram: The slight increase in fibrinogen could be compatible with mild inflammation. While the site of the inflammation cannot be determined from this value alone, there may be residual inflammation from the colic. Acute phase reactants such as fibrinogen may be more sensitive indicators of inflammation in some species, therefore the normal leukogram does not rule out inflammation.

Serum Biochemical Profile

Azotemia: Azotemia with isosthenuria usually suggests renal failure, as long as extrarenal factors that could impair renal concentrating ability are ruled out (for example osmotic diuresis, medullary washout, and some endocrinopathies, see Chapter 5). Some authors describe a relatively high BUN/creatinine ratio of greater than 10:1 with chronic renal failure in horses versus a ratio less than 10:1 with acute renal failure. It is common for pre-renal azotemia to become superimposed on primary renal failure in dehydrated patients. The colic episode may have exacerbated previously subclinical chronic renal disease in this patient, causing fluid deficits.

Hypercalcemia with normal phosphorus: Hypercalcemia with normal to low phosphorus is often described in equine patients with chronic renal failure. This is in contrast to small animal patients, who generally have hyperphosphatemia and a somewhat unpredictable calcium status. PTH does not appear to be responsible for the hypercalcemia in horses. Rather it appears to be related to dietary intake of calcium and may reflect inability of the dysfunctional kidneys to eliminate dietary calcium. Hypercalcemia in horses with chronic renal failure is often worse on alfalfa hay and may improve on grass hay. Therefore, not all horses with chronic renal failure will have hypercalcemia. Horses with acute renal failure may be more likely to have low total serum calcium.

Mild hypochloremia with low normal sodium: Hyponatremia and hypochloremia may be noted in horses with both acute and chronic renal failure. Previous isotonic or hypertonic fluid losses associated with colic and replaced with oral intake of water may further depress serum electrolytes. Pain associated with colic can result in sweating, which can be another significant source of sodium and chloride loss. Mild hyperkalemia has been described in horses with chronic renal failure or severe acute renal failure, but was not present in Nevada at presentation.

Increased GGT: In an adult horse, increased GGT is evidence of liver damage or cholestasis. Liver damage may be attributed to the previous episode of colic, or associated with hepatic lipidosis from the recent anorexia. Severe cholestasis is unlikely with the normal bilirubin.

Increased AST and CK: AST is present in multiple tissues and elevations can be difficult to interpret. Nevada's increased GGT and AST suggests some liver pathology, however the concurrent increase in CK indicates that muscle damage is also likely and may be responsible for some of the increase in AST. Like GGT, elevations in AST are not specific as to the etiology of the tissue damage. Increases in CK can be associated with intramuscular injection, trauma during transportation, and muscle damage with down or rolling animals.

Urinalysis: Normal horse urine is often cloudy because of high mucus content and the presence of calcium carbonate crystals, while horses with renal failure may have clear urine because of the production of high volumes of dilute urine and relative calcium retention (Figure 6-3). Herbivore urine is generally alkaline, however, the urine pH may decrease with uremic or lactic acidosis.

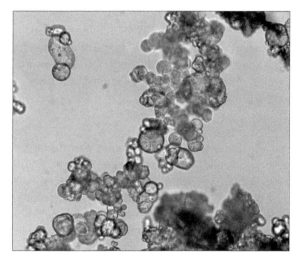

Figure 6-3. Normal equine urine with calcium carbonate crystals.

Case Summary and Outcome
Nevada was treated with intravenous fluids and his azotemia resolved. The combination of laboratory abnormalities and clinical signs, including polyuria/polydipsia and increased dental plaque, were considered to be consistent with chronic renal failure. His episode of colic resulted in temporary decompensation and the development of pre-renal azotemia superimposed on his more chronic renal disease.

Nevada may be compared with Margarite (Chapter 5, Case 9). Margarite had more advanced disease than Nevada, and in addition to the abnormalities shared with Nevada, had hypophosphatemia, and hyperkalemia. As with small animal patients, anemia may be present in horses with renal failure, although it was not present in either Nevada or Margarite at presentation.

Nevada may also be contrasted with Faith (Chapter 5, Case 19) or General (Case 8), cases of pre-renal azotemia. Note that Faith had hypocalcemia and hyperphosphatemia, which is more common in horses with pre-renal azotemia or acute renal failure than in horses like Nevada or Margarite with chronic renal failure. Faith had concentrated urine at the time of presentation, which would suggest that she had adequate renal function. However, she was treated with high doses of non-steroidal anti-inflammatory medications, which can be nephrotoxic under some circumstances. Other cases of renal disease in large animals include Forsythia (Chapter 5, Case 20, llama) and Lucinda (Chapter 5, Case 25, goat).

Case 10 – Level 2

"Austin" is a 6-year-old Labrador Retriever/Beagle mix, castrated male dog. He presented with a 2 week history of lethargy and poor appetite and a 3 day history of vomiting. His owners have noted dark stool over the past few days. Three years previously, Austin had been evaluated for elevated liver enzymes, and chronic active hepatitis and fibrosis was found on biopsy. Austin was treated at the referring clinic with intravenous fluids and antibiotics. He was transferred to the referral institution after he developed ascites. On physical examination, Austin has mild icterus and moderate ascites. While he is very lethargic, he does not appear to be showing clinical signs of hepatic encephalopathy.

White blood cell count:	12.3 x 10⁹/L	(4.9-16.8)
Segmented neutrophils:	10.8 x 10⁹/L	(2.8-11.5)
Band neutrophils:	0.0	(0-0.3)
Lymphocytes:	↓ 0.6 x 10⁹/L	(1.0-4.8)
Monocytes:	0.7 x 10⁹/L	(0.1-1.5)
Eosinophils:	0.2 x 10⁹/L	(0-1.4)

WBC morphology: No abnormalities noted.

Hematocrit:	↓ 37%	(39-55)
Red blood cell count:	↓ 4.94 x 10¹²/L	(5.8-8.5)
Hemoglobin:	↓ 12.8 g/dl	(14.0-19.1)
MCV:	72.4 fl	(60.0-75.0)
MCHC:	34.6 g/dl	(33.0-36.0)
Nucleated RBC/100 WBC	1	

RBC morphology: There is slightly increased anisocytosis and polychromasia with occasional basophilic stippling.

Platelets:	↓ 134 x 10⁹/L	(181-525)

Occasional macroplatelets are seen.

Plasma is icteric

Glucose:	↓ 59 mg/dl	(67.0-135.0)
BUN:	↓ 6 mg/dl	(8-29)
Creatinine:	0.6 mg/dl	(0.6-2.0)
Phosphorus:	3.4 mg/dl	(2.6-7.2)
Calcium:	↓ 8.8 mg/dl	(9.4-11.6)
Magnesium:	1.7 mEq/L	(1.7-2.5)
Total Protein:	↓ 5.3 g/dl	(5.5-7.8)
Albumin:	↓ 2.2 g/dl	(2.8-4.0)
Globulin:	3.1 g/dl	(2.3-4.2)

A/G Ratio:	0.7	(0.7-2.1)
Sodium:	144 mEq/L	(142-163)
Chloride:	115 mEq/L	(106-126)
Potassium:	↓ 3.0 mEq/L	(3.8-5.4)
HCO3:	18 mEq/L	(15-28)
Anion Gap:	14 mEq/L	(8-19)
Total Bili:	↑ 2.50 mg/dl	(0.1-0.3)
ALP:	↑ 2954 IU/L	(20-320)
GGT:	↑ 20 IU/L	(2-10)
ALT:	↑ 579 IU/L	(18-86)
AST:	↑ 221 IU/L	(16-54)
Cholesterol:	129 mg/dl	(82-355)
Triglycerides:	188 mg/dl	(30-321)
Amylase:	426 IU/L	(409-1203)

Coagulation Profile

PT:	↑ 11.1s	(6.2-9.3)
APTT:	↑ 18.3s	(8.9-16.3)
FDP:	↑ >20 µg/ml	(<5)

Urinalysis: Voided

Appearance: Yellow and clear

Specific gravity: 1.008

Protein, glucose, ketones: negative

Bilirubin: 2+

Sediment: Occasional white blood cells were seen. No red blood cells, casts, bacteria, epithelial cells, or crystals seen.

Interpretation

CBC

Leukogram: The mild lymphopenia is compatible with a corticosteroid/stress effect. There is currently no mature neutrophilia or monocytosis, but these can be less consistent features of the corticosteroid leukogram.

Erythrogram: The mild normocytic normochromic anemia may reflect the effects of chronic disease or liver disease. The recent onset of dark stools and the hypoalbuminemia suggest the potential for gastrointestinal blood loss as well. Blood loss anemias are typically regenerative, however if the blood loss is mild, acute, or if other factors such as chronic disease are blunting a response, they may appear non-regenerative. The anisocytosis, polychromasia, and basophilic stippling could be compatible with some marrow response and serial CBC's with reticulocyte counts may demonstrate some marrow activity. The clinical significance of a single nucleated erythrocyte/100 WBC is questionable and may be encountered in a normal animal. Endothelial damage of any cause or lesions of the hematopoietic tissues could result in premature release of nucleated erythroid precursors.

Thrombocytopenia: In combination with data from the coagulation profile, the thrombocytopenia could be compatible with disseminated intravascular coagulation (DIC). Because there is also a non-regenerative anemia, primary marrow disorders could be considered, however extramarrow causes can explain Austin's CBC abnormalities.

Serum Biochemical Profile

Hypoglycemia: Artifactual hypoglycemia was ruled out in this case. Given the chronic history of liver disease, decreased liver function and inadequate gluconeogenesis should be evaluated as a potential cause for low blood glucose. Other abnormalities that would support this cause include low BUN and albumin with evidence of ongoing liver disease (increased liver enzymes), however specific tests of liver function such as serum bile acids and blood ammonia should be performed (See Chapter 2). Nutritional factors are unlikely to cause hypoglycemia unless the body condition score is low, and there are other signs of starvation. Paraneoplastic hypoglycemia is possible, but not supported by the physical examination.

Low BUN: As described above, decreased liver function should be investigated as a cause for low BUN in this case. Polyuria and polydipsia, which is likely in this case given the low urine specific gravity, can also contribute to low BUN because of rapid tubular flow rates and inadequate time for urea reabsorption (See Chapter 5, Case 22). The dark stools suggest gastrointestinal bleeding, which conversely may increase BUN. It appears that the degree of hemorrhage is insufficient to offset the decreases in BUN produced by the other mechanisms.

Hypocalcemia: Because a significant amount of total serum calcium is protein bound, low serum protein is expected to decrease total serum calcium. The biologically active ionized fraction is not expected to change, therefore clinical signs of hypocalcemia are unlikely. Correction formulas have been developed for the dog, however their clinical application in disease may be questionable (Schenck).

Hypoproteinemia with hypoalbuminemia: The low albumin with normal globulins suggests selective loss or decreased production of albumin. Routes of protein loss include skin, third space, the gastrointestinal tract, and the kidneys. Renal losses are most likely to be selective for albumin; other types of protein loss are more likely to result in nonselective loss of both albumin and globulins. Renal losses of protein are less likely in the absence of measurable amounts of proteinuria, however Austin's urine is dilute and a urine protein:creatinine ratio may be a more sensitive measure of urine protein content. Inadequate production of albumin by a poorly functional liver can also result in disproportionately low albumin and is likely in this case. While some globulin proteins are produced in the liver, immunoglobulin production is unaffected because it is extrahepatic. Globulins may even increase in patients with liver failure as generalized immune stimulation can result from inadequate Kupffer cell surveillance of portal blood and increased systemic exposure to bacteria and toxins from the gut. Some gastrointestinal protein loss is suspected because of the dark stool, however if globulin values were initially high because of the decreased liver function, the decrease attributable to GI losses may merely bring previously increased values back into the normal range.

Hypokalemia: Poor intake combined with third space losses (ascites) and possible gastrointestinal losses of potassium explain the hypokalemia.

Hyperbilirubinemia: The major causes of hyperbilirubinemia are decreased liver function, cholestasis, hemolysis or sepsis. Decreased liver function with or without cholestasis are likely based on the serum biochemical profile. Hemolysis is possible because of the anemia, however specific morphologic abnormalities of the erythrocytes such as spherocytes or Heinz bodies that would explain hemolysis are not described. Like blood loss anemias, hemolytic anemias are generally regenerative, however if mild or acute, there may be no evidence of regeneration (see discussion of erythrogram above). There is no evidence of sepsis in the CBC as a cause for increased serum bilirubin.

Increased ALP and GGT: While there are many nonspecific causes of increased ALP and GGT in the dog (See Chapter 2), cholestasis and liver disease are the most likely source of the increased enzymes in this case.

Increased ALT and AST: Increases in these enzymes indicate hepatocellular damage, but do not imply a cause. The previous histologic diagnosis of chronic active hepatitis is sufficient to account for hepatocellular damage. It is important to note that while increased liver enzymes do provide evidence of hepatic pathology, they are not liver function tests. If sufficient numbers of hepatocytes are lost, liver enzyme levels may return to baseline levels despite continuing liver disease and decreased liver function. An acute decrease in PCV with associated hypoxia could further damage liver cells. AST is less liver specific than the ALT and may increase with muscle damage. Measurement of creatine kinase would help determine if muscle damage could account for some of the increase in AST.

Coagulation profile: The prolonged clotting times, thrombocytopenia, and increased FDPs are compatible with disseminated intravascular coagulation (DIC). Alternatively, sufficiently impaired liver function will prevent production of adequate amounts of coagulation factors and prolong the PT and APTT. In addition, because the liver is responsible for clearance of fibrin degradation products, decreased liver function will also result in increased FDPs. Regardless, the patient is still considered to have a coagulopathy.

Urinalysis: Polyuria can characterize liver failure (See Chapter 2 for details, also see Chapter 2, Case 10; Chapter 3, Case 7; Chapter 5, Case 12). The significance of small numbers of leukocytes in the absence of bacteria in a voided sample is unclear, however urine culture could be considered to rule out the possibility of a urinary tract infection.

Case Summary and Outcome

A repeat ultrasound of the liver revealed a small, irregularly nodular liver, compatible with cirrhosis. Blood ammonia concentration was within the reference interval, however serum bile acids were not measured. Blood ammonia is a less sensitive test of decreased liver function than serum bile acids, and the preponderance of other laboratory data is compatible with decreased liver function. Because of the availability of the previous liver histopathology result and the abnormal coagulation data, another biopsy was not performed. Austin was hospitalized and treated with intravenous fluids, antibiotics, gastroprotectants, and small doses of diuretics to reduce the ascites. Minimal improvement was noted in the laboratory values, however Austin appeared brighter and his ascites was reduced. He was discharged to his owners on medical management with a guarded to poor long term prognosis.

Other cases of hypocalcemia and hypoalbuminemia related to decreased liver function include hepatic lipidosis (Chapter 2, Case 11) and portosystemic shunt (Chapter 2, Case 12). Recall that extrahepatic causes of hypoalbuminemia also can result in low total serum calcium. Although low total serum calcium is often attributed to hypoalbuminemia, some patients have significantly low serum albumin associated with a variety of conditions and yet maintain total serum calcium concentrations within reference intervals. This is true for YapYap (Chapter 3, Case 7), who presented with a portosystemic shunt and more severe hypoalbuminemia than Austin (1.8 g/dl compared with 2.2 g/dl), yet his total serum calcium was within reference intervals. A variety of physiological influences including pH and competitive binding of calcium or albumin with other substances in the blood can influence the relationship of total serum calcium and albumin in individual patients.

Schenck PA, Chew DJ. Prediction of serum ionized calcium by use of total serum calcium concentration in dogs. Am J Vet Res 2005;66:1330-1336.

Case 11 – Level 2

"Star" is an 8-year-old spayed female Cairn terrier presenting with a several month history of increased water consumption and urination. Over the last week, Star has become anorexic and started vomiting. On physical examination, Star is quiet, depressed, and dehydrated. Her blood pressure was elevated, and on ultrasound examination, her kidneys were small.

White blood cell count:	10.8 x 10⁹/L	(4.9-16.9)
Segmented neutrophils:	9.0 x 10⁹/L	(3.0-11.0)
Band neutrophils:	0 x 10⁹/L	(0-0.3)
Lymphocytes:	1.1 x 10⁹/L	(1.0-4.8)
Monocytes:	0.4 x 10⁹/L	(0.2-1.4)
Eosinophils:	0.3 x 10⁹/L	(0-1.3)
WBC morphology: No abnormalities noted.		

Hematocrit:	↓ 31%	(37-55)
MCV:	69.7 fl	(60.0-75.0)
MCHC:	33.9 g/dl	(33.0-36.0)
RBC morphology: Slightly increased anisocytosis		

Platelets: Appear adequate

Glucose:	86 mg/dl	(65.0-120.0)
BUN:	↑ 212 mg/dl	(8-29)
Creatinine:	↑ 27.6 mg/dl	(0.5-1.5)
Phosphorus:	↑ 15.6 mg/dl	(2.6-7.2)
Calcium:	↑ 15.6 mg/dl	(8.8-11.7)
Magnesium:	↑ 3.0 mEq/L	(1.4-2.7)
Total Protein:	6.5 g/dl	(5.2-7.2)
Albumin:	3.3 g/dl	(3.0-4.2)
Globulin:	3.2 g/dl	(2.0-4.0)
Sodium:	151 mEq/L	(142-163)
Chloride:	↓ 110 mEq/L	(111-129)
Potassium:	↓ 3.6 mEq/L	(3.8-5.4)
HCO3:	↓ 12 mEq/L	(15-28)
Anion Gap:	↑ 32.6 mEq/L	(8-19)
Total Bili:	0.20 mg/dl	(0.10-0.50)
ALP:	42 IU/L	(12-121)
GGT:	4 IU/L	(3-10)
ALT:	27 IU/L	(10-95)
AST:	33 IU/L	(15-52)
Cholesterol:	↑ 360 mg/dl	(110-314)
Triglycerides:	47 mg/dl	(30-300)
Amylase:	↑ 2629 IU/L	(400-1200)

Urinalysis: Cystocentesis

Appearance: Straw and clear	Sediment:
Specific gravity: 1.014	rare RBC/hpf
pH: 5.5	occasional WBC/hpf
Glucose, ketones, bilirubin: negative	0-5 transitional epithelial cells
Heme: trace	
Protein: 100 mg/dl	

Interpretation

CBC: There is a normocytic, normochromic anemia, that is likely nonregenerative. The anemia may be more severe once fluid deficits are corrected. Anemia of chronic disease is possible, however the azotemia and relatively dilute urine in a dehydrated patient suggests renal disease as a cause for non-regenerative anemia.

Serum Biochemical Profile

Azotemia and dilute urine with dehydration: This combination of laboratory abnormalities is suggestive for renal failure, but there are exceptions when extra-renal factors interfere with renal concentrating ability. If the patient is dehydrated, a pre-renal component may be superimposed on the other causes of azotemia.

Hyperphosphatemia and hypercalcemia: The hyperphosphatemia is most likely attributable to decreased glomerular filtration rate, whether due to renal or pre-renal factors. Calcium changes unpredictably in renal failure, and total calcium may be high, low or normal. In middle-aged and older patients, hypercalcemia of malignancy should also be considered because cancer is an important cause of increased calcium in this demographic.

Hypermagnesemia: Decreased glomerular filtration rate causes increased serum magnesium.

Hypokalemia: Decreased intake associated with anorexia and increased losses via the gastrointestinal tract combine with increased renal losses due to polyuria to lower serum potassium values.

Mild hypochloremia: This is likely due to loss through vomiting.

Mild acidemia (decreased HCO3) with increased anion gap: These changes may be related to uremic acidosis. Lactic acidosis from anemia and poor tissue perfusion secondary to dehydration may also contribute to these laboratory abnormalities.

Hypercholesterolemia: Hypercholesterolemia has been described in canine patients with glomerulonephritis and glomerular amyloidosis. Increases in cholesterol have been attributed to a combination of increased hepatic synthesis and decreased catabolism of lipoproteins. Decreased plasma albumin may stimulate hepatic synthesis of some lipoproteins, and lipoprotein lipase required for lipid metabolism is decreased due to absence of stimulation by heparin sulfate, which is often low in patients with nephrotic syndrome. Although cholesterol levels are said to vary inversely with albumin, some renal disease patients with hypoalbuminemia have normal cholesterol levels (Chapter 5, Case 5), while others have normal serum albumin but elevated cholesterol (Chapter 5, Cases 10 and 17).

Hyperamylasemia: The most likely cause for this change is the decreased GFR, supported by the azotemia and hyperphosphatemia. Clinical signs are vague and include gastrointestinal abnormalities, so pancreatic disease cannot be completely ruled out.

Urinalysis: Because white blood cells were noted in a urine sample collected by cystocentesis, the potential for a urinary tract infection should be evaluated by urine culture. The finding of 100 mg/dl of protein in a poorly concentrated urine sample is also of concern. A urine protein:creatinine ratio is recommended as a more sensitive way to evaluate the proteinuria. It is important to consider that the proteinuria may be the result of lower urinary tract disease rather than glomerular lesions if there is evidence of inflammatory/infectious processes.

Case Summary and Outcome

Star was treated with intravenous fluids, antihypertensive medication, and gastroprotectants. Her urine culture was negative and the urine protein:creatinine ratio was markedly elevated, compatible with glomerular disease. The clinicians decided against performing a renal biopsy to confirm this impression because they did not feel that additional information that would alter the treatment plan would be gained and they were concerned about complications from the procedure. Star was discharged from the hospital, however she returned a week later after developing diarrhea. On presentation she was very weak, and had pale mucous membranes and melena. It was thought that Star had developed gastrointestinal ulceration from uremia and she was humanely euthanized because of her poor prognosis.

Hypoalbuminemia is often used as a criterion for the diagnosis of glomerular disease, however several factors may influence serum albumin levels. At presentation, Star was dehydrated, which increased her serum albumin. In addition, patients with healthy livers and an adequate diet can often maintain serum albumin concentrations for some period of time despite significant losses. Patients that do have hypoalbuminemia associated with glomerular disease may have total serum hypocalcemia, however this is not always the case. For example, Sheba (Chapter 5, Case 5) presented with hypoalbuminemia that was attributed to renal disease, however her total serum calcium was within reference intervals. The unpredictable effects of renal disease on calcium may contribute to complexity in the relationship between total serum calcium and albumin. As always with renal disease, serum ionized calcium must be measured for optimal evaluation of calcium status (Schenck).

Schenck PA, Chew DJ. What's new in assessing calcium disorders-Part 1. In 21st Annual American College of Veterinary Internal Medicine Proceedings. June 4-8, 2003, Charlotte, NC. pp 517-518.

Case 12 – Level 3

"Jill" is a 3-year-old spayed female indoor/outdoor domestic short haired cat. She presented recumbent and poorly responsive to stimuli. When the cat came inside last night, she was lethargic and vomited. On physical examination, Jill is bradycardic, hypothermic, and obtunded. The urinary bladder could not be located on abdominal palpation.

Glucose:	↑ 304 mg/dl	(70.0-120.0)
BUN:	↑ 185 mg/dl	(15-32)
Creatinine:	↑ 10.2 mg/dl	(0.9-2.1)
Phosphorus:	↑ 22.6 mg/dl	(3.0-6.0)
Calcium:	↓ 4.8 mg/dl	(8.9-11.6)
Magnesium:	↑ 3.1 mEq/L	(1.9-2.6)
Total Protein:	5.5 g/dl	(5.5-7.6)
Albumin:	2.4 g/dl	(2.2-3.4)
Globulin:	3.1 g/dl	(2.5-5.8)
Sodium:	149 mEq/L	(149-164)
Chloride:	↓ 102 mEq/L	(119-134)
Potassium:	↑ 9.1 mEq/L	(3.9-5.4)
HCO3:	↓ 11 mEq/L	(13-22)
Anion Gap:	↑ 45 mEq/L	(13-27)
Total bili:	0.2 mg/dl	(0.10-0.30)
ALP:	42 IU/L	(10-72)
GGT:	<3 IU/L	(3-10)
ALT:	↑ 190 IU/L	(29-145)
AST:	↑ 129 IU/L	(12-42)
Cholesterol:	97 mg/dl	(77-258)
Amylase:	791 IU/L	(496-1874)

Urinalysis: Urine could not be obtained

Interpretation

No CBC was performed because of financial limitations

Serum Biochemical Profile

Hyperglycemia: The most likely cause for the hyperglycemia in this case is stress. Concurrent illness may exacerbate the effects of stress on blood glucose concentration (Rand).

Azotemia: The azotemia in this patient is difficult to categorize as pre-renal, renal, or post-renal because there is no information about urinary concentrating ability. The absence of a palpable urinary bladder could be compatible with failure of urine production or ruptured bladder secondary to urethral blockage or trauma such as being hit by a car. The electrolyte abnormalities are compatible with uroabdomen (see Chapter 5, Case 18), however there is no description of fluid accumulation in the peritoneal cavity. Because the cat goes outdoors, the history provided by the owners may be incomplete.

Hyperphosphatemia and hypocalcemia: Hyperphosphatemia in this case is most likely due to decreased glomerular filtration rate and the inability to eliminate urine from the body. Calcium levels are variable in renal failure and total values may not correlate with ionized calcium as they often do in patients with normal renal function. Hypocalcemia may occur secondary to hyperphosphatemia, and acute renal failure can result in more pronounced hypocalcemia than chronic renal failure because of inadequate time for physiologic compensation. Early effects of ethylene glycol intoxication can include hyperphosphatemia because of the high content of this mineral in the antifreeze fluid. Calcium may be chelated by metabolites of ethylene glycol resulting in hypocalcemia. The owners should be questioned about access to anti-freeze.

Hypochloremia and increased anion gap: Hypochloremia in the absence of hyponatremia may be due to disproportionate loss of chloride with vomiting, which was noted in the clinical history. Hypochloremia can also be associated with acid/base abnormalities. The low bicarbonate supports the presence of acidemia, however the markedly elevated anion gap suggests a greater acid/base disturbance than the mildly low HCO3 would suggest. Uremic acidosis may combine with vomiting induced alkalosis to create a mixed acid/base disorder. Candidates for unmeasured anions contributing to the high anion gap in this case include uremic acids, lactic acid (poor perfusion and dehydration), or exogenous acids, including metabolites of ethylene glycol.

Hyperkalemia: Hyperkalemia is most often present in acute or acute-on-chronic renal failure patients with low urine output and reflects inadequate renal elimination of potassium.

Increased ALT and AST: The elevated ALT is compatible with hepatocellular damage; AST is less tissue specific and could also reflect cellular damage of other tissues such as muscle. Inadequate perfusion of many tissues is likely in a patient presenting with bradycardia and hypothermia.

Case Summary and Outcome

Jill was treated with a bolus of fluids and calcium gluconate, however there was little response and no urine production was observed. She was euthanized due to poor prognosis. After further questioning, the owner did recall leakage of anti-freeze from one of the family cars, but no necropsy was performed to pursue a definitive diagnosis.

This case should be compared with Brianna (Chapter 5, Case 21), a dog with renal failure secondary to ethylene glycol ingestion. Both Jill and Brianna had the classical azotemia with hypocalcemia and hyperphosphatemia that may characterize ethylene glycol toxicity, however a more complete data base was obtained for Brianna that was able to document isosthenuria. Characteristic calcium oxalate crystals were not noted in either patient. Electrolyte patterns were similar in these two cases, however Jill also had liver enzyme elevations, probably attributable to her more serious perfusion deficits on presentation.

Based on the calcium/phosphorus pattern, other differentials for Jill could have included renal disease of other etiologies including urethral obstruction (see Chapter 5, Case 7 with hypocalcemia and hyperphosphatemia), acute pancreatitis with decreased glomerular filtration rate, and hypoparathyroidism (Case 3). Remember that amylase is a poor indicator of pancreatitis in cats, so the normal value in this patient should not be used to rule out this diagnosis, however most cats have a more chronic and indolent form of the disease. Hypoparathyroidism by itself is unlikely to account for the azotemia.

Rand JS, Kinnaird E, Baglioni A, Blacksahw J, Priest J. Acute stress hyperglycemia in cats is associated with struggling and increased concentrations of lactate and norepinephrine. J Vet Intern Med 2002;12:123-132.

Case 13 – Level 3

"Isabelle" is a 2-year-old spayed female Cocker Spaniel presenting for a two week history of lethargy, weight loss, intermittent trembling and anorexia. She has been vomiting yellow liquid three times a day. She responded temporarily to intravenous fluid therapy however she is now ill again. On physical examination, Isabelle is thin (2/5 body condition score), approximately 12% dehydrated, and has bradycardia with thready pulses. Muscle tremors are noted.

White blood cell count:	↑ 15.0 x 10⁹/L	(4.1-13.3)
Segmented neutrophils:	↑ 11.8 x 10⁹/L	(3.0-11.0)
Band neutrophils:	0 x 10⁹/L	(0-0.3)
Lymphocytes:	1.8 x 10⁹/L	(1.0-4.8)
Monocytes:	0.9 x 10⁹/L	(0.2-1.2)
Eosinophils:	0.5 x 10⁹/L	(0-1.3)

WBC morphology: No significant abnormalities noted.

Hematocrit:	50%	(37-55)
MCV:	67.3 fl	(60.0-77.0)
MCHC:	35.5 g/dl	(31.0-34.0)

Platelets:	254 x 10⁹/L	(200-450)

Glucose:	96mg/dl	(65.0-120.0)
BUN:	↑ 98 mg/dl	(8-33)
Creatinine:	↑ 6.4 mg/dl	(0.5-1.5)
Phosphorus:	↑ 11.6 mg/dl	(3.0-6.0)
Calcium:	↑ 12.5 mg/dl	(8.8-11.0)
Magnesium:	↑ 3.9 mEq/L	(1.4-2.7)
Total Protein:	↑ 7.9 g/dl	(5.2-7.2)
Albumin:	↑ 4.3 g/dl	(3.0-4.2)
Globulin:	3.6 g/dl	(2.0-4.0)
Sodium:	↓ 128 mEq/L	(140-151)
Chloride:	↓ 97 mEq/L	(105-120)
Potassium:	↑ 9.4 mEq/L	(3.8-5.4)
HCO3:	↓ 13.5 mEq/L	(16-25)
Anion Gap:	↑ 26.9 mEq/L	(15-25)
Total Bili:	0.5 mg/dl	(0.1-0.5)
ALP:	67 IU/L	(20-320)
GGT:	4 IU/L	(3-10)
ALT:	63 IU/L	(10-95)
AST:	42 IU/L	(15-52)
Cholesterol:	305 mg/dl	(110-314)
Amylase:	↑ 1732 IU/L	(400-1200)

Interpretation

CBC: There is a mild mature neutrophilic leukocytosis that could reflect mild inflammation, although no bands or toxic features are present to confirm this impression. A corticosteroid leukogram is unlikely since the lymphocyte numbers are within the reference range.

Serum Biochemical Profile

Azotemia: Isabelle is significantly dehydrated on physical examination, therefore a component of the azotemia is pre-renal. No urine specific gravity is available, so renal azotemia cannot be excluded at this time.

Hyperphosphatemia and hypercalcemia: Renal failure, vitamin D toxicity, and hypoadreno-corticism can produce these changes. Both renal failure and hypoadrenocorticism are compatible with the other laboratory data. In both these conditions, inadequate glomerular filtration rate decreases elimination of phosphorus and leads to its accumulation in the blood. Hypoadrenocorticism is a common cause of hypercalcemia in dogs, but is not associated with increases in ionized calcium and is therefore not pathogenic. Diminished renal excretion of calcium due to cortisol deficiency and hemoconcentration are potential mechanisms for the hypercalcemia. The calcium level should normalize quickly after initiation of therapy. Hypercalcemia of malignancy is common in dogs and should always be considered, however malignant neoplasia is less likely in young dogs.

Hypermagnesemia: Decreased glomerular filtration rate is the cause for the high magnesium.

Hyperproteinemia with hyperalbuminemia: Because the liver does not produce excess albumin (see Chapter 4), hyperalbuminemia is evidence for hemoconcentration. This is compatible with the dehydration described in the physical examination.

Hyponatremia and hypochloremia: Even though Isabelle has been anorexic, inadequate intake is rarely the cause of low sodium and chloride in small animal patients on commercial diets. Given her history, gastrointestinal losses are possible. Electrolytes may also be lost through the skin or into body cavities, however potassium is often lost as well, and Isabelle is hyperkalemic. Renal losses of sodium and chloride can be quantified by performing urinary fractional excretions. Patients with hyponatremia should have low urinary fractional excretion of sodium as the body attempts to conserve the electrolyte. Normal to increased fractional excretion of sodium under these circumstances would be abnormal and reflect either renal disease or hypoadrenocorticism. With Addisonians, the lack of aldosterone release from the adrenal gland results in a failure to conserve sodium by the kidney.

Hyperkalemia: Hyperkalemia is most often the result of inability to eliminate adequate amounts of potassium through the kidneys. In combination with hyponatremia and hypochloremia, it is characteristic of hypoadrenocorticism. Potassium may also accumulate with anuric/oliguric renal failure or in association with post-renal azotemia due to urethral blockage or uroabdomen. Discriminating between these differential diagnoses requires a thorough physical examination and history with ancillary laboratory data such as urinalysis and ACTH stimulation testing.

Low HCO3 and high anion gap: The acidemia and elevated anion gap in this case may be related to either uremic acidosis or lactic acidosis secondary to poor tissue perfusion. Because most of the anion gap in health is due to negatively charged proteins, the hyperal-buminemia could also contribute to increased anion gap.

Increased amylase: The mild change in this value is most compatible with the decreased glomerular filtration rate, although gastrointestinal disease can also be associated with increased amylase and is compatible with the clinical history. Pancreatic disease cannot be ruled out, but is not required to explain this data.

Case Summary and Outcome

Isabelle was treated with shock doses of intravenous fluids to correct her dehydration and to help decrease her serum potassium levels by increasing renal excretion via diuresis. An adrenocorticotropin hormone (ACTH) stimulation test did not demonstrate any response. Her baseline cortisol was 0.3 μg/dl (0.5-4.0 reference interval) and her post-ACTH stimulation cortisol was 0.2 μg/dl (8.0-20.0 reference interval). Isabelle was treated for hypoadrenocorticism (Addison's disease). The abnormalities on her serum biochemical profile normalized over the next few days and she was discharged from the hospital.

Isabelle can be compared with other cases of hypoadrenocorticism, including Kazoo (Chapter 3, Case 12) and Miranda (Chapter 5, Case 23). In contrast to Isabelle and Miranda, Kazoo did not initially have the classical electrolyte abnormalities that usually characterize hypoadrenocorticism. In addition, his protein values were low because Kazoo had a history of a gastrointestinal foreign body and surgery that resulted in hypoproteinemia. These factors may have contributed to his normal calcium value, although only about one third of patients with hypoadrenocorticism are hypercalcemic. Miranda's serum biochemical profile abnormalities more closely approximate Isabelle's, however like Kazoo, Miranda was hypoglycemic. While sepsis may have contributed to Kazoo's hypoglycemia, low blood glucose is a feature of hypoadrenocorticism that Isabelle did not have.

Case 14 – Level 3

"Deputy" is a 10-year-old castrated male English Springer Spaniel presenting with a history of severe pyoderma and allergic dermatitis. On presentation, Deputy is dull and depressed and is in lateral recumbency in his kennel. He is dehydrated, has abdominal distension, and icteric mucous membranes. Crusted, ulcerative lesions extend along Deputy's entire dorsal surface and down the length of all four limbs.

White blood cell count:	8.7 x 10⁹/L	(6.0-17.0)
Segmented neutrophils:	7.3 x 10⁹/L	(3.0-11.0)
Band neutrophils:	0.0 x 10⁹/L	(0-0.3)
Lymphocytes:	↓ 0.4 x 10⁹/L	(1.0-4.8)
Monocytes:	0.9 x 10⁹/L	(0.2-1.4)
Eosinophils:	0.1 x 10⁹/L	(0-1.3)
WBC morphology: No abnormalities noted		

Hematocrit:	↓ 34%	(37-55)
MCV:	71.9 fl	(64.0-73.0)
MCHC:	33.6 g/dl	(33.6-36.6)
RBC morphology: Appears within normal limits.		

Platelets:	↓ 62 x 10⁹/L	(200-450)

Glucose:	99 mg/dl	(65-120)
BUN:	↑ 48 mg/dl	(8-33)
Creatinine:	↑ 3.1 mg/dl	(0.5-1.5)
Phosphorus:	↑ 7.9 mg/dl	(3.0-6.0)
Calcium:	↑ 13.9 mg/dl	(8.8-11.0)
Magnesium:	2.2 mEq/L	(1.4-2.2)
Total Protein:	4.9 g/dl	(4.7-7.3)
Albumin:	↓ 1.8 g/dl	(3.0-4.2)
Globulin:	3.1 g/dl	(2.0-4.0)
A/G Ratio:	↓ 0.6	(0.7-2.1)
Sodium:	144 mEq/L	(140-163)
Chloride:	110 mEq/L	(105-126)
Potassium:	4.8 mEq/L	(3.8-5.4)
HCO3:	22.8 mEq/L	(15-25)
Anion Gap:	18 mEq/L	(5-18)
Total Bili:	↑ 2.7 mg/dl	(0.1-0.5)
ALP:	↑ 663 IU/L	(20-320)
GGT:	↑ 21 IU/L	(2-10)
ALT:	↑ 220 IU/L	(10-86)
AST:	↑ 218 IU/L	(15-52)
Cholesterol:	↓ 108 mg/dl	(110-314)
Amylase:	408 IU/L	(400-1200)

Coagulation Profile

PT:	↑ 12.8s	(6.2-7.7)
APTT:	11.8s	(9.8-14.6)
FDP:	↑ >20 μg/ml	(<5.0)

Interpretation

CBC: Deputy has a mild normocytic normochromic, likely nonregenerative anemia that could be compatible with chronic disease. The anemia may be worse once fluid deficits are corrected. If renal azotemia is documented, renal failure should be considered as a contributor to nonregenerative anemia. In combination with the thrombocytopenia, a primary marrow disorder is possible, and marrow evaluation should be considered if peripheral factors cannot account for the cytopenias. A thorough drug history should be taken to ensure that no myelo-suppressive medication has been administered. Alternative causes for the anemia include acute blood loss with insufficient time for marrow response. This is possible if there is hemorrhage associated with the thrombocytopenia. Hemolysis is a consideration because of the presence of icterus, however there are no morphologic abnormalities of the erythrocytes described that might suggest a stimulus for hemolysis (spherocytes, agglutination, Heinz bodies, etc.). Hemolytic anemias also are typically regenerative unless the patient presents in very acute stages or there are other factors suppressing marrow response.

Given the severe skin lesions, the lack of an inflammatory leukogram is surprising. An inflammatory response may be masked by increased tissue migration of neutrophils. The lymphopenia is likely associated with endogenous corticosteroid effects or may potentially be related to therapeutic corticosteroid use for the skin disease. Protein losing enteropathy may also be associated with a lymphopenia.

The thrombocytopenia may be related consumption of platelets secondary to immune-mediated clearance, hemorrhage, endothelial damage, or as part of disseminated intravascular coagulation. DIC would be be compatible with the results of the coagulation profile. Viral infections and neoplasia should also be ruled out. As noted above, a primary marrow disorder may account for thrombocytopenia if production of platelets is suppressed.

Serum Biochemical Profile

Azotemia: The azotemia cannot be definitively classified without a urine specific gravity. Deputy is dehydrated on presentation, so at least a component of the azotemia is attributable to pre-renal factors.

Hypercalcemia with hyperphosphatemia: Older small animal patients with hypercalcemia should be evaluated for the presence of neoplasia. In this case, ultrasound with cytology or biopsy of the liver should be a top priority because of the icterus and enzyme elevations. Hypercalcemia of malignancy usually causes a compensatory decrease in phosphorus, however this may be complicated by decreased renal phosphorus excretion secondary to the decreased glomerular filtration rate suspected in this dog. Renal failure could also result in this combination of abnormalities. Ionized calcium is more likely to be elevated in patients with hypercalcemia of malignancy than renal failure. Parathyroid hormone related protein (PTHrP) is often elevated in hypercalcemia of malignancy, but would expected to be normal in patients with renal failure. Primary hyperparathyroidism can cause increases in total and ionized calcium, but generally causes hypophosphatemia unless renal issues complicate the presentation (See Case 6, Picasso). Less likely differential diagnoses include Vitamin D toxicosis and hypoadrenocorticism. Hypoadrenocorticism is less likely given the normal electrolytes and lymphopenia, but an atypical presentation is possible. If there is evidence of lameness or bone pain, the patient should be examined for osteolytic lesions.

Hypoalbuminemia: Because Deputy is dehydrated, both albumin and globulin levels may decrease after fluid therapy. Both decreased production and increased losses should be evaluated as contributors to low serum albumin. Decreased liver function can lead to inadequate production of albumin. With liver disease, other laboratory abnormalities would be expected such as hypoglycemia (inadequate hepatic gluconeogenesis), low BUN, hypocholesterolemia, hyperbilirubinemia, prolongation clotting times (inadequate production of clotting factors or vitamin K absorption), mildly increased FDPs (decreased hepatic clearance), and the production of poorly concentrated urine (multiple mechanisms, see Chapter 2, Case 10). While Deputy has some of these abnormalities, none are specific for liver failure. Serum bile acids or blood ammonia measurements should be considered if liver function requires further evaluation. Albumin production may also decrease in patients with significant inflammatory disease because albumin is a negative acute phase reactant. Nutritional factors may impair albumin synthesis, but this is rare and generally associated with severe or prolonged starvation and poor body condition (See Chapter 5, Case 3).

Hypoalbuminemia may also occur with increased losses of albumin. In this case, loss of protein via exudative skin lesions is likely. Additional protein could be lost into the abdominal effusion or with hemorrhage, although bleeding is not described in the clinical history. Protein also may be lost via the gastrointestinal tract or kidneys. Most types of protein loss result in wasting of both albumin and globulins, but glomerular protein losses are relatively selective for albumin. Because the hypoalbuminemia is associated with normal globulins in this patient, glomerular disease is possible, but cannot be evaluated adequately because urinalysis data is not available. Because Deputy likely has significant inflammatory disease, he is likely to be hyperglobulinemic but nonspecific protein losses may have reduced the globulin levels back to within reference intervals.

Hyperbilirubinemia: Hemolysis is a possible cause for increased serum bilirubin and is discussed in the CBC section. Liver disease is another important consideration. The potential for cholestasis is supported by elevations in ALP and GGT, though they may also be elevated due to enzyme induction if Deputy has been treated with corticosteroids for his skin lesions. Decreased liver function could impair hepatocellular uptake of bile (see section on hypoalbuminemia), and sepsis may interfere with bile uptake (See Chapter 2, Case 8). Expected leukogram abnormalities associated with sepsis are not present, however Deputy presents in poor condition with extensive compromise of the skin barrier that could predispose him to bacteremia. The abnormalities of the coagulation profile are compatible with either liver failure or DIC secondary to sepsis.

Increased ALP and GGT: Elevations in ALP and GGT are supportive of cholestasis. There are numerous extrahepatic causes of liver enzyme elevations that should also be considered, however the concurrent hyperbilirubinemia makes liver disease more likely. Liver enzyme elevations alone are not helpful in identifying a specific cause for liver disease. Liver damage may occur secondary to numerous systemic processes, including sepsis and disseminated intravascular coagulation. Cholestasis also may occur secondary to cell swelling associated with hepatocellular damage.

Increased ALT and AST: These enzyme elevations indicate hepatocellular damage. ALT is more liver specific than AST, which originates from many tissues. As stated above, primary liver disease must be distinguished from numerous other potential causes of hepatocellular insult. The toxic effects of bile retention associated with cholestasis can cause hepatocellular damage. In this case, cholestatic and hepatocellular enzyme elevations are of similar magnitude, so a predominant process cannot be presumed.

Hypocholesterolemia: This abnormalitiy is of limited clinical significance, but can occur with poor liver function (See Chapter 3, Case 7), hypoadrenocorticism (See Chapter 3, Case 12), or protein-losing enteropathy (also compatible with lymphopenia).

Coagulation profile: The combination of thrombocytopenia, prolonged coagulation times, and >20 µg/dl FDPs is compatible with DIC. Increased FDPs are often used to support a diagnosis of DIC, although they are neither sensitive nor specific and may increase with liver failure due to decreased clearance or be associated with hemorrhage. In liver failure, both prothrombin time (PT) and normal activated partial thromboplastin time (APTT) are usually prolonged, however this can be inconsistent early in the course of disease. The prolonged PT and normal APTT may be seen early in cases of Vitamin K antagonist poisoning because of the short half-life of Factor VII, which is in the extrinsic pathway. Ultimately, both the PT and APTT usually become prolonged with Vitamin K antagonism.

Case Summary and Outcome

Two liters of fluid were removed from Deputy's abdomen, and he was treated with plasma, crystalloids, and antibiotics. Abdominal ultrasound revealed abnormal nodules throughout the liver and spleen. Multiple lymph nodes throughout the abdomen were enlarged, and the stomach wall was thickened. Cytology samples from the liver were diagnostic for lymphoma, and impression smears from the skin indicated pyogranulomatous inflammation of unknown cause. Deputy was euthanized due to deteriorating condition and poor prognosis. On necropsy, the liver, lymph nodes, and adrenal glands contained evidence of lymphoma, however the spleen was histologically normal. Unfortunately, bone marrow was not evaluated to assist with interpretation of the CBC abnormalities. The cause of the dermatitis was not determined.

The cause for the hypercalcemia was interpreted to be lymphoma, although measurement of PTHrP was not performed. Deputy's case may be compared with Chapter 2, Case 21 (Snoopy), who also had hepatic lymphoma but was not hypercalcemic. Most animals presenting with malignant neoplasia have normal serum calcium, however when the serum calcium is elevated, neoplasia should be considered. Deputy can also be compared with Cleopatra (Case 7), who had hypercalcemia accompanied by hyperglobulinemia and bone pain which led to diagnostic evaluation for multiple myeloma. The development of a diagnostic plan for evaluation of patients suspected to have hypercalcemia of malignancy is frequently guided by clinical signs or other laboratory data suggesting involvement of particular organs (bone in Cleopatra's case and the liver in Deputy's case).

Case 15 – Level 3

"Zinger" is an 11-year-old neutered male domestic short haired cat. Zinger was diagnosed with hypertrophic cardiomyopathy and mild left-sided congestive heart failure one month ago, for which he is being treated with diuretics (furosemide) and aspirin. Historical laboratory abnormalities at the time of diagnosis included prerenal azotemia (urine specific gravity 1.056) and mild elevations of ALT and AST that were interpreted to be compatible with the cardiac disease. His thyroid panel was within normal limits. Two weeks ago, Zinger presented with thrombosis of his right front foot, which was managed successfully with anticoagulants. Today, Zinger presents with a four day history of anorexia, vomiting, and decreased urinations. He is dehydrated, depressed, and has a very small bladder. Zinger's respiratory rate and effort are increased.

Hematocrit:	38%	(28-45)
Glucose:	↑ 235 mg/dl	(70.0-120.0)
BUN:	↑ 320 mg/dl	(15-32)
Creatinine:	↑ 22.7 mg/dl	(0.9-2.1)
Phosphorus:	↑ 24.9 mg/dl	(3.0-6.0)
Calcium:	8.9 mg/dl	(8.9-11.6)
Magnesium:	↑ 4.1 mEq/L	(1.9-2.6)
Total Protein:	6.2 g/dl	(5.5-7.6)
Albumin:	2.2 g/dl	(2.2-3.4)
Globulin:	4.0 g/dl	(2.5-5.8)
A/G Ratio:	0.55	(0.5-1.4)
Sodium:	↓ 130 mEq/L	(149-164)
Chloride:	↓ 91 mEq/L	(119-134)
Potassium:	↑ 7.6 mEq/L	(3.9-5.4)
HCO3:	↓ 9.6 mEq/L	(13-22)
Anion Gap:	↑ 37 mEq/L	(13-27)
Cholesterol:	↑ 235 mg/dl	(50-150)
CK:	↑ 1034 IU/L	(55-382)

Urinalysis: Catheter

Appearance: Yellow and clear	Sediment:
Specific gravity: 1.015	0 RBC/high power field
pH: 6.5	Rare WBC/high power field
Protein: 2+	No casts seen
Glucose: negative	No squamous or transitional epithelial cells are seen
Ketones: negative	No bacteria or crystals present
Bilirubin: negative	Trace fat droplets and debris
Heme: 1+	

Interpretation

Serum Biochemical Profile

Hyperglycemia: The hyperglycemia is likely stress-induced, although no supportive leukogram findings are available. The absence of glucose in the urine makes diabetes mellitus less likely.

Azotemia: Azotemia should be categorized as pre-renal, renal, or post-renal. The minimally concentrated urine supports the possibility of renal failure, and there is no evidence of post-renal disease (fluid in the abdomen or a large, firm bladder). In this case, Zinger's medical history includes therapy with diuretics, which are expected to decrease his urine specific gravity. Prior to diuretic use, Zinger had good urinary concentrating ability. At this time, it is not possible to determine the extent of the urinary concentrating ability in this patient, however he is extremely azotemic and evidence of continuing azotemia once any fluid deficits are corrected should be considered evidence of decreased renal function. In addition to dehydration, compromised cardiac function is a cause of pre-renal azotemia because of inability to maintain adequate perfusion pressure for glomerular filtration. Diuretics can subvert the body's attempt to maintain perfusion pressure through volume loading.

Hyperphosphatemia and normal calcium: The most likely cause of hyperphosphatemia in this patient is decreased glomerular filtration rate, regardless of whether the decreased glomerular filtration rate is due to pre-renal, renal, or post-renal causes. Tissue necrosis can also increase serum phosphorus by releasing intracellular phosphorus. Small animal patients in renal failure may have high, normal, or low serum calcium levels, and ionized calcium levels may not correlate with total calcium levels. The calcium as well as the albumin are at the low end of the reference range, and may reflect protein binding of the calcium to albumin. The presence of proteinuria in dilute urine without evidence of inflammation is suggestive for glomerular protein loss and urine protein:creatinine ratios can help quantify the losses.

Hypermagnesemia: Like phosphorus, serum magnesium levels will increase as glomerular filtration rate declines. In general, furosemide causes decreased serum magnesium. Severe rhabdomyolysis can lead to extracellular release of magnesium.

Hyponatremia and hypochloremia: The most likely cause of the hyponatremia in this case is the diuretic therapy and resultant water and electrolyte wasting by the kidneys. The corrected chloride indicates that the proportional decrease in chloride is greater than that of sodium, suggesting the potential for an acid/base disturbance.

Hyperkalemia: Both diuretics and the polyuric phase of chronic renal failure usually result in increased renal losses of potassium and hypokalemia. Hyperkalemia may develop when urine production decreases in oliguric or anuric renal failure, which is possible with the history of decreasing frequency of urinations and a small urinary bladder despite diuretic therapy. Because of the history of thromboembolic disease and the concurrent elevations in phosphorus, magnesium, and CK, tissue necrosis should be considered a potential cause for the hyperkalemia in this patient. An unlikely possibility is hypoadrenocorticism, which can be characterized by hyponatremia, hypochloremia and hyperkalemia with azotemia and inadequately concentrated urine (See Chapter 5, Case 23).

Decreased HCO3 and increased anion gap: This is compatible with metabolic acidosis associated with accumulation of unmeasured anions, such as uremic acids. In general, the chloride will vary inversely with the HCO3, which is not the case in this patient and a mixed acid/base disorder may be present. Blood gas analysis may be required for full characterization of the acid/base status. The history of cardiopulmonary disease and thromboembolic disease indicates that a respiratory component is likely.

Hypercholesterolemia: There are numerous potential causes for hypercholesterolemia in small animal patients, including metabolic disorders and endocrinopathies. In this case, hypercholesterolemia is probably associated with the renal disease.

Increased Creatine Kinase: This is evidence for muscle degeneration or necrosis, and raises the possibility of another episode of thromboembolic complications of the cardiac disease.

Urinalysis: The 2+ protein in dilute urine with an inactive sediment is compatible with glomerular loss of protein. A urine protein:creatinine ratio is recommended to further evaluate urinary protein losses. Given the inactive sediment in this case, the proteinuria is unlikely to be the result of blood contamination or lower urinary tract disease. Significant glomerular protein loss is not always associated with hypoalbuminemia because of the capacity of a healthy liver for compensatory upregulation of albumin production. Dehydration can also mask hypoproteinemia, which may be the case in this patient since the serum albumin is just at the lower end of the reference interval.

Case Summary and Outcome

Despite aggressive therapy, Zinger stopped producing urine and was euthanized. No necropsy was performed, but it was strongly suspected that acute renal failure could have been precipitated by additional thromboembolic episodes. The presence of hyperphosphatemia, hypermagnesemia, and hyperkalemia could be explained by the oliguric renal failure alone, however they are also compatible with tissue necrosis associated with ischemic damage to tissues. The high CK supports this interpretation, however CK can also be elevated in cats with urinary obstruction. If Zinger did develop a protein-losing nephropathy, loss of endogeneous anticoagulant proteins such as antithrombin III could have contributed to his predisposition to the abnormal formation of blood clots within his vasculature. This case can be compared with Lolita (Case 4), in which rhabdomyolysis resulted in elevated serum phosphorus and CK. Lolita had no evidence of renal disease at presentation, however.

Case 16 – Level 3

"Diva" is 5-year-old spayed female domestic short haired cat. After being missing for seven weeks, she was found in a garage. On presentation, she is obtunded, hypothermic (<90°F), bradycardic (30 bpm), and has very slow respiratory rate. Diva is cachectic and has lost approximately half of her previous body weight. Diva is profoundly dehydrated and blood pressure cannot be measured. She was immediately intubated for ventilation, and an intraperitoneal bolus of warmed physiologic saline was administered. Diva was extubated when she became responsive, and it was possible to collect blood samples for analysis and begin intravenous fluid therapy. However, generalized seizures and tetany followed, culminating in respiratory arrest with resuscitation. She was placed on a ventilator and weaned off over night. Parenteral nutrition was initiated on Day 2, at which time Diva was very weak but more stable. A transfusion was given on Day 3.

	Day 1	Day 3	Day 4	
White blood cell count:	↓ 1.8 x 10⁹/L	11.2	11.4	(4.9-16.8)
Segmented neutrophils:	↓ 0.6 x 10⁹/L	10.5	9.1	(2.8-11.5)
Band neutrophils:	0.1 x 10⁹/L	0.0	0.0	(0-0.3)
Lymphocytes:	1.0 x 10⁹/L	↓ 0.5	1.5	(1.0-4.8)
Monocytes:	↓ 0.0 x 10⁹/L	0.2	↓ 0.0	(0.1-1.5)
Eosinophils:	0.1 x 10⁹/L	0.0	0.8	(0-1.4)
Hematocrit:	↓ 27%	↓ 19	↓ 25	(39-55)
Hemoglobin:	↓ 9.3 g/dl	↓ 6.0	↓ 7.9	(14.0-19.1)
MCV:	49.7 fl	49.9	48.1	(39.0-56.0)
MCHC:	34.4 g/dl	33.0	33.0	(33.0-36.0)
Platelets:	218 x 10⁹/L	adequate	clumped	(181-525)

RBC morphology: Small Heinz bodies are present on Day 1

	Day 1	Day 3	Day 4	
Glucose:	83 mg/dl	↑ 200	↑ 348	(70.0-120.0)
BUN:	↑ 47 mg/dl	16	23	(15-32)
Creatinine:	1.2 mg/dl	↓ 0.5	↓ 0.4	(0.9-2.1)
Phosphorus:	5.6 mg/dl	4.0	↓ 1.9	(3.0-6.0)
Calcium:	9.4 mg/dl	↓ 8.0	8.9	(8.9-11.6)
Magnesium:	↑ 3.4 mEq/L	↓ 1.4	2.5	(1.9-2.6)
Total Protein:	↓ 5.2 g/dl	↓ 4.2	↓ 5.0	(6.0-8.4)
Albumin:	2.9 g/dl	↓ 2.3	2.6	(2.4.3.9)
Globulin:	↓ 2.3 g/dl	↓ 1.9	↓ 2.4	(2.5-5.8)
Sodium:	162 mEq/L	↓ 146	↓ 140	(149-164)
Chloride:	127 mEq/L	↓ 102	↓ 93	(119-134)
Potassium:	4.4 mEq/L	↓ 3.5	↓ 2.0	(3.6-5.4)
HCO3:	17 mEq/L	↑ 37	↑ 39	(13-22)
Total Bili:	0.2 mg/dl	↑ 0.9	↑ 0.4	(0.1-0.3)
ALP:	↑ 94 IU/L	↑ 118	↑ 123	(10-72)
GGT:	3 IU/L	<3	<3	(0-4)
ALT:	91 IU/L	76	66	(29-145)
AST:	↑ 135 IU/L	↑ 156	↑ 79	(12-42)
Cholesterol:	106 mg/dl	119	144	(50-150)
Triglycerides:	141 mg/dl	↑ 211	88	(25-191)
Amylase:	717 IU/L	487	559	(362-1410)

Manual of Veterinary Clinical Chemistry: A Case Study Approach

Interpretation

CBC: At presentation, Diva has marked neutropenia, secondary to margination of neutrophils associated with hypothermia. On day 3, there is a mild lymphopenia that could be attributable to corticosteroid effects. The monocytopenia is of no clinical significance. There is a normocytic normochromic anemia of variable severity throughout Diva's hospitalization. Some of the decrease between Day 1 and 3 is because of dilution following correction of fluid deficits and dehydration. Anemia of chronic disease and chronic malnutrition are the most obvious causes for this anemia, although the patient should also be evaluated for fleas/ticks and gastrointestinal parasites that could further depress the PCV. There also may be a hemolytic component as Heinz bodies were noted on Day 1. The clinical significance of Heinz bodies in cats depends on the number and size of the Heinz bodies. Sick cats frequently have small Heinz bodies that do not contribute significantly to development of anemia. A transfusion on Day 3 caused the increased in PCV on Day 4.

Serum Biochemical Profile Day 1

Increased BUN with normal creatinine: Because of Diva's extreme dehydration and poor perfusion, no urine could be obtained prior to initiating therapy. Given the fluid deficits, the increased BUN is very likely to reflect pre-renal factors. She should be monitored carefully for signs of decreased renal function because her kidneys may have been damaged by circulatory compromise of unknown duration. The marked muscle wasting associated with starvation may result in a lower creatinine measurement than would be expected for the degree of dehydration and pre-renal azotemia present in this patient.

Hypermagnesemia: This abnormality reflects the decreased glomerular filtration rate secondary to dehydration.

Hypoproteinemia with hypoglobulinemia: These values are likely to be even lower once fluid deficits are corrected, as seen on Day 3. Extreme food deprivation can result in hypoproteinemia, and is likely the cause of Diva's hypoproteinemia. Although most patients with starvation have hypoalbuminemia and normal globulins (see Chapter 5, Case 3), this is quite variable, and reversible hypoglobulinemia may occur (Kaneko). Other causes of decreased globulin proteins include various immunodeficiency states that are unlikely in this case. Increased losses of globulin proteins are generally commensurate with albumin wasting associated with hemorrhage, body cavity effusions, gastrointestinal lesions, or diffuse exudative dermal lesions (See Deputy, Case 14).

Increased ALP: There are fewer nonspecific causes of increased ALP in cats than dogs, and liver pathology is possible in this patient. Given the extreme weight loss and normal GGT, some degree of hepatic lipidosis is possible. Many cats with clinically significant hepatic lipidosis also will have elevations in bilirubin and ALT, which Diva does not have. Other considerations for this increase include poor perfusion, sepsis, trauma, or hyperthyroidism. The latter is not as likely in a relatively young cat.

Increased AST: Increased AST most often indicates liver or muscle pathology, however the ALT is not elevated to support hepatocellular damage. No CK levels are available to further evaluate muscle status. As with the ALP, poor perfusion, trauma, sepsis, and hyperthyroidism could elevate AST.

Serum Biochemical Profiles Days 3 and 4

Hyperglycemia: Carbohydrate intolerance and insulin resistance are frequently described consequences of introducing nutritional support after a period of starvation, however the mechanisms are not well understood (Brooks, Miller).

Low serum creatinine: This abnormality is likely related to the low muscle mass and correction of dehydration.

Hypophosphatemia: Hypophosphatemia is the most consistent and classical abnormality associated with the refeeding syndrome. Important mechanisms include decreased dietary intake, ineffective gastrointestinal absorption (decreased absorptive surface area with villous atrophy), and transcellular shift of phosphorus into cells (Miller). Respiratory, but not metabolic alkalosis will also exacerbate transcellular shifts of phosphorus because of an increased intracellular pH that activates glycolysis. Hypophosophatemia also has been reported with diabetes mellitus and hepatic lipidosis in addition to enteral alimentation in cats (Justin).

Hypocalcemia: This abnormality on Day 3 may be associated with the decreased albumin. Hypoalbuminemia is not a consistent feature of refeeding syndrome.

Hypomagnesemia: Low magnesium is related to dietary deficiency in combination with renal losses during catabolism of lean body mass. When nutritional support is implemented, magnesium requirements will increase as tissues are repaired and replenished, further draining already depleted body magnesium.

Hyponatremia may be the result of dilutional hyponatremia secondary to hyperglycemia in which osmotic forces from the glucose pull water into the circulation. Starvation causes sodium and water retention, however if water retention exceeds sodium retention, serum sodium will decline. Fluid retention in combination with reduced heart mass secondary to starvation can precipitate congestive heart failure in human patients. Obvious routes of excessive sodium loss are not present.

Hypochloremia and increased HCO3: Some of the decrease in chloride parallels changes in sodium. The degree of hypochloremia is greater than the degree of hyponatremia, however, suggesting the potential for acid/base abnormalities. The corrected chloride for Day 3 is 109 mEq/L and for Day 4 is 104 mEq/L. Diva has a hypochloremic alkalosis that could be associated with gastric vomiting or diuretic therapy. Alkalosis has been described in human patients with refeeding syndrome, however the mechanism is not clear.

Hypokalemia: Decreased dietary intake combined with insulin-stimulated cellular translocation can cause severe hypokalemia in starved patients that are provided with nutritional support.

Hyperbilirubinemia with increased ALP and AST: See Day 1 interpretation. The development of hyperbilirubinemia could be related to cholestasis with hepatic lipidosis. This is associated with a progressive rise in ALP. Severe hypophosphatemia may lead to hemolytic anemia, however this generally occurs when the serum phosphorus levels are less than 1.0 mg/dl.

Case Summary and Outcome

By Days 3 and 4, the classical laboratory abnormalities of hypophosphatemia, hypomagnesemia, and hypokalemia signaled the development of refeeding syndrome, and nutritional support was withdrawn until mineral and electrolyte imbalances could be corrected. At that time a more conservative rate of support was reinitiated with thiamine supplementation. By the second week of hospitalization, Diva was able to accept enteral feeding and occasionally ate small amounts of food on her own and began physical therapy. By the third week, Diva was still extremely weak, but was able to take a few steps on her own and was discharged from the hospital to her owners to continue supportive care at home. A recheck examination 10 days after discharge revealed progressively improved mobility and appetite, however Diva was still slightly weak in her rear limbs.

Diva's presentation illustrates the relatively mild serum biochemical abnormalities that accompany even profound starvation. During starvation in humans, metabolism shifts from being primarily dependent on carbohydrates to fat, with ketone bodies and free fatty acids supplying most of the energy in the body. Insulin levels drop. When carbohydrates are reintroduced during institution of nutritional support or "refeeding", phosphorus, magnesium, and potassium quickly translocate into cells, precipitating clinical signs related to musculoskeletal and nervous system dysfunction. Thiamine depletion is also exacerbated by increased demand associated with carbohydrate refeeding and this contributes to the development of clinical signs (Crook). The extent to which these pathophysiologic processes may be extrapolated to cats, which have a more protein-based metabolism is unclear (Zoran), however this case does illustrate many similarities to what is reported in the human literature.

Brooks MJ, Melnik G. The refeeding syndrome: An approach to understanding its complications and preventing its occurrence. Pharmacotherapy. 1995;15:713-726.

Crook MA, Hally V, Panteli JV. The importance of the refeeding syndrome. Nutrition. 2001;17:632-637.

Justin RB, Hohenhaus AE. Hypophosphatemia associated with enteral alimentation in cats. J Vet Intern Med 1995;9:228-233.

Kaneko JJ. Serum proteins and the dysproteinemias. In: Clinical Biochemistry of Domestic Animals, 5th ed. JJ Kaneko, JW Harvey, and ML Bruss, eds. Academic Press, San Diego, CA, 1997. pp 117-138.

Miller CC, Bartges JW. Refeeding syndrome. In: Kirk's Current Veterinary Therapy Small Animal Practice XIII. JD Bonagura, ed. W.B. Saunders Company, Philadelphia, PA. 2000. pp 87-89.

Zoran DL. The carnivore connection to nutrition in cats. J Am Vet Med Assoc 2002;221:1559-1567.

Case 17 – Level 3

"June" is a 10-year-old spayed female Soft Coated Wheaten Terrier presenting with a history of severe watery diarrhea. The diarrhea is associated with weight loss and anorexia, although no vomiting has been observed. Owners report that June has been drinking a lot of water. On presentation, June is bright and responsive but weak and is 5% dehydrated. June is thin with some muscle wasting. Auscultation is unremarkable, but she has a slightly tense abdomen on palpation.

Glucose:	↑ 127 mg/dl	(75.0-117.0)
BUN:	↓ 7 mg/dl	(9-31)
Creatinine:	↓ 0.3 mg/dl	(0.6-1.6)
Phosphorus:	↓ 3.0 mg/dl	(3.3-6.8)
Calcium:	↓ 6.9 mg/dl	(9.3-11.5)
Magnesium:	↓ 1.6 mEq/L	(1.7-2.4)
Total Protein:	↓ 3.0 g/dl	(5.0-6.9)
Albumin:	↓ 1.5 g/dl	(2.7-3.7)
Globulin:	↓ 1.5 g/dl	(1.9-3.3)
Sodium:	↓ 141 mEq/dL	(145-153)
Chloride:	116 mEq/dL	(109-118)
Potassium:	5.2 mEq/dL	(3.6-5.3)
Anion gap:	18.2	(15-28)
HCO3:	↓ 12 mEq/dL	(15-25)
Total Bili:	0.2 mg/dl	(0.1-0.5)
ALP:	↑ 352 IU/L	(8-139)
GGT:	↑ 17 IU/L	(2-10)
ALT:	↑ 617 IU/L	(22-92)
AST:	↑ 138 IU/L	(16-44)
Cholesterol:	↓ 85 mg/dl	(143-373)
Amylase:	438 IU/L	(275-1056)

Urinalysis (cystocentesis)

Appearance: Yellow and slightly cloudy
Specific gravity: 1.009
pH: 6.0
Glucose, bilirubin, ketones: negative
Occult blood: 2+
Protein: 1+
Sediment: Inactive other than small numbers of erythrocytes

Interpretation

No CBC was performed.

Serum Biochemical Profile

Hyperglycemia: This mild elevation may be post-prandial or related to stress or corticosteroid treatment. Diabetes mellitus is expected to be associated with greater deviations from the reference interval in most cases.

Low BUN: The small decrease in BUN could be associated with inadequate liver function, which could also explain the low serum albumin and cholesterol. Increased liver enzymes could also be compatible with hepatic pathology. Specific liver function tests such as serum bile acids are indicated. Alternatively, the low BUN could be related to low protein diet or the clinical history of polydipsia and poorly concentrated urine.

Low serum creatinine: This value may be attributed to the low muscle mass described in the history. Fluid loading and volume expansion also could contribute, however June is noted to be dehydrated on clinical examination.

Hypocalcemia and hypophosphatemia: Some proportion of the hypocalcemia is likely associated with the hypoalbuminemia, however ionized hypocalcemia has been reported in dogs with protein losing enteropathy (Kimmel, Kull, Melzer). It is speculated that low calcium and phosphorus levels may be related to poor intestinal absorption or impaired absorption of Vitamin D. Prolonged diuresis may also contribute to renal losses of phosphorus.

Hypomagnesemia: Low serum magnesium may reflect poor absorption and gastrointestinal losses, although renal losses cannot be excluded. Hypovitaminosis D, if present, could also contribute to low serum magnesium levels. Like calcium, the biologically active fraction of magnesium is ionized. Measurement of ionized magnesium is recommended if suspicious clinical signs develop.

Panhypoproteinemia: Decreases in both albumin and globulins suggests nonselective protein losses. In June's case, this most likely is occurring through the gastrointestinal tract. Inadequate food intake could exacerbate these losses. Additional losses of albumin may be occurring via the kidney, since both protein losing nephropathy and protein losing enteropathy have been identified as clinical syndromes in the soft coated wheaten terrier (Littman). Proteinuria is present. Because of the dilute urine, further quantification of urine protein losses should be performed by calculating a urine protein:creatinine ratio.

Mild hyponatremia with normal chloride: The decrease in sodium may be due to losses via the GI tract or the kidney. Anorexia rarely plays a significant role in the development of hyponatremia. Free water retention can dilute serum sodium, however, dehydration makes this unlikely.

Low HCO3 (acidemia): This abnormality likely reflects loss of bicarbonate containing fluid in the diarrhea. Poor perfusion associated with dehydration could result in lactic acidosis, however this is less likely with the anion gap within reference intervals.

Increased ALP and GGT: As discussed in Chapter 2, increased ALP in the dog is a nonspecific change that may be associated with drug effects, endocrinopathies, circulatory disorders, bone pathology, and cholestatic liver disease. Severe cholestatic liver disease is unlikely with a normal bilirubin. Further questioning of the owner revealed that June had been receiving a low dose of corticosteroids. However, the change in GGT is relatively greater than that for ALP, which is not typical for corticosteroid effects alone. June may have underlying liver disease, or liver enzyme elevations may occur secondary to intestinal pathology. Liver enzyme elevation with and without corresponding histopathologic changes have been reported in association with intestinal lymphangiectasia (Melzer).

Increased ALT and AST: These enzyme elevations suggest some degree of hepatocellular damage. The precise causes cannot be determined and are similar to those described for ALP and GGT.

Hypocholesterolemia: Gastrointestinal losses of cholesterol through compromised bowel and ruptured lacteals causes hypocholesterolemia.

Case Summary and Outcome

The liver appeared normal on ultrasonographic examination. Endoscopic biopsies of the stomach revealed mild infiltration of the lamina propria by lymphocytes, plasma cells and eosinophils. Multiple sections of small intestine contained a similar inflammatory cell population and dilated lacteals, which were also evident on endoscopic examination. Dilation of the lacteals may be secondary to the inflammation and could improve with immunomodulation. As a result, June's prednisone dose was increased, and another immunosuppressive drug was added to the treatment regimen.

Familial protein-losing enteropathy of soft coated wheaten terriers was considered as a potential diagnosis, however most of these dogs present at an earlier age, usually around 5 years old (Littman). The basis for this enteropathy is unclear, and evaluation of dietary factors including gluten sensitivity have produced equivocal data (German). It may be important to distinguish the familial syndrome from spontaneous protein-losing enteropathy because of the poor prognosis associated with the familial disease (Littman). Scoring indices to grade the severity of inflammatory bowel diseases have been described in an attempt to measure response to therapy and facilitate comparison between patients, however these do not always include laboratory parameters in the evaluation (Jergens).

German AJ, Hall EJ, Day MJ. Chronic intestinal inflammation and intestinal disease in dogs. J Vet Intern Med 2003;17:8-20.

Jergens AE, Schreiner CA, Frank DE, Niyo Y, Ahrends FE, Eckersall PD, Benson TJ, Evans R. A scoring index for disease activity in canine inflammatory bowel disease. J Vet Intern Med 2003;17:291-297.

Kimmel KJ, Waddell LS, Michel KE. Hypomagnesemia and hypocalcemia associated with protein-losing enteropathy in Yorkshire Terriers: five cases (1992-1998). J Am Vet Med Assoc 2000;217:703-706.

Kull PA, Hess RS, Craig LE, Saunders HM, Washabau RJ. Clinical, clinicopathologic, radiographic, and ultrasonagraphic characteristics of intestinal lymphangiectasia in dogs: 17 cases (1996-1998). J Am Vet Med Assoc 2001;219:197-202.

Littman MP, Dambach DM, Vaden SL, Giger U. Familial protein-losing enteropathy and protein-losing nephropathy in soft coated wheaten terriers: 222 cases (1983-1997). J Vet Intern Med 2000;14:68-80.

Melzer KJ, Sellon RK. Canine intestinal lymphangiectasia. Compendium Cont Educ Sm Anim Pract. 2002;24:953-960.

Case 18 – Level 3

"Glamor" is a 1-year-old Paint mare who presents with diarrhea. She is extremely depressed and her mucous membranes are dark red. She has ulcers on the muzzle and mucocutaneous junctions of the mouth. There is a marked swelling of the intermandibular region and large quantities of purulent discharge are draining from both nares and her mouth. Both submandibular lymph nodes have draining tracts. Loud crackles could be ausculted from all lung fields, but were worst ventrally. She has an elevated heart rate with a prolonged capillary refill time. A large corneal ulcer covered approximately half of her right eye. Her medical history included treatment with excessive quantities of non-steroidal anti-inflammatory medications.

White blood cell count:	↑ 18.5 x 10⁹/L	(5.9-11.2)
Segmented neutrophils:	↑ 15.9 x 10⁹/L	(2.3-9.1)
Band neutrophils:	0.0	(0-0.3)
Lymphocytes:	2.2 x 10⁹/L	(1.0-4.9)
Monocytes:	0.4 x 10⁹/L	(0-1.0)
Eosinophils:	0.0 x 10⁹/L	(0.0-0.3)
WBC morphology: Neutrophils are slightly toxic		

Hematocrit:	43%	(30-51)
Red blood cell count:	12.3 x 10¹²/L	(6.5-12.8)
Hemoglobin:	16.5 g/dl	(10.9-18.1)
MCV:	35.0 fl	(35.0-53.0)
MCHC:	38.0 g/dl	(34.6-38.0)
RBC morphology: Slight poikilocytosis		

Platelets: Clumped but appear adequate

Plasma color: Normal

Fibrinogen:	400 mg/dl	(100-400)

Glucose:	↑ 117 mg/dl	(75-115)
BUN:	↑ 143 mg/dl	(11-26)
Creatinine:	↑ 5.6 mg/dl	(0.9-1.9)
Phosphorus:	↑ 14.3 mg/dl	(1.9-6.0)
Calcium:	↓ 10.0 mg/dl	(11.0-13.5)
Magnesium:	↓ 1.5 mEq/L	(1.7-2.4)
Total Protein:	↑ 7.7 g/dl	(5.6-7.0)
Albumin:	↓ 2.1 g/dl	(2.4-3.8)
Globulin:	↑ 5.6 g/dl	(2.5-4.9)
A/G Ratio:	↓ 0.4	(0.7-2.1)
Sodium:	↓ 118 mEq/L	(130-145)
Chloride:	↓ 71 mEq/L	(97-105)
Potassium:	3.2 mEq/L	(3.0-5.0)
HCO3:	↓ 13 mEq/L	(25-31)
Anion Gap:	↑ 37.2 mEq/L	(7-15)
Total Bili:	2.5 mg/dl	(1.9-3.7)
ALP:	255 IU/L	(109-352)
GGT:	16 IU/L	(5-23)
AST:	↑ 602 IU/L	(180-570)
LDH:	↑ 622 IU/L	(140-440)
CK:	↑ 1081 IU/L	(80-350)

Urine specific gravity: 1.013

Tracheal wash: Smears consist of large numbers of poorly preserved neutrophils with a scant to moderate amount of mucus. Large numbers of bacteria of mixed morphology are present intracellularly and extracellularly. Both Gram negative and positive forms are present (Figure 6-4).

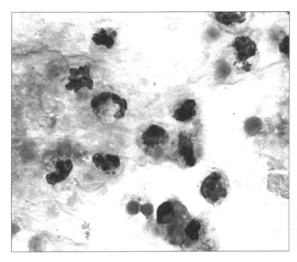

Figure 6-4. Equine tracheal wash with mucus and septic suppurtive inflammation.

Interpretation

CBC: Glamor has a neutrophilic leukocytosis with toxic changes compatible with inflammation.

Serum Biochemical Profile
Very mild hyperglycemia: This change is compatible with stress.

Azotemia with poorly concentrated urine: Poorly concentrated urine with increased BUN and creatinine in a dehydrated patient indicates renal azotemia, likely with a pre-renal component superimposed. Glamor does have electrolyte abnormalities that suggest that medullary washout may impair her ability to maximally concentrate her urine. The BUN, creatinine, and urine specific gravity should be re-evaluated after electrolyte abnormalities have been corrected.

Hypocalcemia with hyperphosphatemia: Glamor's total calcium concentration may be decreased by the concurrent low serum albumin. Large doses of NSIADS, especially in a dehydrated horse, can precipitate acute renal failure, characterized by azotemia, hypocalcemia and hyperphosphatemia. Hypoparathyroidism is unlikely, however poor parathyroid function can be associated with hypomagnesemia. Glamor's total serum magnesium is low, however the biologically active ionized fraction should be measured to assess the potential for magnesium-related hypoparathyroidism.

Hypomagnesemia: Low intake and increased gastrointestinal losses likely combine to cause the hypomagnesemia. Because significant amounts of serum magnesium are protein bound, hypoproteinemia may impact total serum magnesium values.

Hyperproteinemia with hypoalbuminemia and hyperglobulinemia: Low albumin with increased globulins suggests either decreased production of albumin or selective loss of albumin. Decreased production of albumin occurs with inflammation because albumin is a negative acute phase reactant. Severe or prolonged starvation can increase albumin utilization and decrease production, but is unlikely in this case if Glamor's body condition is adequate. Alternatively, severely decreased liver function can lead to deficits in albumin production. This cannot be ruled out in this patient because specific and sensitive tests of liver function such as blood ammonia and serum bile acids were not performed, however normal serum bilirubin,

ALP, and GGT make this less likely. Selective loss of albumin can result from glomerular disease; losses can be quantified by measuring urine protein:creatinine ratios. Although renal disease is strongly suspected in this case, there has been no evaluation of urine protein. Other potential routes for protein loss include the gastrointestinal tract (there is a history of diarrhea) and the draining tracts. Concurrent losses of globulins may be masked by markedly increased production associated with inflammation (acute phase reactants and immunoglobulins).

Hyponatremia and hypochloremia: Excessive electrolyte losses via the kidney or gastrointestinal tract are likely, although third spaces losses into the thorax or via exudative lesions are also possible. The decrease in chloride is disproportionately greater than that of the sodium. This can be seen if chloride is being preferentially lost or sequestered in a segment of the GI tract, but this is generally associated with alkalemia. Typically, HCO3 and chloride vary inversely unless there is a mixed acid/base disorder, which is likely in this case.

Decreased HCO3 with increased anion gap: High anion gap acidemia is associated with accumulation of unmeasured organic acids. In this case, uremic acidosis or lactic acidosis seem likely based on the clinical history and laboratory data. Because significant respiratory disease exists and there is data compatible with a mixed acid/base disorder, blood gas analysis is needed to fully characterize the abnormalities.

Increased AST, LDH, and CK: The increased AST and LDH could be compatible with liver disease. Intestinal disease alone can cause secondary hepatic pathology because portal blood delivers high quantities of bacteria, bacterial toxins, and inflammatory mediators to the liver. These enzymes are not liver specific and also may originate from muscle. Since the bilirubin, ALP, and GGT are within reference intervals and the elevated CK suggests muscle damage, liver disease may not be present. Muscle damage may be the result of poor perfusion secondary to dehydration and sepsis, hypoxemia secondary to respiratory disease, or muscle injury during transportation or with intramuscular injections.

Tracheal wash: This is compatible with septic suppurative inflammation.

Case Summary and Outcome

Glamor was treated with intravenous fluids, antibiotics, and topical ophthalmic medications. Her eye lesions did not respond to medical therapy, and the cornea eventually perforated and was treated surgically. Glamor's condition remained critical with decreasing serum protein levels, so total parenteral nutrition was instituted along with plasma transfusions. Her breathing and azotemia were improving with treatment, but several days later, Glamor began to bleed excessively from venipuncture sites. Her coagulation times were within reference intervals, but she was thrombocytopenic. Glamor died later that day. On necropsy, Glamor had multiple pulmonary abscesses, severe small intestinal enteritis, and ulcerative colitis. Multiple foci of necrosis were noted in both kidneys, compatible with the clinical suspicion of acute renal failure.

Multiple cases of renal failure in various species have been presented in previous chapters and can be compared with Glamor. In particular, the calcium and phosphorus data can be contrasted with Nevada (Case 9), who experienced temporary exacerbation of more chronic renal failure. Glamor's hypocalcemia and hyperphosphatemia is more compatible with acute renal disease in horses, while Nevada's low-normal phosphorus and hypercalcemia is characteristic of chronic renal failure. Nevada's pattern is repeated in Margarite (Chapter 5, Case 9). Horses in this book suspected of having pre-renal azotemia (Case 8 and Chapter 5, Case 19) had hyperphosphatemia and normal to high total serum calcium. The presence of concentrated urine is important in differentiating chronic renal failure from pre-renal azotemia. Dietary content of calcium may also influence the serum calcium data in patients with compromised renal function.

Overview

The regulation of calcium, phosphorus, and magnesium is very complex and diseases of many unrelated systems can influence the data.

Step 1: In the absence of clinical signs, it is recommended to verify any abnormal value by repeat measure. **Rule out artifacts,** such as collection of the sample in EDTA or the occasional spurious hypophosphatemia of unknown origin that is not repeatable with resampling (Case 1).

Step 2: Evaluate the serum protein level. Increases or decreases in serum protein may influence total serum calcium or magnesium values because of protein binding (Case 7, 10, 13, 16, 17, 18).

Step 3: Consider the effects of age or reproductive status. Young animals may have increased serum calcium or phosphorus associated with bone growth; this is sometimes associated with increased ALP. Bone remodeling for other reasons including infectious disease and neoplasia may cause similar changes in older animals. The demands of fetal development or lactation may lower serum calcium (Case 2 and Chapter 2, Case 1).

Step 4: Evaluate the patient for evidence of renal disease. The effects of renal disease on calcium and phosphorus levels vary with the type of renal disease and species. In general, phosphorus will increase with decrements in glomerular filtration rate (Case 8), while changes in total and ionized calcium are less predictable, especially in small animal species. In horses, chronic renal failure is often associated with hypercalcemia with or without hypophosphatemia (Case 9), while acute renal failure is more likely to be characterized by hypocalcemia and hyperphosphatemia (Case 17). Cats with urethral obstruction also sometimes have hypocalcemia (Chapter 5, Case 7). In some cases, hypercalcemia may be the cause rather than the result of renal dysfunction (Case 6, 7, 14). In other cases, intoxication (ethylene glycol) may cause both renal disease and abnormalities of calcium and phosphorus (Case 12). Protein losing nephropathy can be associated with hypocalcemia because of hypoalbuminemia (see Step 2).

Step 5: Consider the effects of gastrointestinal or pancreatic disease. Both colic in horses and pancreatitis in small animal patients can cause hypocalcemia and may be associated with pre-renal changes in glomerular filtration rate that influence phosphorus homeostasis (Chapter 5, Case 19). Diseases that alter gastrointestinal permeability can also influence calcium, phosphorus, and magnesium homeostasis (Case 17).

Step 6: Consider the potential for parathyroid disease. Primary hypoparathyroidism should be considered if there is true ionized hypocalcemia that cannot be attributed to another cause. Measurement of parathyroid hormone (PTH) can be helpful (Case 3). Primary hyperparathyroidism should be considered if other causes of ionized hypercalcemia are ruled out. Evaluation of the neck for the presence of masses in the area of the parathyroid gland helps to confirm this diagnosis (Case 5).

Step 7: Evaluate the patient for extra-parathyroid endocrinopathies that can alter calcium and phosphorus. Feline hyperthyroidism can increase serum phosphorus, and adrenal disease can alter total serum calcium (Case 13). Some malignant neoplasms produce PTHrP or other factors that can cause hypercalcemia (Case 14).

Step 8: Determine if there is a cause for cellular translocation of phosphorus. Cytoplasmic levels of phosphorus are high, and may leak from injured or necrotic tissue (Case 4, 15). Alternatively, phosphorus may translocate into cells due to the action of insulin (Case 16).

Chapter 7

Electrolyte and Acid/Base Evaluation

General Background

The regulation of electrolyte and acid/base balance is extremely complex. While a few basic mechanisms clearly influence this balance, it may be very difficult to determine the exact cause for an abnormality in an individual patient when multiple or complex disorders are present. Some pathophysiologic mechanisms reported in the veterinary medical literature appear to be species specific or are extrapolated from the human literature with no documentation of their significance in domestic animal species. Therefore, some of the mechanisms for abnormalities in the cases that follow may be somewhat speculative. As we have seen with many other analytes, the interpretation of indicators of electrolyte and acid/base status is dependent on history, physical examination findings, and other clinical laboratory data. It may be impossible to say with certainty what electrolyte abnormalities accompany a particular condition because of the influence of so many variables, including food intake, duration and severity of disease, or effects of treatment. Multiple examples of some entities are included in this chapter to demonstrate the variability of clinical chemistry abnormalities in patients with the same primary diagnosis.

Electrolyte concentrations in the blood reflect the electrolyte content of the extracellular fluid and do not accurately reflect intracellular content or total body stores of that electrolyte. **Serum electrolyte values are the sum of gains and losses** from the gastrointestinal tract, kidney, skin, third space (body cavities and interstitium), and intracellular space. In addition, serum electrolyte concentrations are influenced by the addition or loss of free water from the vascular space, so they should be interpreted in the context of the hydration status of the patient. For example, a bleeding patient proportionately loses both water and electrolytes, so initially the serum electrolyte values will be normal despite volume depletion in the intravascular space. Compensatory water retention by the kidney and increased thirst (presuming the patient is drinking water) may transiently dilute the remaining serum sodium until other mechanisms replace the needed electrolyte. The packed cell volume and total protein may provide additional information about free water balance, however primary or secondary disease processes may influence the production and/or losses of erythrocytes and protein. In some cases, multiple abnormalities combine to result in a normal value, which may mask underlying pathologic changes.

Acid/base status may be evaluated using parameters on the routine serum biochemical profile. HCO3, anion gap, and chloride can give information about acid/base status, but in some cases, a blood gas analysis will be required for further evaluation. Acid/base and electrolyte regulation are interconnected, so the data should be interpreted as an integrated whole. Patients with gastrointestinal and/or renal disease are particularly likely to have acid/base and electrolyte abnormalities because of the central roles of these organs in the uptake and elimination of these analytes. A complete discussion of the physiology of electrolyte and acid/base biochemistry is beyond the scope of this book, and the reader is encouraged to review any of the several excellent texts included in the recommended resources section prior to working the cases in this chapter.

Sodium

Sodium is the major cation in the extracellular fluid, including the serum. Sodium is often used by the body to drive cellular transport systems and water reabsorption. Serum sodium may be measured either by ion specific electrode or flame photometry. Ion specific electrode measurements are preferred because they less likely to be affected by the presence of hyperlipidemia or hyperproteinemia, which may artifactually depress electrolyte measurements performed using flame photometry. With direct potentiometric methods using ion specific electrodes, there is no dilution of the samples and lipemic interference with measurement of electrolyte concentrations is not anticipated. However, if an analyzer employs indirect potentiometry with ion specific electrodes in which the sample is diluted as part of the assay, artifactual lowering of electrolyte concentrations may be observed with severe lipemia. If both sodium and chloride are decreased in an obviously lactescent sample, another methodology should be used to confirm concentrations of these electrolytes. This underscores the need to be familiar with the laboratory that you use to run your samples.

As referred to above, serum sodium concentration reflects the ratio of sodium to water in the vascular space and so may be affected by alterations in free water balance independent of real changes in total body sodium. Likewise, proportional loss of both water and sodium will result in normal serum sodium concentrations despite dehydration and low total body sodium. Serum sodium is primarily regulated by the renin-angiotensin-aldosterone system and by regulation of plasma osmolality via central mechanisms including release of antidiuretic hormone.

Hypernatremia
1. ↑ sodium intake

2. ↓ renal excretion of sodium

3. Water depletion with concentration of remaining sodium

Normal Serum Sodium
Proportional gain or loss of water and sodium

Hyponatremia
1. ↓ sodium intake

2. ↑ sodium loss

3. Accumulation of free water with dilution of sodium

Chloride
Like sodium, there is abundant chloride in the extracellular fluid, while there is a smaller amount in the intracellular space dependent on the resting potential of the cell. Chloride is the principal anion filtered by the glomeruli and participates in acid/base balance in addition to being an important regulator of osmolality. Like sodium, movement of chloride across membranes can drive transcellular transport. In many patients, changes in serum chloride will mirror proportional changes in sodium based on gains and losses or fluid shifts. When there is a disproportionate change in chloride, acid/base status should be evaluated. To determine if the change in chloride is proportional to that of sodium, a corrected chloride can be calculated using the formula $(Cl^-)_{corrected}=(Cl^-) \times$ midrange normal sodium$/(Na^+)$. In uncomplicated acid/base disorders, chloride will often vary inversely with the serum bicarbonate (also an anion). If this is not the case, a mixed acid base disorder should be suspected. Methodologic considerations are similar to those described for sodium. Additionally, bromide from potassium bromide may be measured as chloride by some analyzers resulting in artifactual increases in Cl^-.

Hyperchloremia
1. With a proportional change in sodium, see hypernatremia

2. With a disproportionte change in sodium consider acid/base disorder

Normal Serum Chloride
1. See normal serum sodium

2. If the patient is hypernatremic or has a low serum bicarbonate, normal serum chloride may be inappropriate

Hypochloremia
1. With a proportional change in sodium, see hyponatremia

2. With a disproportionate change in sodium, consider acid/base disorder, sequestration or diuretic use.

Potassium

Potassium is the major intracellular cation, however serum levels are approximately equivalent to the extracellular fluid concentration, which is much lower. Therefore, the majority of potassium is in the cell and is not routinely measured, making serum potassium concentration a poor indicator of total body potassium. Potassium is required for the normal function of many enzymes and is critical in generating the normal resting cell membrane potential. Some clinical signs associated with hyper- and hypokalemia are the result of altered membrane excitability because of changes in the resting potential of cells. Like sodium and chloride, serum potassium may be measured using ion specific electrode or flame photometry methods. Also like the other electrolytes, the serum potassium level reflects the sum of intake and loss, however serum potassium concentration is further modulated by transcellular shifts. This is quantitatively more important than with the other electrolytes because of its predominantly intracellular location. Intracellular shifts of potassium can be triggered by insulin and catecholamines, while tissue damage can result in the release of intracellular potassium. Inorganic acidosis associated with some types of diarrhea or renal disease may cause hyperkalemia because potassium shifts out of cells to accommodate the influx of hydrogen ion that occurs to compensate for the acidosis. This does not appear to be a significant issue with organic acidosis or respiratory acid/base imbalances. In general, dietary potassium intake is matched by urinary output. A smaller amount of potassium is lost in feces, however colonic secretion can increase if the kidney is not able to excrete adequate amounts of potassium to maintain homeostasis.

Hyperkalemia
1. ↑ intake

2. ↓ excretion

3. Cellular translocation

Normal Serum Potassium
The cumulative effects of abnormalities in intake, excretion, and translocation can result in a normal value despite significant alterations in potassium homeostasis.

Hypokalemia
1. ↓ intake

2. ↑ losses

3. Cellular translocation

Bicarbonate

Bicarbonate is a major body buffer participating in acid/base homeostasis. It is produced from water and carbon dioxide by red blood cells, renal tubular cells, and cells in the stomach lining.

Increased Serum Bicarbonate (alkalosis)

1. Loss of hydrogen ion

2. Gain of bicarbonate

Decreased Serum Bicarbonate (acidosis)

1. Loss or depletion of bicarbonate

2. Increased production of acid

3. Decreased excretion of acid

Anion Gap

The anion gap is a calculated value used to approximate anions that are not specifically measured on the serum biochemical profile. Because electrochemical neutrality must be achieved, the "anion gap" may be estimated by the difference in measured cations and anions.

Anion gap=$([Na^+] + [K^+]) - ([Cl^-] + [HCO3^-])$

Normal components of the anion gap include negatively charged proteins, organic anions, phosphates and sulfates. Fluctuations in the serum content of these components can influence the anion gap, as can accumulation of a variety of anionic organic acids such as lactic acid, ketoacids, or metabolites of compounds such as ethylene glycol. Therefore, increased anion gap often implies acidemia.

Increased Anion Gap

1. Increased production or accumulation of endogenous acids

2. Increased exogeneous anions as a result of toxicity or metabolism of toxic compounds

3. Hyperalbuminemia associated with dehydration

Decreased Anion Gap (nonspecific change that does not often impact clinical decision making)

1. Increased cationic proteins such as gammaglobulins

2. Hypoalbuminemia

Case 1 – Level 1

"Devo" is an 8-year-old castrated male Golden Retreiver presenting for inability to rise from a sternal position. He is dull and unresponsive with brief periods of aggression. Devo has a history of seizures.

White blood cell count:	↑ 17.9 x 10⁹/L	(6.0-17.0)
Segmented neutrophils:	↑ 16.3 x 10⁹/L	(3.0-11.0)
Band neutrophils:	0 x 10⁹/L	(0-0.3)
Lymphocytes:	1.1 x 10⁹/L	(1.0-4.8)
Monocytes:	0.5 x 10⁹/L	(0.2-1.4)
Eosinophils:	0.0 x 10⁹/L	(0-1.3)

WBC morphology: No significant abnormalities noted.

Hematocrit:	38%	(37-55)
MCV:	70.4 fl	(60.0-75.0)
MCHC:	35.0 g/dl	(33.0-36.0)

RBC morphology: No significant abnormalities noted.
Platelets: Appear adequate

Glucose:	71 mg/dl	(65.0-120.0)
BUN:	22 mg/dl	(8-29)
Creatinine:	0.7 mg/dl	(0.5-1.5)
Phosphorus:	3.9 mg/dl	(2.6-7.2)
Calcium:	11.2 mg/dl	(8.8-11.7)
Magnesium:	2.2 mEq/L	(1.4-2.7)
Total Protein:	7.2 g/dl	(5.2-7.2)
Albumin:	3.6 g/dl	(3.0-4.2)
Globulin:	3.6 g/dl	(2.0-4.0)
Sodium:	150 mEq/L	(142-163)
Chloride:	↑ 153 mEq/L	(111-129)
Potassium:	5.1 mEq/L	(3.8-5.4)
HCO3:	24 mEq/L	(15-28)
Total Bili:	0.10 mg/dl	(0.10-0.50)
ALP:	72 IU/L	(12-121)
GGT:	4 IU/L	(3-10)
ALT:	36 IU/L	(10-95)
AST:	34 IU/L	(15-52)
Cholesterol:	242 mg/dl	(110-314)
Triglycerides:	54 mg/dl	(30-300)
Amylase:	599 IU/L	(400-1200)

Urinalysis: Collection method not indicated

Appearance: Yellow and hazy	Sediment:
Specific gravity: 1.027	0-5 WBC/hpf
pH: 5.0	Occasional RBC/hpf
Glucose, ketones, bilirubin: negative	0-5 transitional epithelial cells
Heme: 1+	
Protein: trace	

Interpretation
CBC: Mild mature neutrophilic leukocytosis that could be compatible with mild inflammation.

Serum Biochemical Profile
Marked hyperchloremia: Physiologic explanations for the abnormality would be difficult to formulate. Some type of artifact or interference is suspected based on the absence of other abnormalities. In this case, consultation with clinicians regarding any potential effects of treatment revealed that the patient had received a loading dose of potassium bromide used for his seizure disorder. This was detected by the ion specific electrode as chloride.

Case Summary and Outcome
Continued monitoring was suggested and diagnostic imaging was recommended to rule out intracranial lesions. The owners elected euthanasia because of cost and guarded prognosis, and necropsy was allowed. Unfortunately, gross and microscopic examination of the central nervous system failed to reveal lesions, which may have been biochemical or metabolic in nature, and thus not visible.

Case 2 – Level 1
Serum is submitted on a 2-year-old male Nubian goat. No history is provided.

Glucose:	↓ 26 mg/dl	(6.0-128.0)
BUN:	22 mg/dl	(17-30)
Creatinine:	1.2 mg/dl	(0.6-1.3)
Phosphorus:	↑ 17.0 mg/dl	(4.1-8.7)
Calcium:	8.7 mg/dl	(8.0-10.7)
Magnesium:	3.5 mEq/L	(2.8-3.6)
Total Protein:	↓ 5.5 g/dl	(6.1-8.3)
Albumin:	3.2 g/dl	(3.1-4.4)
Globulin:	2.3 g/dl	(2.2-4.3)
Sodium:	144 mEq/L	(140-157)
Chloride:	108 mEq/L	(102-118)
Potassium:	↑ 15.9 mEq/L	(3.5-5.6)
HCO3:	23 mEq/L	(22-32)
Anion Gap:	↑ 28.9	(14-20)
Total Bili:	0.2 mg/dl	(0.1-0.2)
ALP:	↑ 526 IU/L	(40-392)
GGT:	37 IU/L	(28-70)
AST:	↑ 918 IU/L	(40-222)
CK:	↑ 181,713 IU/L	(74-452)

Interpretation
Serum Biochemical Profile
Hypoglycemia: This value is difficult to interpret in the absence of any clinical data. As always, artifacts should be considered. In this case delayed separation of serum from cells may artifactually depress glucose levels. A profoundly low glucose such as this is likely to be associated with clinical signs, including seizures. Causes of true hypoglycemia include insulinoma and less frequently other tumors that produce insulin-like substances, and sepsis. Starvation usually results in mild hypoglycemia and then only with severe or prolonged deprivation.

Hyperphosphatemia with normal calcium: Hyperphosphatemia is often associated with low glomerular filtration rate, although this goat is not azotemic. Age related increases in phosphorus may be noted in young growing animals, however this goat is mature. Hypoparathyroidism should be considered, although the calcium may be decreased in these patients. If hypoparathyroidism is compatible with the clinical presentation, ionized calcium may be performed as a superior indicator of the biologically active form of the mineral. Finally, phosphorus may be released from cells with trauma or necrosis, which appears possible based on the hyperkalemia, elevated AST, and marked increase in CK. Rhabdomyolysis and tumor lysis syndrome are two specific conditions in which tissue destruction may lead to marked hyperphosphatemia.

Hypoproteinemia: Although the total protein is low, both the albumin and globulin levels are within reference intervals. Because both are at the lower end of the intervals, these values should be monitored.

Hyperkalemia: This value is extremely high and may be incompatible with life. The combination of hyperphosphatemia and hyperkalemia may be associated with anuric/oliguric renal failure, however this patient is not azotemic. Additional clinical history could provide more information about the potential for urinary obstruction, which is common in goats. As described above, the concurrent hyperphosphatemia and hyperkalemia can also reflect tissue destruction; this diagnosis is supported by other data. Hemolysis can increase potassium levels in the serum of some species or breeds characterized by red blood cells with high potassium content. Iatrogenic hyperkalemia may be caused by excessive potassium supple- mentation, or by treatment with potassium sparing diuretics, drugs that inhibit the renin- angiotensin-aldosterone system, heparin, or potassium penicillin G. Hyperkalemia may be associated with diabetes mellitus because of failure of insulin mediated uptake of potassium by cells. Hypoaldosteronism prevents adequate renal elimination of potassium, and some gastrointestinal disorders are characterized by potassium accumulation.

Increased ALP: Increased ALP may be associated with hepatobiliary disease, however the normal GGT makes this less likely. In this case, bone pathology or intestinal pathology also could be considered, and it was later determined that this goat had undergone an orthopedic surgical procedure prior to death.

Increased AST: This abnormality indicates tissue damage. The marked elevation of CK and normal GGT suggest extrahepatic damage, likely muscle.

Increased CK: The massive increase in this enzyme suggests severe muscle damage.

Increased Anion Gap: Increases in unmeasured anions may be due to poor tissue perfusion or from release from damaged tissue.

Case Summary and Outcome

Upon further inquiry into the clinical history of this patient, it was discovered that the sample collection was post-mortem. This explains the marked increase in intracellular constituents (cellular translocation), which are released as tissues breakdown after death. This makes interpretation of clinical chemistry data collected after death very difficult, so samples should be collected prior to death whenever possible. Similar but less dramatic increases in intracellular constituents were present in Chapter 6, Case 15 (Zinger), a cat with renal failure and thromboembolic episodes that led to tissue necrosis. Interpretation of abnormalities was less clear in Zinger, however, since the renal disease itself could have resulted in failure of renal excretion of phosphorus and potassium and the elevation in CK.

Case 3 – Level 1

"Serengeti" is an 8-year-old intact male German Shepherd presenting with a history of eating garbage many days ago. Since then, Serengeti has been vomiting once a day, and has been anorexic and lethargic. He had diarrhea the day he ate the garbage, but after that has had no feces and has been straining to defecate. He was treated with antibiotics yesterday. On physical examination, Serengeti has a pendulous abdomen and muscle wasting with a prominent spine. He is extremely depressed with increased respiratory rate. An oral examination is not possible because, despite his depression, Serengeti still has the energy to try to bite. His owners are concerned about cost of medical care.

White blood cell count:	↑ 21.2 x 10⁹/L	(4.0-13.3)
Segmented neutrophils:	↑ 20.4 x 10⁹/L	(2.0-11.2)
Band neutrophils:	0.0 x 10⁹/L	(0-0.3)
Lymphocytes:	↓ 0.4 x 10⁹/L	(1.0-4.5)
Monocytes:	0.4 x 10⁹/L	(0.2-1.4)
Eosinophils:	0.0 x 10⁹/L	(0-1.2)
WBC morphology: Within normal limits		

Hematocrit:	↑ 60.0%	(39-55)
Red blood cell count:	↑ 9.14 x 10¹²/L	(5.5-8.5)
Hemoglobin:	↑ 21.3 g/dl	(12.0-18.0)
MCV:	62.0 fl	(60.0-77.0)
MCHC:	↑ 35.5 g/dl	(31.0-34.0)

Platelets:	421 x 10¹²/L	(181-525)

Glucose:	77 mg/dl	(67.0-135.0)
BUN:	27 mg/dl	(8-29)
Creatinine:	0.7 mg/dl	(0.5-1.5)
Phosphorus:	7.1 mg/dl	(2.6-7.2)
Calcium:	10.6 mg/dl	(9.5-11.5)
Magnesium:	2.5 mEq/L	(1.7-2.5)
Total Protein:	5.7 g/dl	(4.8-7.2)
Albumin:	3.1 g/dl	(2.5-3.7)
Globulin:	2.6 g/dl	(2.0-4.0)
Sodium:	↓ 127 mEq/L	(140-151)
Chloride:	↓ 87 mEq/L	(105-120)
Potassium:	↑ 5.8 mEq/L	(3.6-5.6)
Anion Gap:	18.8 mEq/L	(15-25)
HCO3:	27 mEq/L	(15-28)
Total Bili:	0.2 mg/dl	(0.10-0.50)
ALP:	29 IU/L	(20-320)
GGT:	6 IU/L	(2-10)
ALT:	50 IU/L	(10-95)
AST:	36 IU/L	(10-56)
Cholesterol:	157 mg/dl	(110-314)
Amylase:	804 IU/L	(400-1200)

Abdominal Fluid Analysis

Pre-spin appearance: orange and cloudy	
Post-spin appearance: colorless and clear	
Total protein: 3.6 gm/dl	
Total nucleated cell count: 24,300/µl	

Cytologic description: Smears consist of 88% nondegenerate neutrophils, 2% small lymphocytes, and 10% large mononuclear cells. No etiologic agents are seen. Large numbers of round to oval cells are present at the feathered edge of the smears (Figure 7-1). These cells are characterized by scant to abundant deeply basophilic to clear cytoplasm. Most have numerous small clear vacuoles in the perinuclear area and cytoplasmic blebbing is noted. Each cell contains a single large round to oval nucleus with coarsely stippled chromatin. The nucleus is often peripheralized by the vacuoles. Occasional ballooning signet ring cells are present. Anisocytosis and anisokaryosis are marked; the nuclear to cytoplasmic ratio is moderate but variable. Signet ring cells have large and prominent nucleoli.

Interpretation

CBC: Serengeti has a mature neutrophilic leukocytosis and lymphopenia compatible with a corticosteroid response. Mild concurrent inflammation is also possible due to the inflammatory nature of the abdominal fluid; however no toxic changes or left shift are noted at this time. Serengeti is also polycythemic. In this case, a history of vomiting and diarrhea with poor food intake is compatible with dehydration and a relative polycythemia. Hyperproteinemia and hypernatremia may accompany relative polycythemia, but are inconsistent findings because of concurrent protein and electrolyte losses that can occur with diseases leading to dehydration. In this case, both gastrointestinal losses by vomiting and diarrhea and third space sequestration with abdominal fluid accumulation obscured the effects of dehydration. Polycythemia may also occur as a rare neoplastic condition with autonomous proliferation of erythroid precursors (polycythemia vera) or may occur in compensation for renal oxygen deficits with cardiopulmonary disease or some kidney lesions.

Serum Biochemical Profile
Hyponatremia and hypochloremia: Likely sources of electrolyte loss in this patient include losses from the gastrointestinal intestinal tract and third space sequestration in the abdominal cavity effusion. If hypertonic fluids are lost, this will lead to relatively greater losses of electrolytes than water, resulting in low serum electrolytes. When isotonic fluids containing proportional amounts of water and electrolytes are lost, fluid losses are frequently replaced by water consumed by the patient, further diluting remaining electrolytes. Disproportionate decreases in chloride (the corrected chloride is 99 mEq/L) are compatible with vomiting or fluid sequestration. Currently, there are no abnormalities in the serum bicarbonate, although it is approaching the upper limit of the reference interval. Serum chloride and bicarbonate usually vary inversely, and loss of fluid from the upper GI tract is often associated with alkalosis attributed to loss of hydrogen. Concurrent metabolic alkalosis and acidosis could combine to result in a serum bicarbonate value within the reference interval if a mixed acid/base disorder is present. Blood gas analysis may be required for more complete information about Serengeti's acid/base status. In addition to increased losses, serum electrolyte levels may be low due to decreased intake, though this usually does not result in significant lowering of serum sodium and chloride.

Hyperkalemia: Hypoadrenocorticism should be considered, given the combination of hyperkalemia, hyponatremia and hypochloremia in this patient. The corticosteroid leukogram would be unusual in a patient with adrenal insufficiency, while the history of gastrointestinal signs and weakness is compatible with Addison's disease. Some types of gastrointestinal disease or effusions may also be associated with the electrolyte pattern seen in Serengeti. The mechanism is not always clear, but it is speculated that volume depletion and low renal tubular flow rates may contribute to the development of hyperkalemia. Unless there is impaired renal excretion, increased intake of potassium rarely causes hyperkalemia, although this may be seen if intravenous fluids are administered that contain excessive amounts of potassium. Treatment with beta-blockers or angiotensin converting enzyme inhibitors interferes with potassium excretion in the absence of renal disease. There is no evidence of tissue trauma or acid/base abnormalities that would trigger translocation of potassium from cells. In the context of the clinical history, uroabdomen seems unlikely, however measurement of abdominal fluid creatinine could be performed to rule out this possibility.

Case Summary and Outcome

Serengeti's owners elected euthanasia because of financial concerns and the potential for incurable disease. The clinical impression was that Serengeti's effusion may have been due to neoplasia, possibly carcinomatosis, however a primary mass could not be identified at necropsy (Figure 7-1). Other findings at necropsy included membranoproliferative glomerulonephritis (apparently subclinical, although no urinalysis was performed), choleliths, benign prostatic hyperplasia, and massive fibrosis in the omentum. The fibrosis was accompanied by neovascularization, necrosis, inflammation, and prominent atypical mesothelial cells. The anatomic pathologist felt that this lesion was most likely related to a previous penetrating wound of the gastrointestinal tract, however no injury or septic focus could be located.

This case illustrates two important principles. The first is that electrolyte abnormalities classically associated with hypoadrenocorticism (see Chapter 5, Case 23; Chapter 6, Case 13; Chapter 7 Case 3) or uroabdomen (Chapter 5, Case 18; Chapter 7, Cases 12 and 21) may occur secondary to cavity effusions or gastrointestinal disease. The second is the difficulty distinguishing reactive hyperplasia from neoplasia in tissues that are predisposed to marked reactive changes. The final diagnosis in this case remained uncertain despite necropsy.

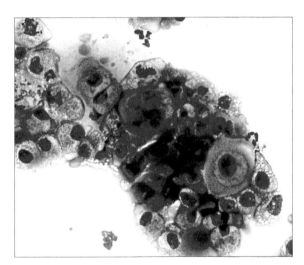

Figure 7-1. Cytology of canine abdominal fluid with atypical epithelial cells consistent with carcinomatosis.

Case 4 – Level 1

"Cinder" is an 8-year-old neutered male Labrador Retriever presenting for progressive lethargy, anorexia, and vomiting. Last month, the owners noticed that he had difficulty getting up and down the stairs, so the referring veterinarian recommended aspirin. Cinder began vomiting when he was treated with aspirin, so the medication was changed to carprofen, which seemed to work better. Two weeks ago, Cinder became anorectic and has not been drinking much water. This morning he was very weak, began to vomit, and have diarrhea. On physical examination, Cinder's mucous membranes are markedly icteric, and he is salivating. Capillary refill time and auscultation are normal. He does appear to be ataxic and very weak.

White blood cell count:	↑ 17.3 x 10⁹/L	(4.0-13.3)
Segmented neutrophils:	↑ 15.7 x 10⁹/L	(2.0-11.2)
Band neutrophils:	0.0 x 10⁹/L	(0-0.3)
Lymphocytes:	↓ 0.2 x 10⁹/L	(1.0-4.5)
Monocytes:	1.4 x 10⁹/L	(0.2-1.4)
Eosinophils:	0.0 x 10⁹/L	(0-1.2)
WBC morphology: Appears within normal limits		
Nucleated RBC/100 WBC:	6	

Hematocrit:	43%	(37-60)
Red blood cell count:	5.8 x 10¹²/L	(5.8-8.5)
Hemoglobin:	14.6 g/dl	(14.0-19.0)
MCV:	77.0 fl	(60.0-77.0)
MCHC:	34.0 g/dl	(31.0-34.0)
RBC morphology: Small numbers of Howell-Jolly bodies are present. Polychromasia is slightly increased, and scattered schistocytes are seen.		

Platelets: Appear adequate in number

Glucose:	71 mg/dl	(67.0-135.0)
BUN:	↓ 7 mg/dl	(8-29)
Creatinine:	Invalid: interference from bilirubin	(0.5-1.5)
Phosphorus:	3.7 mg/dl	(2.6-7.2)
Calcium:	10.0 mg/dl	(9.5-11.5)
Magnesium:	2.4 mEq/L	(1.7-2.5)
Total Protein:	↓ 5.3 g/dl	(5.5-7.8)
Albumin:	3.1 g/dl	(2.8-4.0)
Globulin:	↓ 2.2 g/dl	(2.3-4.2)
Sodium:	157 mEq/L	(141-158)
Chloride:	126 mEq/L	(106-126)
Potassium:	↓ 2.9 mEq/L	(3.8-5.4)
Anion Gap:	14.9 mEq/L	(6-16)
HCO3:	19 mEq/L	(15-28)
Total Bili:	↑ 42.9 mg/dl	(0.10-0.50)
ALP:	↑ 365 IU/L	(20-320)
GGT:	10 IU/L	(2-10)
ALT:	↑ 601 IU/L	(10-95)
AST:	↑ 171 IU/L	(10-56)
Cholesterol:	83 mg/dl	(82-355)
Amylase:	357 IU/L	(400-1200)

Coagulation Profile

PT:	↑ 16.6s	(6.0-9.0)
APTT:	↑ 18.0s	(9.0-16.0)
FDP:	↑ 5-20 µg/ml	(<5)

Urinalysis: Sampling method not indicated.

Specific gravity: 1.032
Bilirubin: 3+
Protein: 1+
Glucose, ketones: negative
Sediment: ammonium biurate crystals are seen

Interpretation

CBC: Cinder has a mature neutrophilic leukocytosis and lymphopenia compatible with corticosteroid effects with or without mild inflammation. The cause for nucleated erythrocytes in this case is difficult to ascertain. Increased nucleated RBCs may accompany a regenerative response, however, Cinder is not anemic. Nucleated RBCs may be present in the circulation in association with endothelial cell damage or lesions in hematopoietic tissues such as the bone marrow or spleen (Figure 7-2). They may also be seen in cases of lead intoxication. When present in sufficient numbers, schistocytes indicate vascular pathology such as disseminated intravascular coagulation (possible with the prolonged coagulation times and slightly increased FDPs) or hemangiosarcoma, although they may also be noted with more benign conditions such as iron deficiency.

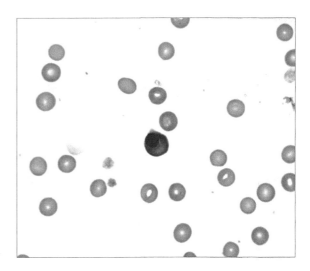

Figure 7-2. Canine blood film showing nucleated red blood cell.

Serum Biochemical Profile

Low BUN: Low BUN often reflects polyuria and polydipsia with increased renal tubular flow rates, however Cinder's clinical history does not include PU/PD. Low protein diets may also contribute. Alternatively, decreased liver function can lower BUN. Other abnormalities of the serum biochemical profile that sometimes accompany poor liver function include hypoglycemia, hypoalbuminemia, and hypocholesterolemia. While all of these analytes are at the lower end of their reference intervals, none are low at this time. Examination of other laboratory data shows prolonged coagulation times, which could also support a diagnosis of impaired liver function. Since none of these parameters are good indicators of liver function, measurement of blood ammonia or serum bile acids is recommended. Ammonia would be preferred when there is concurrent hyperbilirubinemia, because serum bile acid concentrations are expected to increase with cholestasis regardless of liver function.

Hypoproteinemia with hypoglobulinemia: Hypoglobulinemia is most often associated with concurrent hypoalbuminemia and reflects non-selective protein losses into the gut, third space, through the skin, or with hemorrhage. In this case, the albumin (and hematocrit) remains within the reference intervals, although the abnormal coagulation profile suggests the potential for blood loss. Rarely, congenital immunodeficiency syndromes can result in failure of globulin production, but this is unlikely in an 8-year-old dog.

Hypokalemia: Gastrointestinal losses of potassium coupled with inadequate intake combine to cause Cinder's hypokalemia.

Marked hyperbilirubinemia: The presence of schistocytes in the peripheral blood suggests the potential for some hemolysis, however the normal hematocrit argues that hemolysis is minor and could not account for all of the increase in bilirubin. The other major differential diagnosis for hyperbilirubinemia is cholestasis, which is corroborated by the increased ALP, although this change is mild and not accompanied by an increase in GGT. Decreased liver function and sepsis may also cause increased serum bilirubin. Because of the low BUN and prolonged clotting times, the potential for decreased liver function deserves further consideration.

Mildly increased ALP: There are many extrahepatic causes for increased ALP in the dog, including corticosteroid effects which are suggested by the lymphopenia. Other considerations include bone disease, endocrinopathies, and cholestatic liver disease. The clinical history does not indicate a high degree of suspicion of bone disease, nor is the other laboratory work compatible with endocrinopathies implicated in causing elevated ALP such as hyperadrenocorticism or diabetes mellitus. Cholestatic liver disease seems logical given the marked increase in bilirubin, however the minor elevation in ALP and normal GGT seem inordinately low for cholestatic liver disease.

Increased ALT and AST: ALT generally suggests hepatocellular damage, but does not indicate cause. AST is less liver specific and can reflect more generalized tissue damage, especially if the ALT does not change proportionally. Hepatocellular damage could be secondary to gastrointestinal pathology, however the high bilirubin suggests primary liver disease must also be considered.

Coagulation profile: PT and APTT indicate a defect of secondary hemostasis. Common considerations include decreased liver function, anticoagulant rodenticide intoxication, or disseminated intravascular coagulation. All of these may be associated with mildly to moderately increased fibrin degradation products because of either failure of clearance by a dysfunctional liver or increased production associated with excessive breakdown of blood clots.

Urinalysis: Ammonion biurate crystals suggest liver dysfunction in dogs.

Case Summary and Outcome

Cinder's blood ammonia levels were within reference intervals. Because treatment with carprofen has been associated with acute hepatic necrosis in dogs (MacPhail), a toxicity was considered. Cinder was treated with plasma transfusions and vitamin K to prevent abnormal bleeding. Abdominal ultrasound revealed a small, bright liver suggesting a chronic process rather than acute toxicity. Progressive neurological signs developed, culminating in a comatose state. Cinder's owners elected euthanasia due to the poor prognosis. Necropsy revealed marked progressive bridging portal fibrosis and stromal collapse with nodular regeneration and intrahepatic cholestasis, compatible with the marked hyperbilirubinemia documented on the serum biochemical profile. Autolysis precluded evaluation for acute necrosis and documentation of any role for the nonsteroidal anti-inflammatory treatment in the progression of hepatic disease. In this case, the relatively minor elevations in both cholestatic and hepatocellular enzymes may have reflected the small amount of residual hepatic tissue.

Cinder's only electrolyte abnormality was isolated hypokalemia, which is relatively common in domestic animal species with gastrointestinal disease because of the combination of increased losses and decreased intake, but may also be seen with polyuria and anorexia for similar reasons (Chapter 3, Case19).

MacPhail CM, Lappin MR, Meyer DJ, Smith SG, Webster CRL, Armstrong J. Hepatocellular toxicosis associated with administration of carprofen in 21 dogs. J Am Vet Med Assoc 1998;212:1895-1901

Case 5 – Level 1

"Fiero" is a 12-year-old spayed female Dachshund presenting for a one day history of vomiting during which she could not hold down food or water. For the past 3-4 years, Fiero has been treated with an angiotensin-converting enzyme inhibitor because of a heart murmur. Her history also includes parathyroidectomy performed four months ago to correct hypercalcemia. She has always shown a marked interest in garbage eating. On physical examination, Fiero appears painful when her abdomen is palpated and is slightly dehydrated. In the hospital, she has blood-tinged vomitus.

White blood cell count:	13.3 x 10⁹/L	(4.0-13.3)
Segmented neutrophils:	↑ 11.4 x 10⁹/L	(2.0-11.2)
Band neutrophils:	0.0 x 10⁹/L	(0-0.3)
Lymphocytes:	↓ 0.8 x 10⁹/L	(1.0-4.5)
Monocytes:	0.8 x 10⁹/L	(0.2-1.4)
Eosinophils:	0.3 x 10⁹/L	(0-1.2)

WBC morphology: Within normal limits

Hematocrit:	↑ 60%	(39-55)
Red blood cell count:	↑ 9.45 x 10¹²/L	(5.8-8.5)
Hemoglobin:	↑ 20.6 g/dl	(14.0-19.0)
MCV:	61.1 fl	(60.0-77.0)
MCHC:	34.0 g/dl	(31.0-34.0)

Platelets: Appear adequate in number

Glucose:	↓ 57 mg/dl	(90.0-140.0)
BUN:	15 mg/dl	(6-24)
Creatinine:	0.5 mg/dl	(0.5-1.5)
Phosphorus:	4.6 mg/dl	(2.6-7.2)
Calcium:	9.6 mg/dl	(9.5-11.5)
Magnesium:	1.9 mEq/L	(1.7-2.5)
Total Protein:	7.2 g/dl	(5.5-7.8)
Albumin:	3.5 g/dl	(2.8-4.0)
Globulin:	3.7 g/dl	(2.3-4.2)
Sodium:	149 mEq/L	(140-151)
Chloride:	↓ 100 mEq/L	(105-120)
Potassium:	4.0 mEq/L	(3.6-5.6)

Anion Gap:	23 mEq/L	(15-25)
HCO3:	↑ 30 mEq/L	(15-28)
Total Bili:	0.2 mg/dl	(0.10-0.50)
ALP:	↑ 1164 IU/L	(20-320)
GGT:	7 IU/L	(2-10)
ALT:	↑ 127 IU/L	(10-95)
AST:	51 IU/L	(10-56)
Cholesterol:	307 mg/dl	(110-314)
Amylase:	↑ 3547 IU/L	(400-1200)

Interpretation

CBC: Fiero has a mild mature neutrophilia and lymphopenia, which suggests corticosteroid effects. Eosinopenia is another relatively consistent feature of the steroid leukogram, however some eosinophils were noted on the differential cell count. Given the dehydrated state of the patient, the polycythemia is thought to be relative. This is not accompanied by an increase in total protein. It is possible for dehydration to mask hypoproteinemia, and this should be re-evaluated once the patient is rehydrated. Splenic contraction also is a possible cause of an increase in PCV that would not be associated with an increase in total protein.

Serum Biochemical Profile

Hypoglycemia: If this finding is verified by repeat analysis to rule out processing errors, several other possibilities for hypoglycemia should be considered. Hypoglycemia may be associated with poor nutrition, and some sources indicate that small dogs are more prone to develop hypoglycemia secondary to decreased food intake. In most cases, however, food deprivation must be chronic and severe to cause hypoglycemia. Decreased production associated with liver failure is possible, however other analytes produced by the liver such as urea, albumin, and cholesterol remain within reference intervals at this time. Sepsis is another potential cause for hypoglycemia, but not supported by changes on the leukogram. Neoplasia is also a consideration in an older patient.

Hypochloremic alkalosis: With the clinical history of vomiting and Fiero's affinity for trash can dining, gastric vomiting could be a source of chloride and acid loss. The angiotensin-converting enzyme inhibitor may potentiate losses of sodium or chloride and promote retention of potassium. Patients receiving medications that interfere with the function of the renin angiotensin system should have their serum electrolytes periodically monitored and the dose adjusted if necessary.

Increased ALP: As discussed in Chapter 2, increased ALP in the dog is a nonspecific change that may be associated with drug effects, endocrinopathies, circulatory disorders, bone pathology, and cholestatic liver disease. Severe cholestatic liver disease is less likely with a normal bilirubin and GGT, and the history does not suggest a bone disorder, so drug/endocrine effects or milder liver disease (possibly secondary to intestinal pathology) are most likely in this patient.

Increased ALT: Although this is a mild elevation, it does indicate the potential for hepatocellular damage and suggests that the increased ALP may reflect some hepatic disease. The liver damage still may be secondary to intestinal inflammation, since liver enzyme elevations do not distinguish between primary and secondary processes. Endocrinopathies may cause increases in multiple hepatic enzymes.

Hyperamylasemia: Increased amylase is frequently interpreted to signal pancreatic disease such as pancreatitis. This certainly could be compatible with Fiero's clinical history, although the clinical chemistry abnormalities are not classic for pancreatitis. Alternatively, serum amylase may also increase in association with intestinal disease, which may be the case in this patient. Two to three-fold increases in amylase can be the result of decreased glomerular filtration rate. Although Fiero is not azotemic, she appears dehydrated, which may result in pre-renal decreases in glomerular filtration rate.

Case Summary and Outcome

Abdominal radiographs showed foreign material in the pylorus and proximal duodenum. Thoracic radiographs were unremarkable. Fiero was stabilized with fluids prior to surgery for the removal of the foreign material, which turned out to be plastic food wrapping. Because of her liver enzyme elevations, liver biopsy samples were collected at the time of gastrotomy. Microscopic examination revealed chronic active peri-portal hepatitis that was interpreted to be secondary to the recent history of gastrointestinal disease. Steroid hepatopathy was superimposed on the inflammatory process and may have accounted for the relatively pronounced elevation in ALP compared to the other liver enzymes. Although corticosteroids had not been prescribed for Fiero, increased endogenous steroids could have contributed to the hepatopathy. The owners also stated that she may have inadvertently been given prednisone that had been prescribed for two other dogs in the household that have skin disease. Fiero recovered uneventfully at home. The owners put the garbage can in the closet.

Case 6 – Level 2

"Francesca" is an 8-year-old spayed female Beagle presenting for evaluation of vomiting and electrolyte abnormalities. Two weeks ago, she was initially evaluated by the referring veterinarian following a few days of vomiting, lethargy, and diarrhea. At that time, she was noted to be dehydrated and was treated with fluids, antibiotics, and a bland diet. She presented to the referring veterinarian again 10 days later for progression of symptoms and weakness. She has been vomiting after ingestion of any food, water, or medications, but is polydipsic. She has not passed feces for several days. She was subsequently treated with with corticosteroids, and when she did not respond, she was referred to the University. The owner was not aware of any exposure to toxins or foreign material. He was somewhat concerned that someone may have tried to poison Francesca because she occasionally barks at night. Francesca has been generally healthy prior to this episode and is not taking any medications. On presentation, Francesca is quiet but responsive and 10% dehydrated. She is tachycardic and hypothermic with prolonged capillary refill times. Thoracic ausculatation was unremarkable, but she was painful on abdominal palpation. A tubular object was palpable in the mid-abdomen.

White blood cell count:	↑ 28.7 x 10⁹/L	(6.0-17.0)
Segmented neutrophils:	↑ 27.2 x 10⁹/L	(3.0-11.0)
Band neutrophils:	0.0 x 10⁹/L	(0-0.3)
Lymphocytes:	↓ 0.6 x 10⁹/L	(1.0-4.8)
Monocytes:	0.9 x 10⁹/L	(0.2-1.4)
Eosinophils:	0.0 x 10⁹/L	(0-1.3)
WBC morphology: No abnormalities noted.		
Hematocrit:	53.4%	(37-55)
Red blood cell count:	8.11 x 10¹²/L	(5.5-8.5)
Hemoglobin:	↑ 18.4 g/dl	(12.0-18.0)
MCV:	65.8 fl	(60.0-77.0)

MCHC:	↑ 34.4 g/dl	(31.0-34.0)
RBC morphology: Appears within normal limits		

Platelets:	268 x 10¹²/L	(200-450)

Glucose:	↑ 212 mg/dl	(80.0-125.0)
BUN:	↑ 44 mg/dl	(6-24))
Creatinine:	1.1 mg/dl	(0.5-1.5)
Phosphorus:	4.3 mg/dl	(3.0-6.0)
Calcium:	9.9 mg/dl	(8.8-11.0)
Magnesium:	↑ 2.6 mEq/L	(1.4-2.2)
Total Protein:	6.3 g/dl	(4.7-7.3)
Albumin:	3.1 g/dl	(2.5-4.2)
Globulin:	3.2 g/dl	(2.0-4.0)
Sodium:	↓ 120 mEq/L	(140-151)
Chloride:	↓ 59 mEq/L	(105-120)
Potassium:	↓ 1.9 mEq/L	(3.8-5.4)
HCO3:	↑ 34.2 mEq/L	(16-28)
Anion Gap:	↑ 28.7 mEq/L	(15-25)
Total Bili:	0.3 mg/dl	(0.10-0.50)
ALP:	47 IU/L	(20-320)
GGT:	6 IU/L	(2-10)
ALT:	27 IU/L	(5-65)
AST:	47 IU/L	(15-52)
Cholesterol:	220 mg/dl	(110-314)
Amylase:	757 IU/L	(400-1200)

Urine specific gravity: 1.030	

Interpretation

CBC: Francesca has a mature neutrophilic leukocytosis and a lymphopenia compatible with a corticosteroid leukogram. She has been treated with corticosteroids and may have increased levels of endogenously produced steroids due to her illness. Concurrent inflammation could contribute to the mature neutrophilic leukocytosis. No toxic change or left shift are described at this time, however these changes are not always present with inflammatory disease.

Serum Biochemical Profile

Hyperglycemia: Both endogeneous and exogenous corticosteroids can cause hyperglycemia. Diabetes mellitus could be compatible with the clinical signs, although abdominal pain is not typical for diabetic patients unless there is concurrent gastroenteritis or pancreatitis.

Elevated BUN with normal creatinine: The urine specific gravity suggests adequate urinary concentrating ability. BUN may increase prior to creatinine with decreased tubular flow rates associated with dehydration. Sepsis may also cause an increase in BUN with no corresponding change in creatinine. Gastrointestinal hemorrhage or a high protein diet can elevate BUN but the latter is unlikely in patient unable to eat.

Hypermagnesemia: Given the dehydration, this abnormality likely reflects pre-renal decreases in glomerular filtration rate.

Hyponatremia with disproportionately greater hypochloremia: Hyponatremia is rarely dietary in origin even during periods of anorexia. Hyponatremia generally reflects a relative gain of water compared to sodium and chloride or excessive loss of electrolytes. The pathophysiology of Francesca's hyponatremia likely involves both mechanisms. She is experiencing gastrointestinal losses of electrolytes associated with vomiting and diarrhea. In response to the volume depletion, glomerular filtration rate declines. This results in increased isosmostic reabsorption of sodium in the proximal tubule and decreased fluid flow in the distal tubules, impairing water excretion. In addition, volume depletion will encourage release of antidiuretic hormone, leading to further impairment in water excretion. Lastly, fluid losses are often replaced with consumption of water because of increased thirst (note Francesca is polydipsic), further diluting electrolyte levels in the circulation. Vomiting of the contents of the proximal gastrointestinal tract associated with structural or functional obstruction is associated with excessive loss of chloride (HCl), causing a hypochloremic metabolic alkalosis.

Hypokalemia: Francesca's low serum potassium is caused by inadequate intake to compensate for ongoing gastrointestinal losses. Hypokalemia in association with metabolic alkalosis is compatible with vomiting of stomach contents or diuretic use, while hypokalemia in association with metabolic acidosis is more frequently attributable to small intestinal diarrhea, chronic renal failure, or distal renal tubular acidosis.

Increased HCO3 (alkalemia): Loss of hydrogen in addition to electrolytes because of the vomiting of anterior gastrointestinal tract contents is causing the alkalosis.

Increased anion gap: Alkalosis and dehydration are potential causes for the increased anion gap. In this case, a mixed acid/base disorder could develop secondary to lactic acidosis associated with dehydration and poor tissue perfusion. Blood gas analysis may be indicated to follow the acid/base status of this patient.

Case Summary and Outcome

Francesca was taken to surgery and a corn cob was removed from her proximal small intestine. The owners observed that it may have originated from a recently melted snow man their children had made in the yard. Francesca was discharged and had an uneventful recovery at home. Note that both Francesca and Fiero (this chapter, Case 5) had a history of vomiting associated with foreign body ingestion with evidence of hypochloremia and metabolic alkalosis, however Francesca had more pronounced electrolyte abnormalities. This is probably the result of Francesca's more protracted clinical course prior to surgical correction of the small intestinal blockage, although in theory, Fiero's angiotensin converting enzyme inhibitor treatment could have helped maintain her serum potassium levels. Despite Francesca's more serious clinical signs, there are no liver enzyme elevations that suggest steroid hepatopathy, though she does have a corticosteroid leukogram.

Case 7 – Level 2

"Snow" is an 11-year-old spayed female Bichon Frise presenting for a few days of lethargy, decreased appetite, and 2 episodes of vomiting. For the past 8 months, she has had a chronic cough. This was attributed to heart disease based on radiographs and echocardiogram. She was subsequently treated with furosemide and cough suppressants. On physical examination, Snow is icteric, dehydrated, and has a 3/6 heart murmur.

Glucose:	97 mg/dl	(90.0-140.0)
BUN:	12 mg/dl	(6-24)
Creatinine:	0.8 mg/dl	(0.5-1.5)
Phosphorus:	2.8 mg/dl	(2.6-7.2)
Calcium:	9.8 mg/dl	(9.5-11.5)
Magnesium:	2.3 mEq/L	(1.7-2.5)
Total Protein:	6.7 g/dl	(5.5-7.8)
Albumin:	2.9 g/dl	(2.8-4.0)
Globulin:	3.8 g/dl	(2.3-4.2)
Sodium:	↓ 137 mEq/L	(140-151)
Chloride:	↓ 98 mEq/L	(105-120)
Potassium:	↓ 3.5 mEq/L	(3.6-5.6)
Anion Gap:	19.5 mEq/L	(15-25)
HCO3:	23 mEq/L	(15-28)
Total Bili:	↑ 8.1 mg/dl	(0.10-0.50)
ALP:	↑ 4515 IU/L	(20-320)
ALT:	↑ 2359 IU/L	(10-95)
AST:	↑ 1038 IU/L	(10-56)
Cholesterol:	↑ 464 mg/dl	(110-314)
Amylase:	508 IU/L	(400-1200)

Interpretation

CBC: not available

Serum Biochemical Profile

Hyponatremia and hypochloremia: The use of diuretics will contribute to increased renal losses of electrolytes (See Chapter 7, Case 11). The corrected chloride is still slightly low (104 mEq/L), which may be observed in patients taking furosemide. Replacement of fluids and electrolytes lost through the gastrointestinal tract with oral water intake can dilute remaining serum electrolytes. Congestive heart failure will evoke mechanisms of renal fluid retention and increased thirst to increase intravascular water in an attempt to restore circulation to tissues that are not adequately perfused because of poor cardiac function. This will further dilute remaining serum electrolytes.

Hypokalemia: Similar to sodium and chloride, some types of diuretics cause renal potassium wasting. This drain on potassium may be compounded by gastrointestinal losses and low intake.

Hyperbilirubinemia: Major diagnostic considerations for hyperbilirubinemia include hemolysis and cholestatic liver disease. Sepsis and decreased liver function often cause milder hyperbilirubinemia. Evaluating the potential for hemolytic disease requires at least a packed cell volume and preferably a complete CBC. The marked elevation in ALP is compatible with cholestasis, supported by the hypercholesterolemia. Significant increases in the ALT and AST support concurrent hepatocellular damage while severely impaired liver function seems less likely because the BUN, glucose, and albumin are normal and the cholesterol is increased. Serum bile acids would be a more sensitive way to evaluate liver function deficits.

Increased ALP: As described above, markedly increased ALP is suggestive for cholestatic disease, which would be supported by an increased GGT if available. There are numerous potential causes for elevated ALP including some medications and endocrinopathies such as diabetes or hyperadrenocortocism, which are not consistent with the history, physical examination findings, and other clinical chemistry data.

Increased ALT and AST: Elevations in these enzymes indicate hepatocellular damage, although muscle damage also could contribute to the increases. A creatine kinase measurement could help determine if concurrent muscle damage is occurring.

Case Summary and Outcome

Abdominal ultrasound revealed a small liver, a moderate sized gall bladder with no evidence of blockage, and a hypoechoic, slightly enlarged pancreas. Biopsy of the liver showed chronic active hepatitis with a mixed inflammatory infiltrate, piece-meal necrosis, and moderate portal fibrosis. Food was withheld from Snow due to the vomiting, and she was treated with antibiotics, fluids and gastrointestinal protectants. When she was eventually fed, she exhibited decreased mentation compatible with hepatic encephalopathy. At that time, a low protein diet was implemented and ursodeoxycholic acid and lactulose were added to her treatment plan. A cardiology consult was requested by the owner, and Snow was found to have 4+ mitral regurgitation and mild tricuspid regurgitation without evidence of heart failure and excellent contractility. Cardiology recommended changing the treatment of her cardiac disease to an angiotensin converting enzyme inhibitor with furosemide as needed to control clinical signs once her liver disease was better controlled. Eight weeks after discharge, Snow was re-evaluated and was doing very well with no clinical signs of liver disease and a normal serum bilirubin. The owners had noted an increase in her coughing, however radiographic evaluation showed clear lung fields and reduced heart size compared to her last evaluation.

Snow's case demonstrates the interaction between the effects of medication and multiple disease processes. Like Fiero (Chapter 7, Case 5), the diuretic therapy may have potentiated the development of electrolyte abnormalities associated with vomiting and anorexia. Patients taking medications that could influence electrolyte homeostasis should have their serum electrolyte levels monitored periodically. In some cases, doses of medications must be adjusted or alternative therapies instituted in response to laboratory abnormalities.

Case 8 – Level 2

"Delaney" is a 13-year-old Morgan mare presenting with signs of colic. On presentation, Delaney was quiet and her vital parameters were within normal limits. Abdominal palpation revealed a markedly distended cecum. She was taken to surgery on Day 1 to relieve a cecal impaction. An incomplete cecal bypass was performed in which the jejunum was anastomosed to the right ventral colon. Delaney recovered from anesthesia uneventfully. However 4 days post-surgery, she was in pain and had a fever, so additional laboratory work was performed.

Laboratory Data from Day 1, prior to surgery:

Glucose:	108 mg/dl	(60-130)
BUN:	15 mg/dl	(10-26)
Creatinine:	1.1 mg/dl	(1.0-2.0)
Phosphorus:	3.2 mg/dl	(1.5-4.5)
Calcium:	11.4 mg/dl	(10.8-13.5)
Magnesium:	↑ 2.6 mEq/L	(1.7-2.4)
Total Protein:	7.5 g/dl	(5.7-7.7)
Albumin:	3.4 g/dl	(2.6-3.8)
Globulin:	4.1 g/dl	(2.5-4.5)
Sodium:	135 mEq/L	(130-145)
Chloride:	98 mEq/L	(97-110)
Potassium:	4.0 mEq/L	(3.0-5.0)
HCO3:	29 mEq/L	(25-33)
Anion Gap:	12 mEq/L	(7-15)
Total Bili:	2.60 mg/dl	(0.30-3.0)
ALP:	148 IU/L	(109-352)
GGT:	21 IU/L	(4-28)
AST:	↑ 410 IU/L	(190-380)
CK:	↑ 1072 IU/L	(80-446)

Abdominal fluid on Day 1

Appearance: light yellow and clear
Total protein: 2.5 gm/dl
Total nucleated cells: 1,359/µl
Neutrophils are nondegenerate, no etiologic agents are seen.

Data obtained 4 days after the surgery:

White blood cell count:	↓ 3.4 x 10⁹/L	(5.4-14.3)
Segmented neutrophils:	↓ 1.6 x 10⁹/L	(2.3-8.6)
Band neutrophils:	0.0 x 10⁹/L	(0-0.3)
Lymphocytes:	↓ 1.3 x 10⁹/L	(1.5-7.7)
Monocytes:	0.5 x 10⁹/L	(0.0-1.0)
WBC morphology: Some neutrophils contain Döhle bodies		

Hematocrit:	47%	(32-53)
MCV:	50.6 fl	(37.0-58.5)
MCHC:	36.6 g/dl	(31.0-38.6)
RBC morphology: Appears within normal limits		
Platelets: Appear adequate in number		

Fibrinogen:	↑ 500 mg/dl	(100-400)

Glucose:	↑ 148 mg/dl	(60-130)
BUN:	10 mg/dl	(10-26)
Creatinine:	1.1 mg/dl	(1.0-2.0)
Phosphorus:	2.1 mg/dl	(1.5-4.5)
Calcium:	11.7 mg/dl	(10.8-13.5)
Magnesium:	↑ 2.8 mEq/L	(1.7-2.4)
Total Protein:	↑ 7.9 g/dl	(5.7-7.7)
Albumin:	3.2 g/dl	(2.6-3.8)
Globulin:	↑ 4.7 g/dl	(2.5-4.5)
Sodium:	↑ 152 mEq/L	(130-145)
Chloride:	↑ 117 mEq/L	(97-110)
Potassium:	↑ 5.2 mEq/L	(3.0-5.0)
HCO3:	26 mEq/L	(25-33)
Anion Gap:	14.2 mEq/L	(7-15)
Total Bili:	↑ 7.3 mg/dl	(0.30-3.0)
ALP:	328 IU/L	(109-352)
GGT:	24 IU/L	(4-28)
AST:	↑ 870 IU/L	(190-380)
CK:	↑ 1379 IU/L	(80-446)

Abdominal fluid on Day 4

Appearance: orange/red and opaque

Total protein: 4.3 gm/dl

Total nucleated cells: 270,000/μl

The fluid contains numerous erythrocytes and nucleated cells. Neutrophils predominate and rare neutrophils appear degenerate. Some neutrophils contain intracellular debris, although bacteria are not readily apparent. Rare, small plant fibers are seen along the feathered edge (Figure 7-3).

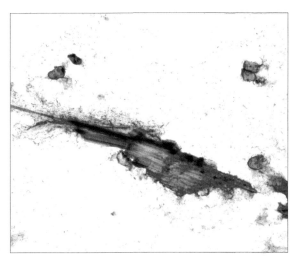

Figure 7-3. Equine abdominocentesis with plant fibers.

Interpretation

Day 1

No CBC was performed. Serum biochemical changes are mild. The slight hypermagnesemia may be due to a pre-renal decrease in glomerular filtration rate associated with dehydration. However, other evidence of dehydration such as azotemia is lacking. The increased bilirubin is mostly likely due to anorexia given the normal ALP and GGT, while the elevated AST and CK suggest muscle damage incurred during transport or treatment (intramuscular injections, etc). The abdominal fluid analysis was within normal limits.

Day 4

CBC: The neutropenia, mild toxic change (Döhle bodies), and hyperfibrinogenemia are compatible with acute inflammation or endotoxemia. This is most likely related to the inflammatory exudate in the abdomen. The lymphopenia may reflect corticosteroid effects.

Serum Biochemical Profile

Hyperglycemia: The hyperglycemia in this case is related to stress, supported by the lymphopenia.

Hypermagnesemia: This may be due to decreased glomerular filtration rate secondary to dehydration or circulatory impairment. There is no azotemia present and a urine specific gravity would be useful in interpretation of these findings.

Hyperproteinemia: The increase in protein is due to an increase in globulins, secondary to inflammation.

Hypernatremia, hyperchloremia: Increased intake of sodium and chloride via diet or fluid therapy is a rare cause of hypernatremia and hyperchloremia. Likewise, hyperadrenocorticism/hyperaldosteronism can cause excessive retention of these electrolytes but are uncommon. Increased sodium and chloride are more often associated with disproportionate losses of water compared to electrolytes via the kidney, gut, or skin. Restriction of water intake may also be a factor, as could replacement of hypotonic fluid losses with isotonic fluid. "Delaney may be experiencing both decreased postsurgical fluid intake as well as hypotonic fluid loss into the gastrointestinal tract, especially if there is ileus with reflux following surgery."

Hyperkalemia: Excessive fluid losses could combine with decreased urinary excretion of potassium to cause hyperkalemia. At this time, Delaney is not azotemic, so impaired renal excretion is less likely. Altered acid/base balance can also impact cellular translocation of potassium, however the HCO3 and anion gap are not abnormal at this time. Intracellular potassium can also be released with tissue damage. A small to moderate amount of damage is likely based on the increase in AST and CK, but this is not likely to significantly impact the serum potassium levels.

Increased AST and CK: This combination of enzymes indicates muscle damage. The increases over that seen on the first day may be secondary to tissue trauma from surgery or additional medical procedures such as intramuscular injections. Poor perfusion associated with sepsis could also contribute to muscle damage.

Case Summary and Outcome

Delaney's septic abdomen was treated by placement of indwelling abdominal drains and serial abdominal lavages. Later, both jugular veins developed thromboses and Delaney's abdominal incisions became infected. Despite these complications, her serum biochemical profiles normalized and she responded well to treatment. She was discharged on antibiotic therapy and with a wound care plan to complete her recovery at home.

Delaney experienced loss of water in excess of electrolytes, leading to increased serum electrolyte concentrations. Replacement of this water with appropriate intravenous fluids or even just increased oral water intake can correct the imbalances. Sometimes water loss alone or even restricted access to water leads to increased serum electrolytes (See Chapter 5, Case 1). Delaney can be compared with previous cases (6, 7) in which the relative losses of water and electrolytes were reversed and excess water was consumed or retained. This illustrates the importance of considering water balance in addition to electrolyte balance when interpreting serum electrolyte data.

Case 9 – Level 2

"Humphrey" is a 16-year-old neutered male domestic short hair cat presenting for lethargy. Four days ago, he vomited a large hairball. The following day, he ate and drank, but vomited three times. For the last 2 days, he has not been eating except for a small amount of baby food and he has become recumbant. On physical examination, Humphrey has normal auscultation and a tense abdomen. An oral examination is not possible because Humphrey wants to bite.

Glucose:	101 mg/dl	(70.0-120.0)
BUN:	↑ 215 mg/dl	(15-32)
Creatinine:	↑ 22.0 mg/dl	(0.9-2.1)
Phosphorus:	↑ 10.8 mg/dl	(3.0-6.0)
Calcium:	9.2 mg/dl	(8.9-11.6)
Magnesium:	2.4 mEq/L	(1.9-2.6)
Total Protein:	↓ 4.9 g/dl	(6.0-8.4)
Albumin:	2.2 g/dl	(2.2.3.4)
Globulin:	2.7 g/dl	(2.5-5.8)
Sodium:	↓ 143 mEq/L	(149-163)
Chloride:	↓ 107 mEq/L	(119-134)
Potassium:	↑ 6.9 mEq/L	(3.6-5.4)
HCO3:	18.5 mEq/L	(13-22)
Cholesterol:	106 mg/dl	(50-150)

Urinalysis: Cystocentesis

Appearance: Yellow and clear	Sediment:
Specific gravity: 1.009	0 RBC/high power field
pH: 7.5	No WBC seen
Protein: negative	No casts seen
Glucose/ketones: negative	No epithelial cells seen
Bilirubin: negative	No bacteria seen
Heme: negative	

Interpretation

A CBC was not done.

Serum Biochemical Profile

Azotemia with isosthenurina: Failure to concentrate urine in an animal with increased BUN and creatinine is compatible with renal azotemia. Although the hydration status was not specifically evaluated, Humphrey's azotemia may be complicated by pre-renal factors.

Hyperphosphatemia: This is most likely due to decreased glomerular filtration rate resulting in failure of the kidney to eliminate phosphorus.

Hypoproteinemia: Serum albumin and globulin are within the reference intervals, however, they are both at the lower end of normal resulting in a lower total protein. Because the serum albumin is at the lower limit of the reference interval, decreased production or increased losses of albumin are possible. Although the dipstick evaluation of protein in the urine was negative, further evaluation of the dilute urine by performing a urine protein:creatinine ratio would be more sensitive. Decreased liver function also may result in decreased production of albumin, but additional tests would be needed to evaluate this possibility. Failure to eliminate water may dilute proteins. These values should be monitored.

Hyponatremia and hypochloremia with normal HCO3: The decrease in chloride is slightly greater than that of sodium. Because decreased intake of these electrolytes rarely results in low serum values, the diagnostic focus is on increased losses, including gastrointestinal, renal, third space, and cutaneous. Humphrey's damaged kidneys likely cannot regulate sodium balance, which could lead to increased renal losses. This could be quantified by performing a urinary fractional excretion of sodium. Disproportional losses of chloride may be related to acid/base abnormalities, however the serum bicarbonate is currently within the reference intervals. Blood gas analysis is needed to uncover a mixed acid/base abnormality when the chloride and bicarbonate do not vary inversely as they typically do.

Hyperkalemia: Polyuric renal failure is often associated with hypokalemia, because the renal tubular flow rate of remaining functional nephrons is high, promoting kaliuresis. In contrast, anuric/oliguric renal failure is often accompanied by hyperkalemia because of low single nephron glomerular filtration rate. Oversupplementation is another cause of hyperkalemia, as is cellular translocation associated with profound tissue trauma, both of which are unlikely in this case.

Case Summary and Outcome

Humphrey was treated with intravenous fluids and gastroprotectants. Despite therapy, his laboratory abnormalities did not improve, and he produced progressively smaller amounts of urine over time. Because of his poor response to therapy and the likely chronic and irreversible nature of his disease, Humphrey was euthanized. At necropsy, Humphrey's tissues were diffusely edematous, suggesting fluid retention and the inability of his kidneys to eliminate a fluid load. Tubulointerstitial nephritis, fibrosis, and mineralization were evident in both kidneys. The lesions were worse in the right kidney, which had severe degeneration of remaining tubules. The cause of the renal failure could not be determined due to the chronic nature of the lesions.

Electrolyte abnormalities associated with renal disease may be quite variable depending on fluid and food intake, use of medications, other concurrent disease processes, and the stage of renal failure (polyuric vs. oliguric/anuric). Although not emphasized in this book, many animals with chronic renal disease who are eating well and have access to water will have normal serum electrolyte levels. Obstruction of urine flow, uroabdomen, or anuric renal failure are often associated with hyperkalemia (Chapter 5, Cases 7, 9, 18). In contrast, patients with polyuric renal failure are predisposed to hypokalemia, particularly if they are anorexic (Chapter 5, Case 10) or have concurrent third space or gastrointestinal losses (Chapter 5, Case 11, 20). Marked and potentially dangerous fluctuations in serum potassium may occur in renal failure patients that undergo rapid changes in glomerular filtration rates associated with relief of severe dehydration or urinary blockage. Alterations in serum sodium and chloride with renal failure are somewhat less predictable than potassium and reflect changes in these electrolytes relative to water. Note that because of fluctuations in water as well as electrolytes and the potential for cellular translocation, serum electrolytes values are not reliable indicators of total body electrolyte stores. Damaged kidneys may be somewhat less able to excrete a sodium load, or to conserve sodium (Chapter 5, Cases 15, 17, 19).

Note that the pattern of hyponatremia, hypochloremia, and hyperkalemia was present in a patient with abdominal effusion (Serengeti, Chapter 7, Case 3), and could be compatible with hypoadrenocorticism. Because patients with adrenal insufficiency often have azotemia and poorly concentrated urine for their degree of dehydration (See Chapter 5, Case 23 and Astra, Chapter 7, Case 13), it may be very difficult to distinguish renal failure from hypoadrenocorticism based on electrolyte abnormalities alone. In Humphrey's case, age and species prioritized renal disease over an endocrinopathy.

Case 10 – Level 2

"Darla" is an 8-year-old spayed female Beagle presenting for hematuria and weakness. On physical examination, Darla is pale, tachycardic and tachypneic. She has no petechiae or ecchymoses, however, 10 to 15 minutes after phlebotomy, a large hematoma forms at the venipuncture site.

White blood cell count:	12.5 x 10⁹/L	(4.0-13.3)
Segmented neutrophils:	11.1 x 10⁹/L	(2.0-11.2)
Band neutrophils:	0.0 x 10⁹/L	(0-0.3)
Lymphocytes:	↓ 0.5 x 10⁹/L	(1.0-4.5)
Monocytes:	0.9 x 10⁹/L	(0.2-1.4)
Eosinophils:	0.0 x 10⁹/L	(0-1.2)
WBC morphology: Appears within normal limits		

Hematocrit:	38%	(37-60)
Red blood cell count:	↓ 5.41 x 10¹²/L	(5.8-8.5)
Hemoglobin:	↓ 12.6 g/dl	(14.0-19.0)
MCV:	66.0 fl	(60.0-77.0)
MCHC:	33.2 g/dl	(31.0-34.0)

Platelets: Clumped, can not estimate

Glucose:	136 mg/dl	(90.0-140.0)
BUN:	19 mg/dl	(6-24)
Creatinine:	0.5 mg/dl	(0.5-1.5)
Phosphorus:	5.1 mg/dl	(2.6-7.2)
Calcium:	↓ 8.6 mg/dl	(9.5-11.5)
Magnesium:	2.3 mEq/L	(1.7-2.5)
Total Protein:	↓ 4.9 g/dl	(5.5-7.8)
Albumin:	↓ 2.5 g/dl	(2.8-4.0)

Globulin:	2.4 g/dl	(2.3-4.2)
Sodium:	↓ 135 mEq/L	(140-151)
Chloride:	↓ 97 mEq/L	(105-120)
Potassium:	↓ 3.2 mEq/L	(3.6-5.6)
Anion Gap:	11.2 mEq/L	(6-16)
HCO3:	↑ 30 mEq/L	(15-28)
Total Bili:	0.2 mg/dl	(0.10-0.50)
ALP:	↑ 393 IU/L	(20-320)
GGT:	<3 IU/L	(2-10)
ALT:	↑ 348 IU/L	(10-95)
AST:	46 IU/L	(10-56)
Cholesterol:	157 mg/dl	(110-314)
Amylase:	481 IU/L	(400-1200)

Interpretation

CBC: Darla is lymphopenic, which suggests corticosteroid effects, although there is no mature neutrophilia or monocytosis. Lymphopenia is one of the most consistent features of the corticosteroid leukogram, while other characteristic changes are not always present. Decreased lymphocyte counts may also be the result of viral mediated lysis or loss via the gastrointestinal tract.

The hematocrit is low normal, while the red blood cell count and hemoglobin are decreased. Darla has evidence of hemorrhage including hematuria and hypoproteinemia, as well as clinical signs which could be related to anemia such as weakness, tachycardia, and tachypnea. Therefore, even though her hematocrit is within the reference interval, it may not be "normal". Although baseline data was not available for Darla, a rapid drop in hematocrit from the upper end of the reference interval to the lower end could have significant physiological effects. While clinical signs may be related to the degree of anemia, they also reflect the rate of decrease in erythrocyte mass. Also, keep in mind that following acute hemorrhage, it may take up to 24 hours to manifest the full decrease in PCV and total protein as these occur subsequent to replacement of intravascular volume by internal fluid shifts, renal conservation of water, and drinking.

Serum Biochemical Profile

Hypocalcemia: Hypocalcemia with normophosphatemia may be associated with hypoalbuminemia, which is present in this case. Darla is spayed, so pregnancy and lactation are not affecting calcium metabolism, nor is there evidence of pancreatic or gastrointestinal disease.

Hypoproteinemia with hypoalbuminemia and low-normal globulins: Low protein values are associated with both increased losses and decreased production. In this case, we are already suspicious of blood loss. There is no evidence of other routes of protein loss such as third space fluid accumulation, skin lesions, or gastrointestinal disease at this time. Because serum albumin is relatively lower than serum globulin levels, selective glomerular loss of albumin is possible. A urinalysis could be performed to quantify protein loss in the urine, however this test will not distinguish proteinuria due to glomerular lesions from protein associated with hematuria originating in other parts of the urinary tract. In these cases, it is often most practical to manage the hematuria prior to attempting to document protein losing nephropathy. Decreased production of protein, predominantly albumin, can be the result of starvation but requires prolonged or severe food deprivation and poor body condition would be evident. Liver failure may also result in decreased synthesis of albumin. Although two liver enzymes are elevated, most analytes on the routine clinical chemistry panel that reflect liver function appear to be within reference intervals (BUN, glucose, and cholesterol). Because these analytes are neither sensitive nor specific indicators of liver function, serum bile acids or blood ammonia measurements should be performed in patients with suspected liver failure. Albumin is a negative acute phase reactant, and its production may be downregulated as part of the inflammatory response. However, there is no evidence of inflammation on the CBC.

Hyponatremia with proportional hypochloridemia: Both increased losses and dilution are likely factors contributing to low serum sodium and chloride. Hemorrhage results in loss of electrolytes proportional to the loss of fluid. Like the fall in PCV and total protein, hyponatremia and hypochloridemia often follow hemorrhage as fluid losses are replaced with water by drinking and as hypotension results in the retention of free water by the kidney due to the action of antidiuretic hormone. Similar mechanisms also may occur when fluids are lost via the gastrointestinal tract, skin, kidney, or into third spaces. Retention of free water can dilute sodium and chloride during pregnancy or congestive heart failure, while the osmotic effects of hyperglycemia can draw water into the circulation from the extravascular space in diabetic patients. Low sodium and chloride are rarely the result of dietary deficiency in small animal patients on commercial diets, even if there is a history of anorexia.

Hypokalemia: The mechanism for Darla's hypokalemia is likely the same as for the abnormalities in sodium and chloride. There is loss of potassium due to hemorrhage with dilution of remaining electrolyte as water accumulates to compensate for the resultant hypovolemia. Inadequate intake of potassium during periods of anorexia may exacerbate hypokalemia.

Increased HCO3: Alkalemia may be associated with the hyperventilation as excessive carbon dioxide is lost when Darla increases her respiratory rate to compensate for the developing anemia and hypoxia.

Mildly increased ALP: There are many extrahepatic causes for increased ALP in the dog, including corticosteroid effects which are suggested by the lymphopenia. This abnormality is mild and not accompanied by a change in GGT, so a thorough medication history should be taken to rule out drug induction. Other considerations include bone disease, endocrinopathies, and cholestatic liver disease. Liver disease is unlikely with the normal GGT and bilirubin. This analyte should be re-evaluated and further work-up is indicated if the increases are persistent or increasing over time. Chapter 2 may be consulted for a complete discussion of hepatic and extrahepatic causes of increased ALP.

Increased ALT: ALT generally suggests hepatocellular damage, but does not indicate cause. In Darla's case, hypoperfusion or poor oxygenation of the liver should be considered as a potential cause for hepatocyte damage. Because the ALP also is elevated, primary liver disease cannot be ruled out. Repeat serum biochemical profile after Darla's anemia is addressed will help determine the appropriate clinical course.

Case Summary and Outcome

The combination of hematuria and hematoma formation at the venipuncture site was considered evidence of coagulopathy, which was confirmed by prolonged prothrombin (PT) and partial thromboplastin times (APTT). After further questioning of the owner it was discovered that Darla had consumed an anticoagulant rodenticide, so she was treated with a plasma transfusion and vitamin K. She was discharged when her clotting times normalized and had an uneventful recovery at home.

Darla developed electrolyte abnormalities because she had been losing isotonic fluids through hemorrhage and replacing them with water, a hypotonic fluid.

Case 11 – Level 2

"Isis" is an 8-year-old spayed female domestic short-haired cat. She was hit by a car 10 days ago and experienced a degloving wound of the right front limb. She has been hospitalized for wound management and is being treated with intravenous fluids and antibiotics. Today, she has tachypnea with harsh lung sounds and tachycardia with a gallop rhythm. On radiographs, Isis has an enlarged liver, cardiomegaly, and pulmonary edema, compatible with congestive heart failure. She began treatment with furosemide earlier in the day, when the doctors noted her tachypnea and harsh lung sounds.

White blood cell count:	↑ 28.4 x 10⁹/L	(5.5-19.5)
Segmented neutrophils:	↑ 25.2 x 10⁹/L	(2.1-10.1)
Bands:	0.3 x 10⁹/L	(0.0-0.3)
Lymphocytes:	2.3 x 10⁹/L	(1.5-7.0)
Monocytes:	0.6 x 10⁹/L	(0-0.9)
WBC morphology: No significant abnormalities noted.		

Hematocrit:	↓ 19%	(28-45)
Red blood cell count:	↓ 4.41 x 10¹²/L	(5.0-10.0)
Hemoglobin:	↓ 5.4 g/dl	(8.0-15.0)
MCV:	↓ 37.0 fl	(39.0-55.0)
MCHC:	↓ 28.4	(31.0-35.0)
RBC morphology: Increased anisocytosis including microcytes		
Platelets: Clumped, but appear adequate in number		

Glucose:	↑ 210 mg/dl	(70.0-120.0)
BUN:	20 mg/dl	(15-32)
Creatinine:	↓ 0.8 mg/dl	(0.9-2.1)
Phosphorus:	↓ 2.7 mg/dl	(3.0-6.0)
Calcium:	↓ 7.3 mg/dl	(8.9-11.6)
Magnesium:	1.6 mEq/L	(1.6-2.6)
Total Protein:	6.4 g/dl	(6.0-8.4)
Albumin:	2.7 g/dl	(2.4-4.0)
Globulin:	3.7 g/dl	(2.5-5.8)
Sodium:	↓ 132 mEq/L	(149-163)
Chloride:	↓ 82 mEq/L	(119-134)
Potassium:	↓ 3.2 mEq/L	(3.6-5.4)
HCO3:	↑ 32 mEq/L	(13-22)
Anion Gap:	21.2 mEq/L	(13-27)
Total Bili:	↑ 0.4 mg/dl	(0.10-0.30)
ALP:	↑ 85 IU/L	(10-72)
GGT:	1 IU/L	(0-5)
ALT:	48 IU/L	(29-145)
AST:	↑ 79 IU/L	(12-42)
Cholesterol:	256 mg/dl	(77-258)
Amylase:	↑ 3323 IU/L	(496-1874)

Interpretation

CBC: Isis has a neutrophilic leukocytosis compatible with inflammation from the leg wound. She also has a microcytic, hypochromic anemia that may be related to chronic blood loss and iron deficiency from the degloving wound.

Serum Biochemical Profile

Hyperglycemia: The increased serum glucose is attributed to pain and/or stress.

Hypophosphatemia: The increased HCO_3 and alkalosis are contributing to an intracellular shift of serum phosphorus. Primary hyperparathyroidism and hypercalcemia of malignancy may also cause hypophosphatemia, however these conditions generally are associated with hypercalcemia, while Isis has hypocalcemia.

Hypocalcemia: Hypocalcemia is frequently associated with low serum albumin, which is not the case here. There is no evidence of renal disease, nor does hypoparathyroidism seem likely with the low serum phosphorus. Cats receiving infusions of bicarbonate or treatment with diuretics such as furosemide can develop hypocalcemia. These treatments may result in a failure to develop a sodium gradient that is adequate to drive passive reabsorption of calcium in the ascending limb of the renal tubule.

Hyponatremia with disproportionate hypochloremia: If the chloride is corrected for the degree of hyponatremia ($82 \times 146/132$), it becomes 90.7, still significantly below the reference interval. Increased losses of sodium and chloride may be occurring through the skin because of the degloving injury. Because diuretic therapy is being used, further sodium wasting may occur in the kidney. In circumstances characterized by renal hypoperfusion such as congestive heart failure, total body sodium may increase because activation of the renin-angiotensin system stimulates increased proximal tubular reabsorption of sodium and water. Because of this, less fluid arrives at the distal parts of the tubule responsible for free water excretion. In addition, non-osmotic stimulation of antidiuretic hormone release further impairs water excretion, leading to dilution of electrolytes in the plasma. Diuretics like furosemide inhibit chloride reabsorption and can slightly increase bicarbonate as well. Hypochloremia is associated with alkalosis.

Hypokalemia: If Isis has a poor appetite, decreased intake may compound increased losses associated with renin-angiotensin system activation. Inadequate delivery of sodium to the distal tubule can predispose to kaliuresis, and diuretic use will exacerbate renal losses of potassium. The diuretic effect may be worse in cats than other species and is more pronounced if electrolyte intake is decreased because of anorexia.

Increased HCO_3 (alkalemia): The effects of the diuretic therapy and chloride depletion contribute to the increased HCO_3. Because of the potential for concurrent respiratory issues in this patient, a blood gas analysis may provide further information about the acid/base status.

Increased AST: This abnormality is mild and probably reflects tissue damage associated with perfusion deficits.

Hyperamylasemia: Increased serum amylase in this case is attributed to decreased glomerular filtration rate. Concurrent pancreatic disease cannot be ruled out, however amylase is not a good indicator of pancreatitis in cats.

Case Summary and Outcome

Intravenous fluid treatment was discontinued and Isis was treated with diuretics to correct the fluid load that was thought to have precipitated the congestive heart failure. She responded well and ultimately recovered from her wound. Various diuretics influence electrolyte homeostasis (See Snow, Chapter 7, Case 7), so the specific medication should be chosen carefully and serum electrolyte values should be monitored.

This case is similar to Darla (Chapter 7, Case 10), who was experiencing isotonic fluid losses that were replaced with water, leading to low serum electrolyte concentrations. Isis's electrolyte abnormalities were further complicated by intravascular volume expansion due to iatrogenic fluid overload and secondary heart failure.

Case 12 – Level 2

"Weasel" is a 10-year-old neutered male Collie dog presenting with a 4 month history of hematuria. Four months ago, he had an initial episode of hematuria that cleared after two cycles of antibiotic treatment. At that time, abdominal radiographs were unremarkable. Two months ago, the hematuria recurred but did not resolve despite prolonged antibiotic therapy. Four days ago, Weasel was presented for further work up for the hematuria. The owners noted that Weasel does not appear to strain, but will urinate, move a few feet, and then urinate a smaller amount which is usually bloodier than the initial urine. He seems to be urinating at the same frequency as he always has. Other than the hematuria, he seemed to be normal and healthy. On physical examination, Weasel appeared well hydrated with normal vital signs and auscultation. However, he was tense on abdominal palpation, and abdominal ultrasound revealed a mass along the ventral aspect of the bladder wall close to the neck. Surgical removal of the mass was scheduled for the following week. However, Weasel's condition deteriorated over the past 4 days, and he returned to the hospital due to lethargy, vomiting, anorexia, straining to urinate and abdominal distension. On this presentation, Weasel is depressed and weak, and there is melena on rectal examination.

White blood cell count:	↑ 17.3 x 10⁹/L	(6.0-17.0)
Segmented neutrophils:	↑ 15.8 x 10⁹/L	(3.0-11.0)
Band neutrophils:	0.0 x 10⁹/L	(0-0.3)
Lymphocytes:	↓ 0.6 x 10⁹/L	(1.0-4.8)
Monocytes:	0.9 x 10⁹/L	(0.2-1.4)
Eosinophils:	0.0 x 10⁹/L	(0-1.3)
WBC morphology: No abnormalities noted		

Hematocrit:	53%	(37-55)
Red blood cell count:	8.11 x 10¹²/L	(5.5-8.5)
Hemoglobin:	18.0 g/dl	(12.0-18.0)
MCV:	65.8 fl	(60.0-77.0)
MCHC:	34.4 g/dl	(31.0-34.0)
RBC morphology: Appears within normal limits		

Platelets:	268 x 10⁹/L	(200-450)

Glucose:	↑ 177 mg/dl	(80.0-125.0)
BUN:	↑ 160 mg/dl	(6-24)
Creatinine:	↑ 12.8 mg/dl	(0.5-1.5)
Phosphorus:	↑ 17.7 mg/dl	(3.0-6.0)

Calcium:	↑ 11.3 mg/dl	(8.8-11.0)
Magnesium:	↑ 3.6 mEq/L	(1.4-2.2)
Total Protein:	7.2 g/dl	(4.7-7.3)
Albumin:	3.6 g/dl	(2.5-4.2)
Globulin:	3.6 g/dl	(2.0-4.0)
Sodium:	↓ 133 mEq/L	(141-151)
Chloride:	↓ 90 mEq/L	(108-121)
Potassium:	5.3 mEq/L	(3.8-5.4)
HCO3:	↓ 13.1 mEq/L	(15-26)
Anion Gap:	↑ 35.2 mEq/L	(15-25)
Total Bili:	↑ 0.6 mg/dl	(0.10-0.50)
ALP:	↑ 666 IU/L	(20-320)
GGT:	5 IU/L	(2-10)
ALT:	↑ 154 IU/L	(5-65)
AST:	↑ 64 IU/L	(15-52)
Cholesterol:	↑ 376 mg/dl	(110-314)
Amylase:	↑ 1572 IU/L	(252-988)

Abdominal fluid analysis

Appearance: Red and turbid

Total nucleated cell count: 8,900 cells/μl

Total protein: <2.5 g/dl

Description: Smears contain small numbers of erythrocytes. The predominant nucleated cell is a nondegenerate neutrophil, which occurs with smaller numbers of large mononuclear cells and reactive mesothelial cells.

Interpretation

CBC: Weasel has a mature neutrophilic leukocytosis and a lymphopenia compatible with a corticosteroid leukogram.

Serum Biochemical Profile

Hyperglycemia: Both endogeneous and exogenous corticosteroids can cause hyperglycemia. Diabetes mellitus should also be considered. Diabetic patients may present with signs of urinary tract disease because of polyuria/polydipsia or concurrent urinary tract infections, however the degree of hyperglycemia is mild at this time.

Marked azotemia: Azotemia should be classified as pre-renal, renal, or post-renal, however a urine specific gravity was not reported in this case. A pre-renal component to the azotemia cannot be ruled out at this point, however the clinical history does not include a clear evaluation of the hydration status. Other indications of dehydration such as polycythemia and hyperproteinemia are not present. Renal failure is possible, however the presence of a mass in the urinary bladder suggests a post-renal cause for azotemia. The recent onset of abdominal distention could be compatible with a ruptured urinary bladder. Weasel has melena and digestion of blood in the intestinal track that may contribute to a mild increase in BUN.

Hyperphosphatemia: This abnormality is due to failure of elimination of phosphorus in the kidney.

Hypermagnesemia: Like phosphorus, retention of magnesium is attributed to failure of elimination through the kidney.

Hyponatremia with disproportionately greater hypochloremia and acidemia: The corrected chloride is 98 mEq/L, so not all of the decrease in chloride may be accounted for by forces acting on sodium concentration. Given the distended abdomen, third space loss of both electrolytes is likely, and inability to eliminate water in the urine can cause dilutional effects. This shift in sodium may be exacerbated by free water retention stimulated by hypotension or low plasma osmolality. Vomiting may contribute to chloride loss. Corrected hypochloremia is typically associated with alkalosis, however Weasel has a low bicarbonate and increased anion gap compatible with a metabolic acidosis, therefore a mixed acid/base disorder is suspected. A blood gas analysis will further characterize the acid/base status. Hyponatremia and hypochloremia can characterize hypoadrenocorticism, however evaluation of the urinary bladder should be the diagnostic priority at this time due to the clinical history.

Increased anion gap: The increased anion gap may be associated with accumulation of uremic acids.

Very mild hyperbilirubinemia: This value is just outside the reference interval, and as an isolated finding it would be of questionable clinical significance. The high normal PCV makes hemolysis an unlikely cause for the increased bilirubin, while the elevations in liver enzymes would suggest the potential for liver disease.

Increased ALP: ALP is a very sensitive indicator of liver disease, but may increase in response to a large number of extrahepatic influences, including metabolic and hormonal disorders. The hyperbilirubinemia and increased ALT and AST support some liver pathology, however severe cholestasis is unlikely given the normal GGT and relatively mild change in bilirubin. The corticosteroid leukogram is compatible with some degree of hormonal induction of ALP.

Increased ALT and AST: The elevation in ALT roughly mirrors the two-fold increase in ALP noted above. It suggests hepatocellular damage, however the etiology is unclear. While ALT may be slightly less sensitive to extrahepatic processes than ALP, it may still increase in the absence of primary liver disease, including in response to corticosteroids. Elevations in AST are less liver-specific than ALT.

Hypercholesterolemia: Because dogs are have a predominance of high density lipoproteins, hypercholesterolemia is unlikely to cause clinical disease but is often used as an indicator of other pathologic processes. Among the things that can promote high cholesterol in dogs are hyperadrenocorticism (possible because of the hyperglycemia, corticosteroid leukogram, and increased ALP), diabetes mellitus (possible because of the hyperglycemia, but not likely), liver disease (possible because of the hyperbilirubinemia and elevated liver enzymes), and renal disease (possible because of the azotemia). Post-prandial effects should be considered, but Weasel has been anorectic.

Hyperamylasemia: The change in this analyte is less than two-fold, thus may be explained by decreased glomerular filtation rate. Pancreatic or intestinal pathology may also contribute.

Abdominal fluid analysis: Despite the low protein, the increased nucleated cell count and predominance of neutrophils suggests suppurative inflammation, which appears to be sterile at this time. Consideration should be given to chemical peritonitis such as uroabdomen (most likely) or bile peritonitis (less likely with clinical history and absence of bile pigment). Comparision of abdominal fluid and serum creatinine measurements can help confirm the presence of urine in the abdomen.

Case Summary and Outcome

Weasel was sent to surgery for abdominal lavage and surgical correction of suspected urinary bladder rupture. Four liters of urine were removed from his abdomen at surgery and a liver biopsy was collected to investigate the potential for liver disease suggested by the liver enzyme elevations. The day after surgery, Weasel appeared brighter and was producing normal amounts of urine. The next day, however, he became lethargic and began vomiting. A positive contrast cystogram revealed urinary bladder leakage through the ventral bladder wall. He went back to surgery, where one liter of serosanguinous fluid was removed and a puncture wound was repaired that was assumed to be the result of stay sutures or the needle used to leak test the incision. Weasel recovered well, and was discharged on piroxicam for the transitional cell carcinoma that was diagnosed by cytology of his bladder mass.

Weasel's data should be compared with Sloop's (Chapter 5, Case 18). Sloop also had a diagnosis of uroabdomen, with a distended abdomen, azotemia, hyperphosphatemia, hyponatremia, hypochloridemia and increased anion gap. Unlike Weasel, Sloop was hyperkalemic and had normal serum bicarbonate compared with Weasel's acidemia. This variation reflects the interindividual differences that often occur between individuals with similar or identical diagnoses. It is likely that Sloop was less able to pass significant amounts of urine for a more prolonged period, leading to accumulation of greater amounts of potassium, while Weasel is less able to compensate for the developing acidosis. Weasel's azotemia is significantly more severe than Sloop's. One possible interpretation of this data is that Weasel has underlying renal disease that interferes with renal regulation of acid/base status, although differences in the pre-renal contribution to azotemia may also influence the data. It should be noted that the degree of azotemia does not correlate with glomerular filtration rate in a linear fashion, and direct comparison of glomerular filtration rates between individual animals using the BUN and serum creatinine is problematic (see the introduction to Chapter 5 for further discussion of interpretation of BUN and serum creatinine).

Case 13 – Level 2

"Astra" is a 4-year-old spayed female Boxer dog presenting with recent weight loss of 22 pounds and exercise intolerance. She has been anorexic with intermittent vomiting, but has not had diarrhea. Astra has had two to four episodes of weakness and collapse. Astra had a positive Lyme snap-test and was treated with antibiotics for two weeks. On physical examination, she is very thin and has marked muscle atrophy. Her capillary refill time is prolonged at 4 seconds, and her eyes are sunken. One of Astra's owners instructs you to do everything necessary to make her better, the other does not wish to pursue diagnostics "because she's a Boxer and she's going to die anyway."

White blood cell count:	14.3 x 10⁹/L	(6.0-17.0)
Segmented neutrophils:	7.6 x 10⁹/L	(3.0-11.0)
Band neutrophils:	0 x 10⁹/L	(0-0.3)
Lymphocytes:	↑ 6.0 x 10⁹/L	(1.0-4.8)
Monocytes:	0.4 x 10⁹/L	(0.2-1.4)
Eosinophils:	0.3 x 10⁹/L	(0-1.3)

WBC morphology: No significant abnormalities seen.

Hematocrit:	↓ 29%	(37-55)
MCV:	66.4 fl	(60.0-77.0)
MCHC:	↑ 37.9 g/dl	(31.0-34.0)

RBC morphology: There is slightly increased anisocytosis. Small numbers of schistocytes, spherocytes, Howell-Jolly bodies, and acanthocytes are present.

Platelets:	400 x 10⁹/L	(200-450)

Plasma appears markedly hemolyzed.

Glucose:	78 mg/dl	(65.0-120.0)
BUN:	↑ 84 mg/dl	(8-33)
Creatinine:	↑ 2.2 mg/dl	(0.5-1.5)
Phosphorus:	↑ 7.9 mg/dl	(3.0-6.0)
Calcium:	↑ 11.8 mg/dl	(8.8-11.0)
Magnesium:	↑ 3.0 mEq/L	(1.4-2.7)
Total Protein:	6.3 g/dl	(5.2-7.2)
Albumin:	↓ 2.6 g/dl	(3.0-4.2)
Globulin:	3.7 g/dl	(2.0-4.0)
Sodium:	↓ 133 mEq/L	(140-151)
Chloride:	↓ 106 mEq/L	(108-120)
Potassium:	↑ 7.0 mEq/L	(3.8-5.4)
HCO3:	20 mEq/L	(16-25)
Anion Gap:	↓ 14 mEq/L	(15-25)
Total Bili:	0.2 mg/dl	(0.10-0.50)
ALP:	180 IU/L	(20-320)
GGT:	3 IU/L	(3-10)
ALT:	47 IU/L	(10-95)
AST:	↑ 67 IU/L	(15-52)
Cholesterol:	107 mg/dl	(110-314)
Triglycerides:	62 mg/dl	(30-300)
Amylase:	↑ 1806 IU/L	(400-1200)

Urinalysis: Method of collection not indicated
Appearance: Yellow and hazy
Specific gravity: 1.016
pH: 9.0
Protein, glucose, ketones, bilirubin, heme: negative
Sediment:
No cells, casts, or crystals
3+ bacteria

Interpretation

CBC: There is a mild lymphocytosis with no associated morphologic abnormalities. This may be attributable to the effects of epinephrine. Alternatively, antigenic stimulation can increased lymphocyte numbers in the circulation. This interpretation would be strengthened if reactive lymphocytes were present. Lymphoid neoplasia could be considered but is less likely given that no atypia is described. Absence of a steroid leukogram in a severely ill dog with appropriate history and serum biochemical data can suggest hypoadrenocortism.

There is a mild normocytic anemia with evidence of hemolysis. Because erythropoiesis never results in excessive hemoglobin content in cells, the increase in MCHC is interpreted to be artifactual and related to the hemolysis. It cannot be determined whether the hemolysis is in vitro or in vivo, however the presence of small numbers of schistocytes and spherocytes is compatible with some in vivo hemolysis. Spherocytes are often associated with immune mediated damage to erythrocytes. Less frequent causes include zinc toxicity, snake or bee envenomation, and erythrocyte metabolic abnormalities. In small numbers, this finding may be non-specific and not diagnostically useful. The same is true for schistocytes, which can be associated with abnormal vasculature, hemostatic abnormalities, or iron deficiency. Howell-Jolly bodies may reflect decreased splenic function, immunosuppression, or increased erythrocyte production. The anisocytosis may be due to small numbers of immature macrocytic erythrocytes that are too few in number to impact the MCV. Additionally, it may be associated with the presence of spherocytes, which appear smaller because of their change from discoid to spherical shape. In fact, the actual volume of spherocytic erythrocytes is minimally affected. Usually hemolysis is associated with a macrocytic, regenerative anemia. It may be that the process is too acute and there has been insufficient time for a regenerative response to become apparent. Erythropoietic response should be assessed with a reticulocyte count, and it takes at least 3-4 days for a significant reticulocytosis to develop following hemorrhage or hemolysis. It is possible that the anemia is non-regenerative and may be related to chronic disease or malnutrition. However, there is no inflammatory leukogram to suggest inflammation.

Serum Biochemical Profile

Azotemia: Astra's urine is not optimally concentrated, suggesting that there may be a renal cause for the azotemia, although a pre-renal component is almost certainly superimposed. Low glomerular filtration rate is also supported by the hyperphosphatemia, hypermagnesemia, hyperamylasemia, and possibly the hyperkalemia. Before renal azotemia can be confirmed, other extra-renal causes of poor urinary concentrating ability should be considered. Liver failure is unlikely given the normal bilirubin, cholesterol and high BUN, however the albumin is low. Serum bile acids or blood ammonia are required to confirm liver dysfunction. Osmotic diuresis is also unlikely with normal urinalysis, and there is no history of diuretic usage. Medullary washout is possible given the hyponatremia and hypochloremia. If medullary washout is the reason for the poorly concentrated urine, appropriate electrolyte supplementation and fluid therapy should correct the problem.

Hyperphosphatemia and hypercalcemia: Renal failure, vitamin D toxicity, and hypoadreno-corticism can lead to these changes. Both renal failure and hypoadrenocorticism are compatible with the other laboratory data and in both, inadequate glomerular filtration rate for elimination of phosphorus leads to its accumulation in the blood. Hypoadrenocorticism is a cause of hypercalcemia in dogs, but is not associated with increases in ionized calcium and the increased calcium is therefore not pathogenic. Diminished renal excretion because of cortisol deficiency and hemoconcentration are potential mechanisms for the hypercalcemia and the calcium level should normalize quickly after initiation of therapy. The most common cause of hypercalcemia in dogs is hypercalcemia of malignancy, which cannot be ruled out in this case. Increases in ionized calcium can cause both reversible and irreversible renal dysfunction, predisposing to the development of hyperphosphatemia. Measurement of parathyroid hormone (PTH) and parathyroid hormone related protein (PTHrP) can help differentiate various causes of hypercalcemia, but is not necessary in this case.

Hypermagnesemia: Decreased glomerular filtration rate is the cause for the high magnesium.

Hypoalbuminemia: Albumin may be decreased because of inadequate production or excessive losses. Because albumin is produced in the liver, poor liver function can result in low serum albumin. Other laboratory abnormalities that may also occur with poor liver function are not present (see above), however serum bile acid measurement could be considered if other explanations for hypoalbuminemia are not applicable. The liver may decrease albumin production in response to inflammation, however the globulin levels are not elevated, nor is there evidence of inflammation in the CBC. Nutritional factors are an uncommon cause of hypoalbuminemia, however Astra has experienced significant weight loss and is in poor body condition, suggesting that albumin may be low because of inadequate protein intake and body stores. Albumin may be diluted in patients with accumulation of fluid in the circulation, which could also result in hyponatremia and hypochloremia. This is most often seen with excessive accumulation of an osmole such as glucose in the circulation, which is not the case here. Excessive selective loss of albumin from the glomerulus is unlikely given the negative protein on urinalysis, however urine protein:creatinine ratio may be a better measure of this in a patient with relatively dilute urine. Nonselective loss of protein into body cavity effusion, via exudative skin lesions, or into the gut is not suspected based on the absence of compatible clinical findings and the normal serum globulin.

Hyponatremia and hypochloremia: Low sodium and chloride in small animal patients on commercial diets are rarely related to inadequate intake. Accumulation of free water with dilution of these electrolytes is a potential mechanism. This can be present in association with congestive heart failure and excessive accumulation of free water due to the effects of antidiuretic hormone. This potentially could explain the prolonged capillary refill time and could cause a pre-renal azotemia as well as syncopal episodes, but it would not easily explain the gastrointestinal signs. Increased losses are the most likely cause for Astra's hyponatremia and hypochloremia, which are approximately proportional. Given her history, gastrointestinal losses are possible. The potential for third space and dermal losses should be evaluated in the context of the clinical information. Renal losses should also be considered, and can be quantified by performing urinary fractional excretions. Patients with hyponatremia should have low urinary fractional excretion of sodium as the body attempts to conserve the electrolyte. Normal to increased fractional excretion under these circumstances would be abnormal and reflect either renal disease or hypoadrenocorticism (lack of aldosterone to signal the need to conserve sodium by the kidney).

Hyperkalemia: Polyuric renal failure is often associated with hypokalemia because of enhanced urinary potassium loss. It is only when glomerular filtration is markedly limited or when urine cannot be eliminated from the body that hyperkalemia ensues. Astra has marked dehydration and clinical evidence of poor perfusion, including weak femoral pulses and prolonged capillary refill time. This could severely reduce glomerular filtration rate. Her other laboratory abnormalities also are suggestive for hypoadrenocorticism, which could lead to hyperkalemia because of aldosterone deficiency. Cellular translocation in response to acidosis is also possible, however this appears to be less important with organic acidosis than mineral acidosis.

Decreased anion gap: The low albumin and abnormal electrolyte values may decrease the anion gap.

Increased AST: This most likely reflects tissue damage secondary to poor perfusion.

Increased amylase: The mild change in this value is most compatible with the decreased glomerular filtration rate. Gastrointestinal disease also can be associated with increased amylase and is compatible with the clinical history. Pancreatic disease cannot be ruled out, but is not required to explain this data.

Urinalysis: The bactiuria indicates either contamination or a urinary tract infection.

Case Summary and Outcome

Based on the suspicion of hypoadrenocorticism, an ACTH stimulation test was performed. Both pre and post-stimulation values were <1.00 μg/dl, compatible with a diagnosis of hypoadrenocorticism. A cardiology consult was not pursued based on normal auscultation and thoracic radiographs. Astra was successfully treated with hormone supplementation and antibiotics for the urinary tract infection.

These electrolyte abnormalities are classic for hypoadrenocorticism, however they are not present in all cases of hypoadrenocorticism (Sadek). Therefore, any dog with a suggestive history including weakness, lethargy, gastrointestinal signs, or collapse with hypovolemia could potentially have hypoadrenocorticism. In some cases, the absence of any features of the corticosteroid leukogram despite signs of severe illness may be a clue. Hyponatremia, hypochloremia and hyperkalemia may also characterize other processes in addition to hypoadrenocorticim. These conditions include primary gastrointestinal disease (DiBartola), cavity effusions (Chapter 7, Case 3) including uroabdomen (Chapter 5, Case 18), or renal failure (Chapter 7, Case 9). Astra is a good example of extra-renal factors resulting in laboratory data that could suggest primary renal disease. Astra is azotemic with relatively dilute urine, hyperphosphatemia, hypermagnesemia, and hyperkalemia. All of these changes may result from decreased glomerular filtration rate as was the case for Humphrey (Chapter 7, Case 9). Low sodium and chloride could be attributable to primary renal dysfunction, in which case urinary fractional excretions of these electrolytes would be high. Typically, appropriate fluid therapy will correct electrolyte abnormalities and temporarily restore urinary concentrating ability in patients with hypoadrenocorticism, while patients with renal failure will continue to produce dilute urine.

DiBartola SP, Johnson SE, Davenport DJ, Prueter JC, Chew DJ, Sherding RG. Clinicopathologic findings resembling hypoadrenocorticism in dogs with primary gastrointestinal disease. J Am Vet Med Assoc. 1985;187:60-63.

Sadek D, Schaer M. Atypical addison's disease in the dog: a retrospective survey of 14 cases. J Am Anim Hosp Assoc 1996;32:159-163.

Case 14 – Level 3

"Twix" is a 2-week-old Brown Swiss/Holstein mix calf presenting with a three day history of diarrhea and lethargy. Originally, the diarrhea was yellow and runny, and she was treated with antibiotics and electrolyte solutions. Over the past 2 days, the diarrhea became white and watery. On physical examination, Twix had a good suckle reflex, though she was dull, lethargic, and reluctant to stand. Ausculatation was normal, and she was mildly dehydrated. Twix was not febrile or bloated. The diarrhea now has a dark brown mucoid, pudding-like consistency. One other calf in the herd also may be affected. This farm has had documented infections with *Cryptosporidium, Salmonella,* and corona virus in the past.

White blood cell count:	↑ 17.3 x 10⁹/L	(4.1-11.3)
Segmented neutrophils:	5.7 x 10⁹/L	(0.8-7.2)
Band neutrophils:	↑ 3.1 x 10⁹/L	(0-0.1)
Lymphocytes:	4.5 x 10⁹/L	(1.1-7.1)
Monocytes:	↑ 4.0 x 10⁹/L	(0.0-0.9)

WBC morphology: 1+ toxic change in the neutrophils and rare reactive lymphocytes

Hematocrit:	36%	(24-39)
MCV:	↓ 36.4 fl	(39.2-52.5)
MCHC:	35.5 g/dl	(33.5-35.7)

RBC morphology: Scattered acanthocytes and echinocytes

Platelets:	↑ 754 x 10⁹/L	(222-718)

Glucose:	↑ 101 mg/dl	(56-83)
BUN:	↑ 32 mg/dl	(6-20)
Creatinine:	↑ 1.7 mg/dl	(0.5-1.1)
Phosphorus:	6.6 mg/dl	(4.0-7.7)
Calcium:	9.5 mg/dl	(8.4-10.1)
Magnesium:	2.5 mEq/L	(1.7-2.5)
Total Protein:	↓ 5.6 g/dl	(6.9-9.4)
Albumin:	2.5 g/dl	(2.5-3.5)
Globulin:	3.1 g/dl	(2.5-4.5)
Sodium:	↑ 163 mEq/L	(134-144)
Chloride:	↑ 136 mEq/L	(95-106)
Potassium:	5.1 mEq/L	(3.9-5.5)
HCO3:	↓ 14 mEq/L	(26-33)
Anion Gap:	18.1 mEq/L	(14-20)
Total Bili:	↑ 0.8 mg/dl	(0.10-0.4)
ALP:	↑ 223 IU/L	(29-101)
GGT:	↑ 333 IU/L	(5-34)
AST:	↑ 424 IU/L	(190-380)
SDH:	15 IU/L	(4-55)
CK:	↑ 1224 IU/L	(63-294)
AST:	↑ 95 IU/L	(26-93)
	(Reference intervals are for adult cows)	

Interpretation

CBC: Twix has a leukocytosis with increased band neutrophils, toxic change, and monocytosis, indicating inflammation (Figure 7-4). The microcytosis may be due to age associated differences in red blood cell size (Adams). Thrombocytosis is often associated with inflammation in large animal species.

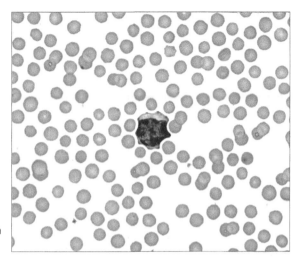

Figure 7-4. Reactive lymphocyte in bovine blood film.

Serum Biochemical Profile

Hyperglycemia: Stress is the most likely explanation for the hyperglycemia, however since the transition to ruminal digestion does not occur in calves until 3 to 4 weeks of age, serum glucose levels may be somewhat higher than in the adult.

Azotemia: Twix is mildly azotemic. Without a urine specific gravity, the azotemia is difficult to classify, however the history and physical examination suggest pre-renal azotemia due to dehydration.

Hypoproteinemia: Both albumin and globulin levels are within the reference intervals, making the significance of the low total protein difficult to interpret. Neonatal animals often have lower serum total protein values because of relatively greater total body water content and naïve immune systems. The protein values may be elevated by dehydration, and should be reassessed after fluid deficits are corrected.

Hypernatremia and hyperchloremia: In this case, isotonic or hypotonic fluid losses combined with supplementation with hypertonic to isotonic fluids leads to relative water deficit and accumulation of excessive electrolytes. Most patients that have access to water and have adequate renal function will still be able to regulate serum electrolyte concentrations. Unfortunately, Twix did not have access to water, but it is likely that she has normal renal function and the mild azotemia is pre-renal.

Decreased bicarbonate (acidemia): Loss of bicarbonate containing fluids in the diarrhea is the likely cause of the low bicarbonate.

Increased ALP: While an increase in the ALP could be compatible with hepatobiliary disease, bone growth in young animals also will elevate this value and complicate interpretation.

Increased GGT: Elevation in serum GGT is a more specific indicator of liver disease in large animal species than ALP, however it may also be influenced by age-related phenomena such as peripartum elevations following colostrum ingestion. In addition, liver damage may occur secondary to intestinal disease and/or hypoperfusion. The normal SDH suggests that increases in ALP and GGT may be due to extra-hepatic causes such as bone growth and colostrum ingestion, respectively. While less likely, it is possible that liver damage occurred transiently in the past but is not ongoing and thus is no longer reflected by changes in SDH, which has a very short serum half life and rapidly decreases after cessation of injury.

Increased AST and CK: These enzyme elevations suggest muscle damage, potentially related to medical intervention or transport. The AST is less tissue-specific than the CK and could also be related to hepatocellular damage.

Case Summary and Outcome

Twix was treated with intravenous fluids containing bicarbonate until the acidosis resolved, then she received oral milk replacer. Sodium and chloride supplementation was gradually decreased until her electrolyte abnormalities were corrected. She was also treated with antibiotics. Fecal samples were evaluated for *Salmonella,* corona virus, rota virus, and *Escherichia coli,* and a non-hemolytic *E. coli* was cultured. Twix responded well to therapy and was released from the hospital.

Like Delaney (Chapter 7, Case 8), Twix likely experienced loss of hypotonic fluids, leading to concentration of remaining electrolytes in a smaller volume of intravascular water. Generally, this will stimulate thirst and water intake, so in both patients, restricted access to water may have contributed to the electrolyte abnormalities. Loss of isotonic fluids can also result in hypernatremia and hyperchloridemia if electrolytes are over-supplemented as was the case for Twix. This is roughly the opposite process that occurred with Darla (Chapter 7, Case 10), where isotonic fluid loss associated with hemorrhage was replaced by increased intake of water, diluting remaining electrolytes in the blood. These cases show that gains and losses of both electrolytes and water must be considered when evaluating serum electrolyte data.

Adams R, Garry FB, Aldridge BM, Holland MD, Odde KG. Hematologic values in newborn beef calves. Am J Vet Res. 1992;53:944-950.

Case 15 – Level 3

"Jason" is a 3-year-old Staffordshire Terrier presenting with anorexia and lethargy after consuming 1/3 of the Thanksgiving turkey carcass 2 weeks ago. He previously was diagnosed with diabetes mellitus. Jason is being treated with insulin, but he has had worsening polyuria and polydipsia despite increasing doses of insulin. Several weeks ago, hematuria was noted and Jason was treated with antibiotics. Jason typically has an excellent appetite, but had been eating less prior to the turkey episode. On presentation to the referring veterinary practice 2 days ago, mineral opacities were seen on survey radiographs. A subsequent abdominal exploratory merely revealed an area of ileus, which was evacuated with no evidence of obstruction. At that time, the liver was enlarged and fatty in appearance. A biopsy was taken, however no results are yet available. Two days after surgery, Jason was referred to the teaching hospital because of declining status and inability to maintain hydration despite fluid therapy. On presentation, Jason appears obtunded, dehydrated and shocky. He has bilateral diabetic cataracts and a non-painful but doughy abdomen. He has numerous decubital ulcers, with a large decubital ulcer over his left lateral hock.

White blood cell count:	↑ 39.1 x 10⁹/L	(6.0-17.0)
Segmented neutrophils:	↑ 35.9 x 10⁹/L	(3.0-11.0)
Band neutrophils:	↑ 0.4 x 10⁹/L	(0-0.2)
Lymphocytes:	↓ 0.8 x 10⁹/L	(1.0-4.8)
Monocytes:	↑ 1.6 x 10⁹/L	(0.2-1.2)
Eosinophils:	0.4 x 10⁹/L	(0-1.3)
WBC morphology: No significant abnormalities noted		

Hematocrit:	↓ 25%	(37-55)
MCV:	↓ 62.7.4 fl	(64.0-77.0)
MCHC:	↓ 30.8 g/dl	(31.0-34.0)
RBC morphology: Mild anisocytosis and polychromasia, rare Howell-Jolly bodies		

Platelets:	↑ 585 x 10⁹/L	(200-450)

Glucose:	↑ 194 mg/dl	(65.0-120.0)
BUN:	↓ 4 mg/dl	(8-33)
Creatinine:	0.5 mg/dl	(0.5-1.5)
Phosphorus:	4.3 mg/dl	(3.0-6.0)
Calcium:	↓ 8.8 mg/dl	(9.5-11.5)
Magnesium:	1.9 mEq/L	(1.4-2.7)
Total Protein:	5.3 g/dl	(5.2-7.2)
Albumin:	↓ 2.4 g/dl	(2.5-3.7)
Globulin:	2.9 g/dl	(2.0-4.0)
Sodium:	↑ 163 mEq/L	(140-151)
Chloride:	↑ 130 mEq/L	(105-120)
Potassium:	4.6 mEq/L	(3.8-5.4)
HCO3:	22.4 mEq/L	(16-25)
Anion Gap:	15.2 mEq/L	(15-25)
CK:	↑ 3220	(55-309)
Cholesterol:	266 mg/dl	(110-314)

Interpretation

CBC: Jason has a moderate neutrophilic leukocytosis with a mild regenerative left shift, lymphopenia, and monocytosis. Corticosteroid effects could contribute to the increased mature neutrophils, lymphopenia and monocytosis, while the regenerative left shift suggests inflammation is also playing a role in the leukogram changes. Jason has a microcytic hypochromic anemia, which suggests the potential for an iron deficiency anemia, especially in combination with the thrombocytosis. A portosystemic shunt may be accompanied by microcytosis but is unlikely with the other clinical and laboratory data. Some Japanese breeds normally are microcytic (Akita or Shiba Inu).

Serum Biochemical Profile

Hyperglycemia: Although this level of blood glucose is compatible with other causes of hyperglycemia such as stress, corticosteroid treatment, or pancreatitis, diabetes mellitus is the most likely cause given Jason's history.

Decreased BUN: The low BUN may be related to the polyuria/polydipsia and increased tubular flow rates. A low protein diet could contribute. Decreased liver function is possible given the microcytosis and hypoalbuminemia, however it is not specifically evaluated here. The creatinine is at the lower limit of the reference interval and may reflect polyuria/polydipsia or muscle wasting.

Hypocalcemia with normal phosphorus: The low serum albumin may account for some of the hypocalcemia but will not impact ionized calcium. Laboratory error does occur, so the test could be repeated to verify the abnormality. Other considerations in this case include acute pancreatitis, which is possible with the history of dietary indiscretion. Primary hypoparathyroidism or Vitamin D deficiency are possible, however they are rare and often associated with hyperphosphatemia, which is not present here. Ionized calcium could be measured to further clarify Jason's calcium status.

Mild hypoalbuminemia: Decreased intake, decreased production or selective losses result in hypoalbuminemia. Jason has been anorexic with muscle wasting, suggesting that poor nutritional status could impair albumin production. There is some potential for decreased liver function, however further testing is required to assess this possibility. Selective loss of albumin through the glomerulus could be occurring, and a urinalysis or urine protein:creatinine ratio should be performed to quantify proteinuria. It is important to remember that urine protein may be elevated in association with occult urinary tract infections, which are common in diabetic patients.

Hypernatremia with proportional hyperchloremia: These electrolyte abnormalities occur when there is a disproportionate deficit of free water and may be associated with hypotonic fluid losses (renal, gastrointestinal, third space, cutaneous). Restricted access to water alone, or in concert with the hypotonic losses could also cause these elevations. In Jason's case, glucose in the urine causes osmotic diuresis and fluid loss. Gastrointestinal fluid losses are also likely, while no mention is made of an effusion or significant skin disease. Jason's pressure sores suggest that he was unable to move adequately to drink water, and his access to water may have been restricted associated with the enterotomy. Intravenous fluid therapy appears to have been inadequate to maintain hydration, and replacement of hypotonic fluid losses with isotonic fluids could exacerbate the electrolyte excesses.

Increased CK: The elevated CK may be related to muscle damage from inability to move and the development of pressure sores. Other potential causes include iatrogenic manipulation such as surgery and intramuscular injections.

Case Summary and Outcome

Jason was treated with antibiotics and intravenous fluids appropriately adjusted for his electrolyte abnormalities. He also received insulin and medication to control pain. His decubital sores were treated and he was frequently repositioned. By the next day, Jason was able to roll over on his own and was supported to drink small bowls of water every 2 hours. He was also given frequent small meals. Jason was hospitalized for almost two weeks, but had a remarkable recovery with normal electrolytes, improving strength and a glucose curve showing moderately well controlled diabetes. The wound on his left hock was also healing, but required continuing care at home. The liver biopsy collected at surgery showed fatty change compatible with the history of diabetes.

Like Twix, the calf in the Case 14, this chapter, fluid losses (renal due to osmotic diuresis in this case, gastrointestinal in the previous case) combined with restricted access to water led to hypernatremia and hyperchloremia. Serum electrolyte data and acid/base status can be quite variable in diabetic patients depending on food intake, degree of polyuria, and any associated gastrointestinal signs. In some diabetics, serum electrolyte values fall within the reference interval (Hooligan, Chapter 3, Case 20), while other patients may have hyponatremia and hypochloridemia associated with relative water excess because of the osmotic effects of hyperglycemia (Marion, Chapter 3, Case 18). It is likely that Hooligan and Marion had free access to water during their illness.

Case 16 – Level 3

"Decker" is an 11-year-old neutered male domestic short haired cat that presents with a several year history of diabetes mellitus that usually is well managed. This morning, Decker was vomiting and lethargic. On presentation, he is thin, with an unkempt coat.

Glucose:	↑ 327 mg/dl	(70.0-135.0)
BUN:	↑ 58 mg/dl	(8-29)
Creatinine:	↑ 2.3 mg/dl	(0.9-2.0)
Phosphorus:	↑ 8.1 mg/dl	(3.0-7.2)
Calcium:	↓ 9.2 mg/dl	(9.4-11.6)
Magnesium:	↑ 3.1 mEq/L	(1.9-2.6)
Total Protein:	6.7 g/dl	(5.5-7.6)
Albumin:	3.6 g/dl	(2.8-4.0)
Globulin:	3.1 g/dl	(2.3-4.2)
Sodium:	155 mEq/L	(149-164)
Chloride:	↓ 109 mEq/L	(119-134)
Potassium:	4.0 mEq/L	(3.8-5.4)
HCO3:	↓ 8 mEq/L	(13-22)
Anion gap:	↑ 42 mEq/L	(15.0-28.0)
Total bili:	0.1 mg/dl	(0.10-0.30)
ALP:	↑ 995 IU/L	(10-72)
GGT:	↑ 25 IU/L	(3-10)
ALT:	↑ 373 IU/L	(29-145)
AST:	↑ 114 IU/L	(12-42)
Cholesterol:	↑ 789 mg/dl	(77-258)
Triglycerides	↑ 425 mg/dl	(25-321)
Amylase:	↑ 3568 IU/L	(496-1874)

Urinalysis: Catheter

Appearance: Red and cloudy	Sediment:
Specific gravity: 1.025	Occasional RBC/high power field
pH: 6.0	Rare WBC/high power field
Protein: 2+	No casts seen
Glucose: 4+	No squamous or transitional
Ketones: 3+	epithelial cells seen
Bilirubin: negative	No bacteria or crystals present

Interpretation

No CBC was performed

Hyperglycemia: Given the history of diabetes mellitus, the hyperglycemia is attributed to this previously diagnosed condition. Exacerbation by stress cannot be ruled out.

Mild azotemia: Increased BUN and creatinine indicate a decrease in glomerular filtration rate. However, ruling out a potential renal component of azotemia in diabetic patients can be complicated by the osmotic diuresis caused by the presence of glucose and ketones in the urine, which prevent proper concentration of urine by normally functional kidneys. Some degree of pre-renal azotemia is also expected.

Hyperphosphatemia: Phosphorus is not being eliminated at normal rates because of the decreased glomerular filtration rate.

Hypocalcemia: The cause for the mild decrease in total serum calcium is not apparent here. Mild deviations from normal may be the result of laboratory error, and should be verified. If Decker does have renal disease, this is the most likely cause of a true hypocalcemia, however ionized calcium may be normal and should be measured if clinically indicated.

Hypochloremia with normal serum sodium: Like the low calcium level, the deviation of chloride from the reference interval is minimal and may not be clinically significant. There is a history of vomiting, which could lead to loss of chloride.

Low serum bicarbonate (acidemia) with increased anion gap: This combination of abnormalities suggests an accumulation of unmeasured anions. Ketoacidosis accounts for much of this, however uremic acidosis or lactic acidosis secondary to dehydration and poor perfusion cannot be ruled out. Other unmeasured anions may include exogenous compounds. For example, ethylene glycol toxicity, while unlikely given other laboratory data and clinical information, could present with some similar changes on the profile, including increased anion gap, azotemia, hypocalcemia, and hyperphosphatemia.

Increased ALP and GGT: These enzymes often indicate cholestasis. Liver disease is common in older cats and cannot be ruled out here, although no hyperbilirubinemia or bilirubinuria is present at this time. Various endocrinopathies, including diabetes mellitus and hyperthyroidism, also may cause increased serum activities of these enzymes.

Increased ALT and AST: Elevations in these enzymes suggest hepatocellular damage, but they also may increase with endocrinopathies.

Hypercholesterolemia and hypertriglyceridemia: Postprandial effects are unlikely in this patient because of anorexia and vomiting. Endocrinopathies and renal disease can increase serum lipids. In diabetes mellitus, inadequate insulin action reduces lipoprotein lipase activity in addition to the generalized recruitment of lipids as an energy source during perceived tissue "starvation."

Case Summary and Outcome

Decker was stabilized in the hospital and sent home, where he continued to do well on a higher dose of insulin. As discussed in the previous case, some patients with diabetes mellitus have normal or nearly normal serum electrolyte values, especially if there are no accompanying gastrointestinal issues and the patient is able to drink water. Decker's hypochloremia was more likely due to the vomiting than the actual hyperglycemia. Likewise, dehydration secondary to osmotic diuresis can cause prerenal azotemia in some patients like Decker and Hooligan (Chapter 3, Case 20), but not others (Jason, Chapter 7, Case 15; Marion and Amaryllis, Chapter 3, Cases 18 and 19). Still others may have low BUN and serum creatinine as a result of compensated polyuria/polydipsia and/or muscle wasting (Decker and Gerhardt, Chapter 5, Case 22). Other laboratory abnormalities that can be commonly associated with diabetes mellitus include liver enzyme elevations (Chapter 3, Cases 18, 19, 20; Chapter 5, Case 22), hypercholesterolemia (Chapter 3, Cases 18, 19; Chapter 5, Case 22) and hypertriglyceridemia (Chapter 3, Cases 18, 19; Chapter 5, Case 22).

Case 17 – Level 3

"Smooch" is a 4-year-old spayed female Bichon Frise presenting for lethargy, anorexia, and tachypnea. One month ago, she presented with hematemesis and was diagnosed with immune-mediated thrombocytopenia. She was subsequently treated with corticosteroids and cyclosporine. At this presentation, Smooch is slightly dehydrated with pale pink mucous membranes. Smooch's abdomen is distended and is somewhat painful on palpation. She has cranial organomegaly with thin skin and alopecia. She has increased bronchovesicular sounds compatible with pneumonia.

White blood cell count:	↑ 79.5 x 10⁹/L	(4.0-13.3)
Segmented neutrophils:	↑ 66.1 x 10⁹/L	(2.0-11.2)
Band neutrophils:	↑ 0.8 x 10⁹/L	(0-0.3)
Lymphocytes:	2.4 x 10⁹/L	(1.0-4.5)
Monocytes:	↑ 10.2 x 10⁹/L	(0.2-1.4)
Eosinophils:	0.0 x 10⁹/L	(0-1.2)
WBC morphology: Toxic change		
Hematocrit:	↓ 28.7%	(39-55)
Red blood cell count:	↓ 4.41 x 10¹²/L	(5.8-8.5)
Hemoglobin:	↓ 10.0 g/dl	(14.0-19.0)
MCV:	65.1 fl	(60.0-77.0)
MCHC:	34.0 g/dl	(31.0-34.0)
Platelets:	323 x 10⁹/L	(160-425)
Glucose:	↑ 499 mg/dl	(90.0-140.0)
BUN:	↑ 36 mg/dl	(6-24)
Creatinine:	↓ 0.5 mg/dl	(0.6-1.5)
Phosphorus:	↓ 2.4 mg/dl	(2.6-7.2)
Calcium:	↓ 8.7 mg/dl	(9.5-11.5)
Magnesium:	2.0 mEq/L	(1.7-2.5)
Total Protein:	6.2 g/dl	(5.5-7.8)
Albumin:	3.2 g/dl	(2.8-4.0)
Globulin:	3.0 g/dl	(2.3-4.2)
Sodium:	↓ 142 mEq/L	(145-151)
Chloride:	113 mEq/L	(105-120)
Potassium:	↓ 2.4 mEq/L	(3.6-5.6)
Anion Gap:	24.4 mEq/L	(15-25)
HCO3:	↓ 7.0 mEq/L	(15-28)
Total Bili:	↑ 2.9 mg/dl	(0.10-0.50)
ALP:	↑ 17,433 IU/L	(20-320)
GGT:	↑ 149 IU/L	(2-10)
ALT:	↑ 216 IU/L	(10-95)
AST:	↑ 175 IU/L	(10-56)
Cholesterol:	↑ 461 mg/dl	(110-314)
Amylase:	↑ 3235 IU/L	(400-1200)

Urinalysis: Free catch
Appearance: Dark yellow and cloudy
Specific gravity: 1.021
pH: 6.5
Glucose: 3+
Ketones: 4+
Bilirubin: 3+
Protein: 3+
Sediment: 5-20 erythrocytes/hpf

Interpretation

CBC: Smooch has a marked neutrophilic leukocytosis with a mild left shift and toxic change, and monocytosis, compatible with marked inflammation (Figure 7-5A and B). In her case, this may be secondary to pneumonia or pancreatitis. Her steroid therapy is likely contributing to the neutrophilia and monocytosis, however a lymphopenia characteristic of a steroid leukogram is not present. The platelet numbers have normalized since the initiation of treatment for immune mediated thrombocytopenia (ITP). However Smooch now has a normocytic normochromic anemia, likely non-regenerative. A reticulocyte count is needed to confirm this. Given the inflammatory leukogram, a nonregenerative anemia of chronic disease/inflammation is possible.

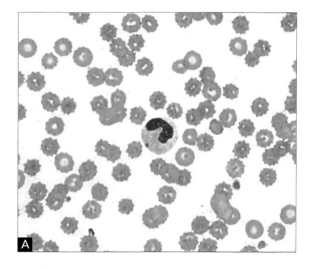

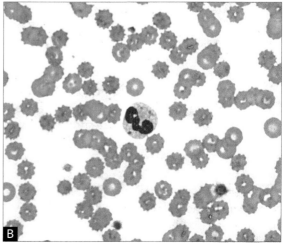

Figure 7-5A & B. Band neutrophil A. and segmented neutrophil B. in canine blood film.

Serum Biochemical Profile

Hyperglycemia: This blood glucose level is very high, and in combination with the ketonuria, indicates diabetes mellitus. Corticosteroid treatment causes insulin resistance and could exacerbate or precipitate clinical diabetes.

Increased BUN with low creatinine: Increased BUN with normal or low creatinine may occur with mild pre-renal or renal decreases in glomerular filtration rate. The increased BUN in this case may be due to gastrointestinal hemorrhage. Muscle wasting could contribute to the low creatinine.

Hypophosphatemia and hypocalcemia: Translocation of phosphorus into cells can be stimulated by insulin therapy, although it is not clear if Smooch has received insulin at the time of this sample collection. Diabetic patients may have total body phosphorus deficits because of muscle wasting, loss of phosphorus in urine, and impaired tissue phosphorus utilization. Smooch is tachypneic, which also may trigger translocation of phosphorus into cells. Both the low phosphorus and low calcium may be related to increased renal losses associated with iatrogenic hyperadrenocorticism. Hypovitaminosis D or gastrointestinal disease are possible but less likely causes. Hypocalcemia may be associated with pancreatitis, which may also explain the increased amylase and inflammatory leukogram.

Hyponatremia: The hyponatremia is likely dilutional as a result of the osmotic draw of water into the circulation by the hyperglycemia. An alternative possibility is loss of sodium with hemorrhage and replacement of lost fluid with free water by drinking. Given the heart murmur, assessment of cardiac function should be considered as congestive heart failure and fluid loading may also produce hyponatremia.

Hypokalemia: Multiple causes for hypokalemia are present in this patient. Decreased intake makes it more difficult for Smooch to replace ongoing losses associated with polyuria and osmotic diuresis. Vomiting could further contribute to potassium loss, and insulin therapy may lead to translocation of potassium into cells.

Decreased serum bicarbonate (acidemia): The production of organic acids such as ketoacids is the likely cause of the acidemia. In most cases, this would cause an increased anion gap, however the accumulation of unmeasured anions is counterbalanced by electrolyte abnormalities. Large amounts of ketoacids also may be eliminated in the urine, so polyuria helps minimize their accumulation, particularly in animals that can take in enough fluid to maintain normal hydration status.

Hyperbilirubinemia: There are several potential causes for increased serum bilirubin in this patient. Sepsis can interfere with hepatocellular uptake of bile, and is possible given the significant inflammatory response in the leukogram. The anemia could be caused by hemolysis, however specific morphologic abnormalities that would corroborate that interpretation were not noted on the blood film examination. Cholestasis appears likely given the marked elevations in ALP and GGT, although some portion of these increases are likely due to diabetes mellitus and treatment with corticosteroids. Primary liver disease remains a consideration.

Increased ALP and GGT: As discussed in Chapter 2, increased ALP in the dog is a nonspecific change that may be associated with drug effects, endocrinopathies, circulatory disorders, bone pathology, and cholestatic liver disease. In this case, increased ALP and GGT is due to a combination of endocrinopathy and cholestatic liver disease. It is likely that corticosteroid induced ALP is increased due to the therapy for ITP. Although the corticosteroid induced fraction of ALP can be measured, it may not be possible to sort out the relative combinations of multiple factors until Smooch can be weaned off corticosteroid therapy and her diabetes better controlled.

Increased ALT and AST: Elevated ALT and AST indicate hepatocellular damage. The relative increases in hepatocellular enzymes are less severe than the cholestatic enzymes, however this may be due to contributions from corticosteroid therapy and diabetes rather than reflecting more severe cholestatic versus hepatocellular disease.

Hypercholesterolemia: Smooch is experiencing numerous potential problems that could cause increased serum cholesterol. Hypercholesterolemia is associated with diabetes mellitus and hypercortisolism. It may also occur with pancreatitis, suggested by the increased amylase.

Hyperamylasemia: Minor elevations of amylase (2-3 fold) may occur with decreased glomerular filtration rate. Although Smooch is dehydrated, her serum creatinine is low, making this difficult to assess. Pancreatitis can occur concurrently with diabetes and may be associated with other laboratory abnormalities such as hypercholesterolemia, hypocalcemia and an inflammatory leukogram.

Urinalysis: Osmotic diuresis due to glucose and ketones in the urine will result in a low specific gravity. Glucose and ketones at very high concentrations can contribute minimal increases in the urine specific gravity because standard methodology evaluates numbers of particles in the urine and their size. Although the sediment appears inactive, urine culture should be considered as diabetic patients are predisposed to the development of occult urinary tract infections (McGuire).

Case Summary and Outcome

Smooch was treated with antibiotics and gastroprotectants along with insulin therapy for her diabetes. Although becoming regenerative, her anemia worsened and she became hypoproteinemic secondary to gastrointestinal hemorrhage. As a result, she required a blood transfusion. Her pneumonia gradually improved during her hospitalization. In addition, her ketosis eventually resolved, and she was discharged on insulin with a nasogastric tube for nutritional support. The dose of corticosteroids was reduced in order to minimize its effects on the gastrointestinal tract and to improve sensitivity to insulin therapy.

The interpretation of Smooch's laboratory work is more difficult because of her pre-existing conditions and medications. Corticosteroid therapy may increase blood glucose levels and induce liver enzymes as well as cause hypercholesterolemia. However, the glucose value here would be too high for corticosteroid effects alone. Futhermore, some hepatobiliary disease and/or hemolysis also could contribute given the anemia and hyperbilirubinemia. Pancreatitis also may be associated with increased liver enzymes, hypercholesterolemia, hypocalcemia, and hyperglycemia. In some cases, pancreatic disease can contribute to the development of diabetes mellitus if insulin producing beta-cells are damaged as part of the process.

The pathogenesis of the electrolyte abnormalities is similarly murky because of the potential for multiple contributing factors. As noted above, dilution of sodium is possible with diabetes or cardiovascular disease, while increased losses through hemorrhage or third space effusions cannot be ruled out. Unlike the previous two cases of diabetes (Jason and Decker, Chapter 7, Cases 15 and 16), Smooch is hypokalemic. Some diabetics may have hyperkalemia (Chapter 3, Case 18; Chapter 5, Case 22) if insulin action is inadequate to promote the movement of potassium into cells, while others have hypokalemia (Chapter 3, Case 19). Potassium may be low because of decreased intake if Smooch is anorexic. Also, Smooch likely has increased renal losses of potassium as tubular flow rates increase with glucose/ketone or glucocorticoid induced diuresis. Because Smooch is already hypokalemic, her serum potassium values should be monitored carefully when insulin therapy is instituted because insulin will cause some translocation of serum potassium into cells. Rapid and dangerous fluctuations in potassium may occur during treatment for diabetes even if the initial serum potassium values are within reference intervals, so levels should be monitored carefully during initial stabilization.

McGuire NC, Schulman R, Ridgway MD, Bollero G. Detection of occult urinary tract infections in dogs with diabetes mellitus. J Am Anim Hosp Assoc 2002; 38:541-544.

Case 18 – Level 3

"Zippy" is a 10-year-old castrated male schnauzer mix dog presenting for polyuria and polydipsia. He has a history of arthritis that has been managed with glucosamine. Last month he was diagnosed with Lyme disease and treated with doxycycline. After doxycycline therapy was initiated, Zippy began urinating in the house. Blood work performed 2 weeks ago showed marked hyperglycemia, however the owners did not want to treat this problem until they returned from a two week vacation. When they returned from vacation yesterday, the pet-sitter indicated that Zippy had decreased appetite and had been lethargic over the last week. This morning, Zippy was not ambulatory. On presentation, Zippy is recumbent and tachypneic with pale mucous membranes. He is hypothermic and has melena on rectal examination.

White blood cell count:	5.7 x 10⁹/L	(4.0-13.3)
Segmented neutrophils:	4.7 x 10⁹/L	(2.0-11.2)
Band neutrophils:	0.2 x 10⁹/L	(0-0.3)
Lymphocytes:	↓ 0.2 x 10⁹/L	(1.0-4.5)
Monocytes:	0.6 x 10⁹/L	(0.2-1.4)
Eosinophils:	0.0 x 10⁹/L	(0-1.2)

WBC morphology: Neutrophils show slight toxic changes

Hematocrit:	↓ 25.0%	(37-60)
Red blood cell count:	↓ 4.38 x 10¹²/L	(5.5-8.5)
Hemoglobin:	↓ 8.8 g/dl	(12.0-18.0)
MCV:	↓ 58.8 fl	(60.0-77.0)
MCHC:	33.2 g/dl	(31.0-34.0)

Platelets: Appear adequate in number

Glucose:	↑ 1009 mg/dl	(90.0-140.0)
BUN:	↑ 90 mg/dl	(6-24)
Creatinine:	1.4 mg/dl	(0.5-1.5)
Phosphorus:	3.2 mg/dl	(2.2-6.6)
Calcium:	↓ 6.1 mg/dl	(9.5-11.5)
Magnesium:	2.5 mEq/L	(1.7-2.5)
Total Protein:	↓ 3.2 g/dl	(4.8-7.2)
Albumin:	↓ 1.9 g/dl	(2.5-3.7)
Globulin:	↓ 1.3 g/dl	(2.0-4.0)
Sodium:	↓ 130 mEq/L	(140-151)
Chloride:	↓ 97 mEq/L	(105-120)
Potassium:	↓ 1.6 mEq/L	(3.6-5.6)

Anion gap:	↑ 29.6 mEq/L	(15-25)
HCO3:	↓ 5 mEq/L	(15-28)
Total Bili:	0.4 mg/dl	(0.10-0.50)
ALP:	↑ 2232 IU/L	(20-320)
GGT:	↑ 17 IU/L	(2-10)
ALT:	62 IU/L	(10-95)
AST:	86 IU/L	(10-56)
Cholesterol:	153 mg/dl	(110-314)
Amylase:	↑ 5420 IU/L	(400-1200)

Urinalysis: Catheterized sample

Appearance: Dark yellow and hazy	Sediment:
Specific gravity: 1.031	Occasional erythrocytes/hpf
	Occasional WBC/hpf
pH: 5.0	>10 granular casts/hpf (Figure 7-6)
Glucose: 4+	trace bacteria
Ketones: 3+	
Bilirubin: 1+	
Protein: 100 mg/dl	

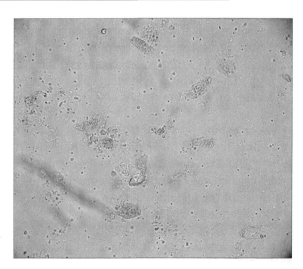

Figure 7-6. Granlar casts in canine urine.

Intepretation

CBC: Zippy has a mild lymphopenia that could be compatible with corticosteroid effects, although other elements characteristic for the corticosteroid leukogram such as a mature neutrophilia and monocytosis are not present. A viral infection causing lympholysis cannot be ruled out, and the toxic changes in the neutrophils suggests some underlying inflammation. But, based on the clinical history and other laboratory data, other processes such as a gastrointestinal lesion allowing loss of lymphocytes appear possible. Gastrointestinal loss of lymphocytes is possible based on the panhypoproteinemia, as nonselective protein loss occurs through the gut. With lymphangiectasia, cholesterol is also lost with lymph, usually resulting in hypocholesterolemia. However, Zippy's cholesterol currently is within reference intervals. In addition, classical lymphangiectasia is not associated with melena.

Zippy has a microcytic, normochromic anemia. Microcytosis can be a normal characteristic of some breeds (Akita, Shiba Inu), however it also is associated with portosystemic shunting and iron deficiency. With the exception of albumin, serum biochemical parameters that may decrease with impaired liver function such as glucose, BUN and cholesterol appear to be increased or within the reference interval. Liver function tests such as serum bile acids would be needed to rule out liver dysfunction. Iron deficiency may be a more likely explanation of the anemia. Zippy has melena, which is a common cause of iron deficiency in older dogs. Morphologic abnormalities of the erythrocytes that can accompany iron deficiency such as hypochromasia and schistocytes are not reported, however they may occur later in the course of disease than microcytosis. Thrombocytosis may also occur in iron deficient patients, but is not noted here. Anemia of chronic disease may contribute to the anemia, however this is typically normocytic and normochromic. Anemia due to hemorrhage is most often regenerative, however occasionally the blood loss is too acute to show signs of regeneration at the time of initial presentation.

Serum Biochemical Profile

Severe hyperglycemia: There are numerous potential causes for mild increases in blood glucose. Hyperglycemia of this magnitude is almost certainly associated with diabetes mellitus and is compatible with the clinical history of urinating in the house and polydipsia/polyuria. A urinary tract infection may accompany diabetes mellitus and contribute to changes in patterns of urination.

Increased BUN with normal creatinine: Elevated BUN may be related to the presence of gastrointestinal hemorrhage, resulting in digestion of large amounts of protein. This may be compounded by the potential for dehydration and low renal tubular flow rates if water intake has not been sufficient to compensate for fluid losses due to osmotic diuresis. The presence of large numbers of granular casts is very concerning because they contain the remains of sloughed renal tubular epithelial cells, indicating the potential for serious kidney damage. In this case, profound hyperglycemia may have been associated shock and hypoperfusion.

Hypocalcemia: Some of this change may be due to the hypoalbuminemia and decreases in the protein bound fraction of calcium. Hypoalbuminemia-associated hypocalcemia should not result in clinical signs because ionized calcium remains normal. However, this is a very low total calcium value, and measurement of the biologically active ionized calcium is warranted. Because of the increased amylase, pancreatitis should be considered as a potential cause for hypocalcemia as well.

Panhypoproteinemia: Concurrent hypoalbuminemia and hypoglobulinemia most often suggests nonselective protein losses. In this case, the melena suggests hemorrhage or gastrointestinal protein loss. There is mild proteinuria, however this may be related to the presence of urinary tract inflammation and is unlikely to significantly impact serum levels. Other sources of nonselective protein loss are similar to routes of electrolyte loss and include cutaneous and third space losses.

Hyponatremia: Increased losses of sodium may be occurring with gastrointestinal disease or hemorrhage, and will be exacerbated if losses of electrolyte containing fluids are replaced with water. The severe hyperglycemia draws fluid into the vascular space by osmosis, further diluting out remaining sodium.

Hypochloremia: The corrected chloride is 108 mEq/L, indicating that changes in chloride are of similar etiology to those described for sodium.

Hypokalemia: A number of factors are influencing Zippy's potassium status. Low intake because of anorexia compounds the potential for loss in the gastrointestinal tract. The presence of glucosuria and ketonuria suggest that osmotic diuresis and increased tubular flow rates are increasing urinary potassium losses. The negatively charged ketones also promote potassium loss in the urine to preserve electrical neutrality. Impaired insulin activity could increase extracellular fluid potassium content.

Increased anion gap and low bicarbonate: Zippy has a hypochloremic metabolic acidosis. In his case, the increased anion gap may be attributable to the presence of ketoacids, although poor perfusion associated with dehydration or circulatory compromise could cause a superimposed lactic acidosis.

Increased ALP: Diabetes mellitus is one of the endocrinopathies that may be associated with elevations in some liver enzymes. A concurrent corticosteroid induction cannot be ruled out. Given the normal bilirubin and ALT, primary liver disease seems less likely at this time.

Increased AST: This elevation is a nonspecific indicator of tissue damage. If there is hepatocellular damage, the ALT usually will also be increased, but is not the case here. Perfusion deficits could contribute to tissue damage.

Hyperamylasemia: Decreased glomerular filtration rate is a common cause of increased amylase in the dog, however elevations in amylase attributable to GFR are generally limited to two to three fold elevations. Alternatively, there is evidence of intestinal disease, which can also cause elevations in amylase. Finally, pancreatitis is possible.

Urinalysis: The urine is concentrated at this time. However, the presence of granular casts (see Figure 7-6) can be a sign of renal tubular damage, and concentrating ability may decline over time. Significant amounts of glucose and ketones in the urine will contribute to the urine specific gravity measurement and may suggest greater concentrating ability than the dog is truly capable of. Glucosuria can reflect tubular dysfunction or can occur when the tubular maximum for reabsorption of glucose has been exceeded, which is clearly the case for this patient. As discussed previously, the proteinuria could be compatible with glomerular damage or with infectious/inflammatory urinary tract disease. Urinary tract infection is a common complication of diabetes mellitus because of glucosuria and immune dysfunction and is suggested by the presence of leukocytes and bacteria.

Case Summary and Outcome
Despite therapy, Zippy's clinical condition continued to deteriorate after presentation, and he became anuric. The marked difficulty breathing suggested the potential for pulmonary thromboembolism. His melena continued, and he began to vomit large amounts of blood. He was euthanized due to poor response to therapy and grave prognosis.

The degree of Zippy's hyperglycemia is unusual compared with the other cases of diabetes in this book (Chapter 3, Cases 18, 19, 20; Chapter 5, Case 22, and the preceeding three cases in this chapter), and is the most likely to cause significant shift of fluids from the interstitial to the intravascular space, diluting electrolytes. Refer back to the Case Summary and Outcome for the previous case (Smooch) for further discussion and comparison of variable electrolyte abnormalities in the diabetes cases presented in several chapters of this book. Like Decker (Chapter 7, Case 16), Zippy has an increased anion gap acidosis, likely due to the accumulation of ketoacids associated with the diabetes mellitus. Based on the recumbency, hypothermia, and casts in the urine, Zippy may have generalized tissue hypoperfusion and lactic acidosis may complicate the ketoacidosis. Once he became anuric, uremic acidosis also would have been present.

Case 19 – Level 3

"Stowaway" is a 3-year-old female alpaca presenting with a one week history of lateral recumbency, bruxism, decreased appetite, and dullness. Several months ago, Stowaway gave birth to a cria, was down for 2 days, and did not produce milk. At that time, she was hospitalized for several days, diagnosed with gastrointestinal parasitism and treated. Three months later she had another episode of recumbency and fecal flotation revealed parasitism. Stowaway again responded well to treatment and gained weight. At this presentation, the alpaca is depressed and in sternal recumbency. Stowaway is thin and has bilateral gut sounds but no distinct compartmental contractions are noted. Fecal flotation is negative.

White blood cell count:	↑ 23.2 x 10⁹/L	(7.5-21.5)
Segmented neutrophils:	16.0 x 10⁹/L	(4.6-16.0)
Band neutrophils:	0	(0-0.3)
Lymphocytes:	3.0 x 10⁹/L	(1.0-7.5)
Monocytes:	↑ 2.8 x 10⁹/L	(0.1-0.8)
Eosinophils:	1.4 x 10⁹/L	(0.0-3.3)
WBC morphology: Appears within normal limits		

Hematocrit:	37%	(29-39)
RBC morphology: Appears within normal limits		

Platelets: Appear adequate in number

Fibrinogen:	400 mg/dl	(100-400)

Glucose:	↑ 563 mg/dl	(90-140.0)
BUN:	↑ 150 mg/dl	(13-32)
Creatinine:	↑ 6.4 mg/dl	(1.5-2.9)
Phosphorus:	6.8 mg/dl	(4.6-9.8)
Calcium:	9.9 mg/dl	(8.0-10.0)
Total Protein:	↓ 5.2 g/dl	(5.5-7.0)
Albumin:	↓ 2.8 g/dl	(3.5-4.4)
Globulin:	2.4 g/dl	(1.7-3.5)
Sodium:	↓ 132 mEq/L	(147-158)
Chloride:	↓ 82 mEq/L	(106-118)
Potassium:	↓ 2.8 mEq/L	(4.3-5.8)
HCO3:	↑ 31 mEq/L	(14-28)
Total Bili:	0.1 mg/dl	(0.0-0.1)
ALP:	180 IU/L	(30-780)
GGT:	18 IU/L	(5-29)
LDH:	↑ 491 IU/L	(14-70)
AST:	↑ 324 IU/L	(110-250)
CK:	↑ 913 IU/L	(30-400)

Urinalysis: Method of sampling is not indicated.	
Appearance: Yellow and clear	
Specific gravity: 1.017	
pH: 6.0	
Protein, glucose, ketones, bilirubin: negative	
Sediment: Occasional erythrocytes, leukocytes, and epithelial cells seen	

Abdominal fluid

Total nucleated cell count: 500/µl

Total protein: 4.0 gm/dl

Description: The fluid contains small numbers of nucleated cells with a predominance of macrophages. Occasional nondegenerate neutrophils and a few small lymphocytes can also be seen. No etiologic agents are seen.

Intepretation

CBC: Stowaway has a leukocytosis characterized by a monocytosis, compatible with inflammation. Monocytosis also may accompany tissue necrosis. Both neutrophil numbers (Figure 7-7) and fibrinogen are at the upper limit of the normal ranges.

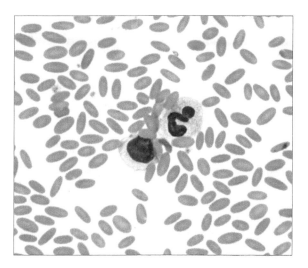

Figure 7-7. Normal neutrophil, lymphocyte and elliptical erythrocytes in Alpaca blood film.

Serum Biochemical Profile

Hyperglycemia: This is likely a pronounced stress response, common in camelids (See Chapter 2, Case 14 for references).

Azotemia: While the hydration status of this alpaca is not indicated, the urine is not well concentrated, suggestive for renal azotemia. Given the low serum electrolyte concentrations, medullary washout could interfere with renal concentrating ability in addition to any concurrent renal disease.

Hypoproteinemia with hypoalbuminemia: Hypoalbuminemia with normal globulins often implies either selective glomerular loss of albumin or decreased production of albumin associated with liver failure or malnutrition. Liver failure cannot be ruled out, but is less likely with normal serum bilirubin, ALP and GGT. Stowaway is thin, so nutritional factors may impact protein balance. Proteinuria was not detected on the urinalysis, however with relatively dilute urine, a urinary protein:creatinine ratio would be a more sensitive test for glomerular protein loss. The history of parasitism indicates the potential for gastrointestinal losses of protein, however these are often nonselective losses. In some cases, increased production of globulin proteins associated with an acute phase reaction or immune stimulation may be masked by simultaneous nonselective protein loss, resulting in serum globulin value within the reference interval.

Low sodium and chloride: The corrected chloride remains below the reference interval at 94 mEq/L. Dilution or increased losses are the most likely mechanism as malnutrition seldom results in hyponatremia and hypochloremia. Hyperglycemia may cause some osmotic draw of fluid into the intravascular space, however this should dilute sodium and chloride approximately equally. Loss of electrolytes by both renal and gastrointestinal routes are possible in this case. Renal losses could be quantified by calculation of urinary electrolyte fractional excretions. Patients with renal disease may be less able to conserve sodium when there is decreased intake and/or increased losses by other routes such as the gastrointestinal tract. Disproportionate hypochloremia could occur if there is stasis of fluids in the proximal gastrointestinal tract, which would also be compatible with the increased serum bicarbonate.

Hypokalemia: Decreased intake is more likely to influence the serum potassium level than sodium and chloride levels. Potassium losses via the kidney and gut may also contribute to the hypokalemia. Hypokalemia is further potentiated by alkalosis as potassium ions shift intra-cellularly in exchange for hydrogen ions.

Increased bicarbonate (alkalosis): Sequestration or loss of acid containing gastrointestinal secretions due to upper gastrointestinal stasis is the likely cause for this abnormality.

Increased LDH, AST, and CK: The combination of enzyme elevations in the absence of a change in bilirubin, ALP, or GGT suggests muscle damage, which may result from recumbency or associated with medical procedures.

Urinalysis: This patient appears to have paradoxical aciduria, whereby the conservation of sodium and chloride is prioritized at the expense of hydrogen loss in the urine.

Abdominal fluid: Because of the relatively low cell count consisting of macrophages and high protein, this fluid is compatible with a modified transudate. The protein exceeds the 3.5 gm/dl value typically used for exudate, and repeat sampling may be justified to rule out the possibility of an early inflammatory reaction.

Case Summary and Outcome

Treatment with intravenous fluids, gastroprotectants, and pain medication resulted in normalization of the electrolyte and acid/base abnormalities, however Stowaway was persistently azotemic. Radiographs showed distended and gas filled small intestines with a severely dilated intestinal segment in the caudal abdomen. Increased opacity in the second and third gastric compartments was also noted. The radiologist concluded there was a mechanical or functional obstruction, which would be compatible with the clinical chemistry data. Because she continued to be anorexic and recumbent, Stowaway was euthanized. At necropsy, Stowaway had an annular, sharply demarcated and narrow focus of necrosis in the spiral colon that was compatible with ischemic necrosis secondary to thrombosis or focal strangulation. The potential for embolic disease was supported by the presence of multifocal acute thromboemboli in the lungs. Renal tubular proteinosis with hyaline casts was noted in the kidney. Protein losing nephropathy can be associated with depletion of endogenous anticoagulants such as antithrombin III, contributing to development of thromboembolic disease.

While Stowaway's hyperglycemia and electrolyte abnormalities would be compatible with diabetes mellitus in other species, the degree of hyperglycemia that can be associated with stress or illness is exaggerated in camelids. The marked degree of hyperglycemia makes osmotic dilution of electrolytes possible (See Zippy, Chapter 7, Case 18). However in Stowaway's case, gastrointestinal sequestration is an important mechanism underlying the electrolytes changes and best explains the disproportionate hypochloridemia. Finally, diabetes mellitus is most often associated with acidosis (Chapter 7, Cases 16, 17, 18), while the metabolic alkalosis present in this case is more compatible with loss or sequestration of fluid in the upper gastrointestinal tract.

Case 20 – Level 3

"Simba" is a 9-year-old neutered male domestic shorthaired cat presenting with a one day history of hiding. Prior to this, Simba has been a healthy cat, though lately, he has been gaining weight from eating special food left out for another cat in the household. He is not on any medications, and he is current on vaccinations. On presentation, Simba is obtunded and hypothermic. He is estimated to be 8-10% dehydrated with poor femoral pulses, and his urinary bladder is distended. Blood was drawn for an initial chemistry panel (Day 1). Because abdominal radiographs revealed possible uroliths in the bladder, Simba was taken to surgery for stone removal and to restore patency to the urinary tract. A second chemistry panel was performed the day after surgery (Day 2).

	Day 1	Day 2	
Glucose:	101 mg/dl	↑166	(70.0-120.0)
BUN:	↑192 mg/dl	↑34	(15-32)
Creatinine:	↑14.3 mg/dl	1.6	(0.9-2.1)
Phosphorus:	↑11.6 mg/dl	3.1	(3.0-6.0)
Calcium:	↓6.9 mg/dl	↓8.3	(8.9-11.6)
Magnesium:	↑3.0 mEq/L	2.4	(1.9-2.6)
Total Protein:	↓5.2 g/dl	↓4.6	(5.5-7.6)
Albumin:	↓2.0 g/dl	↓1.9	(2.2-3.4)
Globulin:	3.2 g/dl	2.7	(2.5-5.8)
Sodium:	↓148 mEq/L	151	(149-164)
Chloride:	↓114 mEq/L	↓110	(119-134)
Potassium:	↑7.7 mEq/L	↓2.6	(3.9-5.4)
Anion gap:	26.7 mEq/L	↓9.8	(13-27)
HCO3:	15 mEq/L	↑33.8	(13-22)
Total bili:	↑2.6 mg/dl	↑0.7	(0.10-0.30)
ALP:	26 IU/L	29	(10-72)
GGT:	3 IU/L	3	(3-10)
ALT:	70 IU/L	38	(29-145)
AST:	↑145 IU/L	↑98	(12-42)
Cholesterol:	↑232 mg/dl	↑178	(50-150)
Amylase:	815 IU/L	1842	(496-1874)

Urinalysis: sampled from a urinary catheter on Day 2
Specific gravity: 1.011

CBCs were not performed.

Day 1 Serum Biochemical Profile
Azotemia: Azotemia should be categorized as pre-renal, renal, or post-renal. The clinical findings of distended urinary bladder and uroliths on radiographs suggest that post-renal azotemia is likely. Urinary obstruction would also explain the hyperkalemia present on Day 1. The concurrent dehydration makes it likely that pre-renal factors are exacerbating the azotemia.

Hyperphosphatemia and hypocalcemia: The most likely cause of hyperphosphatemia in this patient is decreased glomerular filtration rate, regardless of whether this is due to pre-renal, renal, or post-renal causes. Other potential causes of hyperphosphatemia include severe tissue damage. Small animal patients in renal failure may have high, normal, or low serum calcium levels, and ionized calcium levels may not correlate with total calcium levels as they often do in healthy animals. In a small study of cats with urethral obstruction, 75% had low ionized calcium, and 27% had low total calcium (Drobatz). More information on the mechanisms for these changes is available in Chapter 5, Case 7 (Ringo). The low albumin may make a small contribution to the decrease in total calcium due to a decrement in protein bound calcium.

Hypermagnesemia: The increase in magnesium is due to decreased renal function.

Hypoproteinemia: The hypoproteinemia is due to a selective decrease in albumin, which may occur with glomerular damage. A complete urinalysis is needed to determine if there is proteinuria. Decreased production is unlikely as there is no clear evidence of liver disease, nor is the cat malnourished.

Hypochloremia and hyponatremia: Given the clinically apparent dehydration, the slight hyponatremia and hypochloremia are likely due to loss of electrolytes in marginal excess of water. This may occur with acute renal failure or vomiting. Third space losses such as uroabdomen can also result in these electrolyte changes and the integrity of the urinary bladder should be evaluated. The decrease in chloride on Day 1 is slightly greater than the decrease in sodium, suggesting that the acid/base status should be evaluated. The combination of hyponatremia, hypochloremia and hyperkalemia is compatible with hypoadrenocorticism, but this syndrome is rare in cats and not in keeping with the history and physical examination.

Hyperkalemia: Hyperkalemia is associated with renal disease characterized by inability to eliminate urine, whether from urethral blockage, uroabdomen, or oliguric/anuric renal failure. Increased intake, oversupplementation, or drug effects are not compatible with the clinical history. Translocation due to acute inorganic acidosis also appears unlikely. Translocation from damaged tissue is possible given the concurrent increase in AST and phosphorus.

HCO3 and anion gap: HCO3 is still within the normal reference interval but near the lower end. Blood gas analysis indicated a persistent acidemia which is likely due to decreased renal excretion of hydrogen ions secondary to obstruction or possibly uroabdomen. Lactic acidosis may also contribute to the acidemia.

Hyperbilirubinemia: The cause for the hyperbilirubinemia is not apparent; its significance is unclear given the substantial decrease observed in 24 hours. In general, causes for hyperbilirubinemia include hemolysis, cholestatic liver disease, liver failure, and sepsis. The potential for hemolytic disease cannot be assessed in the absence of CBC data. CBC data would also help determine if sepsis is an important differential diagnosis. Poor perfusion of the liver secondary to dehydration and impaired circulation may contribute to liver hypoxia and impaired function. At this point, significant liver disease seems unlikely given the normal ALP, GGT, and ALT, although no specific tests of liver function have been performed.

Increased AST: This increase is mild and is not accompanied by an increased ALT, making liver a less likely source of this enzyme. Hemolysis or muscle damage are possible sources of the increased AST. Measurement of CK could help substantiate the presence of muscle damage, which may result from a variety of causes including damage/trauma to the urinary tract, invasive medical procedures, or hypoperfusion.

Hypercholesterolemia: The hypercholesterolemia is mild, however it may be a marker for various metabolic derangements, endocrinopathies, and hepatic or renal disease (See Chapter 3). Like hyperbilirubinemia, this abnormality appears to be resolving and should be monitored over time.

Additional Clinical Information and Case Outcome
A urinary catheter was placed with some difficulty because of accumulation of gritty

crystalline material in the urethra. Simba underwent surgery to remove three 2 mm calculi from the urinary bladder and was treated post-operatively with fluids and antibiotics. Simba did not eat well in the hospital and was discharged a day early because of concern that he might be developing hepatic lipidosis.

Day 2 Serum Biochemical Profile:
Hyperglycemia: The mild hyperglycemia present on Day 2 is likely due to stress or may be secondary to supplementation in intravenous fluids.

Azotemia: While serum creatinine has decreased into the normal range, BUN is still mildly increased, and there may be some renal parenchymal damage post obstruction. The minimally concentrated urine is compatible with a post-obstructive diuresis.

Hypocalcemia: By Day 2, the phosphorus has normalized due to the diuresis. The calcium is still slightly low which may be due to the hypoalbuminemia and a subsequent a decrement in protein bound calcium.

Hypoproteinemia: The hypoalbuminemia has worsened by Day 2 and may reflect dilution of an already low protein by intravenous fluids. Because of the potential proteinuria and residual renal parenchymal damage following obstruction, urinalysis and urine protein:creatinine ratios should be monitored in the future.

Hypochloremia: By Day 2, the mild hyponatremia has been corrected, and there is a dispro-portionate hypochloremia. If there is not apparent cause of excessive loss of chloride via gastric vomiting, an acid/base derangement may be the cause of the low chloride.

Hyperkalemia followed by hypokalemia: Serum potassium does not accurately reflect total body potassium, and rapid changes in potassium over time may occur associated with changes in renal tubular flow rates and fluctutations in acid/base status. On Day 2, urine flow has been re-established, and Simba is experiencing post-obstructive diuresis with kaliuresis.

HCO3 and anion gap: The increased HCO3 in combination with hypochloremia could indicate a mixed acid/base disorder. The low anion gap on day 2 probably reflects hypopro-teinemia, while the markedly increased HCO3 suggests alkalemia. The dramatic change in acid/base status over one day in this case is due to overzealous administration of sodium bicarbonate in response to the previous acidemia.

Case Summary
Simba can be compared with Ringo (Chapter 5, Case 7). Both cats had clinical signs compatible with urinary obstruction, hyperphosphatemia, hypocalcemia, similar degrees of azotemia, and dilute urine. Both cats were hyperkalemic because the urinary obstruction prevented adequate potassium excretion. Both cats also had low serum chloride, with serum sodium values low or near the lower limit of the reference interval. Both cats also had serum bicarbonate levels near the lower limit of the reference interval initially (possibly uremic acidosis or lactic acidosis), but Simba's treatment with bicarbonate induced an iatrogenic alkalosis on Day 2. Another significant change in Simba's blood work on Day 2 is the rapid drop in serum potassium level that is associated with relief of the urinary tract obstruction and subsequent diuresis. It is likely that Ringo experienced a similar decline, however serial data was not available. This rapid fluctuation in potassium status could be seen in any patient that experiences a marked increase in glomerular filtration rate, for example after correction of extreme dehydration.

Drobatz KJ and Hughes D. Concentration of ionized calcium in plasma from cats with urethral obstruction. J Am Vet Med Assoc 1997;211: 1392-1395.

Case 21 – Level 3

"José" is a 1.5-year-old miniature donkey that was castrated three weeks ago. After surgery, there appeared to be excessive swelling around the incision. He has been straining to urinate since then. At presentation, José has bilateral abdominal distention with moderate swelling of the sheath of the penis and in the dependent inguinal areas. He is tachypneic, tachycardic, and depressed. No gut sounds are detected. He has not urinated for several days and stopped passing manure two days ago. (The reference intervals provided are for horses and are not specific for donkeys.)

White blood cell count:	↑ 24.6 x 10⁹/L	(5.4-14.3)
Segmented neutrophils:	↑ 19.4 x 10⁹/L	(2.3-8.6)
Band neutrophils:	0.0 x 10⁹/L	(0-0.3)
Lymphocytes:	2.5 x 10⁹/L	(1.5-7.7)
Monocytes:	↑ 2.7 x 10⁹/L	(0.0-1.0)
WBC morphology: No abnormalities noted.		
Hematocrit:	44%	(32-53)
MCV:	51.5 fl	(37.0-58.5)
MCHC:	34.3 g/dl	(31.0-38.6)
RBC morphology: No abnormalites noted.		
Platelets: Clumped but appear adequate		
Fibrinogen:	↑ 1000 mg/dl	(100-400)
Plasma is slightly lipemic		
Glucose:	↑ 484 mg/dl	(60-130)
BUN:	↑ 114 mg/dl	(10-26)
Creatinine:	↑ 12.5 mg/dl	(1.0-2.0)
Phosphorus:	4.3 mg/dl	(1.5-4.5)
Calcium:	↓ 9.6 mg/dl	(10.8-13.5)
Magnesium:	↑ 8.4 mEq/L	(1.7-2.4)
Total Protein:	↑ 8.3 g/dl	(5.7-7.7)
Albumin:	2.6 g/dl	(2.4-3.8)
Globulin:	↑ 5.7 g/dl	(2.5-4.5)
Sodium:	↓ 117 mEq/L	(130-145)
Chloride:	↓ 72 mEq/L	(97-110)
Potassium:	↑ 6.8 mEq/L	(3.0-5.0)
HCO3:	↑ 39 mEq/L	(25-33)
Anion Gap:	12.8 mEq/L	(7-15)
Total Bili:	0.3 mg/dl	(0.30-3.0)
ALP:	↑ 505 IU/L	(109-352)
GGT:	↑ 53 IU/L	(4-28)
AST:	↑ 424 IU/L	(190-380)
CK:	↓ 74 IU/L	(80-446)
Triglycerides:	↑ 1288 mg/dl	(90-52)

Abdominocentesis

Appearance: Tan and cloudy	
Total nucleated cell count: 16,700/µl	
Total protein: 2.0 gm/dl	
Description: The predominant cells are nondegenerate neutrophils and lesser numbers of macrophages. Scattered erythrocytes are present and some macrophages are erythrophagic. No etiologic agents are seen.	

Abdominal fluid creatinine: 20.6 mg/dl.

Interpretation

CBC: José has a neutrophilic leukocytosis and monocytosis with hyperfibrinogenemia, indicating inflammation.

Serum Biochemical Profile

Hyperglycemia: Common causes of hyperglycemia in horses include stress or excitement associated with transport or pain, corticosteroid therapy, or Cushing's syndrome. Diabetes mellitus is rare in equids.

Azotemia: Because of the anuria, no urine specific gravity is available to classify the azotemia on the basis of urinary concentrating ability. The abdominal fluid analysis and creatinine points to uroabdomen and a post-renal azotemia. Intravascular fluid volume contraction may result in a pre-renal component as well.

Hypocalcemia: Gastrointestinal disease, renal disease, and sepsis may be associated with hypocalcemia in Equidae (Toribio). José has evidence of urinary obstruction. Hypocalcemia is most typical of acute renal failure and is often accompanied by hyperphosphatemia, which is not present here. Sepsis is possible given the inflammatory leukogram. Poor gastrointestinal absorption is possible with decreased gut sounds. Ionized calcium measurement would provide more information about the likelihood that José will develop clinical signs of hypocalcemia, but at this point the calcium may normalize with correction of the underlying disorders.

Hypermagnesemia: In this case, the hypermagnesemia is due to the anuria and subsequent failure to eliminate magnesium in the urine. Hypermagnesemia is rare in large animal species and is more often the result of oversupplementation or treatment with magnesium containing products.

Hyperproteinemia with hyperglobulinemia: Increased production of acute phase reactants such as fibrinogen and/or increased production of immunoglobulins in response to antigenic stimulation are causing the changes in serum proteins.

Mild hyponatremia with disproportionately greater hypochloremia: Multiple mechanisms are contributing to the hyponatremia and hypochloremia. There is loss of electrolytes into the abdominal effusion as a result of a ruptured bladder. Horses produce hypertonic sweat with a relatively high concentration of chloride, and this may be an additional route for loss of electrolytes if José has been sweating due to pain. Osmotic draw of additional fluid from extracellular spaces into the circulation by excessive amounts of glucose could dilute the remaining sodium. There may be an artifactual lowering of sodium and chloride with severe lipemia if the chemistry analyzer employs indirect potentiometry with ion specific electrodes in which the sample is diluted as part of the assay. The corrected chloride is 84 mEq/L, which indicates that additional forces are acting on chloride. Hypochloremia is often noted in association with metabolic alkalosis, which is present in this case. Digestive disturbances resulting in loss or sequestration of chloride containing fluid can lower serum chloride, and this may be possible considering the decreased gut sounds and failure to pass manure.

Hyperkalemia: Accumulation of potassium in the serum can occur when glomerular filtration rate drops sufficiently to prevent elimination of potassium in the urine. In this case, pooling of urine in the abdomen allows translocation of potassium back into the circulation from the abdominal cavity to re-establish equilibrium of potassium concentrations across the semi-permeable serosal lining.

Increased bicarbonate (alkalemia): Sequestration or loss of acid or chloride containing fluids will precipitate alkalosis. Alkalosis also may be perpetuated by the need to conserve sodium and the relative deficit of chloride. When sodium is resorbed in the proximal tubule, an anion must follow to maintain electrical neutrality. When chloride is not available in adequate quantities, increased amounts of sodium are present in the distal tubule. Sodium resorption will be coupled with hydrogen loss and generation of bicarbonate, maintaining the alkalosis.

Increased ALP and GGT: The combination of elevations in ALP and GGT suggest hepatobiliary disease. Severe cholestasis seems unlikely because the serum bilirubin is within reference intervals. In large animal species, the GGT is considered a more reliable indicator of liver disease, and it is compatible with liver damage associated with hyperlipidemia. The GGT value should be interpreted with caution, however, because the upper limit of the GGT reference interval for donkeys and burros may be two to three times greater than that of horses. Horse reference ranges are often used for these species as they were in this case, potentially leading to errors of interpretation.

Increased AST: This enzyme is a nonspecific indicator of tissue damage, possibly liver in this case. As with GGT, the upper limit of the reference interval may be higher for donkey's.

Decreased CK: This individual value is not diagnostically significant, but does suggest that the increase in AST is more likely to be associated with liver damage than muscle injury.

Hypertriglyceridemia: Increased serum triglycerides can be associated with metabolic disorders, particularly hyperlipemia in horses, ponies, and donkeys. Note that serum triglyceride values may be slightly higher in healthy donkeys compared to horses. Fasting precipitates excessive fatty acid mobilization from adipose with subsequent increased triglyceride synthesis and fatty infiltration of organs, including the liver. In this case, the urinary tract disease may have depressed food intake and caused disease.

Case Summary and Outcome

José was taken to surgery for correction of his uroabdomen. Nutritional support was instituted and he recovered from his hyperlipidemia. Like Simba, the obstructed cat (Chapter 7, Case 20), the inability to excrete urine from the body leads to excess potassium accumulation and azotemia. In José's case, the cause of the hyponatremia and hypochloremia is somewhat clearer than for Simba. In addition to loss of electrolytes into the effusion, the same osmotic effects that cause intravascular fluid shifts that diluted sodium and chloride in the hyperglycemic alpaca (Chapter 7, Case 19) and cases of diabetes occur here as well. Sweating is also a route for electrolyte loss in Equidae. The secondary hyperlipidemia could cause artifactually low values for electrolytes if indirect potentiometry or flame photometry methodology were used. Secondary metabolic disease may develop in anorexic horses, resulting in complications not directly related to the primary disease. This was observed with the hyperlipidemia and elevated liver enzymes that were not directly due to urinary tract obstruction.

Toribio RE. Parathyroid Gland Function and Calcium Regulation in Horses. American College of Veterinary Internal Medicine Forum 2003. Charlotte, NC.

Case 22 – Level 3

"Pat" is a 6-year-old neutered male Cockapoo presenting for an episode of lethargy, vomiting, and difficulty breathing. He was seen one day ago and the referring veterinarian noted an enlarged heart and liver on radiographs. Pericardiocentesis yielded 185 ml of hemorrhagic fluid. Pat was treated with antibiotics and vitamin K. On presentation to the referral institution, Pat is weak but alert. He has injected sclera and bright pink mucous membranes with prolonged capillary refill time. He is not febrile. His heart and respiratory rates are elevated, and he has a grade III/VI systolic murmur.

White blood cell count:	↑ 19.5 x 10⁹/L	(4.0-13.3)
Segmented neutrophils:	↑ 15.8 x 10⁹/L	(2.0-11.2)
Band neutrophils:	0.2 x 10⁹/L	(0-0.3)
Lymphocytes:	2.8 x 10⁹/L	(1.0-4.5)
Monocytes:	0.7 x 10⁹/L	(0.2-1.4)
Eosinophils:	0.0 x 10⁹/L	(0-1.2)
Nucleated RBC/100 WBC:	3	
WBC morphology: Appears within normal limits		

Hematocrit:	50.0%	(37-60)
Red blood cell count:	7.52 x 10¹²/L	(5.5-8.5)
Hemoglobin:	17.2 g/dl	(12.0-18.0)
MCV:	61.8 fl	(60.0-77.0)
MCHC:	34.0 g/dl	(31.0-34.0)

Platelets: Appear adequate in number.

Glucose:	↓ 55 mg/dl	(90.0-140.0)
BUN:	↑ 50 mg/dl	(6-24)
Creatinine:	1.5 mg/dl	(0.5-1.5)
Phosphorus:	↑ 7.9 mg/dl	(2.6-7.2)
Calcium:	↓ 8.3 mg/dl	(9.5-11.5)
Magnesium:	2.3 mEq/L	(1.7-2.5)
Total Protein:	5.1 g/dl	(4.8-7.2)
Albumin:	↓ 2.0 g/dl	(2.5-3.7)
Globulin:	3.1 g/dl	(2.0-4.0)
Sodium:	↓ 130 mEq/L	(140-151)
Chloride:	↓ 95 mEq/L	(105-120)
Potassium:	4.6 mEq/L	(3.6-5.6)
Anion gap:	16.6 mEq/L	(15-25)
HCO3:	23 mEq/L	(15-28)
Total Bili:	↑ 1.0 mg/dl	(0.10-0.50)
ALP:	↑ 300 IU/L	(20-121)
GGT:	6 IU/L	(2-10)

ALT:	↑ 107 IU/L	(10-95)
AST:	↑ 150 IU/L	(10-56)
Cholesterol:	161 mg/dl	(110-314)
Amylase:	553 IU/L	(400-1200)

Coagulation Profile

PT:	↑ 10.7s	(6.2-9.3)
APTT:	↑ 21.9s	(8.9-16.3)
FDP:	<5 µg/ml	(<5.0)

Pericardial Fluid Analysis

Pre-spin appearance: red and cloudy
Post-spin appearance: yellow and hazy
Total protein: 4.0 gm/dl
Total nucleated cell count: 110,000/µl

Description: Direct smears are markedly cellular, consisting of 98% degenerate neutrophils and 2% monocytes. Many RBCs are present. Many bacteria are present, most of which appear to be rods. Organisms are present intra- and extracellularly and include Gram positive and Gram negative forms (Figure 7-8).

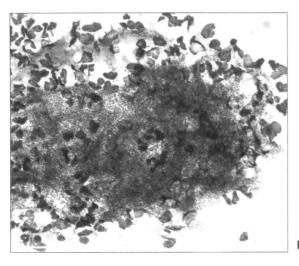

Figure 7-8. Septic pericardial fluid.

Interpretation

CBC: Pat has a mature neutrophilic leukocytosis that is attributable to inflammation, although the numbers of band neutrophils remain within the reference interval. Small numbers of nucleated erythroid precursors are also noted in the circulation. These are often present as a result of endothelial injury or lesions in hematopoietic tissues. In this case, hypoxemia associated with diminished cardiac function or sepsis may cause endothelial damage and release of erythroid precursors.

Serum Biochemical Profile

Hypoglycemia: Because of the inflammatory leukogram and the cytologic appearance of the pericardial fluid, sepsis is an important differential diagnosis for the hypoglycemia, assuming that no processing errors occurred. The hypoglycemia is mild and may not be associated with clinical effects.

Increased BUN with normal creatinine: Because a urine specific gravity is not available for this patient, renal function is difficult to evaluate. BUN may increase prior to creatinine early in renal compromise or with decreased tubular flow rates associated with dehydration or other causes of pre-renal azotemia such as decreased cardiac output. Sepsis may also cause an increase in BUN but no change in creatinine. Consumption of a high protein diet can elevate BUN.

Hyperphosphatemia: Decreased glomerular filtration rate is a common cause of hyperphosphatemia and is consistent with pre-renal azotemia in a patient that is dehydrated or has impaired cardiac function. Tissue necrosis may increase serum phosphorus. However, there is little evidence to support this mechanism without a CK, only a mildly increased AST, and the potassium within reference intervals. Because the calcium is also low, hypoparathyroidism also may be considered. The most likely cause of the hypocalcemia is decreased protein bound calcium secondary to the hypoalbuminemia.

Hypoalbuminemia and normal globulin: Isolated hypoalbuminemia may be attributable to decreased production. Liver failure is possible given the hypoglycemia and prolonged coagulation times. However, other substances produced by the liver such as urea and cholesterol are not decreased. Specific tests of liver function such as serum bile acids or blood ammonia could be performed as more sensitive and specific indicators of liver function. Alternatively, the liver may decrease production of albumin in response to inflammation, because this protein is a negative acute phase reactant. This seems likely in the context of the neutrophilia and septic pericardial effusion. Decreased production due to starvation is unlikely in a patient with adequate body condition. Albumin also may be selectively lost via the glomerulus, and could be evaluated by urinalysis. Nonspecific protein losses into third space including the pericardial sac usually result in decreases in both albumin and globulins. Repeated drainage of the pericardial effusion can contribute to the hypoalbuminemia. Loss of globulins by this route may be countered by increased production with inflammation, resulting in globulin values that fall within the reference interval. Lastly, dilution of albumin may occur in fluid loading states such as congestive heart failure, which could be an issue here because of the pericardial effusion.

Hyponatremia and hypochloremia: Similar to protein, serum levels of sodium and chloride reflect the balance of intake, losses, and dilution. Routes of electrolyte losses are similar to protein and include the kidney, gastrointestinal tract, skin, and third space. In Pat's case, third space loss into the pericardial cavity, especially with repeated drainage, could deplete electrolytes. Electrolyte loss via the kidneys may be evaluated by measuring urinary fractional excretions, however these are rarely performed in routine practice. The absence of significant signs of gastrointestinal disease makes this route unlikely. Hemodilution or hemoconcentration also may alter serum electrolyte concentrations if free water changes are disproportionate to gains or losses of electrolytes. In the case of congestive heart failure, poor perfusion pressures trigger antidiuretic hormone release, which will encourage increased water intake and free water retention, effectively diluting sodium and chloride. Most domestic animals on commercial diets will not have dietary deficiency or excess of sodium and chloride.

Hyperbilirubinemia: The septic process described above may be interfering with hepatocellular uptake of bile, resulting in a mild hyperbilirubinemia. Increases in ALP, ALT, and AST support the potential for hepatobiliary disease and cholestasis, which could cause increased bilirubin, although the cholestatic enzyme GGT is not elevated. Hemolysis as a cause of the mild increase in serum bilirubin is unlikely give the normal PCV. If the hyperbilirubinemia persists after successful treatment of the infectious process, further investigation of the potential for liver disease should be considered.

Increased ALP with normal GGT: Extrahepatic causes of liver enzyme elevations should always be considered in addition to the potential for hepatobiliary disease. Both sepsis and cardiovascular disease have the potential to elevate serum liver enzyme activities in the absence of primary liver pathology. A thorough drug history should be taken to rule out effects of medications, and concurrent endocrinopathies need to be considered for their potential to impact liver enzymes.

Increased ALT and AST: ALT is relatively liver specific in small animal species and generally reflects hepatocellular damage. AST is present in the liver, but is less specific and will increase with damage to extrahepatic tissues such as muscle. Sepsis and poor perfusion are expected to cause hepatocellular damage, but may injure other tissues as well.

Coagulation profile: Both the PT and APTT are prolonged, indicating a defect of secondary hemostasis. Both liver disease and sepsis may impair hemostasis. Disseminated intravascular coagulation is not yet occurring based on the normal platelet numbers and fibrin degradation products.

Case Summary and Outcome

Based on the initial data, Pat was treated with fluids and antibiotics. Echocardiography revealed a large volume of fluid still present within the pericardial sac, right atrial collapse, and a small left ventricle with moderate function. Because of the persistent pericardial effusion, a multi-hole catheter was placed for continuous drainage. Later, Pat had surgery to remove a section of the pericardium. Histology revealed severe fibrinopurulent bacterial pericarditis. During surgery, a chest tube was placed to continue drainage of purulent material. Over the five days following surgery, Pat became progressively more bright and alert. Drainage collected from the chest tubes showed diminishing inflammation, and tubes were removed. Pat was discharged on long-term combination antibiotic therapy.

Like Snow (Case 7) and Isis (Case 11) in this chapter, poor perfusion due to cardiovascular compromise could lead to free water retention and dilution of Pat's serum electrolytes. In Pat's case, loss of electrolytes into the pericardial effusion would also potentiate hyponatremia and hypochloremia, while Snow had increased renal loss of electrolytes associated with the use of diuretics for her heart disease. Isis experienced cutaneous loss of electrolytes through her degloving wound. Pat's serum potassium levels are currently within the reference interval. However, serum potassium levels do not accurately reflect total body potassium stores, which may be low due to the effusion, anorexia or vomiting. Poor renal perfusion associated with septic shock may promote higher serum potassium. Serum potassium values may fluctuate rapidly in response to therapy or changes in Pat's medical condition. Unlike Snow, Isis and Pat may have experienced nonselective protein losses as well. Isis was able to maintain serum protein levels while Pat developed hypoproteinemia. Serum protein levels may also be affected by water retention and dilution.

Case 23 – Level 3

"Diamond" is a 2.5-year-old spayed female domestic short haired, indoor/outdoor cat that presented with a history of lethargy, depression, and decreased appetite for three days. On physical examination, Diamond is recumbent, pale and hypothermic, and no menace or blink response can be elicited. She has dyspnea and bradycardia. On auscultation, heart sounds are muffled, and foul smelling brown fluid is obtained via thoracocentesis. Her body condition score is low.

White blood cell count:	↑ 43.8 x 10⁹/L	(4.5-15.7)
Segmented neutrophils:	↑ 42.0 x 10⁹/L	(2.1-10.1)
Band neutrophils:	0.0 x 10⁹/L	(0-0.3)
Lymphocytes:	1.8 x 10⁹/L	(1.5-7.0)
Monocytes:	0 x 10⁹/L	(0-0.9)
Eosinophils:	0 x 10⁹/L	(0.0-1.9)

WBC morphology: Moderate toxic changes are observed in the neutrophils

Hematocrit:	↓ 24%	(28-45)
Hemoglobin:	↓ 8.2 g/dl	(10.5-14.9)
MCV:	41.5 fl	(39.0-56.0)
MCHC:	34.2 g/dl	(30.5-36.2)
Platelets (manual count):	↓ 104 x 10⁹/L	(183-643)

The plasma is icteric.

Glucose:	↑ 161 mg/dl	(70.0-120.0)
BUN:	↓ 12 mg/dl	(15-32)
Creatinine:	↓ 0.5 mg/dl	(0.9-2.1)
Phosphorus:	3.7 mg/dl	(3.0-6.0)
Calcium:	↓ 7.7 mg/dl	(8.9-11.6)
Magnesium:	2.0 mEq/L	(1.9-2.6)
Total Protein:	↓ 3.9 g/dl	(6.0-8.4)
Albumin:	↓ 1.4 g/dl	(2.2.3.4)
Globulin:	2.5 g/dl	(2.5-5.8)
Sodium:	↓ 144 mEq/L	(149-163)
Chloride:	↓ 107 mEq/L	(119-134)
Potassium:	↓ 3.0 mEq/L	(3.6-5.4)
HCO3:	↑ 28 mEq/L	(13-22)
Anion Gap:	↓ 12.0 mEq/L	(13-27)
Total Bili:	↑ 1.2 mg/dl	(0.10-0.30)
ALP:	13 IU/L	(10-72)
GGT:	<3 IU/L	(0-4)
ALT:	57 IU/L	(29-145)
AST:	↑ 61 IU/L	(12-42)
Cholesterol:	108 mg/dl	(50-150)
Amylase:	1145 IU/L	(362-1410)

Coagulation Profile

PT:	9.9s	(7.6-10.4)
APTT:	↑ 53.6s	(11.8-17.4)
FDP:	<5 ug/dl	(<5.0)

Thoracic Fluid Analysis

Appearance: brown and opaque	
Total protein: 3.5 g/dl	
Total nucleated cells: 240,000/μl	

Description: Direct smears contain large numbers of cells, however cells are in very poor condition. The majority of cells that can be identified are extremely degenerate neutrophils that contain numerous bacteria of mixed morphology. Many large foamy macrophages are also present. Bacteria also occur in large extracellular mats. Both Gram positive and negative organisms are present, including small coccobacilli and some long, thin rods that chain.

Interpretation

CBC: There is a marked mature neutrophilic leukocytosis with toxic change compatible with inflammation, the source of which is the thoracic cavity. Diamond also has a normocytic, normochromic anemia that is interpreted to be non-regenerative. A reticulocyte count is needed to confirm this conclusion. Anemia of chronic disease is a likely contributor, however given the relatively low protein, acute hemorrhage should also be considered. Infectious causes of anemia such as panleukopenia (unlikely here with the leukocytosis) and FeLV should always be ruled out, especially in young cats. The concurrent moderate thrombocytopenia also suggests that a bone marrow disorder should be considered, however decreased platelets may be associated with increased consumption secondary to hemorrhage or inflammatory disease rather than failure of production. Patients with a septic focus may develop disseminated intravascular coagulation, which can cause moderate thrombocytopenia due to increased consumption.

Serum Biochemical Profile

Hyperglycemia: This increase may be due to the nonspecific effects of illness or stress. Acute endotoxemia may be associated with hyperglycemia, although some septic patients eventually develop hypoglycemia.

Decreased BUN and creatinine: These analytes may be low due to poor body condition or low protein diet. They are not likely to be clinically significant, other than to rule out azotemia at this point.

Hypocalcemia: The most likely cause for the hypocalcemia is the decrease in albumin. Because the cat is profoundly weak, an ionized calcium should be measured to determine if Diamond would benefit from supplementation.

Hypoproteinemia with hypoalbuminemia and borderline-low globulins: Dilution, decreased production, and increased losses are the basic mechanisms for low serum protein values. No specific evaluation of hydration status was mentioned in the clinical history, however with the history of lethargy and anorexia, Diamond is more likely to be dehydrated than overhydrated. Diamond's poor body condition is potentially compatible with low protein production associated with malnutrition, however the decrease in protein associated with poor intake is usually milder than the seen here. Because there is evidence of inflammation, albumin production may be low because it is an acute phase reactant. Poor liver function also may result in low albumin production, however this seems less likely in the context of the clinical history. Increased losses into the septic effusion in the thorax is a major contributor to the hypoproteinemia and hypoalbuminemia in this case. Third space protein losses are generally non-selective, resulting in loss of albumin and globulin. The globulin may remain within reference intervals despite these losses because of increased production of immunoglobulins and acute phase reactants in response to the inflammation. Other potential nonselective sources of protein loss that are unlikely in this specific patient include gastrointestinal losses and dermal losses. Selective loss of albumin via the glomerulus is not specifically evaluated here because a urinalysis was not performed. Glomerular disease seems less likely because the BUN and Cr are low, however the early phases of glomerular disease may not be always be characterized by azotemia.

Hyponatremia with hypochloremia: The degree of hypochloremia is slightly greater than the degree of hyponatremia (corrected chloride is 115 mEq/L). As discussed above in the protein section, water accumulation is unlikely to account for the decreased sodium and chloride. Decreased intake is also not likely to be important. Loss into the effusion is the most likely cause for the abnormality, although other sources of increased loss cannot be ruled out. The additional decrease in chloride that cannot be accounted for by the change in sodium is attributed to the alkalemia.

Hypokalemia: The decrease in potassium is related to loss into the pleural effusion, however decreased intake may also be a factor for this electrolyte. Acid/base abnormalities are often cited as a cause for cellular translocation of potassium.

Alkalemia (increased HCO3): The alkalemia may be due to metabolic alkalosis or a compensated respiratory acidosis. The presence of dyspnea and evidence of acid/base abnormalities indicate the need for blood gas analysis to further characterize the process.

Low anion gap: The low anion gap is attributed to hypoalbuminemia.

Mild hyperbilirubinemia: Sepsis may interfere with hepatocellular uptake of bile, which can cause slight increases in bilirubin. Because BUN and serum albumin are also low and coagulation times are prolonged, decreased liver function should be considered, but is less likely based on the clinical history. Significant cholestatic disease is unlikely because the ALP and GGT are within reference intervals. The anemia suggests that hemolysis is possible.

Increased AST: This enzyme may originate from hepatocytes, muscle cells, or erythrocytes and is a non-specific indicator of tissue damage. To clarify the tissue of origin, the AST should be interpreted in the context of ALT and CK values. This elevation is mild and may not be very diagnostically significant, however tissue damage may result from sepsis and poor perfusion related to shock.

Abdominal fluid analysis: Septic suppurative inflammation

Coagulation: Thrombocytopenia with prolonged activated partial thromboplastin time could be signs of a mixed hemostatic disorder such as disseminated intravascular coagulation (DIC). The presence of DIC is not corroborated by increases in FDPs. The degree of thrombocytopenia is not sufficiently severe to result in spontaneous bleeding as an isolated abnormality, however in combination with a secondary hemostatic defect, abnormal bleeding is possible. Diamond's APTT is elevated, however the PT is within reference intervals. In general, liver disease or vitamin K antagonists cause both the PT and the APTT to become prolonged. Sometimes the PT is abnormal first because factor VII in the extrinsic pathway has the shortest halflife, however occasionally the APTT will become prolonged first in liver disease. Regardless, the coagulation status of this patient should be monitored.

Case Summary and Outcome

Pleural effusion was documented radiographically, and Diamond experienced respiratory arrest during bilateral chest tube placement. She was successfully resuscitated and placed on a ventilator overnight. She responded to antibiotic treatment for the septic process in her thoracic cavity and was eventually weaned from the ventilator.

Diamond's data may be compared with June (Chapter 4, Case 11), who also had pyothorax. Both cats had hyponatremia and hypochloridemia, but June was able to maintain her serum potassium level while Diamond was hypokalemic. Both experienced significant protein losses along with electrolyte depletion associated with the effusions. Both cats also had mild hyperbilirubinemia and liver enzyme elevations due to sepsis, but June had mild stress or early endotoxin associated hyperglycemia while Diamond had hypoglycemia attributable to sepsis.

Case 24 – Level 3

"Caviar" is a 5-month-old female Bichon Frise presenting with a history of vomiting, diarrhea, and poor appetite since she was adopted 3 months ago. On physical examination, Caviar is weak and dull and very thin. She is tachycardic and has weak pulses. During the examination, she has bloody diarrhea.

White blood cell count:	↑ 38.2 x 10⁹/L	(4.0-13.3)
Segmented neutrophils:	↑ 32.9 x 10⁹/L	(2.0-11.2)
Band neutrophils:	↑ 0.4 x 10⁹/L	(0-0.3)
Lymphocytes:	↑ 4.9 x 10⁹/L	(1.0-4.5)
Monocytes:	↓ 0.0 x 10⁹/L	(0.2-1.4)
Eosinophils:	0.0 x 10⁹/L	(0-1.2)
Nucleated RBC/100 WBC	1	

WBC morphology: Moderate numbers of reactive lymphocytes are present

Hematocrit:	↓ 18.0%	(37-60)
Red blood cell count:	↓ 2.47 x 10¹²/L	(5.5-8.5)
Hemoglobin:	↓ 4.9 g/dl	(12.0-18.0)
MCV:	65.1 fl	(60.0-77.0)
MCHC:	↓ 27.2 g/dl	(31.0-34.0)

Platelets: Appear adequate in number

Glucose:	↓ 26 mg/dl	(90.0-140.0)
BUN:	↓ 7 mg/dl	(8-33)
Creatinine:	↓ 0.2 mg/dl	(0.5-1.5)
Phosphorus:	6.3 mg/dl	(2.2-6.6)
Calcium:	↓ 7.5 mg/dl	(9.5-11.5)
Magnesium:	↓ 1.2 mEq/L	(1.7-2.5)
Total Protein:	↓ 2.4 g/dl	(4.8-7.2)
Albumin:	↓ 1.0 g/dl	(2.5-3.7)
Globulin:	↓ 1.4 g/dl	(2.0-4.0)
Sodium:	↓ 129 mEq/L	(140-151)
Chloride:	106 mEq/L	(105-120)
Potassium:	↑ 6.8 mEq/L	(3.6-5.6)

Anion gap:	↓ 10.8 mEq/L	(15-25)
HCO3:	19 mEq/L	(15-28)
Total Bili:	↑ 0.9 mg/dl	(0.10-0.50)
ALP:	↑ 369 IU/L	(20-320)
GGT:	2 IU/L	(2-10)
ALT:	↑ 851 IU/L	(10-95)
AST:	↑ 225 IU/L	(10-56)
Cholesterol:	↓ 24 mg/dl	(110-314)
Amylase:	472 IU/L	(400-1200)

Coagulation Profile

PT:	↑ 16.2s	(6.2-9.3)
APTT:	↑ 38.4s	(8.9-16.3)

Intepretation

CBC: Caviar has a neutrophilic leukocytosis with a very mild left shift and a reactive lymphocytosis compatible with inflammation and antigenic stimulation. The monocytopenia has no clinical implication. The significance of small numbers of nucleated erythrocytes in a young animal is questionable, however endothelial damage secondary to inflammation or sepsis is a possible cause for these cells to be present in the circulation. Nucleated red blood cells may also appear during a regenerative response to anemia. Caviar has a normocytic hypochromic anemia which is difficult to classify at this time. The hypochromasia could reflect some attempt at regeneration. A reticulocyte count is needed to assess a regenerative response.

Serum Biochemical Profile

Hypoglycemia: Once processing errors have been ruled out, physiologic causes of hypoglycemia may be considered. The inflammatory leukogram and poor clinical condition at presentation are compatible with sepsis. Impaired liver function associated with a congenital portovascular anomaly is possible and supported by other laboratory indicators indicative of poor hepatic function, including low BUN, hypoalbuminemia, hyperbilirubinemia, decreased serum cholesterol and prolonged coagulation times. Evaluation of liver function by measurement of serum bile acids or blood ammonia is strongly recommended. The young age of the patient makes paraneoplastic hypoglycemia unlikely. Although Caviar clearly has poor body condition and nutritional deficits, this is rarely a cause of hypoglycemia by itself (See Belinda, Chapter 4, Case 1; Marsali, Chapter 5, Case 3; Diva, Chapter 6, Case 16).

Decreased BUN and creatinine: Decreased BUN may be related to potentially compromised liver function. Low creatinine is attributed to poor body condition and low muscle mass.

Hypocalcemia with normal phosphorus: Low total serum calcium is probably caused by the low serum albumin. The chronic history of diarrhea suggests the possibility of malabsorption as a cause hypocalcemia (See Red Molly, Chapter 4, Case 4).

Panhypoproteinemia: Most patients with panhypoproteinemia are experiencing increased nonselective losses of protein. In this case, gastrointestinal losses seem the most likely route with the history of chronic diarrhea as well as gastrointestinal hemorrhage. Hemorrhage may be secondary to defects in hemostasis as indicated by the prolonged coagulation times. Given the chronicity of the problem, other causes of diarrhea and protein losing enteropathy need to be evaluated in this patient. Nutritional factors may further compromise Caviar's ability to compensate for ongoing losses and to maintain serum protein levels. Compounding these factors is the the potential for decreased liver function to impair albumin production.

Globulin levels in young animals may be slightly lower than aged animals because they have been exposed to fewer antigens.

Hyponatremia with low normal chloride: Gastrointestinal losses of electrolytes are suspected. Hemorrhage may contribute to the hyponatremia by triggering mechanisms resulting in retention of free water by the kidney in response to hypovolemia and dilutional effects. The chloride is relatively high compared with sodium, however the serum bicarbonate remains within the reference interval. This is compatible with a mixed acid/base disorder, and blood gas analysis should be considered.

Hyperkalemia: Assuming that significant hemolysis or release from damaged tissues is ruled out, decreased urinary excretion of potassium should be evaluated. This commonly occurs if urine cannot be eliminated from the body such as with oliguric/anuric renal failure, urinary tract obstruction, or ruptured urinary bladder. Although a urinalysis is not currently available, Caviar is producing urine and does not have a clinical history compatible with these problems. The electrolyte abnormalities and history of gastrointestinal signs could also be consistent with hypoadrenocorticism, however Caviar would be a very young dog to present with this condition. Alternatively, some dogs with primary gastrointeintal disorders may develop these electrolyte abnormalities, resembling hypoadrenocorticism. This occurs because of diarrhea-induced losses of water, sodium and chloride result in volume contraction and subsequent low renal tubular flow rate and potassium retension. Because whipworm infection has been documented in dogs with this pseudohypoadrenocorticism syndrome, a fecal floatation is warranted.

Decreased anion gap: This abnormality may be explained by the marked hypoproteinemia. Proteins such as albumin are important unmeasured anions.

Hyperbilirubinemia: Both sepsis and decreased liver function seem likely causes for the mild hyperbilirubinemia. The slight elevation in ALP and normal GGT make significant cholestasis less likely. Because Caviar is anemic, the blood film should be evaluated for evidence of hemolysis.

Increased ALP: The cause of this mild abnormality may be difficult to determine in a dog with a complex clinical presentation. Extra-hepatic causes of increased ALP include bone growth in young dogs and the effects of medications and hormones. Mild cholestasis could result from swelling secondary to hepatocellular damage. Liver enzyme elevations also occur in association with intestinal damage because of increased exposure to bacteria and toxins from the damaged gut.

Increased ALT and AST: Elevations in these enzymes reflect hepatocellular damage. Some degree of hepatocellular hypoxia/hypoperfusion is likely given the anemia and potential for sepsis. Primary liver disease should also be considered since other laboratory abnormalities are consistent with decreased liver function.

Hypocholesterolemia: This abnormality is consistent with either decreased liver function or intestinal loss secondary to protein losing enteropathy.

Coagulation profile: Prolongation of coagulation times may occur with decreased liver function due to failure to produce coagulation factors. This may be compounded by impaired gastrointestinal absorption of vitamin K, resulting in vitamin K deficiency and production of inactive coagulation factors.

Case Summary and Outcome

Caviar was treated with antibiotics, intravenous fluids, plasma, and dextrose. Her condition seemed to improve. Further diagnostic work-up included a negative parvovirus test and fecal floatation. Postprandial serum bile acids were 221 µmol/L (reference interval = 0-25), confirming poor liver function. A large extrahepatic vascular shunt was demonstrated by abdominal ultrasound, however there was concern about the possibility of concurrent intestinal disease, including lymphangiectasia or infectious enteritis. Caviar stabilized with medical therapy and underwent surgical correction of the shunt. She began to eat and maintain a normal glucose level after surgery, however a few days after discharge, she developed ascites. Another surgery was performed to attempt to reduce the constriction of the shunt, but it was not possible to remove or enlarge the constrictor. She responded to symptomatic therapy and was discharged to the care of the referring veterinarian.

In Caviar's case, the combination of increased gastrointestinal losses of electrolytes with poor perfusion and inadequate renal excretion of potassium produced electrolyte abnormalities that could be associated with hypoadrenocorticism (Case 13), uroabdomen (Case 21), and other causes of third space losses such as effusion (Case 1). In previous cases of electrolyte depletion associated with hypoglycemia, the decreased blood glucose has been due to sepsis (Pat, Chapter 7, Case 22), but Caviar's hypoglycemia is due to inadequate liver function.

Case 25 – Level 3

"Albus" is 6-month-old Paint stallion presenting with a 2 day history of profuse diarrhea and decreased appetite. On presentation, he is tachycardic and has tacky mucous membranes.

White blood cell count:	↓ 2.7 x 10⁹/L	(5.4-14.3)
Segmented neutrophils:	↓ 0.5 x 10⁹/L	(2.3-8.6)
Band neutrophils:	0.0 x 10⁹/L	(0-0.3)
Lymphocytes:	2.1 x 10⁹/L	(1.5-7.7)
Monocytes:	0.1 x 10⁹/L	(0.0-1.0)

WBC morphology: Neutrophils show mild toxic changes

Hematocrit:	35%	(32-53)
MCV:	↓ 33.7 fl	(37.0-58.5)
MCHC:	34.9 g/dl	(31.0-38.6)

RBC morphology: No abnormalities noted

Platelets: Clumped but appear adequate

Glucose:	↑ 238 mg/dl	(60-130)
BUN:	↑ 31 mg/dl	(10-26)
Creatinine:	↑ 2.4 mg/dl	(1.0-2.0)
Phosphorus:	↑ 12.0 mg/dl	(1.5-4.5)
Calcium:	↓ 10.6 mg/dl	(10.8-13.5)
Magnesium:	↑ 2.8 mEq/L	(1.7-2.4)
Total Protein:	↓ 5.4 g/dl	(5.7-7.7)
Albumin:	3.1 g/dl	(2.6-3.8)
Globulin:	↓ 2.3 g/dl	(2.5-4.5)
Sodium:	↓ 129 mEq/L	(130-145)
Chloride:	↓ 84 mEq/L	(97-110)
Potassium:	↑ 6.1 mEq/L	(3.0-5.0)

HCO3:	↓ 20.0 mEq/L	(25-33)
Anion Gap:	↑ 31.1 mEq/L	(7-15)
Total Bili:	1.25 mg/dl	(0.30-3.0)
ALP:	↑ 552 IU/L	(109-352)
GGT:	15 IU/L	(4-28)
LDH:	↑ 539 IU/L	(122-360)
AST:	321 IU/L	(190-380)
CK:	↑ 1212 IU/L	(80-446)

Urine specific gravity: 1.035

Interpretation

CBC: Albus has leucopenia characterized by marked neutropenia and mild toxic change suggestive for acute inflammation or endotoxemia, likely related to intestinal disease.

Serum Biochemical Profile
Hyperglycemia: Diabetes mellitus is rare in horses, and the hyperglycemia in this case is related to stress or excitement.

Azotemia: The urine specific gravity suggests that the azotemia is of pre-renal origin.

Hyperphosphatemia: The pre-renal decrease in glomerular filtration rate is leading to accumulation of phosphorus.

Hypocalcemia: The mild hypocalcemia is probably related to the presence of gastrointestinal disease (see Faith, Chapter 5, Case 19).

Hypoproteinemia with hypoglobulinemia: Hypoglobulinemia is most often associated with concurrent hypoalbuminemia and reflects non-selective protein losses into the gut, third space, through the skin, or with hemorrhage. In this case, the albumin remains within the reference intervals. Isolated hypoglobulinemia can reflect failure of passive transfer in neonatal animals, but globulins remain somewhat low until antigenic exposure of initially naïve animals increases immunoglobulin production over time. Albus is likely to have had serum globulin levels at the lower end of the reference interval prior to his illness as an age-related phenomenon. Rarely, congenital immunodeficiency syndromes such as combined immunodeficiency syndrome of Arabian foals can result in failure of globulin production.

Mild hyponatremia with disproportionately greater hypochloridemia: Gastrointestinal losses of sodium and chloride are contributing to these abnormalities. Decreases in chloride that are disproportionate to changes in sodium are often associated with alkalemia. When a disproportionate hypochloremia is associated with decreases in HCO3, as in this case, a mixed acid/base disorder is suspected. In Albus, poor perfusion and lactic acidosis may lead to increased amounts of lactate in the urine. Because lactate cannot be resorbed by the renal tubules, sodium excretion in the urine is increased to maintain electrical neutrality. Consequently, chloride resorption in the proximal and collecting tubules does not occur because it depends on the electrochemical gradient established by prior resorption of sodium, which is failing to occur.

Hyperkalemia: Accumulation of potassium in the serum can occur when glomerular filtration rate drops sufficiently to prevent elimination of potassium in the urine. Additionally, inorganic acidosis can cause a transcellular shift of potassium outside of cells. Other potential causes for hyperkalemia that are unlikely in this particular patient based on the clinical history and laboratory work would include massive tissue necrosis or rhabdomyolysis, hypoaldosteronism, and effects of drugs such as angiotensin converting enzyme inhibitors or trimethoprim-sulfa antibiotics. Rhabdomyolysis and tissue necrosis are unlikely given the very mild increases in enzymes such as CK.

High anion gap acidosis: The high anion gap is the result of accumulation of unmeasured anions. Possibilties for Albus include uremic acids, and lactic acidosis secondary to dehydration and poor perfusion.

Increased ALP and LDH: Liver enzymes may increase secondary to intestinal disease due to a variety of mechanisms. These may include hepatocellular injury from increased exposure to bacteria, endotoxin, or inflammatory mediators. Hepatocellular hypoxia may result from systemic inflammation and circulatory imbalances. Ascending biliary infection or regurgitation of intestinal contents into the common bile duct associated with increased luminal pressure can result in cholestasis. In one study, histopathologic evaluation of the liver from five horses with proximal enteritis all had liver lesions that were attributed to the intestinal disease, supporting the interpretation that liver enzyme elevations can occur secondary to enteritis (Davis). While hepatocellular injury is the most likely cause for the increased serum LDH, this enzyme is not liver specific and may also originate from muscle tissue. ALP may also be high in young animals due to bone growth.

Increased CK: This enzyme indicates muscle damage. Muscle damage may occur as a result of transport or medical procedures such as intramuscular injections. If Albus is painful, he may self-traumatize and cause muscle damage. Although connective tissue in general is resistant to the effects of hypoxia, poor perfusion could contribute to muscle damage in some cases.

Case Summary and Outcome

Tests for rotavirus and *Clostridium perfringens* were negative. Albus responded to symptomatic therapy consisting of antiobiotics, fluids and pain medication. Albus may be compared with Delaney (Chapter 7, Case 8), who had much less complicated laboratory data. Delaney illustrates gastrointestinal disease in which electrolyte losses are minimal, while free water loss and restricted access to water lead to hypernatremia and hyperchloremia. In contrast, Albus is experiencing more significant electrolyte losses along with possible free water retention or increased intake to compensate for ongoing fluid losses, resulting in hyponatremia and hypochloremia. Note the low sodium and chloride with high potassium, a pattern that has been seen several times in the previous cases in this chapter. While Delaney has no apparent acid/base abnormalities, enteritis and fluid imbalances contribute to the development of a high anion gap metabolic acidosis in Albus.

Davis JL, Blikslager AT, Catto K, Jones SL. A retrospective analysis of hepatic injury in horses with proximal enteritis. J Vet Intern Med 2003;17:896-901.

Overview

Step 1: If electrolyte levels are high, consider

    Increased input through diet or therapeutic interventions (Case 1, and 14)

    Decreased elimination, particularly through the kidney (Case 9, 13, 20, and 21)

    Cellular translocation, especially for potassium (Case 2, and 17)

    Concentration of electrolytes in a smaller volume of fluid (Case 8, and 15)

    Electrochemical compensation for acid/base abnormalities

Step 2: If electrolyte levels are low, consider

    Decreased input via diet, mostly for potassium (Case 4, and 11)

    Electrolyte loss:

        Gastrointestinal tract (Case 4, 5, 6, 7, 18, 19, 24, and 25)

        Kidneys (Case 9, 13, 18, and 19)

        Third space (body cavities, interstitium) (Case 3, 20, 21, and 23)

        Cutaneous losses (Case 11, and 21)

        Hemorrhage (Case 10, and 24)

    Dilution (Case 9, 10, 12, 17, 18, 21, and 22)

    Electrochemical compensation for acid/base abnormalities

Step 3: If electrolyte values are normal, but the patient has potential sources of retention or loss or has abnormalities of fluid or acid/base regulation, consider the possibility that multiple factors causing opposing abnormalities have cumulatively resulted in a normal value

Step 4: If the patient is alkalotic (high bicarbonate), consider bicarbonate retention, acid sequestration or depletion (Case 5, 6, 10, 11, 19, and 21)

Step 5: If the patient is acidemic (low bicarbonate), consider loss of bicarbonate or acid retention (Case 12, 18 and 25)

Step 6: If the patient has an increased anion gap, consider hyperalbuminemia with dehydration or accumulation of endogenous or exogenous organic acids (Case 6, 12, 17, 18, 20, and 21)

Step 7: If the patient has a decreased anion gap, consider abnormalities of proteins or cations such as calcium and magnesium (Case 13, 23, and 24)

Index

Blood chemistry analysis
  for feline leukemia, 177-178
  for polyclonal gammopathy, 262-263
  in premature foal, 183-184
  for upper airway distress, 186-187
Blood clotting, impaired, 97
Bone
  diseases of, 17
  formation of, 275
  remodeling of in hypercalcemia, 275
Bone demineralization, maxillary and mandibular, 286-287
Bone marrow analysis
  for feline leukemia virus, 179-180
  for polyclonal gammopathy, 262-264
Bone marrow aspirate, 136, 139, 171
  for lymphoid neoplasm, 202
Bowel
  compromised, 97, 159, 189
  distention of, 172-173
  in feline panleukopenia, 97
  protein loss from, 159, 189
  hypocalcemia and absorption in, 274
  ischemic necrosis of, 173
Bromcresol green (BCG), 150
BUN/creatinine levels
  decreased
    in abused horse, 199
    with extrahepatic vascular shunt, 399
    in hypoparathyroidism, 279
    in portosystemic shunt, 226
    in pyothorax, 396
  elevated
    in feline leukemia, 178
    from foreign body in intestines, 344
    in heat stroke, 182
    in pericarditis, 393
    in pre-renal azotemia, 195
    in severe colic, 172-173
    in severe urinary tract disease, 197
    in transitional cell carcinoma, 214
  in gastrointestinal hemorrhage, 376
  in renal tubular dysfunction, 233
BUN levels
  decreased
    in cholestatic liver damage, 57
    in diabetes, 370
    in feline hepatic lipidosis, 38
    in hepatocellular damage with cholestasis, 35
    in impaired liver function, 91-92
    in inflammatory bowel disease, 320-321
    in liver disease, 299
    in pancreatitis, 118
    in portosystemic shunt, 42
    in progressive hepatic disease, 339
  elevated, 193
    in diabetes, 380
    in immune mediate hemolytic anemia, 45
    with seizures, 94

    in starvation, 317
  in renal function, 193

C
Calcitonin, 272
Calcium
  for hypoparathyroidism, 280
  low ionized, 282
  for parturient paresis, 279
  renal toxicity of, 203
  for tying up, 283
Calcium gluconate, 212
Calcium serum levels
  abnormalities in, 272-326
  evaluation of, 273-275
  hyperphosphatemia and, 275
  measurement of, 272
  regulation of, 272-273, 326
Calcium wasting, 248
Canine parvo test, 97
Carbohydrate intolerance, 317
Carbohydrate metabolism tests, 74-148
Carcinomatosis, 337
Cardiac disease, 313
Cardiopulmonary arrest, 146
Cardiopulmonary disease, 313-315
Cecal impaction, 348
Cellophane banding, 227
Cellular translocation, 334
  in hyperkalemia, 352
Cesarean section, for dead fetus, 19
Chelating compounds, 274
Chemotherapy
  for bladder carcinoma, 198
  for lymphoid neoplasm, 203
  for lymphoma and decreased liver function, 70
Chest tube drainage, 394
Chest tube placement, 177
  for respiratory arrest, 398
Chloride serum levels
  function and, 329
  imbalances in, 329-330
  normal, 329-330
  in thromboembolic disease, 383-384
Cholecystoduodenostomy, 118
Cholestasis
  decreased liver function with, 54-59
  elevated liver enzymes in, 376-377
  hepatocellular damage and, 27-30, 30-33, 34-37, 62-67
  hyperbilirubinemia and, 376
  indicators of, 71
  with mild inflammation, 52-55
  in renal azotemia, 60-62
Cholesterol
  homeostasis of in endocrinopathy, 106-107
  impaired production and degradation of, 100
  interpretation of, 74-75
Clinical chemistry profiles

abnormal results in, 7
explaining problems and abnormalities in, 5
grouping into meaningful categories, 4-5
guiding diagnostic work up, 6
indications for, 2
integrating data from, 5
normal with disease presence, 4
steps in, 2-6
Clostridium perfringens test, 403
Coagulation abnormalities
in cholestatic liver disease, 54
in cholestatic liver failure, 58
in extrahepatic vascular shunt, 400
in hepatocellular damage with cholestasis, 36
in hypoadrenocorticism, 105-106
in liver disease, 10
in lymphoma, 312
in pancreatitis, 114
in pericarditis, 394
in progressive hepatic disease, 340
in pulmonary thromboembolism, 188
in pyothorax, 397
in reduced liver function, 139, 141
in transitional cell carcinoma, 215
Coagulation necrosis, 84
Coagulopathy
in liver disease, 39-40, 300
in reduced liver function, 141-142
treatment of, 37
Colic, 247, 294
biochemical profile in, 248-250
severe, 172-173
Complete blood count (CBC)
abnormalities of in liver disease, 10
corticosteroid release and, 15
interpretation of, 13
Computed tomographic scan, pituitary, 99
Congestive heart failure, 356-358
in renal fluid retention, 346
Coombs' test
in immune mediate hemolytic anemia, 46
in zinc toxicosis, 146
Corneal ulceration, 323, 325
Corticosteroids
effects of, 175, 343, 359
in diabetes, 370, 376
in electrolyte abnormalities, 377
lymphopenia and, 379
in progressive hepatic disease, 339
in hepatopathy, 21
in hyperglycemia, 144
hyperglycemia and, 245
for immune-mediated thrombocytopenia, 101-102
liver enzyme levels and, 88-89
in lymphopenia, 15
Creatine kinase (CK) elevation
in acute overwhelming inflammation, 19
in renal disease, 243
in thromboembolism, 315

Creatinine levels. *See also* BUN/creatinine level
decreased
in diabetes, 371
in inflammatory bowel disease, 321
in starvation, 318
elevated, in gastrointestinal disease, 403
measurement of, 193
in renal function, 193
Cystocentesis, 15

D
Degenerative left shift, 214
Dehydration
azotemia and, 146-147, 245, 302
in colic, 248
compromising calcium excretion, 202-203
in electrolyte abnormalities, 353
hyperalbuminemia and, 190
hyperamylasemia and, 145-146
hyperglobulinemia and, 151
indicators of, 267
in renal disease, 242
serum albumin levels and, 173
in severe colic, 173
treatment of, 308
with urinary obstruction, 385
Depression
in pancreatic carcinoma, 110
in renal tubular necrosis, 142
Dermatitis, facial, 47
Dexamethasone, 74
Diabetes
biochemical profile in, 128-130
classification of, 125-126
differential of, 80
hyperglycemia in, 381
long term monitoring of, 126
treatment of, 377
Diabetes insipidus
differential for, 263
Diabetes insipidus-like syndrome, 203
Diabetes mellitus, 256-258
biochemical profile in, 132-133
diagnosis of, 378-381
electrolyte imbalance in, 369-371
hyperglycemia and, 144
hyperglycemia in, 344, 359, 376, 402
with ketosis, 131
liver enzyme elevation in, 23, 377
with near normal electrolytes, 372-373
treatment and outcome of, 134, 371, 378
Diagnostic tests
clinical chemistry profile guiding, 6
prioritizing, 6
sensitivity and specificity of, 4, 6
Diarrhea
bloody, 398
in fluid loss, 366
with foreign body in intestines, 343

in cholestatic liver disease, 24, 32, 58, 64
decreased, 10, 171
elevated
  activities of, 10
  in bladder rupture, 246
  categorizing cause of, 10
  causes of, 134, 176
  in cholestasis, 29, 32, 58
  in chronic hepatitis, 347
  in coagulopathy, 355
  in colic, 249
  degree of, 10
  in diabetes, 125, 133, 257, 373, 381
  disorders related to, 10-70
  in ethylene glycol toxicity, 305
  extrahepatic causes of, 12
  in extrahepatic vascular shunt, 400
  in feline infectious peritonitis, 167
  in feline leukemia, 179
  in fluid loss, 367-368
  from garbage eating, 342
  in gastrointestinal disease, 403
  in glomerulonephritis, 252
  in heat stroke, 183
  in hepatocellular carcinoma, 25-26
  in hepatocellular damage, 157-158
  in hyperbilirubinemia, 128
  in hyperthyroidism, 23, 238
  in hypoadrenocorticism, 261, 365
  in immune mediate hemolytic anemia, 46
  in inflammatory bowel disease, 321
  in intestinal disease, 175
  in liver disease, 134, 155, 235-236, 300, 376-377
  in lymphoma, 311
  in neonatal foal, 293-294
  in pancreatitis, 113-114, 115, 117, 118-119,
    129-130
  in parathyroid adenoma, 285
  in parvovirus infection, 164
  in pericarditis, 394
  in portosystemic shunt, 43, 226
  in postmortem serum sample, 334
  in progressive hepatic disease, 340
  in pulmonary thromboembolism, 188
  in pyelonephritis, 229
  in pyothorax, 397
  in recumbency and anorexia, 384
  in reduced liver function, 141-142
  in renal azotemia, 61
  in renal failure, 268, 296, 324-325
  in renal tubular dysfunction, 232-233
  in renal tubular necrosis, 144, 145-146
  in septic abdomen, 350
  in severe colic, 173
  in starvation, 317, 318
  in tick borne disease, 162
  in transitional cell carcinoma, 215
  in tying up, 283
  in urinary obstruction, 386

  in urinary tract disease, 197, 360
  evaluation of, 10-71
  in hepatocellular injury, 66, 70
  in hypoadrenocorticism, 105
  in immune-mediated thrombocytopenia, 102
  in impaired liver function, 91-92
  in insulinoma, 88-89
  medications, disorders, and extrahepatic
    processes inducing, 10
  in pancreatic carcinoma, 111
  in reduced liver function, 137-140
  with seizures, 94
  tips in interpreting, 10
Liver failure
  albumin downregulation with, 151
  diagnosis of, 297-300
  differential for, 263
  in hypoproteinemia and hypoalbuminemia, 383
Liver function
  decreased with hepatocellular damage and
    cholestasis, 54-59
  hepatocellular damage and, 67-70
  impaired, 71, 90-92
  lethargy and anorexia in, 135
Liver function tests
  in diabetes mellitus, 256-257
  in hepatocellular damage with cholestasis, 36-37
Lumbar spinal pain, 289
Lungs, diffuse nodules in, 111
Lyme disease
  diagnosis of, 204-206
  tests for, 206-207, 362
  treatment and outcome of, 206-207
  treatment of, 378
Lyme snap-test, 362
Lymph node aspirates
  for Lyme disease, 205
  for tick born disease, 161
Lymphadenopathy, generalized peripheral, 160-162
Lymphangiectasia, 401
Lymphocytosis, 363, 399
Lymphoid neoplasm
  malignant, 169-172
  renal function tests for, 201-203
Lymphoma, 309-312
Lymphopenia, 15, 175
  in bladder rupture, 245
  CBC in, 21, 23
  in cholestasis with hepatocellular damage, 35
  in coagulopathy, 354
  corticosteroids and, 128
  in diabetes, 379
  in glomerulonephritis, 251
  in hyperthyroidism, 238
  in progressive hepatic disease, 339
  in renal disease, 242
  in renal failure, 219
  in renal thermal injury, 231

secondary, 16-17
Lytic bone lesions, 17

M
Magnesium
abnormalities of, 272-326
homeostasis of, 326
low ionized, 282
measurement of, 273
regulation of, 326
for tying up, 283
Magnesium abnormalities
case examples of, 276-325
overview of managing, 326
Malabsorption syndromes, 274
Malignancy, hypercalcemia of, 310
Malnutrition, 48-49
Meconium, intra-alveolar, 185
Medication effects
on laboratory values, 4
on serum cholesterol levels, 74
Megakaryocytic hyperplasia, 136-137
Melena
in diabetes, 378, 380, 381
in renal disease, 230, 231-232
Membranoproliferative glomerulonephritis, 337
Metabolic disorders, 49. *See also* Diabetes
Methimazole
for hyperthyroidism, 23
side effects of, 240
for urinary tract infection, 239
Microangiopathic hemolysis, 157-158
Microcytosis, 155
liver dysfunction and, 156
Micronodular hyperplasia, 32
Mineral imbalances, 275, 276-326. *See also*
specific minerals and conditions
Mini-profiles, 4-5
Monoclonal gammopathy
in abused horse, 199-200
diagnosis of, 169-172
Monocytosis, 383
Multiple myeloma, 289-291
diagnosis of, 169-171
treatment of, 171-172
Muscle atrophy, 362
Muscle tremors, 306
Muscle wasting
BUN/creatinine levels in, 376
in diabetes, 370
Myeloid hyperplasia, 37
Myoglobinuria, 283

N
Nasogastric intubation, 247
Neoplasia, 337
biliary, 175-176
bladder, 207-209
diagnosis of, 147

differential for, 264
hyperglobulinemia and, 190
hyperglobulinemia in, 151
Nephropathy
hypercalcemic, 264
protein losing, 315, 326
Nephrotic syndrome, 242
Neutropenia, 181
differentials for, 35
in glomerulonephritis, 251
in multiple myeloma, 170
in parvovirus infection, 164
in septic abdomen, 350
in starvation, 317
with thrombocytopenia, 187
in transitional cell carcinoma, 214
Neutrophil count, 181
Neutrophilia
in bladder rupture, 245
in hyperthyroidism, 238
Neutrophils, degeneration of, 178, 179
Non-steroidal anti-inflammatory drugs (NSAIDs)
in gastrointestinal lesions, 250
in GI ulceration and hemorrhage, 221-222
in renal failure, 269
toxicity of, 223-224
Normally abnormal values, 2
Nutritional status
in hypocalcemia, 274
in impaired albumin synthesis, 311

O
Omentum, fibrosis in, 337
Osteosarcoma, 17
Overhydration, 190
Oxalate toxicity, 269
Oxytocin, 19

P
Pancreas
carcinoma of, 110-111, 176
cytology of, 108-109
tumors of, 107-109
zinc toxicity and, 146-147
Pancreatic disease
amylase elevation in, 308
diagnosis of, 147
elevated amylase in, 365
endocrinopathies and, 131
increased amylase in, 290
in mineral imbalances, 326
Pancreatic enzymes
interpreting serum levels of, 74
tests for, 146
Pancreatic lipase immunoreactivity, 134
Pancreatitis
in calcium and phosphorus balance, 326
case example of, 115-120
in cholestasis, 32

treatment of, 318- 319
Steroid hepatopathy, 21, 343
Stomach, endoscopic biopsy of, 322
Stranguria
  in metastatic neoplasia, 207
  renal function tests for, 196-198
Stress, serum glucose levels and, 76
Suckle reflex, 185

T

Thermal endothelial damage, 183
Thiamin depletion, 319
Thoracentesis, 395
Thrombocytopenia
  in cholestasis, 29, 54
  in feline infectious peritonitis, 166
  in hepatocellular carcinoma, 25
  in hypoadrenocorticism, 104, 105-106
  immune-mediated, 100-103, 374, 375
  in liver disease, 298
  in lymphoma, 310, 312
  mechanisms of, 231
  with methimazole therapy, 240
  in multiple myeloma, 170
  in neutropenia, 187
  in pancreatitis, 116-117
  in portosystemic shunt, 225
  in pulmonary thromboembolism, 188
  in pyothorax, 397
  severity of, 136-137
  in tick borne disease, 161, 162
  in transitional cell carcinoma, 214
Thromboembolism
  in acute renal failure, 313-315
  in recumbency and anorexia, 384
Thyroid hormone testing, 239
Thyroid test, 99
Tick borne disease, 160-162
Tooth, broken, 276-277
Total protein measurement, 150
Tracheostomy, 186
Transfusion, 58
Transitional cell carcinoma, 361
  diagnosis of, 198, 213-215
Traumatic injury, elevated liver enzymes in, 156-158
Triglycerides serum levels
  in hyperlipidemia, 78
  interpretation of, 75
Trypsin-like immunoreactivity (TLI), 65
Trypsin-like immunoreactivity (TLI) test
  for pancreatic disease, 109, 115, 134
  for renal failure, 146
Tubulointerstitial nephritis, 351-353
Tumor associated hypoglycemia, 83-85
Tying up, 280–283
Typhlocolitis, necrotizing and ulcerative, 188-189

U

Ulcerative colitis, 325
Ultrasound
  for cholestatic liver disease, 54, 64
  for enlarged gall bladder, 285
  for hydronephrosis, 218
  for impaired liver function, 92
  for insulinoma, 89
  for liver disease, 236
  for liver masses, 175-176
  for lymphoid neoplasm, 202
  for lymphoma, 312
  for pancreatitis, 109, 112, 117-118
  for portosystemic shunt, 227
  for reduced liver function, 139
  in urinary tract disease, 197-198
Upper airway edema, postsurgical, 186
Uremia, 192
Urethral obstruction, 210-212, 305
Urinalysis
  in cholestasis, 58
  in diabetes, 125, 133, 372, 379, 381
  in feline hepatic lipidosis, 39
  in feline infectious peritonitis, 167-168
  in GI inflammation, 248
  in hepatocellular damage, 15, 36
  in hyperthyroidism, 239
  in hypoadrenocorticism, 261, 363
  in impaired liver function, 91
  in multiple myeloma, 170, 171
  in NSAID poisoning, 223
  in pancreatic disease, 108, 119-120, 130
  in parathyroid adenoma, 285
  for pneumonia and diabetes, 377
  in portosystemic shunt, 226-227
  in pre-renal azotemia, 195
  in progressive hepatic disease, 340
  in pyelonephritis, 229
  in recumbency and anorexia, 384
  in Red Maple leaf toxicity, 52
  in renal disease, 243, 303
  in renal failure, 138-139, 220, 255, 296, 315
  in renal secondary hyperparathyroidism, 288
  for tick born disease, 161
  in tubulointerstitial nephritis, 351
  in tying up, 283
  in urinary tract disease, 197, 212, 365
  in zinc toxicosis, 146-147
Urinary bladder
  cytology of, 208-209
  leakage from, 360-361
  mass in, 208-209
  metastatic neoplasia of, 207-209
  rupture of, 244-246, 359-360
    repair of, 361
  tumors of, 197-198
Urinary bladder stones, 385
Urinary catheterization, 386-387
Urinary tract

disease of, 359-361
infections of
bacteriuria in, 365
treatment of, 239
inflammation of, 210-212
obstruction of, 385-387
prolonged, 209
severe disease of, 196-198
Urine
accumulation or obstruction of, 192
dilute, with azotemia, 212
intercellular yeast in, 208
loss of concentrating ability in, 192
Uroabdomen, 388-390
electrolyte abnormalities with, 337
surgical correction of, 390-391

V
Vitamin D
in calcium and phosphorus homeostasis, 272-273
for hyperparathyroidism, 280
hypercalcemia and, 275
impaired absorption of, 321
Vitamin D toxicity, 307
differential for, 310
electrolyte abnormalities in, 364
in hypercalcemia with hyperphosphatemia, 288
in hyperphosphatemia, 282
hyperphosphatemia and, 144
hyperphosphatemia and hypercalcemia in, 260
Vitamin E, 283
Vitamin K
for coagulopathy, 355
deficiency of in coagulation abnormalities, 400
for feline hepatic lipidosis, 40
Vitamin K antagonist poisoning, 312
Vomiting, 174
in azotemia and renal failure, 241
in chronic hepatitis, 346
in diabetes mellitus, 372
in ethylene glycol toxicity, 304
with foreign body in intestines, 343-345
with garbage eating, 341-343
in hepatocellular damage, 65-66
in hyperamylasemia, 145-146
in hypoadrenocorticism, 259, 362
in hypochloremia, 373
in hypokalemia, 129
in ibuprofen poisoning, 221
in lymphoid neoplasm, 201
in pancreatic carcinoma, 110
in pancreatic disease, 107-109
in parathyroid adenoma, 284
in parvovirus, 163
in pericarditis, 391
in progressive hepatic disease, 338
in pyelonephritis, 227
in renal azotemia, 61
in renal disease, 301

in renal failure, 253

W
Water loss, 351
in electrolyte abnormalities, 403
Weakness
in coagulopathy, 353
hind limb, 292-294
Weight loss, 174, 316
in feline infectious peritonitis (FIP), 165
in hypoadrenocorticism, 306, 362
in Lyme disease, 204
in protein losing enteropathy, 158-159
Wheezing, 34

X
Xylazine, 76

Z
Zinc toxicosis, 143-144
diagnosis of, 146-147
in renal failure, 269